Children's Nursing

For Churchill Livingstone:

Commissioning Editor: Ellen Green
Project Manager: Valerie Burgess
Project Development Editor: Mairi McCubbin
Design Direction: Judith Wright
Illustrator: Marion Tasker
Copy-editor: Sue Beasley
DTU Operator: Janet Smith
Indexer: Liza Weinkove
Sales promotion executive: Hilary Brown

Children's Nursing

Edited by

Linda McQuaid BA DMS MBA RGN RSCN MHSM
Project Manager, Children's Services, BHB Community Healthcare
NHS Trust/Havering Hospitals NHS Trust, Hornchurch, Essex
Formerly Children's Services Manager, Central Middlesex Hospital
NHS Trust, London

Sally Huband BA(Hons) RGN RSCN SCM RNT
Formerly Senior Lecturer, Paediatrics, Sussex and Kent Institute, Brighton

Esther M. Parker MN RGN RSCN NDN PGCE RNT
Programme Coordinator, Child Health, Wolfson School of Health Sciences,
Thames Valley University, London

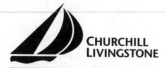
CHURCHILL
LIVINGSTONE

NEW YORK EDINBURGH LONDON MADRID MELBOURNE SAN FRANCISCO TOKYO 1996

CHURCHILL LIVINGSTONE
Medical Division of Pearson Professional Limited

Distributed in the United States of America by Churchill
Livingstone Inc., 650 Avenue of the Americas, New York, N.Y. 10011,
and by associated companies, branches and representatives throughout
the world.

First edition 1996

ISBN 0 443 05087 2

British Library of Cataloguing in Publication Data
A catalogue record for this book is available from the British Library.

Library of Congress Cataloging in Publication Data
A catalogue record for this book is available from the Library of Congress

Medical knowledge is constantly changing. As new information becomes
available, changes in treatment, procedures, equipment and the use of
drugs become necessary. The editors/authors/contributors and the
publishers have, as far as it is possible, taken care to ensure that the
information given in this text is accurate and up to date. However,
readers are strongly advised to confirm that the information, especially
with regard to drug usage, complies with latest legislation and
standards of practice.

The
publisher's
policy is to use
paper manufactured
from sustainable forests

Produced by Longman Singapore Publishers Pte Ltd.
Printed in Singapore.

Contents

Contributors

Jean Bayne RSCN RGN DN
Formerly Community Paediatric Sister,
Central Middlesex Hospital, London
16 The endocrine system

Jean Beattie MA BA RGN RSCN DipN RCNT RNT
CertEd(FE)
Senior Lecturer in Nursing Studies, School of
Nursing and Community Health, Department of
Health and Social Sciences, University of Central
England, Birmingham
7 Morals and ethics in children's nursing

Ginny Colliss SRN RSCN DipN(Lond)
Sister, Oncology Unit, and Senior Nurse Advisor,
Children's Services, Addenbrookes Hospital
NHS Trust, Cambridge
24 Children having oncology treatment

Tracey Coventry RSCN RGN RM
Sister, Intensive Therapy Unit, Royal Hospital
for Sick Children, Yorkhill, Glasgow
26 Critically ill children

Sue Davies MN SRN RSCN
Formerly Clinical Nurse Specialist, Paediatric
Cardiac Unit, University Hospital of Wales,
Cardiff
10 The circulatory system

Jacqueline Denyer RGN RSCN RHV
Clinical Nurse Specialist for Epidermolysis
Bullosa, Paediatrics, Great Ormond Street
Hospital for Children NHS Trust, London
17 The skin

Marcelle E. de Sousa RGN RSCN
Dialysis Sister, Department of Paediatric
Nephrology, Guy's Hospital, London
13 The renal system

Andrew Dickson RMN DMS
Clinical Director, Department of Child and
Family Psychiatry, Yorkhill NHS Trust, Glasgow
23 Children with mental health problems

Mabel G. Doku RN RM RHV DipPsych
Specialist Health Visitor, Child Development
Centre, St Mary's Hospital, Praed Street, London
21 Children with special needs

Nicola M. Eaton BSc RSCN RGN PGCE
Lecturer in Nursing, University of Wales,
Swansea
28 Children at risk

Amanda Field RGN RSCN
Manager, GU/HIV Medicine, St Mary's Hospital
NHS Trust, London
19 Immunity

Diana Forster BA(Hons) MSc RGN RM RHVT RNT
Independent Writer and Consultant in Health
Psychology and Health Promotion, London
2 Promoting health

Douglas Fraser
Nurse Therapist, Yorkhill NHS Trust, Glasgow
23 Children with mental health problems

Lucy Godman SRN RSCN RCNT DipDN
Paediatric Community Sister, Hillview, Bentley
25 Children with chronic illness

Sharon Goodchild RGN RSCN
Senior Staff Nurse, St. Peter's Hospital, Chertsey,
Surrey
22 Adolescents

Sally Huband BA(Hons) RGN RSCN SCM
Formerly Senior Lecturer, Paediatrics, Sussex
and Kent Institute, Falmer, Brighton
3 Patterns of ill health
12 Nutrition and the digestive system
27 Terminally ill children

Sue Linnett RGN RSCN ENB405
Formerly Sister, Neonatal Unit, St. Mary's
Hospital, Paddington; Sister, Special Care Baby
Unit, Queen Mary's Hospital, Roehampton;
National Co-ordinator, Blisslink Parent Support
Network
20 The Special Care Baby Unit

Elizabeth J. Mair BSc(Hons) RGN RSCN RHV
Health Visitor, Leicestershire
18 Hearing and vision

Linda McQuaid BA DMS MBA RGN RSCN MHSM
Project Manager, Children's Services, BHB
Community Healthcare NHS Trust / Havering
Hospitals NHS Trust, Hornchurch, Essex
Formerly Children's Services Manager, Central
Middlesex Hospital NHS Trust, London
6 Professional role of the children's nurse
10 The circulatory system

Stephanie Moulai RSCN RGN ONC DipN
Paediatric Ward Sister, Chelsea and Westminster
Hospital, London
12 Nutrition and the digestive system

Jean S. Neave BA(Hons) MSc RGN RHV FWT PGCEA
Principal Lecturer, Applied Behavioural
Sciences, Thames Valley University, London
4 Sociology and social policy

Dympna O'Grady PGD RGN RSCN RCNT CertEd(FE)
Child Branch Leader, Sister Dora College of
Nursing and Midwifery, Walsall, Burton on Trent
7 Morals and ethics in children's nursing

Jonathan Pagdin MMedSci RSCN RGN
Limb Inequality Service Coordinator and Clinical
Nurse Specialist for Limb Reconstruction,
Sheffield Children's Hospital, Sheffield
15 The musculoskeletal system

Esther M. Parker MN RGN RSCN NDN PGCE RNT
Programme Coordinator, Child Health, Wolfson
School of Health and Sciences, Thames Valley
University, London
5 Development of paediatric nursing

Sue Price MN RGN RSCN CertEd DipN
Lecturer in Paediatric Nursing, Child Branch
Coordinator, Department of Nursing Studies,
University of Birmingham, Birmingham
8 Concepts of individualised care

Penny Reid BSc(Hons) RGN RHV DipNE
Senior Lecturer, Health and Community Studies,
Thames Valley University, London
4 Sociology and social policy

Jim Richardson BA RGN RSCN PGCE
Lecturer in Nursing Studies, School of Nursing
Studies, University of Wales College of
Medicine, Cardiff
14 The nervous system

Philippa Smith BSc(Hons) RN DipHE
Staff Nurse, Host Defence Unit, Hospital for Sick
Children, Great Ormond Street, London
9 General concepts of child care

Jayne Taylor BSc(Hons) RGN RHV DipN(Lond) CertEd
Head of School of Nursing and Midwifery,
Suffolk College, Ipswich
2 Promoting health
27 Terminally ill children

Joanne Trussler RSCN RGN
Senior Sister, Nicholson Ward, Royal Alexandra
Hospital for Sick Children, Brighton
11 The respiratory system

Rosemary Turnbull RSCN
Dermatology Nurse, Great Ormond Street
Hospital for Children NHS Trust, London
17 The skin

Heather Wood BA MN
Research and Development Officer, Frenchay
Hospital, Bristol
1 Normal health

Kevin Woodhams RGN RSCN
Charge Nurse, Royal Alexandra Hospital for Sick
Children, Brighton
11 The respiratory system

Edwina Wooler SRN RSCN
Clinical Nurse Specialist in Paediatric Asthma,
Royal Alexandra Hospital for Sick Children,
Brighton
11 The respiratory system

Reviewers

Karen Booth BSc(Hons) RGN ENB405
Lecturer Practitioner in Neonatology, Trevor
Mann Baby Unit, Royal Sussex County Hospital,
Brighton

Sue Brunner RSCN
Nurse, Child Development, MacKeith Centre,
Brighton

Margaret Coates RSCN RGN RNT Dip(Sister Tutor)
Formerly Paediatric Nurse Tutor, Sheffield and
North Trent College of Nursing and Midwifery
(now University of Humberside), Sheffield

Janet M. Hall RGN RSCN
Senior Sister, Royal Alexandra Hospital for Sick
Children, Brighton

Sonia Harle RGN RSCN
Formerly Nurse Manager, Adolescent Ward,
Westminster Children's Hospital (now Chelsea &
Westminster), London

Fiona Hornby RSCN RGN DMS
Senior Sister, Paediatrics, Northwick Park and St
Marks NHS Trust, Middlesex

Sally Huband BA(Hons) RGN RSCN SCM RNT
Formerly Senior Lecturer, Paediatrics, Sussex
and Kent Institute, Brighton

Morag McCarthy SRD
Paediatric Dietitian, Royal Alexandra Hospital
for Sick Children, Brighton

Sheena A. McClure RGN RSCN
Paediatric Community Staff Nurse, Royal
Alexandra Hospital for Sick Children, Brighton

Helen Mitchell RGN RSCN CertONC
Paediatric Oncology Nurse Specialist, Royal
Alexandra Hospital for Sick Children, Brighton

Jo Nandzo BSc(Hons) RGN RM RSCN DPSN
Sister, Outpatient Department and Casualty,
Royal Alexandra Hospital for Sick Children,
Brighton
28 Children at risk

B Ruston RGN RSCN SCM DNC CPT
Paediatric Community Sister, Royal Alexandra
Hospital for Sick Children, Brighton
27 Terminally ill children

Catherine Shopland MCSP SRP
Senior Paediatric Physiotherapist, Royal
Alexandra Hospital for Sick Children, Brighton
15 The musculoskeletal system

Helene Smith RSCN ONC ENB415
Senior Sister, Lydia Intensive Care Unit, Royal
Alexandra Hospital for Sick Children, Brighton
26 Critically ill children

Caroline Spence RGN RSCN DN
Paediatric Community Sister (Diabetes Specialist
Nurse), Royal Alexandra Hospital for Sick
Children, Brighton
16 The endocrine system

Ethel Trigg MBA RGN RSCN DMS FETC
Outpatients and Medical Records Manager,
Worthing and Southlands Hospital NHS Trust,
Shoreham by Sea, West Sussex
General advisor and coordinator of reviews for chapters 10, 12, 15, 16, 17, 20, 21, 24, 25, 26, 27 and 28.

Preface

Changes in nurse education over the past few years have been more radical than ever before. Student nurses today are encouraged to develop a more-questioning approach to study and, from an early date, are encouraged to utilise nursing research to inform their practice. There has been a growing appreciation of the importance of sociological and psychological factors in the nursing of children, in contrast to the more traditional emphasis on biological factors.

In the past there have been few British textbooks for students wishing to specialise in children's nursing: this book is intended to address that lack. As no single text can attempt to cover the whole spectrum of children's nursing, the aim of this book is to provide a general overview and to direct students to other sources if more in-depth information is required.

Children have needs even when they are well, and children's nurses must have a good knowledge of normal development as well as the specific needs of sick children. Over the past 10 years there has been increasing emphasis on keeping children safe and well, hence the need for health promotion and monitoring of children. There has also been a move away from hospital care, with shorter stays, more day surgery and the spread of paediatric community nursing teams. This text aims to take account of these changes in the provision of care.

Children's Nursing is designed to follow a similar structure to that used in *Common Foundation Studies in Nursing* (Kenworthy, Snowley &

Gilling 1996). Students who have used that text during the common foundation programme should find this continuity helpful. The book is divided into four sections, as follows.

Section 1 The child: self and society

This first section considers the overall development of the child and some of the sociological and environmental influences. There is an emphasis on the role of health promotion and the prevention of ill health.

Section 2 Nursing: fundamental principles

This section looks at the specific role of the children's nurse and the ways in which it is different from the role of the nurse in other specialities. The need for nurses trained to care for children has been acknowledged since the Platt Report (MOH 1959) and the Court Report (DHSS 1976). This section begins with the development of paediatric nursing and follows through to current thinking and practice, and the way in which care is planned to meet the needs of individual children and families.

Section 3 Nursing: principles and skills for practice

This section is divided into 'systems' to provide a logical framework. The section gives some insight into the physiological differences between the child and the adult and also discusses some of the pathological processes that may cause ill health. It is not meant to be a comprehensive guide to all the 'medical conditions' but, rather, indicates the way in which the child may be affected by these processes. The children's nurse needs to be a skilled observer, aware of signs of ill health, and must also develop specific skills in order to care for the sick child effectively. We hope that this section will go some way to assist the student in acquiring these skills.

Section 4 Special client groups

Some children have special needs for a variety of reasons, such as immaturity or disability. This section covers some of these groups. Cross references to other sections have been used where necessary to help the reader.

Other features

Each chapter starts with an introduction, which also identifies the aims of the chapter. Case examples and activities are included, throughout, to involve the reader and invite further study. Care has been taken in designing a layout that will attract and stimulate the reader. End-of-chapter conclusions summarise each chapter's main features. Each chapter is comprehensively referenced and the student is also alerted to other texts for further study in related areas.

Skilled nursing requires both knowledge and practice and as we are fortunate in having contributors from both the clinical field and education, we hope that this book will help to bring the two areas together. We are indebted to all those who have contributed and would like to thank them for their hard work and commitment.

1996   Linda McQuaid
                                          Sally Huband
                                         Esther Parker

REFERENCES

DHSS 1976 Fit for the future: the report of the committee on child health services (Court Report). HMSO, London
Kenworthy N, Snowley G, Gilling C, 1996 Common foundation studies in nursing, 2nd edn. Churchill Livingstone, Edinburgh
Ministry of Health 1959 The welfare of children in hospital. Report of Central Health Services Council (Platt Report). HMSO, London

1

The child:
self and society

This first section introduces the concept of childhood. It considers the development of the child and some of the factors which may affect the health of the child. Children cannot be considered in isolation. Their health and development is influenced by both family lifestyles and by social policies and this section addresses some of these factors

1

Child development

Heather Wood

This chapter considers the growth and
development of children from conception to
puberty, placing particular emphasis on the
development of sensorimotor and cognitive skills
in the young child.

The chapter aims to:
- demonstrate the importance of maternal health
  for normal growth and development in utero
- describe patterns of growth from birth to
  puberty
- consider the newborn infant and early
  development
- give typical developmental stages for various
  ages up to 5 years
- describe some abnormalities in growth and
  development after birth
- discuss ideas about child development.

PRE-BIRTH DEVELOPMENT

GROWTH AS A BIOLOGICAL PROCESS

A knowledge of intrauterine growth is
important for children's nurses because of the
insight it gives into the causes of congenital
difficulties, the care of preterm babies, and the
importance of healthy parents.

   The study of the growth of the embryo
reveals several things that make growth at

this stage of human development different from that of the infant after birth. The speed and changing nature of the growth process itself is more dramatic than at any other time in life and a wide range of types of growth occur:

- multiplicative growth—increase in cell numbers
- auxetic growth—increase in cell size
- differentiation and specialisation of cells into organs
- interstitial increase in intercellular material
- appositional growth of tissues adding more cells.

For example, during the early days of cell division in the blastocyst (the ball of cells which develops following fertilisation of the ovum by the sperm) there is cell division within the zona pellucida around the newly fertilised ovum, but no increase in cell size within it. This type of growth is *multiplicative growth*.

The *auxetic type of growth* occurs throughout the stage when the embryo is implanting in the endometrium of the mother's uterus. It involves growth in cell size, which is independent of the rate of cell division and occurs as the early embryonic cells absorb nutrients and fluids from their environment.

A third type of growth, which takes place just after implantation, is the process of *differentiation* of the embryonic cells into different layers, called ectoderm, endoderm and mesoderm, and the growth of the mesoderm into organs with highly specialised functions.

Another example of auxetic growth can be seen in the growth of the nervous system in the developing fetus. After the sixth month of gestation, it is thought that there are no new neurones produced, but there is a huge increase in the amount of cytoplasm within neurones as peripheral cytoplasmic processes extend to improve communication between them. This kind of growth continues after birth as the neurological system develops.

Effects of cell differentiation into different tissue types

There are some consequences of the specialisation of cells that takes place in the early embryo. Specialised cells behave differently, not only in developing their designated functions, but also as living cells themselves.

The process of differentiation of early embryonic cells into different types that will go on to form skin, internal organs, nervous system, etc. also slows the process of multiplicative cell division because differentiated cells seem to divide less frequently. Some highly differentiated and specialised cells may not divide again, but are replaced from a group of cells—the stem cells—whose main function is to produce other cells which become more differentiated as they age. This can be seen in the skin and mucous membrane cells derived from the outer layer of the very early embryo—the ectoderm. The ectoderm not only gives rise to the skin of the embryo but also folds and invaginates during the formation of the primitive body cavities and ends up as the lining of the gut, including the mouth, and the endometrium of the uterus. These layers of the body are a defence layer between the internal organs and the outside world and need constant replacement due to wear and tear. In the skin, the basal cells of the epidermis actively divide to produce new skin cells which look like the parent cells, but gradually become flattened and move up to replace the dead cells as they flake off the dry outer layer of the skin. They do not divide unless there is a wound to the skin when they may begin to divide during epithelialisation.

Another striking example of the loss of cell division in highly specialised cells is that of the erythrocyte, the red blood cell. These cells are produced by stem cell tissue in the marrow of the bones, but as they age they lose their nuclei and are unable to divide, even if there is severe loss of red blood cells due to disease or damage to the bone marrow, or additional need due to altitude sickness.

In the growing embryo, the body size is increased rapidly and the skin stem cells are very active. Recent research into wound healing has shown that fetal skin cells have exceptionally good healing abilities, leaving no scarring when damage is repaired. The mechanism for this is uncertain at present, but it is clear that it differs from that after birth.

Other recent research into growth in adults shows that the stem cells are quite active and more cells are produced than are destroyed by wear and tear. There appears to be a mechanism by which cells are destroyed by the body's immune system in a programme of cell replacement. The precise cause is yet to be discovered.

ABNORMALITIES IN GROWTH

Abnormal growth in the embryo and fetus has two main groups of causes:

- environmental factors
- genetic abnormalities.

Environmental factors

Since the mother is the fetal environment, her health and welfare are essential to healthy development of the baby. Parents feel considerable anxiety and guilt over the birth of a child with developmental abnormalities and may seek help in understanding what has happened. All nurses have a role in health promotion which involves knowing how to prevent ill health and damage to the developing child.

Growth and development of the fetus can be affected by impaired nutrition or by assaults from radiation, infections or toxic substances within the mother's bloodstream. Some common teratogens are ionising radiation (which is why pregnant women are only X-rayed with great caution), infective organisms such as cytomegalovirus and chemicals such as mercury and some drugs (e.g. thalidomide). The most vulnerable periods for abnormalities to occur during pregnancy are illustrated in Figure 1.1.

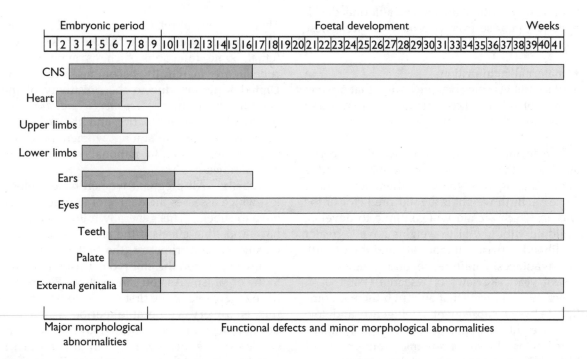

Figure 1.1   Critical periods of organ vulnerability during early development: dark shading indicates high-risk periods, lighter shading lower-risk periods (adapted from Moore 1988).

Brain development is affected at several stages during development. The early stages of neurogenesis when the neural tissues start to differentiate and specialise is the first point of vulnerability. The critical period for brain growth occurs during the first 16 weeks of gestation, and damage during this stage of development will give rise to major morphological defects such as anencephaly, microcephaly, spina bifida, etc. This is usually detected by screening during early pregnancy, using blood tests to determine the amounts of certain proteins that indicate abnormalities, and later by ultrasound examination of the fetus to identify abnormalities visually. The advantage of these tests is that mothers may choose to have the pregnancy terminated by abortion, but if they are unable or unwilling to undertake this course, the effects of knowing in advance that a baby is damaged may not be helpful.

Poor fetal nutrition

Poor fetal nutrition during intrauterine development can arise from two main causes. These are:

- maternal malnutrition
- placental insufficiency (including that arising from blood vessel constriction due to nicotine intake by the mother).

The incidence of low birth weight is correlated with the social class of the mother and is higher among very young mothers aged under 15 years. Birth weight is a good predictor of the way in which a child will continue to develop. Children with low birth weights have a greater likelihood of perinatal mortality and their health disadvantages continue beyond infancy into school years. Reviews of research (Wehmer & Hafez 1975) indicate that although there is some link between subsequent intelligence and low birth weight, this outcome is not equally distributed across the socioeconomic groups and low birth weight children who are brought up in an environment with few material advantages may

have their poor start compounded by the complex effects of a deprived childhood. There are suggestions that the socioeconomic factors may be more important to developmental outcomes than poor nutrition in utero.

Maternal nutrition. Malnutrition and diseases of poor diet are a greater scourge in less-developed countries, but even in developed, wealthier countries anaemia is a condition which is closely related to diet in women who do not have enough iron or folic acid intake. Anaemia makes a pregnant woman more tired and less able to sustain the blood losses of delivery. Severe maternal anaemia is also linked to low birth weight in the baby and to poor immunity to infection. Other maternal nutritional factors also play their part—the link between maternal folic acid deficiency and fetal neural tube defects such as spina bifida has led to mothers being advised to increase their intake of dietary sources of this vitamin, such as green vegetables, during pregnancy.

Environmental assaults

There are several relatively common conditions of pregnancy which may affect the growth of the fetus. Some infections such as syphilis and rubella are mercifully becoming rare in the United Kingdom due to the sensitivity of the syphilis bacterium, *Treponema pallidum*, to commonly used antibiotics and the reduction in cases of rubella among women of childbearing years due to national immunisation programmes.

Rubella. All pregnant women have a blood test which assesses the degree of immunity they have to rubella. This generally mild disease can have appalling effects if the mother contracts it during the first trimester (the first 3 months of pregnancy) when the embryo is very vulnerable to the organism. As you can see from Figure 1.1, the eyes are one of the first organs to be formed; this is a very vulnerable period when eye development may be affected by viruses that can cross the barrier between the mother's bloodstream and that of the embryo. The embryo does not have the kind of immunological defences that would protect it against invasion and it depends upon maternal defences to defeat the virus before it reaches the placenta. If a mother has no immunity, she may catch rubella from an infected person (the disease is spread by droplet infection) and cannot defend the baby. The effects are becoming rarer, but when damage occurs it includes congenital cataracts and blindness, sometimes with abnormally small underdeveloped eyes (microphthalmos).

The early development of the ear at about the seventh week of gestation can also be affected by rubella or syphilis, which damage the developing inner ear, leading to congenital deafness.

Toxoplasmosis. This is one of the more serious commonly encountered infections which can infect the placenta itself and cross the placental barrier to infect the fetus. It is caused by a protozoal parasite found in the faeces of infected domestic cats and in infected meat. The mother herself experiences little or no effect of the infection and may not know that she has been in contact with it.

Timing of infection also makes a difference to the effects on the developing embryo. If the mother is infected with toxoplasmosis during the early stages of pregnancy, the organism is less likely to cross the placental barrier but more likely to have severe effects on the embryo if it does. This may lead to stillbirth, death shortly after birth or damage to the developing eyes or brain, which are very vulnerable during the early weeks of development (see Fig. 1.1). This may appear as hydrocephalus, microcephalus, chorioretinitis or cerebral calcification.

Later infection gives rise to enlarged liver or spleen, jaundice, convulsions or later development of abnormalities—sometimes years after birth. It is important that mothers understand that care to avoid contact with toxoplasmosis must be taken throughout pregnancy. Because the infection is potentially so serious in consequence, and the source of the infection is relatively common, pregnant women are advised to take precautions such as avoiding contact with cat faeces by not cleaning litter trays, wearing gloves when gardening, etc.

AIDS. Human immunodeficiency virus (HIV) which causes AIDS also presents particular risks to the developing fetus, and a proportion of infants born to seropositive mothers are themselves HIV-positive from birth. There is evidence that HIV is also passed from infected mothers to previously uninfected infants in breast milk, but research is still going on to establish the precise risks. In developed countries where there is adequate clean water and mothers can afford artificial milks, it may be better to bottle-feed babies if the mother is HIV-positive, but in developing countries where these facilities are not available, the dangers of bottle-feeding and gastroenteritis may be much greater than the risk of HIV transmission in breast milk.

Listeriosis. This is a food-borne infection that causes gastroenteritis and is commonly associated with the consumption of unpasteurised soft cheeses and undercooked chicken. It is a mild feverish condition in otherwise healthy adults, but gives rise to severe problems in the fetus if the mother contracts it during pregnancy, again because it crosses the placental barrier. Depending upon the stage of development at which infection takes place, listeriosis can cause premature delivery, meningoencephalitis, hydrocephalus and even intrauterine death. Pregnant women should be advised to avoid foods that may be contaminated and to be very careful about hygiene in cooking and preparing meat.

Drug and alcohol abuse during pregnancy is also linked with fetal abnormality. There is a well-recognised pattern of problems which occur in fetuses affected by high maternal alcohol intake—the fetal alcohol syndrome. Babies and children so affected show delayed growth and both physical and mental development are slowed. Severely affected children also show facial characteristics which are thought to be part of this syndrome.

Children whose mothers smoked cigarettes in pregnancy also show delayed growth and may be born prematurely or be very 'light for dates' if born at around full-term gestation. For this reason, would-be mothers should give up smoking, preferably before conception.

The nursing importance of understanding about conditions which affect the child before birth lies in the need to care for affected children after birth and give them and their families the extra support they will need to promote the health of the child. There is also evidence from some follow-up studies that such babies continue for years to show poor growth compared with their unaffected peers and also poorer intellectual development. These factors require careful research and interpretation as the child gets older because, as well as continued environmental influences, there are obvious social issues which are likely to arise when a child is raised by a parent who is a heavy smoker or abuses drugs or alcohol (Corraco et al 1993).

Genetic abnormalities

Genetic abnormalities may arise from abnormal gametes from either parent. Gametes are haploid cells, i.e. they have half the number of chromosomes that are found in ordinary body cells, so each parent contributes half of the chromosomes that the child will inherit. These two 'halves' of genetic material combine at fertilisation when the nuclei of the gametes merge to form a single diploid cell with a full complement of chromosomes. Identical twins are formed during cell division in the early embryo when the ball of cells is split and continues to develop as two separate embryos, each with exactly the same genetic components. Non-identical twins are produced when two separate gamete pairs merge to produce two individual embryos, which have different genetic material and therefore are no more alike than siblings born at different times.

The range of genetic abnormalities and their known mechanisms of inheritance are beyond the scope of this chapter, but scientific knowledge of this sort of problem has suggested that environmental factors have more influence than we had previously supposed, and that adults sometimes encounter chemical or radiological hazards that can affect their children's and even their grandchildren's genetic make-up. These mutagenic factors affect the developing gametes and cause damage to their chromosomes. They do not necessarily need to be encountered during embryonic development in the months of pregnancy, but can affect developing gametes in the parents' reproductive organs long before conception takes place.

DEVELOPMENT AFTER BIRTH

PATTERNS OF GROWTH

Factors affecting growth

The rate of growth of young children is linked to the late maturation of the human species. Similar correlations are found in the wider animal kingdom—the more complex the species, the longer the maturation period of the young tends to be. Children and adolescents mature earlier in our generation than in that of our grandparents and this is thought to be linked to differences in nutritional intake. Growth depends upon a complex mix of genetic inheritance and environmental conditions, chiefly the socioeconomic conditions of the family.

Other differences in growth rates and form are linked to the gender of the child. This is especially true in adolescence, when girls may mature earlier than boys. While these differences occur, they are much less than the difference between the child of taller than average parents and the child of smaller than average parents. These differences can be used to assess the eventual height of children using parent-specific growth charts (see Box 1.1), but if one parent is tall and the other shorter than average, they are less useful.

Growth from birth to puberty

The height and weight of the infant at birth indicates the interaction between the genetic inheritance and the environmental influences

Box 1.1 Establishing standards for growth

The patterns of growth of young children were originally studied through measurements of large numbers of growing children over a period of many years. This is a difficult form of research because it is necessary to enrol many families in the study and follow them and their children over a period of many years. Given the mobility of many families in today's society, this is extremely difficult and costly research. The problems in turn mean that few centres can afford to take on this type of research. This is why we are still using growth charts which were originally prepared in the 1940s.

There are other ways of obtaining growth standards. For example, there have been large-scale cross-sectional studies of children of the same age to identify variations in size and maturity. These are helpful, but statistically less useful than the longitudinal studies, if only because children grow at different rates and single measurements give no guidance on the rates of growth. The data they produce can, however, be compared with data from earlier longitudinal work to identify changes in average size at different ages within particular populations. One example of this is the research on growth of Japanese children and young adults today compared with those of earlier generations in response to changed diets (Micozzi 1987).

There have been changes in our own population since the longitudinal studies of the 1940s and 1950s. Children today are growing taller and maturing earlier than they were 50 years ago. Britain is now a multiracial society, which raises questions about whether a child from another ethnic group can be measured against criteria developed for indigenous children. There are complex patterns of change which affect migrating people who change their diet to match with that of the new host community. This may affect child growth, eventual adult height and patterns of diet-related ill health, and studies are still monitoring these changes among non-indigenous Britons and their children. It is possible that patterns of changed growth rates similar to those observed for indigenous children may be detected in the second and third generations of offspring of immigrants from other areas of the world to the United Kingdom.

The implications for this in practice are that percentile growth charts must be used with due consideration for these potential influences when assessing the growth of infants and children whose parents or grandparents come from another ethnic group. This has been recognised in the USA, where growth charts for different ethnic groups may be used.

Box 1.2 Getting an accurate measurement

Young babies who are unable to support their own weight require special care to measure body length. This is usually done using a special mat marked in inches and centimetres. The mat is placed on a firm surface and the baby laid on it, with the crown of the head against a rigid endpiece. The infant is then gently stretched out to full length by one nurse while the head is kept in place by another nurse or the baby's mother. This enables an accurate length measurement to be made quickly without distress to the child.

Older children and adults also need careful measurement to get accurate results. Proper equipment is important—a fabric tape measure or the door frame is seldom accurate for very small children. In addition to this, the intervertebral discs in the spinal column are compressed under the weight of the head and upper body during the course of the day, which means that we are slightly taller (as much as 2 cm) in the morning than in the evening.

per day in length. Body length is difficult to measure accurately in newborns without special equipment, but at birth, babies are on average about 20 inches (50 cm) long. After birth, the infant grows as much as 6 inches in length during the first 6 months of life alone (Box 1.2). Head circumference in normal newborn infants averages between 33 and 36 cm at its widest point.

Most babies weigh between 5.5 and 9.5 pounds at birth, with an average full-term pregnancy birth weight in the United Kingdom of 7.5 pounds. By the time they are 2 years old, normal toddlers may weigh as much as four times their birth weight (see Apps 1 and 2).

Boys tend to be larger than girls, and this is reflected in the separation of gender in growth charts.

Growth rates are not a smooth progression, but tend to be faster at first until the child reaches 3 years of age, then slower until the adolescent growth spurt around puberty, which starts at about 11 years for girls and about 13 years for boys (see Apps 3 and 4). Between these two periods, growth is steadier and the body shape and relative proportions tend to be fairly stable.

within the womb during gestation. Indeed, the fastest rate of growth at any stage of development is during the fourth month of gestation, when the fetus grows about 1.5 mm

Changes in body proportions

The proportions of the body of a newborn infant are very different from those of an adult or an older child. The head is larger in relation to the size of the body. Sinclair (1989) notes that early European painters sometimes did not adjust for this proportionate difference in their portraits of babies, which have a rather miniaturised appearance. The Renaissance in Europe brought about a more scientific attitude to painting and dissection, and careful anatomical study became more common. It is noticeable that the later painter, Raphael, painted much more realistic infants than his medieval predecessors.

There is an increase in the proportion of body fat in young infants up until 6 months of age, but after this age they become more mobile and energetic and there is a gradual change in their body shape between about 9 months and 2 years. The child is proportionally different from the infant in having less-rounded limbs with more development of muscle as physical activity increases. The proportion of the body which is composed of fat changes to reflect this.

Bone growth

Bone growth is also very fast, with increasing ossification of bones matching the growth in body weight. Where this does not occur due to poor diet, rickets may result in bowing of the long bones of the legs, but most children in western societies have adequate nutrition and this condition is much less common than it was in earlier generations. Active long bone growth continues until puberty

with growth centres called epiphyses near the ends of each bone generating new tissue and a constant breakdown of old bone shape to allow growth to take place. The skull bones close by about 2 years and the soft fontanelles of infancy are protected by bony growth.

Nutrition and energy needs

The energy needs for growth during the first few months of life are supplied entirely by milk from either breast or bottle (Box 1.3). New foods are gradually introduced into the diet during infancy and childhood, and some changes take place within the gastrointestinal tract during development. One of the first to be encountered is the eruption of teeth. It is rare for infants to be born with teeth. The first teeth to erupt are usually the lower (mandibular) incisors, the front biting teeth. This takes place at about 6 months of age. The teeth, both primary ('milk teeth') and secondary dentitions, are present in the gums at birth, but the secondary teeth are mere rudimentary buds and the primary teeth are not fully calcified.

Growing children have high energy needs and a higher basal metabolic rate (BMR) than

Activity 1.2

A mother of a demanding baby of 3 weeks of age tells you that, although she is determined to feed her baby herself, she is very tired by breast-feeding so frequently. She has decided to 'rest' her breasts by giving alternate infant formula bottle feeds in between breast feeds to allow her body to recover and produce more milk. How would you advise her?

Table 1.1 The Mayo Foundation normal standards of basal metabolic rate (kcal/m^2/h) (adapted from Boothbay et al 1936)

Males		Females	
Age in years	BMR	Age in years	BMR
6	53.0	6	50.6
		6.5	50.2
7	52.5	7	49.1
		7.5	47.8
8	51.8	8	47.0
		8.5	46.5
9	50.5	9	45.9
9.5	49.4		
10	48.5	9–10	45.3
10.5	47.7		
11	47.2	11	44.8
12	46.7	12	44.3
		12.5	43.6
		13	42.9
		13.5	42.1
13–15	46.3	14	41.5
		14.5	40.7
		15	40.1
		15.5	39.4
16	45.7	16	38.9
16.5	45.3	16.5	38.3
17	44.8	17	37.8
17.5	44.0	17.5	37.4
18	43.3		
18.5	42.7	18–19	36.7
19	42.3		
19.5	42.0		
20–21	41.4		
22–23	40.8	20–24	36.2
24–27	40.2		
28–29	39.8		
30–34	39.3	25–44	35.7
35–39	38.7		
40–44	38.0		
45–49	37.4	45–49	34.9
50–54	36.7	50–54	34.0
55–59	36.1	55–59	33.2
60–64	35.5	60–64	32.6
65–69	34.8	65–69	32.3

adults (Table 1.1). Boothbay et al (1936) found that the BMR of a 6-year-old child was around 30% higher than in the adult of 30. Children have much smaller stomachs than adults and therefore need to eat more frequent smaller meals with good protein/energy content. This metabolic difference also means that children are more vulnerable than adults to protein/energy malnutrition.

In underdeveloped countries and among poorer populations in developed countries, this is a dangerous age for children and mortality in young children can be high, especially when breast-feeding ceases. The major threat is of protein/energy malnutrition. Some studies have shown high rates of malnutrition among children in poor families and urban areas of developing countries where even the subsistence crops and gathered food of the rural poor are not available (Ahmed 1992, Shetty 1992).

DEVELOPMENT OF SENSORIMOTOR AND COGNITIVE SKILLS

The development of the sensorimotor and cognitive skills of the young child is well illustrated in the Stycar sequences of Mary Sheridan (1980). They do not produce quantified developmental quotients by which children may be compared, but provide a method of simple assessment of the individual child without the need for complex specialised clinics or equipment and form a useful guide for nurses in hospitals or community settings seeking to identify problems in early childhood and to check whether children's performance is broadly above or below the standard for their age.

The Stycar items are grouped as follows:

- posture and large movements
- vision and fine movements
- hearing and speech
- social behaviour and play.

The development of the young child between birth and 5 years is considered within these categories.

Birth and the first year

The first weeks of life

Reflex movements. The young baby at birth is equipped with a number of primitive instinctual movements which assist in the performance of certain activities that are important to survival. These include:

- the ability to suck and swallow milk
- the ability to eliminate waste from bladder and bowels
- a palmar and plantar grasp reflex
- the Moro reflex, which occurs when the infant is startled and involves the arms being flung apart symmetrically and then brought together.

The infant who is placed prone, lying on the face, will be observed to turn the head so that the face is sideways.

Newborn babies will also show other reflex abilities such as primary walking, in which they make 'stepping' movements and extend their legs when supported with their feet resting on a hard surface. Blink and pupil reaction reflexes are also present from birth, and infants will turn towards diffuse light and close their eyes when exposed to a bright light.

Some of these movements are capable of interpretation in the light of evolutionary success. For example, the infant who does not root for the breast and suck at the nipple is unlikely to do well at feeding. The infant who can turn the head to avoid suffocation when placed face down is more likely to survive such an experience. The palmar and plantar reflexes may relate to grasping the mother, or to our simian origins.

The responses to bright light are similar to those of adults, but the turning towards diffuse light does not persist. The Moro and stepping reflexes are harder to interpret in evolutionary terms.

Many of these primitive reflexes disappear over the first few weeks of life, but some persist lifelong (e.g. pupil reaction). In the main, it appears that the disappearing reflexes are replaced by functional abilities such as turning towards sounds, gazing at moving objects, reaching under more or less conscious control for attractive objects, increased manual manipulative skill, weight-bearing through the legs, etc.

Crying. The first sound of the newborn infant is the distinctive birth cry. Thereafter, the cry is the most common sound the infant makes and it has been widely interpreted as the first attempt at audible communication between the infant and care givers. We all find the sound of a baby crying to be attention-grabbing—people turn to look and usually respond with sympathy and comfort. Studies have been undertaken on crying patterns and duration by using 24-hour audio tape recordings of infant sounds.

There are wide variations between babies, and even siblings may have very different crying patterns. Some studies suggest that boys may be more prone to cry than girls (Moss 1987) but this has not been found in other research.

Some 29% or so of babies cry for very long periods of time—as much as 3 hours or even more over a 24-hour period. This is very stressful for their parents, who may be concerned that the infants are ill or that there is something wrong with their care or feeding. Some babies have been changed from breast milk to formula in an attempt to 'satisfy' them, and then subsequently a number of different milk formulae may be tried.

Crying is quickly interpreted by parents as communication and they can make estimates of the child's needs for food, comfort or sleep according to the nature of the cry.

Parent–child interaction. The socialising abilities of the newborn baby are relatively few. Babies seldom smile before about 6 weeks of age, but mothers are very aware of this first response. Babies respond to discomfort or distress by crying, but stop when they are picked up and spoken to, and during feeding they gaze intently at the face of the person feeding them and can even be induced to follow some facial movements when alert. This kind of increasing responsiveness is very satisfying to parents.

Parents are also very alert to their new baby. The baby with sensory difficulties such as deafness will not exhibit a startle reflex to loud noises, only when stimulated by physical disturbance. Babies with severe visual defects do not startle and blink in response to a bright light, but may follow sounds with their eyes. Detection of these sensory difficulties at or around birth is becoming easier with specialised equipment, but few babies are tested this young and usually it is the mother's acute sense of her infant's responses which first alerts her to sensory problems.

Immunisation against poliomyelitis, diphtheria, pertussis and tetanus begins at 2 months and is completed before babies reach 1 year of age. Measles, mumps, rubella and meningitis immunisation follows in the second year (see Ch. 2).

At 3 months

Posture and large movements. By 3 months, the normal baby will have lost more of the early primitive reflexes and is on the way to becoming a much more discriminating and responsive person. Some head control can be expected, likewise kicking and playing with the fingers, all of which show that motor coordination is developing well. There is no sign of the leg extension and early primary walking movements noted in the newborn, and weight-bearing generally does not appear before about 6 months of age.

Vision and fine movements. The baby is also less drowsy and more visually attentive, watching and following moving objects. Eye coordination is not perfect; occasional squints will still be seen. Hand–eye coordination is not usual before about 4 months, but the baby will grasp and shake a rattle briefly.

Social behaviour and play. At 3 months more varied sounds are observed and the baby recognises preparations for feeding and responds eagerly. Enjoyment of caring routines (especially bathtime) is also noticeable.

At 6 months

Posture and large movements. By the time babies are 6 months old, they are more physically able and coordinated and can take their weight through their legs if supported, sit straight, roll and kick. Head control is also good, and babies can raise themselves on their elbows when lying prone. Crawling is well established from around 7 months and so is unsupported sitting.

Vision and fine movements. Manual dexterity is also improved and the child can pass toys from hand to hand, focus on them and manipulate them with a characteristic palmar grasp. The toys and other objects being examined are likely to get further investigation as infants tend to take everything to their mouths.

Hearing and speech. Sounds become more varied in content, and cooing and babbling are added to the repertoire by the time the infant is about 6 months old. Non-vocal communication is also used from about 9 months, with directed gaze, expression and finger-pointing all being used to indicate things which interest the infant.

The good sitting posture and balance of babies at this age mean that distraction hearing testing can be undertaken, using low-volume sound of high and low frequencies to attract the baby to turn towards the sound. The timing of this test takes advantage of the fact that babies of this age are very curious and attentive to quiet sounds and will readily turn to see what is happening. They also babble and vocalise with a wide range of sounds and are generally sociable, even responding to unfamiliar adults without shyness, as long as the parent is present.

Social behaviour and play. The 6-month-old child is not yet mobile, but is very responsive and curious, being generally not too fearful to welcome new people. Children of this age are old enough and alert enough to be entertained by simple play with older siblings, examining toys and passing them from hand to hand to mouth for appraisal.

At 6 months, babies may show early signs of teething and are generally able to take a wide range of foods as well as milk (see Box 1.4). Their ability to tackle some types of family food without liquidising means that they are much more part of the family than the tiny infant. They cannot yet handle a spoon and few will have teeth, but they will gnaw on finger foods and

Box 1.4   Diet at 6 months

There is some debate over diet because many family foods do not contain much iron. The debate still continues over the need to use vitamin- and iron-fortified commercial baby foods such as 'follow on' formulae, rather then family foods, etc. While there is a risk of anaemia in some babies, most infants are well nourished by a good range of family foods, suitably prepared, together with breast milk or cow's milk, but there is a large and profitable baby food industry offering a wide range of convenience products for babies and toddlers.

'teething' toys. Because they have a tendency to put everything in their mouths, safety is an issue to avoid choking or ingestion of unsuitable substances.

At 1 year

Posture and large movements. By the time that normal babies are 1 year old, they are able to support their weight for much longer periods and some will even walk with support or 'cruise' around the furniture. Increasing mobility and stability mean that children need some environmental protection to prevent accidents (see Box 1.5).

Vision and fine movements. Manipulation is increasingly skilled with both hands being used, and finger-pointing is used to indicate interesting items. The former palmar grasp should now be fading to the use of a more developed 'tripod' grasp using fingers rather than the palm area to manipulate objects.

Box 1.5   Safety within the home

Young children just starting to toddle have no appreciation of common dangers in their environment. Falls are very common, but serious injuries are more likely if the home is not safe. Stairs, windows and trailing electrical flexes of kitchen equipment can be very interesting to young children. So are the contents of cupboards. Fireguards, stair gates, safety harnesses, covers for electrical sockets and a watchful eye are all needed! Parents need advice on accident prevention and children's nurses have good opportunities to encourage safe practice.

Hearing and speech. The babble of the younger infant gives way to sounds that are increasingly like speech. Some children will have a few words, but most meaningful communications are very simple and not always comprehensible outside the family. Helen Bee (1989) gives some good examples of these early vocabularies from a study by Scollon (1976).

Social behaviour and play. Toys need to reflect the infant's new-found manipulative skill, and the traditional 'activity centre' toy with its different manipulations is enjoyable. Some visual and cognitive skills are established allowing the child to recognise familiar people, find toys which have rolled out of sight and watch toys cast from a high chair or cot to see where they fall. This group of phenomena are linked cognitively to form a set of ideas about the natural world which includes persistence of objects, relationships with family members and familiar adults, and also the way in which objects behave. Children may also recognise pictures of parents, siblings, etc. This discrimination also means that children of about 8–9 months are much more fearful and shy of strangers and need to see the familiar parent close at hand for comfort and reassurance. Nurses should approach children of this age gently and allow them to 'warm up' gradually to the idea of being friends. Sudden enthusiastic introductions can cause the child distress.

By the time the baby is 1 year old, social skills are also enhanced by the use of more sophisticated vocalisation and obvious understanding of simple words and phrases. The skills of feeding and eating a wider range of food develop in parallel with vocalisation, both being vocal skills. Objects are rarely taken to the mouth for examination, but explored using hand and eye instead. Games involve adults in speech exchange games and 'give and take' of objects, plus pushing of truck and wheeled toys.

The next 4 years

This is a period of massive cognitive development as young children learn to make sense of their environment. Possibly the greatest achievement of children in this age group is human communication through language.

 For information on speech development in children, readers should consult the list of further reading at the end of the chapter.

The main factors which appear to promote the social and intellectual development of children between 1 and 5 years are the degree to which they are stimulated by their environment and the positive attention they receive from adults around them. The mechanism by which these factors are provided varies.

Bee (1989) lists five elements found within families whose children made good progress:

- They provided appropriate play material for the child—Bee considers developmental stage appropriateness to be more important than quantity of toys.
- They are emotionally responsive to and involved with the child, spend time encouraging their child and show warmth in interactions and attitude to the child.
- They talk to their child, using language which is descriptively rich and accurate.
- They avoid excessive punishment, control and restrictions on the child, allowing the child to explore and make mistakes.
- They have high expectations that the child will do well and make good progress.

The young toddler

Posture and large movements. Physical development in the normal child is quite variable, but most children are walking well by 16 months, and by the age of 18 months to 2 years most children can run and cope with stairs, one step at a time.

Vision and fine movements. Manual activities are increasingly skilled by 18–24 months and picture books, paints and brick building are all enjoyed. Children from about 15 months can

drink very well from a cup and use a spoon to feed themselves, provided food is cut up into manageably sized portions.

Hearing and speech. Verbal abilities extend to about 50 words by the age of 2 years, with wide comprehension and obvious verbal 'work' during which the child asks names of objects, repeats words spoken by others and vocalises at length during play.

Social behaviour and play. Whilst toddlers have a reputation for being difficult, it is important to remember that children of this age are individuals and the degree to which they mix and play happily with others is also a function of their individuality.

Socially, 2-year-old children are sometimes difficult to manage because of their negativity and strong need to express their own wishes and their possessiveness about toys and adult attention. Tantrums are frequent and children express their frustrations regularly!

Play is energetic and involves active exploration of the environment. It tends to follow the pattern of parallel play among children under 3; that is they will play similar games alongside other children, but the play does not extend to sharing the toy or engaging in cooperative games. Games with rules are also rather complex for the young toddler.

Toilet training also begins to take place from any time after about 16 months of age, but the age of achievement varies considerably. Boys are said to be slower than girls, but there may be social or practical reasons for this observation.

At 3 years: the older toddler

Posture and large movements. At 3 years, children are very mobile and capable of running, jumping and climbing, and throwing and kicking balls with greater confidence. They are also capable of riding a tricycle. They still have poor appreciation of common dangers and need care when out and about near to traffic.

Vision and fine movements. Fine movements and coordination enable fairly complex block building including copying simple 'bridge' patterns. Children can also copy and match simple letters and make simple drawings of people, which include facial features.

Hearing and speech. Speech skills are developing fast with a large vocabulary and more conventional use of grammar. Stories and rhymes are enjoyed. Children may be able to count, but this is usually just another 'rhyme game' and there is little appreciation of the nature of numbers. Bilingual families are quite common and the process by which children acquire a second language is fascinating (Box 1.6).

Social behaviour and play. Socially, children at 3 years are less frustrated and more amenable than younger toddlers. Play tends to be more cooperative too, involving 'helping' with housework, active make believe and sharing of toys with others. The mixing of fantasy and fact leads to 'tall tales' where everyday people and situations are mixed with the fantastic from stories—a factor which makes working with abused children of this age quite a delicate and skilled process.

By this age, children should have a degree of skill at eating with a spoon and some will manage a small-sized knife and fork. When possible, it is good to encourage this child to take meals with the rest of the family, eating sensibly from the main meal (Box 1.7). It is a pleasant social experience, and children learn by picking up adult ways of behaving at meals.

Most children are reliably dry during the daytime by the time they reach 3 years, but they take longer to be dry overnight. By the time they are

---

Box 1.6 The child of the bilingual family

If parents plan to have their children speak both languages, it is as well to speak both from the beginning. There will be a stage when words from both are confused, but if parents make it clear which words belong with which language, children will gradually sort out the two as their vocabulary and grasp of syntax get better. Nurses caring for the child who is speaking early words in two languages may find this confusing if they are unfamiliar with the second language, but parents can be asked to compile a glossary of special words used by their child and their English equivalents, to avoid frustration for all concerned.

Box 1.7 The diet of young children

Many families do not have family meals and, because of changed lifestyles and eating in front of the television, children tend to eat on the move. This can lead to the consumption of quickly produced finger foods, often high in fat and sugar. Children who consume a lot of snack foods such as crisps and sweets tend to have little experience of eating full meals. The diet of many young children in the United Kingdom requires improvement to avoid many of them becoming obese and unhealthy later in life (see Ch. 2).

3½, toilet training is usually well advanced with many children managing to be dry during both the day and the night (see Ch. 13).

At 4 years: the pre-school child

Posture and large movements. At about 4 years old, a child's normal motor activity shows increased skill. The child shows greater ability at climbing and descending stairs and can usually manage to stand on tiptoe and hop (on the preferred dominant foot). Right or left dominance is usually established by this stage.

Vision and fine movements. The skills of the 4-year-old at brick building and copying letters are more accurate and the opposing thumb can be used with any finger. Pencils are held in adult fashion with the more primitive infantile palmar or tripod grips being rarely used. Figurative drawings show better appreciation of the relative size of body parts and a 4-year-old can also draw a simple house. Children can also name primary colours correctly and match them.

Hearing and speech. Speech by 4 years is generally grammatically correct and intelligible with few infantile phonetic substitutions of sounds. Stories are enjoyed, with fantasy in telling their own stories and accounts of events and appreciation of verbal jokes. Rhymes and songs are learnt by heart.

Social behaviour and play. 4-year-olds can usually eat most foods using a spoon and fork dextrously. Self-care skills are also getting more proficient, including washing, teeth cleaning dressing and undressing with a little help and

Activity 1.3

Using the Stycar book, spend time with three young children of different ages under 5 and observe them closely during play to see if they are able to demonstrate some of the age-appropriate activities and abilities outlined in the developmental areas of gross and fine movement, verbal and social skills.

supervision. Children of this age also need and enjoy the company of others, and playgroups or other pre-school activities are very helpful.

At 5 years: the school-age child

Posture and large movements. By the time the child is 5 years old, mobility is skilled and athletic, including hopping, skipping and balancing, walking along a narrow straight line and some appreciation of the rules of ball games in addition to increased playing skills.

Vision and fine movements. 5-year-olds also show increased dexterity in building and copying tasks and good control of pencils, crayons, etc. Some children will begin to write simple letters, and drawings are increasingly sophisticated with neat colouring and better representation of subjects. Colour matching involves a wider range of colours.

Hearing and speech. Speech includes appreciation of abstract as well as concrete nouns and children enjoy and act out stories. There is some evidence that speech skills on starting school are linked to better performance in learning at school, although the mechanism by which these two are connected is not clear (Calnan & Richardson 1977).

Social behaviour and play. 5 is the age by which most children in this country start school, often full-time classes. They therefore need a range of social and communication skills which will enable them to encounter new people without the support of a parent and to express their needs. It is also helpful for a child to have had experience of playing with others of the same age and level of maturity, rather than adults or older siblings only. The school playground can be an alarming place for a small child who has a very limited social experience.

Behaviour is more cooperative overall and there are fewer quarrels with playmates because the idea of game rules and fair play is comprehended. Children can now enjoy dressing up and acting out stories together and will form friendships, usually with their own gender.

Appreciation of time, date and rules of behaviour is also beginning by this age. Some children pick up additional skills such as numbers and reading, if exposed to these during play or at nursery school. The symbolic nature of numbers is also better understood at this age. 5-year-olds are also gentler and more understanding of the needs of younger siblings and pet animals and will comfort distressed companions.

GROWTH AND DEVELOPMENTAL ABNORMALITIES

There are many reasons why children may fail to reach their apparent growth potential. Some are very rare, such as metabolic disorders which are often due to inherited genetic abnormalities, e.g. mucopolysaccharidosis. Others occur more commonly, and paediatric nurses may expect to encounter some cases either diagnosed as abnormalities or under the broader category of 'failure to thrive'. Some of these conditions affect the growth of the limbs more than overall proportionate growth.

Proportionate smallness of stature

There may be an inherited tendency to proportionate short stature which is familial and can be detected by looking at the family of the small, slow-growing child, comparing the growth of parents and siblings. Failure in intrauterine growth and low birth weight may also affect the subsequent development and growth of children in that they may take several years to 'catch up' with their potential normal growth curve.

Endocrine disorders such as hypothyroidism

produce short stature as well as delay in mental development. Similar stunting of growth and failure to reach full genetic potential height may also be observed in children with untreated cardiac disease, although this is rare with modern early surgical corrections of defects. Cystic fibrosis and coeliac disease may also affect growth potential, but with more effective management of these diseases, affected children live longer and achieve more normal growth patterns than previous generations. A deficiency of growth hormone will also produce small stature without affecting the relative proportions of the body and in this case the general health of the child is likely to remain normal apart from the small stature.

Nutritional failure to thrive is divided into organic and non-organic causes. Organic causes may be due to any of the above diseases or to inadequate or unsuitable feeding. Non-organic failure to thrive may be due to emotional deprivation or abuse.

Failure to maintain normal growth where the relative body proportions are unaffected is detected by careful child health surveillance and the use of growth charts and accurate measurements. The second category of small stature and growth failure where there is disproportionate shortness of the limbs is more easily detected but may have a very serious prognosis for the child.

Disproportionate smallness of stature

The most common of the short-limbed failures to grow is the condition of achondroplasia, a dominantly inherited condition where there is failure of the limbs to grow without the rest of the body proportions being affected. Less common, but with serious effects on development and general health is the condition known as 'brittle bone syndrome' or osteogenesis imperfecta. This varies in severity but may leave a child badly disabled or even lead to death.

Much less common in developed countries than before the last war is the condition of rickets, where nutritional deficiencies lead to bowing of the legs and consequent loss of height. Fortification of bread flour and margarine is still enforced in the United Kingdom to prevent this. Very occasionally some children raised in conditions of poverty and deprivation may still show signs of rickets.

SOME THEORETICAL IDEAS ABOUT CHILD DEVELOPMENT

One of the interesting aspects of studying the developing child is that there are several different theories about how psychological development may be taking place. A theory is a collection of ideas which fit together logically to provide an explanation for what we see in the world around us. No theory is usually the whole story and looking at different theories gives us a number of views of child development which all contribute something to our understanding.

Understanding the ideas about what causes and promotes human development is important to people who have the care of young children because they wish to do whatever they can to help these children. It is helpful to look at a few of the current concepts used in describing the development of the normal child.

The first developmental concept, which is particularly important in the early stages of child development, is the idea of differentiation and hierarchical organisation, initially of embryonic cells into organs. This idea relates to the embryo in that although the cells are initially relatively undifferentiated, they rapidly differentiate into different tissues and organs. This continues after birth in the functional development of nervous and muscular control in motor skills.

Another recent concept in child development study considers the way in which children's early and instinctual behaviour promotes their likelihood of success in tackling new experiences such as feeding. This is called pre-adaptation behaviour and includes the kind of instinctive behaviour which normal infants show at birth, such as sucking and grasping reflexes. These kinds of patterns are likely to be retained because they increase the likelihood of success in feeding.

According to Piaget's studies in child development, children pass through a stage of development called the sensorimotor stage as they learn hand–eye coordination, walking and other major motor skills. The early reflexes of the newborn baby lead to increasing voluntary control of limbs and head, with those patterns of movement which have been most successful being retained; so, from initial reflexes, the infant gradually develops coordinated responses to environmental stimuli.

One of the other major concepts which arises during the observation of the development of the pre-school child is the idea of critical or sensitive periods for the acquisition of important skills. It defines particular age ranges during

---

Box 1.8 The case of Genie (Fromkin et al 1974, Kyle 1980)

An example of a case when it was thought that a child had missed the critical age for acquiring skills was an abused American child known as Genie. Genie was the only child of a couple who appear to have had multiple problems—her mother was blind and her father held bizarre ideas about child rearing. The abuse Genie suffered took the form of confinement to a single room, spending long periods alone, often strapped into a toilet chair or a cot. She was discovered in the early 1970s at the age of 10 years, almost unable to walk, without speech, severely developmentally retarded and unable to sustain any normal interpersonal relationship even to the point of eye contact.

Although there was horror at the extent of her abuse, the scientists found the case very interesting as a rare example of a so-called 'feral' child and also because the extreme deprivation of human contact had apparently not permitted the acquisition of speech in spite of the fact that she could hear. If Genie could acquire speech at 10 years of age, it would cast serious doubt on the critical stage theory of development. In fact, despite years of speech therapy, Genie never learned to speak with normal patterns and lost some of her early communication abilities over time.

Unfortunately, however, there was a major confounding variable in this case; no medical or developmental records had ever been made on Genie, and there was consequently no proof that she had been born normal. If this unfortunate girl had been handicapped from birth, it would have gone some way towards explaining her inability to acquire speech. Without this evidence, the case could not serve as an example of a missed critical period and it would be deeply unethical to risk the development of normal children by deliberately depriving them of human contact in order to test the theory experimentally.

---

which infants and young children can pick up skills because they have reached the point of maturity at which they are equipped to develop them. Conversely, if this critical time is missed, the child may have difficulty in developing the skills later on in life. This idea is frequently applied to speech acquisition, but is very difficult to prove for ethical and methodological reasons (see Box 1.8).

The study of human growth and development shows that there is a balance between the effects of nature (the genetic inheritance of the child) and nurture (the environment in which development takes place) and that these two influences appear to operate in a way in which each affects the other. The factors of a poor heredity can be counteracted by early compensatory measures; for example, children who inherit a tendency towards myopia are provided with glasses which enable them to continue to develop visual skills as if they were quite normal visually. Children who have a difficult environmental experience, such as being born prematurely, may show delayed milestones for a few years and appear small for their age, but by about 6 years nearly all will have caught up with their normally born counterparts and be at the correct height, weight and developmental stage for their age.

THE CHILD WITHIN THE FAMILY

The family is the ecological setting for normal childhood. Even for those children who cannot be brought up within a normal family setting, there are efforts to model a substitute social setting which mirrors the small family group of adults and children rather than the large institutional homes and hospital settings in which children used to be raised before the 1950s and 1960s. Many of the ideas behind this small-scale organisation come from the work of John Bowlby whose book *Child Care and the Growth of Love* was first published in 1953 following a study undertaken for the World Health Organization which linked the quality of maternal care with the future mental health and social adjustment of the child.

One of the most prominent aspects of this influential work is that the role of the mother is seen as central. The role of the father does not have the same salience and little seems to have been expected of fathers traditionally. The Truby King baby care books, which influenced the mothers and health educators earlier this century, suggest that the father's role is mainly one of kindly supervision, ensuring that the mother gets out for some occasional wholesome amusement (with plenty of fresh air!), though he should also attend the odd mothercraft class with her to ensure that she does not forget what she is told. He should refrain from his 'conjugal demands' during pregnancy in order not to provoke a miscarriage and not insist that his wife resume her household duties during the first month after the birth. Apart from these acts of consideration, there is simply the registration of the birth and a prompt christening and the duties of the father are largely accomplished (Truby King 1938). Much of day-to-day child care was considered to be demeaning for a man and competence was not expected.

Spock in the late 1950s suggested that a slightly greater involvement was good to make the father feel important—the occasional feed or napkin change would be sufficient (Spock 1957). Since those days, the role of men as economically active providers and of women as carers has been changed by a combination of feminism and the need for cheaper part-time workers in modern industry. Unemployment has sent many men back to the home, not all of whom were brought up to expect the role of day-to-day caring parent to young children. Nurses need to support fathers in the care of children, particularly when the child is sick or disabled, and enable them to play a part as caring parents.

Increasingly, children are born and raised within single-parent families. This is due to the increasing rate of divorce in western societies and the relative readiness of young women to start their families without being married to the father. Although the idea of mothers going out to work has become more acceptable, there are still many difficulties associated with this pattern of family life. Mothers often have to be both breadwinners and carers, and women still tend to be less well paid than men. These two factors mean that a single mother may have a greater workload than her married counterpart and that her family is likely to suffer a degree of material disadvantage. The single mother with a sick child needs to develop a network of support to enable her to cope, and nurses need to be alert to these needs in caring for the child.

CONCLUSION

The nature of child development is one which is still a major object of scientific study and explanation. All children's nurses need a clear idea of the sequence of the development of young children and the ways in which this can be helped and promoted. They are well placed to advise and support parents and promote the health of the child within the family by discussing their needs and health care.

For adolescent development, see Chapter 22.

REFERENCES

Ahmed F 1992 Nutritional situation of Dhaka. Southeast Asian Journal of Medicine and Public Health 23(Suppl. 3): 59–64

Bee H 1989 The developing child. HarperCollins, New York

Boothbay et al 1936 The Mayo Foundation normal standards of basal metabolic rate. Cited by: Brim O G Jr, Kagan J (eds) 1980 Constancy and change in human development. Harvard College, USA

Bowlby J 1965 Child care and the growth of love. Penguin, Harmondsworth

Brim O G Jr, Kagan J (eds) 1980 Constancy and change in human development. Harvard College, USA

Calnan M, Richardson K 1977 Speech problems among children in a national survey: associations with reading, general ability, mathematics and syntactic maturity. Educational Studies 3(1): 55–66

Corrao G, Busellu G, Valenti M, Lepore A R, Sconci V, Casacchia M, di Orio F 1993 Alcohol-related problems within the family and global functioning of the children: a population-based study. Social Psychiatry and Psychiatric Epidemiology 28(6): 304–308

DHSS Committee on Medical Aspects of Food Policy 1988 Present day practice in infant feeding: third report. HMSO, London

Fromkin V et al 1974 The development of language in Genie: a case of language acquisition beyond the 'critical period'. Brain and Language 1(1): 81–107

Kyle J G 1980 Auditory deprivation from birth—clarification of some issues. British Journal of Audiology 14(1): 34–36

Martin J, White A 1988 Infant feeding 1985. Office of Population Censuses and Surveys, Social Survey Division. HMSO, London

Micozzi M S 1987 Cross cultural correlations of childhood growth and adult breast cancer. American Journal of Physical Anthropology 73(4): 525–537

Moore K L 1988 Essentials of human embryology. B C Decker, Ontario

Moss 1987 Sex, age and state as determinates of mother–infant interaction. Merrill-Palmer Quarterly 13: 19–36

Piaget J 1953 The origins of intelligence in children. Routledge & Kegan Paul, London

Pridham K F 1990 Feeding behaviour of 6–12 month old infants: assessment and sources of parental information. Journal of Paediatrics 117: S174–S180

Pridham K F, Knight C B, Stephenson G R 1989 Mothers' working models of infant feeding: description and influencing factors. Journal of Advanced Nursing 14: 1051–1061

Scollon R 1976 Conversations with a one year old. University Press of Hawaii, Hawaii

Sheridan M D 1980 From birth to five years: children's developmental progress. NFER–Nelson, London

Shetty P S 1992 City studies on nutrition: Bangalore, India. Southeast Asian Journal of Tropical Medicine and Public Health 23(Suppl. 3): 54–58

Sinclair D 1989 Human growth after birth. Oxford University Press, Oxford

Spock B 1957 Commonsense book of childcare. Meredith Press, New York

Truby King 1938 Mothercraft. Whitcombe & Tombs, Melbourne

Wehmer F, Hafez E S 1975 Maternal malnutrition, low birthweight and related phenomena in man. Physiological and behavioural interactions. European Journal of Obstetrics, Gynecolology and Reproductive Biology 4(5): 177–187

FURTHER READING

Speech development in children

Barrett J 1994 Help me speak: parents' guide to speech and language therapy. Souvenir Press, London

Bee H 1992 The developing child, 6th edn. HarperCollins, New York (A classic, readable text which has a very useful section on the development of language in children)

Bruner J 1983 Child's talk: learning to use language. Oxford University Press, Oxford (A small paperback, based on his psychological studies)

Garvey C 1984 Children's talk. (Developing child series) Fontana, London (A clearly written, useful paperback, based on research and written for professionals and parents)

Naremore R C, Hopper R 1990 Children learning language: a practical introduction to communication development, 3rd edn. Harper Row, New York (An American text, designed mainly for teachers and educationalists)

Promoting health

Jayne Taylor   Diana Forster

This chapter considers the vital importance of health promotion—including health protection, health education and disease prevention—in relation to children's nursing. It aims to develop the health-promoting nurse by:

- **emphasising an integrated approach to health promotion**
- **considering the importance of inequalities in health for families and children**
- **outlining the processes, principles and strategies of health promotion**
- **introducing health promotion approaches targeted towards specific age groups.**

INTRODUCTION

Health promotion during childhood and adolescence is vitally important because it is during these critical periods of the life span that the learning of health-related behaviours, attitudes, values and perceptions takes place. The child's environment and quality of life in turn affect later life and its quality. Behaviours learned during these early years provide the basis for health-related behaviours during adulthood. Promoting a healthy lifestyle, preventing disease and optimising recovery from illness during the adult years are by-products of a healthy lifestyle in the early years. This chapter will consider individual behavioural and much wider aspects of health and its promotion.

- Accessibility: health care which is provided close to where people live and work.
- Acceptability: health care which is appropriate and provided in ways which people find acceptable.
- Equity: all people have an equal right to health and health care.
- Self-determination: people have the right and the responsibility to make their own health choices.
- Community involvement: people have the right and the responsibility to participate individually and collectively in the planning and implementation of their health care.
- A focus on health: primary health care concentrates on the promotion of health as well as on the care of people who are sick, frail or disabled.
- A multisectoral approach: housing, food policies, environmental policies and social services have an important part to play.

There is a need for a shift in focus from concentrating only on personal behaviour, such as whether or not children are brought for immunisation, towards external factors which are also capable of influencing health and health-behaviour. This approach is based on the key principles which were set out in the Declaration of Alma Ata (WHO 1978) (Box 2.1).

WHAT IS HEALTH PROMOTION?

Downie et al (1990) offer the following definition of health promotion: 'Health promotion comprises efforts to enhance positive health and prevent ill health, through the overlapping spheres of health education, prevention and health protection' (Fig. 2.1).

Health education

Health education may be defined as 'any activity which promotes health-related learning, i.e. some relatively permanent change in an individual's capabilities or dispositions' (Hall 1991). An example would be the change in parents' awareness of the dangers of letting their child be exposed to too much sun, and knowing how to prevent this, following a paediatric nurse's health education session.

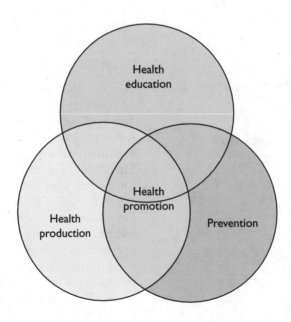

Figure 2.1   Three overlapping spheres of health promotion (adapted from Downie et al 1990).

Prevention

Prevention has three components; primary, secondary and tertiary.

Primary prevention. This involves preventing the occurrence of disease or injury. Immunisation programmes to prevent diseases such as whooping cough, a danger to the health of babies, are examples of primary prevention.

Secondary prevention. This aims to stop the development of disease or handicapping conditions by early detection and appropriate action. For instance, through screening programmes designed to discover deafness in babies, hearing aids, special teaching and parental guidance can be introduced as soon as possible. This leads to the best possible development of speech and quality of life.

Tertiary prevention. This involves preventing deterioration, where possible, and impeding the progress of established disease or disability by appropriate treatment, rehabilitation or palliative care. It involves providing appropriate support—both emotional and practical—advising and information giving. The role of the community nurse in paediatric learning disability for instance involves working with parents by helping them to identify and use services available, discuss hopes, fears and plans for the children's future, and request new services for unmet needs.

Paediatric Macmillan nurses can be very supportive, providing links between cancer treatment centres and among primary health care teams, and establishing optimum home care and quality of life for the child with cancer. One parent is quoted as saying: 'At times I have felt so alone with my child at home that I have looked forward to the visit from my Macmillan nurse for advice and support. She has helped me cope with my child and his illness at the very "lowest" times—I don't know what I would have done without her visits' (Evans & Kelly 1995).

Health protection

The health protection sphere is concerned with legal and fiscal measures, regulations and policies and voluntary codes of practice. The aim in this sphere is to empower people to make healthy choices. Community nurses may for example attempt to influence local policy makers to protect health. One way of protecting health is by providing low-cost housing to prevent homelessness or unsatisfactory living conditions. Current housing policies deny many parents the homes they need for themselves and their children.

The overall goal of health promotion is summed up by Downie et al (1990) as: 'the balanced enhancement of physical, mental and social positive health, coupled with the prevention of physical, mental and social ill-health.' This goal includes the reduction of inequalities in health and improving the quality of life for families and children.

The health-promoting nurse

One of the main aims of this book is to provide a rationale and a research base for nursing children and promoting their health. All nurses, whatever their realm of practice, should be able to justify their actions and have a clear understanding of the research that informs their practice—'nurses and midwives need to develop their own nursing strategy for promoting health' (ENB 1994).

A recent review of both pre- and post-registration educational programmes for nurses, midwives and health visitors (Lask et al 1994) proposed three main recommendations:

• There is a need for nurses, midwives and health visitors to develop their own conceptualisation of health promotion.
• Health promotion needs to be addressed throughout educational programmes.
• Nursing facilitators should be introduced to help students apply health promotion theory to practice.

Health and well-being are the constant goals of children's nursing, rather than focusing solely on immediate clinical problems. This does not mean that clinical problems are unimportant, but that they should be viewed in a broader, holistic context. Nursing activities then become proactive rather than reactive. Thus health promotion within nursing practice is an integral part of nursing care and should relate to the whole range of the child's experience.

'The challenge of paediatric nursing today is in meeting the needs of the whole child. This means not only attending to his physical care, but also paying attention to his thoughts, his feelings and the need for his family' (Jolly 1981).

Health education and health promotion

The traditional approach to health education focused largely upon the prevention of medically defined disease and upon negative aspects of health, e.g. 'you should not smoke, drink, eat too little or too much or have unprotected sex'. This approach does not address positive health, and is mainly limited to physical aspects of ill health. It concentrates upon correcting individual behaviour, while ignoring the influence of political, cultural and societal factors upon children and families and the communities in which they live. The move towards the wider-based activity of health promotion has largely been spurred by recognising that traditional health education has many limitations. Health promotion is an umbrella concept; it covers a broad range of activities and interventions which include health education but also incorporate the overlapping spheres of health protection and the prevention of ill health already considered.

Health education and cognitive development

When communicating with children and young people, their reasoning powers and ability to understand and make sense of information need to be considered. These are facets of development, linked to age and to the kinds of life experiences in the child's background. Coming to hospital for out- or inpatient care is often frightening and unfamiliar for children, adding to their discomfort and requiring skilful interpersonal interaction

from health professionals. Such interaction is based on a knowledge of developmental processes which govern children's increasing understanding and logical reasoning power. For example, at 6–7 months babies normally recognise familiar people and show fear of strangers. Most young children are likely to suffer from separation anxiety if parted from their parents, and worry that parents will not come back. Children between 2 and 5 years old regard the body in terms of its surface only—the parts they can see—so descriptions of what is happening inside them would be hard for them to understand. They may think that illness is their own fault—perhaps a punishment for being naughty. Development of moral judgement and adult logical reasoning is not completed before the age of 10–12 years.

Limited powers of understanding can lead to bewilderment and frightening misinterpretation. If nurses can predict possible difficulties they are more able:

- to help improve explanations of illness and hospitalisation
- to provide sensitive reassurance for children
- to gain greater understanding of what the child is saying and meaning
- to gain some insight into how the child is interpreting all the strange occurrences that can accompany illness (Muller et al 1992).

AN INTEGRATED APPROACH TO HEALTH PROMOTION

It is unrealistic to separate the child's health status from that of the family, the cultural milieu and the environment. Health and health behaviour are affected by parental views, values

Activity 2.1

Plan to explain to a five-year-old what will happen when his tonsillectomy is performed, and afterwards. What misunderstandings might he have? How would you check what he fears and believes?

and beliefs, which in turn are influenced by cultural norms and the parents' own experiences of health and ill health.

The definition and goal of health promotion quoted earlier (Downie et al 1990) point to the need for empowering people, including parents and children, to increase control over and improve their health. Health promotion is not something that is 'done to' a child or parent, like giving an injection or providing advice, but it pervades and informs every aspect of nursing care—whether acute or community care, mental health or learning disabilities or any aspect of child and adult health—becoming an integral part of it (Skinner 1995).

Skinner (1995) discusses the use of nursing models in relation to health promotion. For example, care for a child suffering burns following an accident at home will include planning for the prevention of further accidents. A comprehensive framework for assessing, planning and evaluating care, which is provided by various nursing models, helps nursing outcomes to be measured in a meaningful way, thus enhancing health promotion.

Kelly et al (1993) identify four levels of health promotion which should all be considered as an integrated approach in any health promotion intervention (Box 2.2).

The relationship between these four levels, explored in more detail below, can be linked to the integration of the three spheres of health promotion itself (Fig. 2.1) into nursing practice.

Environmental level

The environment cannot be ignored in health promotion interventions, as it may be health promoting or health protecting in itself or health damaging. It also provides the background within which health promotion activities take place.

The importance of the relationship between the quality of the physical environment and the health of children and their families has long been recognised. Children need to have clean and supportive environments at home and school that nurture their development and protect them from harm. They also need protection from psychological abuse. Article 19 of the United Nations Convention on the Rights of the Child, to which the United Kingdom is a signatory, is shown in Box 2.3.

Poverty and inequality in the United Kingdom

Health strategies for children include the goal of equalising mortality and morbidity rates among different socioeconomic groups and reducing inequalities in health (Victor 1995). A study of trends in the living circumstances of children show that a higher proportion of them were poorer in 1991 than in 1979 (Kumar 1994). Unemployment and low pay are likely to be the most important single factors. Numbers of families affected by unemployment have increased substantially, causing the environment of children to be impoverished. Children whose parents are in low-paid work are also far more likely than others to be living in poverty. The rise in lone-parent families has particularly contributed to increasing child poverty. In 1979, 28% of children who lived with one parent were poor, but by 1991 this had risen to 74% (Kumar 1994).

Box 2.4   A health care charter for children (James 1995)

A comprehensive children's community profile needs to be developed, in partnership with children and young people, as an audit and community development tool. This could form the basis of a local health care charter for children and contribute to the future commissioning of children's services.

Most lone parents are women, and health promotion workers need to take account of the pressures of poverty upon day-to-day living and child care. An example of this is provided by Graham (1993). Her research study demonstrates a clear relationship between mothers who smoke—as a means of coping in difficult circumstances—and a range of housing problems, including damp, insufficient heating, a lack of play space, noise and accommodation needing repair. However, 'Health of the Nation' (DoH 1992) strategies tend not to address wider social questions of eradicating poverty and sharing financial resources more fairly. James (1995) proposes a health care charter for children to promote children's health in the wider environment (see Box 2.4).

Many people, including:

- city planners
- social and health workers
- housing and traffic administrators
- teachers
- environmental health officers
- business employers
- community activists

take part in promoting environmental health. This is especially important in transcultural societies where a rich variety of different life-styles need to be recognised (Parmar 1993). Information is available in the United Kingdom from local health promotion/education departments and environmental health offices.

Preventing childhood accidents

One of the main 'Health of the Nation' targets, identified in a follow-up document (DoH 1993a)

is to reduce the death rate among children aged under 15 by at least 33% by the year 2005, from 6.6 per 100 000 in 1990 to no more than 4.4 per 100 000. It states that the health promotion activities relate:

- to improving awareness and knowledge about the risks involved in everyday behaviour
- to encouraging people, especially parents and carers, to adopt a healthy or safer pattern of behaviour
- to encouraging those at risk to change their behaviour to reduce the risk of accidents.

One example of progress in this direction is the Berkshire Hospital's cycle helmet campaign which was recognised with the Prince Michael award for road safety (DoH 1993a).

Many children die or are injured as a result of road traffic accidents, home accidents, drowning, fires and poisoning. Nursing children back to health after surviving such accidents is one major aspect of children's nursing today, but an awareness of wider issues helps to promote health through accident prevention. Children of parents in social class V (e.g. unskilled manual workers) are four times more likely to suffer accidental death than those in social class I (e.g. professional and upper managerial). Before school age most fatal accidents happen at home, where children spend much of their time. Almost half of accidental deaths in the home are due to fires. Families living in overcrowded accommodation are significantly less likely to have a fitted and working smoke alarm. Nurses should be aware of other particular risk factors, such as the fire risks for families in temporary accommodation who may have to use unsafe heaters without

Activity 2.2

Arrange a visit to your local health promotion unit and ask what children's safety campaigns are being planned. Consider ways in which you might publicise these to parents or teachers and help the campaigns to benefit those in greatest need.

Box 2.5   Safety initiatives planned for an inner-city health authority (Woodroffe & Williams 1994)

- Car seats for babies to be on sale at the general hospital.
- Contract with the local taxi company operating from the hospital to be re-negotiated to ensure that car seats are provided for babies and children.
- The Child Accident Prevention Trust to be commissioned to provide 100 training sessions with local parents.

effective fire-guards. One group of health visitors set up a safety equipment loan scheme, run by parents themselves (Wright 1994). There is a clear responsibility in promoting freedom from accidents to consider wider issues than the behavioural ones concentrated upon in the 'Health of the Nation' strategy (DoH 1992).

Safety initiatives planned by one inner city health authority are shown in Box 2.5.

Nurses can also play their part in influencing policies relevant to health promotion. Many local authorities employ specialist road safety officers, particularly regarding children and older people's safety, and nurses may for example plan to liaise with them. Traffic and highway engineering is concerned with preventing accidents through the careful design of road carriageways, road junctions, pedestrian crossings, speed reduction measures (road humps etc.), parking control schemes and the segregation of traffic, pedestrians and cyclists (Pike D 1995).

Safe play areas

Housing schemes need to incorporate safe play areas for children. In some areas many families, particularly those from ethnic minorities, live in high rise flats or inner city housing where there is little space for children to play. Concern is often expressed about the high number of road traffic accidents among Asian children, for example, in large cities, and this sometimes prompts the circulation of leaflets about road safety. However, many children have nowhere to play other than in the narrow, traffic-filled streets. Pearson (1986) uses this as an example of

a victim-blaming approach, pointing out that health and safety could be promoted far more effectively through the provision of adequate housing and traffic-free play areas. The focus is thus not upon individuals and their behaviour but upon the social, economic and political factors which promote unhealthy environments.

Collaboration between health and local authorities is essential in improving and protecting the environment, particularly concerning:

- air quality
- pollution control
- toxic substances
- waste
- noise and nuisances
- pests and vermin
- dog control (particularly to prevent children ingesting *Toxocara canis* from dog faeces)
- litter
- communicable diseases
- food hygiene

all of which may have an adverse effect on children's health and well-being.

Since the late 1980s for instance there has been increasing concern about rising levels of nitrogen dioxide in the air related to vehicle emissions, and high concentrations of sulphur dioxide. These are particularly likely to have adverse effects on children with asthma, hay fever and chest infections. Children are especially vulnerable because they breathe more air for a given volume of lung tissue than adults, and their airways may be more susceptible to the irritant effects of air pollution. In summer, when children are more often outdoors, they are likely to be more exposed to exhaust fumes and sunlight which react together to form low-level ozone. This substance can damage lung epithelium, increasing susceptibility to the allergens which cause asthma and respiratory infections. Fulton (1994) points out that the 'Health of the Nation' (DoH 1992) targets only concentrate on medical interventions, such as the prescription of peak-flow meters and agreed care plans between doctor and patient. Nurses may collaborate, however, in taking a preventive approach, for example encouraging parents to take the lead in local initiatives to reduce pollution.

Life-skills

Children demonstrate a keen awareness and concern about health at a community level. James (1995) found in her research study that even young children were able to articulate their views and feelings about public health and environmental issues, if they have the opportunity to do so and if appropriate methods are used to elicit their views. Paintings, for example, revealed dark grey and brown surroundings, and children spoke of fears and worries about a range of issues from cockroaches, and noise and dirt from traffic, to anxiety and extreme stress caused by disputes with neighbours.

Research cited by Kalnins et al (1992) describes surveys carried out in cities in Canada and the USA asking children to indicate places and things in their communities that correspond to certain adjectives—dangerous, dirty, happy, peaceful, etc. Health problems for these children were associated with fear of people such as drunks and drug dealers, the dangers of crossing busy streets, lack of recreational facilities, being home alone and coping with stray dogs. The findings suggest that an important element of health promotion for children should be life-skills training which provides children with an understanding of the skills they require to resolve the health problems they encounter and opportunities to practice such skills. Examples of life-skills training are shown in Box 2.6.

Box 2.6   Life-skills—examples (adapted from Hopson & Scally 1980)

- Effective communication
- Making and managing relationships
- Managing conflict
- Being assertive
- Working in groups
- Influencing others
- Managing stress
- Coping with life-changes

Activity 2.3

Reflect upon your own environmental setting—where you live, study or work. Can you identify any aspects which might be damaging to the health and well-being of children? How might these aspects of the environment be improved?

This consideration of some aspects of environmental health reflects the main principles of the World Health Organization's global strategy for health for all by the year 2000 (WHO 1981). These principles include:

- participation by local communities in decisions relating to health and health care provision
- healthy alliances with other agencies whose activities impinge on health
- a commitment to reducing inequalities in health.

Similarly, the health policy for Europe includes targets related to environmental health (see Box 2.7).

Box 2.7   European Target 18—Policy on environment and health (WHO 1993)

By the year 2000, all Member States should have developed, and be implementing, policies on the environment and health that ensure ecologically sustainable development, effective prevention and control of environmental health risks and equitable access to healthy environments.

Social level

The second level of health promotion identified by Kelly et al (1993) is at the level of social structure—patterns of group behaviour. Cultural influences, such as religious customs and family background are examples of a child's social structure. Interventions at this level might involve a variety of ways of influencing group behaviour including education, advertising and propaganda, community development projects (e.g. setting up a nursery or playgroup), demonstrations and media events and changes in legislation.

Collective approaches to health

A community is more than the sum of its individuals—its strength may lie in its unity. By working together, people can make sense of their families' lives through sharing experiences, learning from each other and gaining confidence (Billingham 1994). Examples of collective initiatives include groups facilitated for parents by health visitors, community health groups in which people tackle health issues beyond the medical remit such as safety standards in council housing (Watt & Rodmell 1993) and self-help groups.

Social contexts

Health promotion measures need to take account of the social context in which people live. The major influences on young people's smoking behaviour for instance are parents, peers, friends and the media. Thus for health promotion to be effective it must use social networks and recognise that different social groups respond in different ways. Recent evidence from the 'health and lifestyle' survey (Blaxter 1990) suggests that it is only people in the higher social classes who are likely to improve their and their children's health through changes in taking exercise or smoking, drinking and eating habits. Families and individuals who are disadvantaged through poverty or lack of social support are unlikely to improve their health status by changing their consumption of tobacco, alcohol and certain types of food or by engaging in regular exercise. When people behave in ways which are detrimental to their own or their children's health there may be a tendency to blame them (Bond & Bond 1994). Parents who smoke and whose children have bronchitis, mothers of unvaccinated children with whooping cough, parents of HIV-positive children and women who may have difficulty when

delivering their babies, are sometimes blamed by health workers for their behaviour. Clearly, as Bond & Bond (1994) point out, such people are theoretically in a position to alter their lifestyles and improve their own and their children's health by not smoking, by getting their children vaccinated, by using safe sexual practices or by attending antenatal care. However, there are structural and personal constraints which make it difficult for some people to adopt standards of behaviour acceptable to some health professionals. Graham (1993) asked open-ended questions in her research study, mentioned earlier, to identify why mothers who had tried to give up smoking had started again. The major reasons clustered around the difficulties of managing their lives without cigarettes. It was hard to cope with everyday problems, stress, irritability and boredom. It was also difficult to withstand pressures to smoke—either direct interpersonal pressure from partners, or the indirect pressure of being in the company of smokers. Merely providing information about the risks of smoking is therefore often not effective. Graham also found that 60% of the current smokers in her study of pregnant women and mothers of young babies had not attempted to stop smoking, although they understood the possible effects on their own and their children's health. One mother, a smoker living with her partner, said: 'Before the baby was born, I was in bed and breakfast and I thought when she was born I was going to be put in a hostel with a young baby.' Another smoker told the researcher: 'I quarrelled with my mum when I got pregnant and had to move into a hostel. Since then, I've had the worry about finding somewhere to live and the worry about the new baby.' These mothers had more urgent concerns than giving up the comforts smoking provided.

The variety of influences upon people and their experience of their social structures needs to be considered by nurses and other health promoters. Health professionals, however, often identify pregnancy and early motherhood as times rich in opportunities for initiating behavioural change, but do not take a holistic, integrated approach to health promotion, re-membering all the outside influences on health behaviour there might be.

Group and individual health promotion initiatives need to encourage problem-solving approaches to life in general, not just to items of isolated behaviour.

Deliberate attempts to change society may have unexpected and unplanned results. Trying to prevent narcotic drug use among teenagers for instance through advertising campaigns may actually excite curiosity about the topic and increase drug usage instead. An integrated approach to health promotion would take account of social structure and consider ways of meeting peoples' differing needs for enhancing their health choices, partly perhaps by discussing their views and concerns with them.

Organisational level

Some organisations have an explicit health promotion function—for instance health promotion units or departments, and public health departments. Others, including schools, hospitals and health centres have a commitment to the delivery of health promotion although it is not their main function. In a hospital or other organisation where care is delivered, the wider culture or climate should encourage the development of an equal partnership between the nurse, child and family. Such a reciprocal relationship and partnership is based upon mutual trust and respect for each other's contribution, knowledge and capabilities. Within it, participants are willing to share knowledge, expertise and skills whilst also supporting each other (Smith 1995). A vital component in such an organisational culture is that each member of the caring team feels valued and involved in decision-making and planning. Reflective practice may be encouraged through effective leadership. Swain (1995) discusses the value of regular clinical supervision in providing the space and opportunity to reflect on practice: why the work is being approached in a particular way; what might be difficult; and the nature of

the interaction with clients. Although Swain's discussion relates mainly to community nursing, as she points out, the principle of clinical supervision is now an accepted part of the national agenda for the development of the nursing, midwifery and health visiting professions (DoH 1993b). Professional development in turn enhances the health of patients and clients as it contributes to their empowerment. In the paediatric setting the nurse may empower the child/parent and family through:

- the sharing of knowledge, skills and information
- teaching and education
- developing confidence and competence with support and advice
- promoting self-care and independence

thus building an equal partnership in the caring process (Smith 1995).

The health-promoting school

Schools provide an arena in which positive steps may be taken to encourage good health among young people. A school has a powerful impact on the development of healthy lifestyles, although it is only one factor among many. When developing health promotion policies and health education programmes, other influences including families, the community, peer groups, the media, legislation and pupils' backgrounds need to be taken into account. Ways of promoting the health of children with special educational needs have to be effectively considered. The needs of bilingual children should be accommodated, and differing cultural and

Activity 2.4

Plan a health education session with parents of a sick baby who has not been orally fed for some while because of surgery. How would you encourage parents to introduce a varied diet suited to the baby's age and health status?

ethnic backgrounds and experiences carefully incorporated.

The facilities offered by a school can help to put theories into practice. Tuck shops and school dinner systems which offer a choice of foods encourage pupils to use their knowledge of healthy eating. Sports facilities available for use out of school hours enable children to apply their knowledge about health and exercise, for example:

- knowing that regular exercise promotes well-being and promotes bodily health
- knowing that regular exercise increases the functional capacity of people of all ages and can help those who are disabled or chronically ill
- understanding the advantages of incorporating regular exercise as part of their lifestyle, to improve both their physical and mental health (National Curriculum Council 1990).

Applying ideas of empowerment to children involves changing the ways in which children are traditionally perceived. A shift in attitude may be required, from thinking about children as recipients of health promotion efforts on their behalf, to regarding them as partners in health promotion. Some school health services have introduced pupil-held records—for example the 'health fax' (see Box 2.8).

Children's own views and concerns about health may thus be accepted and considered, and each child's competence to make and implement decisions recognised and respected.

The role of the school nurse

School nurses are in an excellent position to promote health—they are virtually the only health care professionals to have regular contact with large groups of healthy young people. They also work closely with children who have special needs. By profiling their schools and auditing their own work they are able to identify met and unmet needs. Their clients include most of the young population of today and the adult population of tomorrow. Skills of school nursing have been developed beyond the traditional

---

Box 2.8   The school health fax (McAleer & Jackson 1994)

The health fax was piloted in 21 schools in inner London for pupils in year seven (11-plus). It was developed as a focus for health interviews and as a tool to empower young people to share responsibility for their own health. In some pilot schools many pupils used English as a second language, and travelled regularly between England and other countries. A readily accessible, up-to-date health record was expected to be advantageous. Evaluation showed that most pupils liked the fax and appreciated having a comprehensive record of their own health status.

---

routine, task-oriented ones. School nurses are now recognised as:

- managers of health care
- deliverers of health care
- advocates for health
- evaluators of programmes of care
- facilitators of the health-promoting school (DoH 1995).

It is through the identification of need that school nurses can work closely with school staff, competently assessing the health of individuals and discussing health needs with the child, parent and teacher (Bagnall 1994).

Health education and the curriculum

Health education should be an integrated and continuous programme available to all pupils throughout the school years. Key areas such as relationships, personal safety and substance use and misuse may for instance be introduced to pupils at an early age. Progression in learning will involve developing and expanding upon these topics at regular intervals throughout a pupil's school career, encouraging the gradual expansion of knowledge and understanding and the development of skills and values (Kiger 1995).

Schools may identify professionals in the community, including paediatric nurses, who could contribute to the development or teaching of health-related topics, in liaison with school nurses and the rest of the school health team.

Topic areas for health education identified by the National Curriculum Council (1990) include:

- substance use and misuse
- sex education
- family life education
- safety
- health-related exercise
- food and nutrition
- personal hygiene
- environmental aspects
- psychological aspects.

Child abuse

Nurses in collaboration with schools can advise on how to educate children and young people about their right to personal safety. Child abuse prevention programmes can be introduced in schools, although preferably these should be combined with other curriculum topics so that the issue of abuse is placed in a context which is understandable but unalarming to children. Children need to be introduced to such programmes early, at primary school as well as at secondary school level, so that they have the knowledge, skills and language to say 'no' and talk to a trusted adult.

Programme design

Programmes for pupils should be designed to:

- provide opportunities to achieve their physical, psychological and social potential
- help them to know themselves better and to think well of themselves
- provide appropriate health-related knowledge and help pupils to develop the understanding and skills to use it
- promote attitudes and behaviour which contribute to personal, community and family health
- promote positive attitudes towards equal opportunities and life in a multicultural society by dealing sensitively with values and with cultural and religious beliefs (National Curriculum Council 1990).

Bagnall (1994) points out that on average there are three children with asthma in a class of 30. In a health-promoting school such children would not be stigmatised by being constantly monitored by the school health team, but school staff themselves would have access to training in the management of asthma; medication would be easily accessible —in the classroom or in the older child's pocket— and possible triggers would be removed from the environment. A survey was carried out in 79 primary schools in 1991–2 to determine whether an increased knowledge of asthma improved teachers' ability to manage the disease. The level of knowledge was found to be low, but teachers who had received training about asthma and its management were more knowledgeable and likely to take appropriate action in the event of an attack—administering an inhaler, calling parents and seeking medical help when necessary. School nurses are in an ideal position not only to detect children who are undiagnosed or having problems with their asthma, but also to advise, support and educate children, teachers and parents. There needs to be good communication between schools, general practice and hospital paediatric units, with school nurses liaising between them (Carruthers et al 1995).

Individual level

At the individual level of health promotion, the RCN's (1992) philosophy of care for paediatric nurses is highly relevant. In considering the needs of the child as an individual, it states that nurses should:

- recognise each child as a unique, developing individual whose best interests must be paramount

Activity 2.5

Plan to prepare an information pack for teachers in a local school who wish to incorporate a knowledge of asthma and its effects and management into their curriculum. What sources of leaflets, videos and other learning aids can you identify locally and nationally?

- listen to children, attempt to understand their perspectives, opinions and feelings and acknowledge their right to privacy
- consider the physical, psychological, social, cultural and spiritual needs of children and their families
- respect the right of children, according to their age and understanding, to appropriate information and informed participation in decisions about their care.

How do young people change?

Whether young people decide to change their behaviour, as already discussed, will depend on many factors, including:

- their beliefs, for example about how effective the new behaviour is in improving health
- their motivation, for example whether they value their health sufficiently to make changes
- the normative pressures on them, that is the strength of the pressure put on them from influential people around them.

Health education may be needed to support an intention by providing knowledge and skills. For example, an intention to use condoms as protectives against HIV infection will require not merely motivation but also knowledge of where to obtain condoms and the social interaction skills necessary to negotiate use with a partner (Whitehead & Tones 1990).

Primary nursing

The hospital may be seen as a daunting, strange and frightening place for an individual child or adolescent. Primary nursing in conjunction with continuity in patient allocation by a named nurse is one way of reducing this trauma (see Ch. 8). It may be helpful if the child and family are involved in the selection of their primary nurse. Under a system of primary nursing the nurse develops a special relationship with the child and family, and also acquires an in-depth knowledge of their needs, enabling a participative style of health care to develop and promote the child's optimum health.

Integration

To concentrate only on the individual in promoting health may be tinkering on the margins of health improvement. Health education for individual children and families is an important aspect of health promotion, but it needs to be part of a wider action to promote health—taking into account all four levels of health promotion.

The WHO (1978) approach is concerned with empowering individual people and families to have more control over their health through support from public policies and actions that make it easier for them to make choices about health. For example, it is difficult for parents to have control over their families' health where healthy foods are too expensive, where there is traffic pollution, where housing is inadequate or there are too many steps for wheelchairs and prams, or where there are high levels of unemployment. The link between families and the lives they lead is almost indivisible; people have to be seen as being parts of groups and communities as well as just individuals. Health promotion therefore should address all levels (Pike S 1995).

Accident prevention—an example of integration

Accident prevention, discussed earlier, can be used to illustrate three main approaches which reflect the different levels of health promotion identified:

1. The educational approach involves raising awareness and increasing knowledge in an attempt to change attitudes and behaviour.
2. The engineering approach aims to modify the environment so that injuries can be prevented or reduced in severity.
3. The enforcement approach uses legislation, regulations or standards to ensure that educational messages or environmental modifications are complied with.

There is an increasing body of evidence that accident prevention using the educational approach is less effective than that using the engineering or enforcement approaches (Towner et al 1993). In *The Health of the Nation* (DoH 1992), however, the role of the primary health care team is discussed mainly in terms of the educational approach to accident prevention. There is a place for one-to-one health education, for example in advising parents to put cold water into the bath before adding hot; not to leave an infant alone in the bath; to check toys for removable parts or not to drink hot fluids while holding a baby. On the other hand, the introduction of child-resistant containers for all household cleaning products is probably the most effective way of reducing accidental poisonings, as the experience of child-resistant containers for analgesics and antipyretics clearly demonstrated in the 1970s (Woods et al 1994).

Primary health care and health promotion

The basic values set out in the Declaration of Alma Ata (Box 2.1, p. 24) such as the need for services to be available, culturally acceptable, affordable, accessible and professionally and scientifically sound, apply to primary care as well as to secondary care. The usual 'core' primary health care team (PHCT) members are shown in Figure 2.2.

Many other health and social care professionals may also become part of, or liaise with, the PHCT. These include paediatric community or hospital nurses, Macmillan nurses, school nurses, social workers and counsellors. Collaboration with other relevant health experts may be developed by inviting them to meetings, providing the team with a wide range of potential knowledge and skills which help to promote clients' health in the community. In order that PHCTs promote health effectively, team-building exercises are recommended (see Box 2.9).

The scope of activity for primary health care systems is broad. Improvements in standards of care have been targeted at children by means of

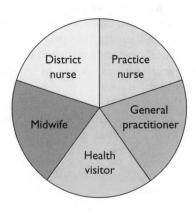

Figure 2.2   The 'core' primary health care team.

incentives for family practitioners in the form of training and remuneration. PHCTs should value the client or patient and family's contributions to care. Effective teams encourage the participation of parents and of self-help groups organised around specific health issues, such as the management of sickle cell disease, diabetes or epilepsy in children, and haemophiliacs' family needs.

Child health surveillance

Child health surveillance is the coordinated assessment of children's health and development. The purpose of surveillance is to identify any problems and ensure that appropriate interventions are made as early as possible, thus

---

Box 2.9   Team building—key considerations (Pritchard & Pritchard 1992)

- What are our goals? What is the task? Does it need teamwork?
- What are our various roles in the team? Who will carry out the task?
- What are the agreed procedures for successful teamwork? How do we evaluate and carry out team tasks?
- Are our interpersonal relationships as good as possible? Is team effectiveness threatened by unresolved conflict?

Activity 2.6

Can you identify any self-help groups for children and their families which meet in your locality? Find out from the local community health council, council for voluntary services or social services department what groups there are. Are there unmet needs for groups to be set up for other families?

reducing later difficulties. A large number of problems identified are minor and may be resolved by relevant advice, support and management in the home or health centre, and if necessary, referral to other professionals. These include speech and language therapists, audiologists, orthoptists, sleep clinic therapists, physiotherapists, occupational therapists and child psychologists.

Parents are usually told that they may discuss their child's development at any stage with the health visitor, GP or community doctor and any concerns raised will be taken seriously, as parents know their own children better than anyone else. Centile or stepladder charts are normally used for recording developmental progress covering four main aspects:

- gross motor development
- speech and language
- vision and fine movement
- social aspects of development (Robertson 1991).

Routine checks are summarised below:

- Neonatal examination—by hospital paediatrician or GP and midwife. This includes a full physical examination, including recording weight, length and head circumference. A check is made for congenital dislocation of the hips (CDH) and testicular descent. Screening is carried out for phenylketonuria and thyroid disease.
- 10–12 days—by health visitor. The physical and emotional health of the mother are discussed and assessed. A full examination is made of the baby, including vision and hearing, and a test for

CDH is carried out; weight, length and head circumference are recorded on a centile chart.
- 6–8 weeks—by GP or community paediatrician. Growth and development are reviewed, and any parental concerns are investigated and discussed thoroughly. The baby is examined and the weight, length and head circumference recorded on a centile chart.
- 8–9 months—by health visitor or GP. A further review of growth and development is made, asking about particular parental concerns. A distraction hearing test is carried out, and the infant's visual behaviour observed, looking for squint. A check is made for evidence of CDH. Weight and length are recorded if concern is indicated.
- 18–24 months—by health visitor. This review of development includes hearing and early language, mobility, manipulative skills, social relationships and a discussion of the range of normal growth and behaviour.
- 36–48 months—pre-school examination. This is a general health and developmental progress review, including vision, squint, hearing, behaviour and language acquisition; any concerns or needs are referred to relevant specialist professionals. Immunisation status should be checked and updated if necessary. Physical examinations by the doctor include checking for testicular descent and heart abnormalities (Hall 1991).

Health education for parents

This includes many topics which parents are likely to want to discuss amongst themselves—in group sessions, using health professionals as a resource for providing information, demonstrations (e.g. baby bathing) and explanations, or in one-to-one encounters with a health worker. Ewles & Simnett (1995) discuss practical aspects of health education in detail.

Examples of topics for parents' health education include:

- promoting breast-feeding; giving bottle-feeding and sterilisation advice if required
- baby care
- sibling management
- crying and sleep problems

- transport in cars
- advice and information about child health clinics and support for parents
- effects of passive smoking
- accident prevention, e.g. bathing, scalding by liquids, fire dangers, sleeping safely in cot
- immunisation schedule explained and discussed
- anticipatory guidance about weaning and sharing family meals
- dental care
- anticipatory guidance covering home safety with increasing mobility, e.g. stair gates
- skin care, preventing sunburn
- developmental needs, e.g. language and play
- social needs, e.g. mixing with other children
- avoidance and management of behaviour problems
- discussion of bladder and bowel control if requested
- preparation for school.

Planning for health education

Having identified needs, the key to the success of any health teaching activity is effective planning and preparation (Kiger 1995). To begin with, overall goals should be established. These are usually expressed in general terms, such as:

- to improve general understanding, general skills or physical coordination
- to modify or change attitudes, beliefs or standards
- to give information, share knowledge, or present ideas
- to stimulate action
- to encourage changes in behaviour.

Goals or aims can be further broken down into more specific objectives. Objectives should be realistic, achievable and able to be measured and evaluated. They should describe an intended result of health teaching—for example, 'the parents should demonstrate how to clean teeth and how much toothpaste to put on to a child's brush'.

Activity 2.7

Plan a health education programme for a small group of parents about the promotion of dental health. Consider how you will 'get the message across' in relation to:

- taking children to the dentist regularly
- keeping sugary food and drinks for meal times only, and in small amounts
- teaching and encouraging effective teeth cleaning
- supporting water fluoridation.

Which of the following methods might you use?

- group discussion so that attitudes, knowledge and beliefs can be explored
- information and advice giving
- demonstration of skills involved
- use of videos, leaflets, tapes and slides.

Learning will be helped by learners taking part in a range of activities through listening, looking, talking and doing. Talks are generally best prepared by a set of notes logically ordered so that the material to be presented is clear and interesting, based upon:

- an opening introduction
- a set of ordered key points
- a concluding summary.

Discussion time and question-and-answer time should be allowed for, and an evaluation, asking people for feedback about the session and how they have benefited, held at the end.

Immunisation

Immunisation schedules are offered as the safest and most effective protection for babies and children against diseases listed in Box 2.10, and are an example of primary prevention. As more children are immunised, the disease in question is prevented from being passed on. Parents need to be fully informed and to have time to consider and raise questions and concerns about their child's immunisation programme.

Box 2.10   Immunisation schedule (HEA 1993)

At 2 months
- Hib (*Haemophilus influenzae* type b)—one injection
- DTP (diphtheria, tetanus, pertussis)—one injection
- Polio—by mouth

At 3 months
- Hib—one injection
- DTP—one injection
- Polio—by mouth

At 4 months
- Hib—one injection
- DTP—one injection
- Polio—by mouth

At 12–15 months
- MMR (measles, mumps, rubella)—one injection

At 3–5 years
- Diphtheria, tetanus—booster injection
- Polio—booster by mouth

Girls at 10–14 years
- Rubella—one injection

Girls and boys at 13 years
- BCG (tuberculosis)—one injection

School leavers 15–19 years
- Tetanus—one injection
- Polio—booster by mouth

HEALTH PROMOTION—OLDER CHILDREN AND ADOLESCENTS

Older childhood and adolescence are usually periods of the life span which are associated with good physical health. The older child and adolescent begin to take more responsibility for their own health as they become less dependent upon parental decisions. They typically spend more time with peers and less time with parents— initially in same-sex peer groups and then in mixed-sex peer groups as they become older.

In terms of health promotion, the older child and adolescent begin needing to make independent choices about a number of important issues which may have short-term or long-term consequences for their health. In addition, they have to develop their own problem-solving strategies, some of which can be seen as adaptive while others are considered maladaptive. Whilst they may still be influenced by family beliefs and values, and their early experiences of health behaviour will form the foundation of health knowledge and problem-solving as they move towards adulthood, these young people are likely to be heavily influenced by peers and the media. It is therefore *always* important that those involved in health promotion with these groups are aware of the latest trends, fashions, cults and pressures which are so influential in their clients' lives. Health messages for adolescents must be tailored to their needs, suitable in style and content and designed for maximum impact while being sensitive to race, culture and gender.

Emotional and social health may be considered in terms of:

- feelings
- emotions
- interests
- motivations
- attitudes
- values.

All of these elements develop and change as adolescents mature. Social well-being is enhanced by considering these factors of emotional and social health, and discussing them with participants as a vital part of health promotion activities.

Health professionals can, for example, help to reduce physical inactivity in adolescents, thus promoting their health in general. Head injuries from road accidents may be reduced by encouraging the use of cycle helmets in teenagers, and lobbying for cycle tracks. The risk factors for suicide in adolescence are complex, but may include substance misuse, which can be prevented. Unwanted pregnancies in young girls may be reduced by sex education, although knowledge by itself may be insufficient. Active participation, through encouraging discussion and exchanging views for instance, is an effective way of imparting health knowledge. It is important to raise self-esteem as well as to provide factual information if lifestyles are to be changed. Life-skills training (see Box 2.6 p. 30) has a valuable part in promoting adolescent health and well-being. Health education may be viewed as 'freeing' people to make health choices for themselves (Greenberg 1992).

Healthy choices

Areas in which health promotion interventions can be effective in enabling young people to make healthy choices include:

- drugs
- alcohol
- volatile substances
- smoking
- sexual health.

Drugs

A wide range of drugs may be readily available to young people, but unlike alcohol and tobacco, the majority of young people never try a drug, and even fewer experiment with drugs or develop a serious drug problem (Home Office 1993).

However, illicit drugs have been used by a significant number of older children and adolescents for a number of years, although the types of drugs used have changed according to availability and 'fashion'. For example, 'ecstasy'—methylenedioxyamphetamine (MDMA)—and 'crack' (a derivative of cocaine) were unheard of 20 years ago.

Cannabis is the most commonly tried drug with 1–2% of 12- and 13-year-old children and 15% of 13- to 16-year-olds admitting usage at some time (Balding 1992). LSD (lysergic acid diethylamide) and magic mushrooms had been tried by 6–7% of 15- to 16-year-olds and 5% had tried amphetamines.

The use of drugs such as cocaine and heroin is small and decreasing—possibly due to the greater availability of ecstasy, which is also considerably cheaper. According to Balding (1992) 4% of 15- to 16-year-olds have tried ecstasy, and its usage seems to be increasing with a small number of fatalities each year, whereas use of cocaine and heroin has fallen to less than 1%.

There are several health education programmes aimed at preventing drug use among young people, based around the knowledge/attitudes approach, the values/decision-making approach and the social competency or life-skills approach. However, there is a lack of informative research identifying the most effective approaches in relation to preventing drug abuse among adolescents. Longitudinal evaluation studies are needed to identify the most efficient ways of ensuring positive behaviour in the long term. Any health promotion strategy should be sensitive to the many influences related to drug use, which include peer pressure, parental factors, gender, personality and age.

Practical problems. Health promotion in preventing drug abuse is an example of primary prevention; at the secondary and tertiary levels there are often pressing problems to be addressed. Counselling and emotional support are likely to have a limited impact if practical problems are not dealt with at the same time. Many young people who become homeless are drug users—there is a reluctance among private landlords and some housing bodies to rent accommodation to them. There may also be legal problems associated with the illegal nature of drug-taking. Drug workers need to maintain good contacts with community law centres and can possibly advise nurses. Similarly, expert advice may be required in relation to urgent financial problems and welfare rights. Drug users tend to neglect their health by not eating an adequate diet for instance. This lack of attention to health care is of particular concern in the case of young people who are infected with HIV; it is desirable that sensible guidelines are followed to maximise the body's immunity. Individual HIV-antibody-positive drug users need help in motivating themselves to change their lifestyle and in solving their problems—particularly homelessness (Anderson & Wilkie 1992). Drug users are at risk of contracting the HIV virus and developing AIDS if they share injecting equipment that is infected, and schemes to provide new equipment—thus limiting damage—have been developed in some areas.

Alcohol

Alcohol, whilst as potentially harmful as illicit drugs if used in excess, presents a different problem for health promoters. Alcohol is an accepted part of almost all sections of society, and is used by adults to relax, to celebrate, to combat shock and as a way of cheering themselves up. The 'pub' serves an important function in British society, and is portrayed by popular soap operas as the centre of all activity and a place where lonely characters can go to find company.

The messages children and adolescents therefore receive are that alcohol is widely used, socially acceptable and capable of making people feel better. It is not surprising that most young people have tried alcohol by late adolescence. For most young people, however, alcohol does not become a problem. An OPCS survey (1986) found that among 11- to 15-year-olds, 40% claimed never to have had a drink, 30% said that they had a drink a few times a year, 18% drank once or twice a month and 13% normally drank once or twice a week. This does not allow for complacency as concern has been expressed about signs of rising trends in alcohol consumption among young people. The dangers of alcohol abuse are many, both short term and long term. Alcohol use has been associated with risk-taking and high-risk sexual activity, and the dangers of drinking and driving are well known. Longer-term consequences include such conditions as hypertension and liver damage.

Health promotion in relation to the use of alcohol is somewhat problematic because of the wide and legal use of alcohol in society. The behavioural outcome of any strategy should focus on the sensible use of alcohol and upon reasons for its use. Helping people to develop healthy problem-solving strategies is clearly important, as is providing information about the potential long- and short-term detrimental effects of alcohol use. Tones & Tilford (1994) emphasise that health promotion activity aimed at enabling effective decision-making, self-empowerment and coping skills will be more effective than taking a didactic

Box 2.11   Action for sound health (East Surrey Health Promotion Unit 1994)

The Action for Sound Health campaign is run by a healthy alliance of 14 local voluntary and statutory organisations. Two major concerns underpin its work:

• the prevention of severe chronic diseases (e.g. cardiovascular disease and certain cancers) by modifying behaviour which leads to increase in the incidence of these diseases, such as smoking, misuse of alcohol, lack of exercise and poor nutritional habits
• reducing more immediate threats to the health of young people (e.g. accidents, alcohol and drug misuse, unprotected sex and unplanned pregnancy).

Initiatives include:

• Informal events, e.g. 'Offbeat Band Nights' where campaign staff set up a stall in the theatre foyer with educational and 'fun' materials for the audience, and hold discussions in groups about smoking, alcohol, drugs and safer sex. Discussing unprotected sex and the question of relationships, for example, had a very immediate impact when standing in the foyer bar. By sponsoring bands, the health promotion team became an integral part of the events, with regular attenders among the young people asking for the free health educational packs.
• Theme evenings on topics such as stress and relaxation, nutrition and take-away food, exercise, smoking, sexual health and accident prevention. Quiz/questionnaire sheets were completed, reaction time test assault courses set up, bio-dots measuring stress by changing colour on the skin were used and participative discussions held. Educational materials included a 'Ten top tips for condom use' poster and a leaflet supporting a smokerlyser test called 'Carbon monoxide and you'. Evaluation (both qualitative and quantitative) showed that 'Offbeat' target groups of young people have developed increasing trust and confidence in health-team members and benefited from the information and activities—sharing knowledge with family and friends, and in some cases managing to stop smoking.

approach (see Box 2.11). As with drug education, it is important that the community takes some responsibility for sensible alcohol use by refusing to serve alcohol to those who are legally under-age. It is also important to reach parents, who have been shown to be influential in the sensible use of alcohol. Children of parents who allow sensible amounts of alcohol to be consumed and who are positive role models are more likely to adopt a healthy attitude towards alcohol. It appears that where alcohol becomes a 'forbidden fruit' and involves deception, the adolescent is more likely to continue drinking in greater quantities and more frequently (OPCS 1991).

Volatile substances

Statistics show that more than 120 people a year die from inhaling glue and other solvents, compared with about 70 per year dying from heroin abuse. While illicit drug use tends to increase with age, the abuse of volatile substances reaches a peak in early adolescence and then decreases with age (Balding 1992). As adolescents grow older they tend to either give up substance abuse or move to more sophisticated (and expensive) forms of abuse, such as the use of drugs and/or alcohol.

The wide range of substances abused by young people includes substances readily available in many homes, for example:

- lighter fuel
- glue
- perfume
- aerosols
- acetone.

The immense dangers of volatile substance abuse are heightened when the user is alone, although the practice is often a group activity. The lone abuser is at particular risk because of the immediate effects of intoxication and dizziness associated with this abuse. When a volatile substance is inhaled from a plastic bag, if the user loses consciousness, potentially fatal risks are evident. It is also possible for long-term damage to liver, kidneys or brain to be caused by prolonged use (ISDD 1995).

There is a strong argument for discouraging the use of volatile substances at a young age, as they are cheap, readily available and tempt older children and young adolescents. As discussed earlier, primary school health education should include these topics sensitively introduced. Prevention of volatile substance abuse should be aimed at two specific types of potential users:

- those who may be coerced by peer group pressure
- friendless children.

Health education strategies with the first group should be aimed at enabling young people to influence their peer groups rather than conform to them, perhaps by concentrating upon life-skills (see Box 2.6, p30). The second group tend to conform to the behaviour of a group indulging in negative behaviour because they desperately need to belong, or who remain alone and use maladaptive ways of coping with loneliness and isolation. These young people are more difficult to help, as they abuse substances as a retreat from adolescence, family or life (Hodgkinson 1995).

Smoking

Whilst cigarette smoking reached a peak in the 1970s and is now decreasing, studies show that nearly one-quarter of 15-year-olds in England in 1992 were regular smokers, smoking at least once a week (Central Statistical Office 1995). The prevalence of cigarette smoking among secondary school children increases dramatically with age. Only 7% of 13-year-olds and 1% of 11-year-olds were found to be regular smokers. Boys tend to start experimenting with smoking earlier than girls, but by the age of 14 girls are more likely to have tried smoking than boys. By the age of 16, 70% of girls have tried smoking compared with 64% of boys. It has been suggested that smoking among adolescent girls may be attributed partly to media advertising, which tends to target young women. It may also be perceived as a way of regulating weight for girls, while boys are more influenced by the fashion to be fit and athletic.

There is a clear link between children's smoking and that of their parents (Central Statistical Office 1995). In 1992, children in England whose parents both smoked were two-and-a-half times more likely to be regular smokers than if neither parent smoked. Differences in smoking habits between social groups have already been discussed in relation to women in Graham's (1993) study (see p. 28). In 1992, men in the unskilled manual group were three times more likely to smoke than those in the professional group, showing that the decline in smoking habits is related to social class (Central Statistical Office 1995). This indicates that inequalities in health may be actually widening, as smoking-related diseases take effect.

There is also a link between children's smoking and drinking habits. Those who smoked regularly were almost 10 times as likely as those who had never smoked to have drunk at least once a week.

As with the use of volatile substances, research points to the need for smoking prevention programmes to begin in primary schools, perhaps with nurses acting as advisers to the teachers. At all ages, didactic forms of teaching are much less effective than participatory methods where children can discuss and consider issues for themselves, with access to information so that misconceptions are explored or avoided. As with other subjects discussed in this chapter, it is important to consider the context within which young people live, and health promotion should be integrated to include the family, the wider school environment and the community. In the health-promoting school (see pp. 32–34), no-smoking policies may be introduced so that staff cannot be seen smoking by young people.

Sexual health—HIV and AIDS prevention

By September 1994 a cumulative total of 9.9 thousand AIDS cases had been reported and 6.7 thousand deaths from AIDS were known to have occurred in the United Kingdom: females accounted for only 8% of cases and 7% of deaths. In the year 1993 there were 1.6 thousand AIDS cases reported in the United Kingdom, a rate of 2.8 per thousand population. This is one of the lowest rates in the European Community (Central Statistical Office 1995). However, in recognition of the potential risks to young people in terms of HIV infection, and the incidence of pregnancy among teenagers, the 'Health of the Nation' strategy (DoH 1992) highlighted sexual health as one of its key targets. Promoting safer sexual practices is one part of the strategy, together with encouraging young people to consider the implications of becoming sexually active.

Empowering young people to delay the age at which they become sexually active may reduce the incidence of risk-taking behaviour. Adolescents are potentially at risk of contracting HIV for a number of reasons, including the association with drug misuse, discussed earlier, and because of risky behaviour. Although widespread campaigns have warned of the dangers of unprotected homosexual and heterosexual intercourse, messages have not reached or been effectively assimilated by target groups.

One study which has implications for nurses involved in promoting sexual health suggests that young people may have significant gaps in their knowledge relating to safe sexual practices (Dilorio et al 1993). Another study also found differences in interpreting some words and terminology, suggesting a lack of understanding. Some young people claimed to practice safer sex but in reality did not always do so, not thinking that they themselves were at risk. Young people sometimes felt that they could tell intuitively whether a potential partner was HIV-positive (Dockrell & Joffe 1992).

Although pregnancy rates for girls under 16 fell in 1991 for the first time in 10 years—to 9.3 per 1000 from the peak of 10.1 per 1000 in 1990—the United Kingdom still has the highest rate in western Europe. The 'Health of the Nation' (DoH 1992) target of 4.8 per 1000 by 1995 is a long way off.

The legal picture:
• The governors of maintained secondary schools are required to provide sex education (including education about HIV/AIDS and other sexually transmitted diseases) to all registered pupils.
• The governing bodies of primary schools are required to decide whether sex education should take place, and if so, in what form.
• Parents have the right to withdraw their children from all or part of sex education outside the National Curriculum in both primary and secondary schools (Education Act 1993).

Guidelines. Guidelines stress that sex education in schools should be contextual and form part of a moral framework which promotes the value of family life, marriage and responsible parenthood. Education should also be appropriate to the cognitive level of pupils. Giving advice to young people in schools about the use of contraceptives, particularly condoms, is problematic. Educational guidelines state that it is inappropriate for teachers to give such advice without parental consent, and yet studies have shown that young people have identified information about condom use as an important component that was missing from sex education classes (Woodcock et al 1992). Despite difficulties, it is essential that young people are given the opportunity to explore their feelings about sex and sexuality. This can best be carried out in discussion sessions and workshops which are sensitively conducted and take into account the cognitive and cultural variations between members of the group. Topics may include the development of relationships; the concept of owning your own body; sexuality; myths about sex; HIV and AIDS; pregnancy and decision-making.

Evaluation

A successful health promotion strategy requires the evaluation of both personal and group outcomes. Interventions may thus be developed further and if necessary refocused, providing valuable opportunities for promoting health at all levels of the community.

CONCLUSION

Health promotion is the process of helping people to improve and increase control over their own and their children's health, working towards the goal of a fulfilling and creative life. An integrated approach to health promotion empowers people and groups to interact at environmental, social, organisational and individual levels, helping to tackle widening inequalities in health.

REFERENCES

Anderson C, Wilkie P 1992 Reflective helping in HIV and AIDS. Open University Press, Milton Keynes

Bagnall P 1994 Investing in school-age children's health. Nursing Times 90(31): 27–29

Balding J 1992 Young people in 1991. Schools Health Education Unit, University of Exeter

Billingham K 1994 Beyond the individual. Health Visitor 67(9): 295

Blaxter M 1990 Health and lifestyles. Tavistock/Routledge, London

Bond J, Bond S 1994 Sociology and health care, 2nd edn. Churchill Livingstone, Edinburgh

Carruthers P, Ebbutt A F, Barnes G 1995 Teacher's knowledge of asthma and asthma management in primary schools. Health Education Journal 54(1): 28–36

Central Statistical Office 1995 Social Trends 25. HMSO, London

Department of Health (DoH) 1992 The health of the nation: a strategy for health in England. Cm 1986. HMSO, London

Department of Health (DoH) 1993a One year on: a report on the progress of the health of the nation. Department of Health, London

Department of Health (DoH) 1993b A vision for the future: the nursing, midwifery and health visiting contribution to health care. HMSO, London

Department of Health (DoH) 1995 School nurses in the new health services structure. HMSO, London

Dilorio C, Parsons M, Lehr S 1993 Knowledge of AIDS and safer sex practices among college freshmen. Public Health Nursing 10(3): 159–165

Dockrell J, Joffe H 1992 Methodological issues involved in the study of young people and HIV/AIDS: a socio-psychological view. Health Education Research 7: 509–516

Downie R S, Fyfe C, Tannahill A 1990 Health promotion: models and values. Oxford University Press, Oxford

East Surrey Health Promotion Unit 1994 Sounding out the young. Healthlines 13: 22–23

Education Act 1993 Chapter 35. HMSO, London

English National Board for Nursing, Midwifery and Health Visiting (ENB) 1994 Project—philosophy of health. RCN, London

Evans M, Kelly P 1995 Bringing support home for families of children with cancer. British Journal of Nursing 4(7): 395–401

Ewles L, Simnett I 1995 Promoting health: a practical guide, 3rd edn. Scutari Press, London

Fulton Y 1994 Emerging impacts. Primary Health Care 4(2): 6–8

Graham H 1993 When life's a drag: women, smoking and disadvantage. Department of Health, London

Greenberg J S 1992 Health education: learner-centered instructional strategies, 2nd edn. Brown, Iowa

Hall D 1991 Health for all children, 2nd edn. Oxford Medical, Oxford

Health Education Authority (HEA) 1993 A guide to childhood immunisations. HEA, London

Hodgkinson L 1995 Drug abuse: your questions answered. Ward Lock, London

Home Office 1993 Statistics of drug addicts notified to the Home Office, United Kingdom 1992. Home Office, London

Hopson B, Scally M 1980 Lifeskills teaching: education for self-empowerment. McGraw Hill, London

Institute for the Study of Drug Dependence (ISDD) 1995 Coping with a nightmare: drugs and your child. ISDD, London

James J 1995 Children speak out about health. Primary Health Care 5(10): 8–12

Jolly J 1981 The other side of paediatrics. Macmillan, London

Kalnins I, McQueen D V, Backett K C, Curtis L, Currie C E 1992 Children, empowerment and health promotion: some new directions in research and practice. Health Promotion International 7(1): 53–59

Kelly M P, Charlton B G, Hanlon P 1993 The four levels of health promotion: an integrated approach. Public Health 107(5): 319–326

Kiger A 1995 Teaching for health: the nurse as health educator, 2nd edn. Churchill Livingstone, Edinburgh

Kumar V 1994 Poverty and inequality in the UK: the effects on children. National Children's Bureau, London

Lask S, Smith P, Masterson A 1994 A curricular review of pre- and post-registration education programmes for nurses, midwives and health visitors in relation to the integration of a philosophy of health: developing a model for evaluation. Institute of Advanced Nursing Education, RCN, London

McAleer M, Jackson P 1994 The school health fax. Nursing Times 90(31): 29–30

Muller D J, Harris P J, Wattley L 1992 Nursing children: psychology, research and practice, 2nd edn. Chapman & Hall, London

National Curriculum Council (NCC) 1990 Curriculum guidance No. 3. The whole curriculum. NCC, York

Office of Population Censuses and Surveys (OPCS) 1986 Adolescent drinking. HMSO, London

Office of Population Censuses and Surveys (OPCS) 1991 Smoking among secondary school children in 1990. HMSO, London

Parmar A 1993 Safety and minority ethnic communities: a preliminary report on the home safety information needs of the Asian, Chinese and Vietnamese communities living in the UK in the 1990s. Royal Society for the Prevention of Accidents, Birmingham

Pearson M 1986 Racist notions of ethnicity and culture in health education. In: Rodmell S, Watt A (eds) The politics of health education: raising the issues. Routledge & Kegan Paul, London, pp 38–56

Pike D 1995 Health and the environment. In: Pike S, Forster D (eds) Health promotion for all. Churchill Livingstone, Edinburgh, pp 171–183

Pike S 1995 Health promotion now: the development of policy. In: Pike S, Forster D (eds) Health promotion for all. Churchill Livingstone, Edinburgh, pp 27–38

Pritchard P, Pritchard J 1992 Developing teamwork in primary health care: a practical workbook. Oxford University Press, Oxford

Robertson C 1991 Health visiting in practice, 2nd edn. Churchill Livingstone, Edinburgh

Royal College of Nursing (RCN) 1992 Paediatric nursing: a philosophy of care. RCN, London

Skinner J 1995 Towards an integrated model of health promotion in nursing practice. In: Pike S, Forster D (eds) Health promotion for all. Churchill Livingstone, Edinburgh, pp 185–196

Smith F 1995 Children's nursing in practice: the Nottingham model. Blackwell, Oxford

Swain G 1995 Clinical supervision: the principles and process. HVA Publications, London

Tones K, Tilford S 1994 Health education: effectiveness, efficiency and equity, 2nd edn. Chapman & Hall, London

Towner E, Dowswell T, Jarvis S 1993 Reducing childhood accidents. HEA, London

United Nations 1992 The United Nations convention on the rights of a child. HMSO, London

Victor C 1995 Inequalities in health and health promotion. In: Pike S, Forster D (eds) Health promotion for all. Churchill Livingstone, Edinburgh, pp 157–170

Watt A, Rodmell S 1993 Community involvement in health promotion: progress or panacea? In: Beattie A, Gott M, Jones L, Sidell M (eds) Health and wellbeing: a reader. Macmillan, Basingstoke, pp 6–13

Whitehead M, Tones K 1990 Avoiding the pitfalls. HEA, London

Woodcock A, Stenner K, Ingram R 1992 'All these contraceptives, videos and that …': young people talking about sex education. Health Education Research 7(4): 517–531

Woodroffe C, Williams J 1994 Accidents. In: Jacobson B (ed) East London and the City: health in the East End. East London & the City Health Authority and City & East London FSHA, London, pp 63–68

Woods A, Kendrick D, Rushton L 1994 Safety practices among parents and children in a primary care setting. Health Education Journal 53(4): 397–408

World Health Organization (WHO) 1978 Primary health care: report of the International Conference on Primary Health Care, Alma-Ata, USSR. WHO, Geneva

World Health Organization (WHO) 1981 Global strategy for health for all by the year 2000. WHO, Geneva

World Health Organization (WHO) 1993 Health for all targets: the health policy for Europe, updated edn. WHO, Regional Office for Europe, Copenhagen

Wright C 1994 Safety equipment loan scheme. Community Nursing Association Newsletter (Autumn 1994): 2–3

FURTHER READING

Ewles L, Simnett I 1995 Promoting health: a practical guide, 3rd edn. Scutari Press, London

Kiger A 1995 Teaching for health: the nurse as health educator, 2nd edn. Churchill Livingstone, Edinburgh

Kumar V 1994 Poverty and inequality in the UK: the effects on children. National Children's Bureau, London

Pike S, Forster D (eds) 1995 Health promotion for all. Churchill Livingstone, Edinburgh

Smith F 1995 Children's nursing in practice: the Nottingham model. Blackwell, Oxford

Patterns of ill health

Sally Huband

This chapter will introduce students to the concepts of ill health in children and examine the changes that have taken place over the past 100 years.

The chapter aims to:
- draw comparisons with developing countries, to identify causes of death and disease in this country at the turn of the century
- demonstrate that although children in this country have never been healthier, 50% of all deaths remain preventable
- illustrate that poverty remains a major cause of ill health and mortality.

To determine what we mean by ill health, we need to consider what we mean by health. The most useful definition for the purpose of this chapter is the definition from the World Health Organization:

Health is not merely the absence of disease, but a state of complete physical, mental and social well being.

(WHO 1958)

CHANGES IN THE PATTERN OF DISEASE OVER THE LAST 100 YEARS

The changing pattern of disease has more to do with environmental factors than the impact of 20th century medicine. The diseases that kill children in developing countries nowadays and killed children in the United Kingdom in earlier times are the diseases of poverty. In the United Kingdom in the late 19th century and early 20th century, children died from infectious diseases, from starvation and from the results of polluted water supplies and poor sanitation. The ability to produce more food and to distribute it more evenly, due to the changes in agriculture and the building of canals and railways, led to a general improvement in nutrition. Public health measures in supplying clean water and sanitation led to a decline in both water-borne and food-borne infections.

In England and Wales, the infant mortality rate (IMR) stood at 150 per 1000 live births in 1900. By 1943, the IMR had fallen to 50 per 1000 and currently stands at 7.4 per 1000. The IMR is the number of infants (per 1000 live births) who die before the age of 1 year and is one of the indicators used to measure the health of the nation (OPCS 1989, OPCS 1991a). Most of this change has been due to the improvement in the standard of living. However, the infant mortality rate is only one measurement and was less relevant in the first part of the century than it is today. In the 1850s, 40 children per 1000 died between the ages of 1 and 19. By 1900, this death rate had been halved. Nowadays it is relatively uncommon for children to die after the age of 1 year and in 1990 the rate had fallen to 0.03% of the population of that age group (OPCS 1991a).

The study of mortality and morbidity in developing countries is helpful in demonstrating the impact of social changes on health. The measurement used to assess the health of the children in these countries is the under-5 mortality rate (U5MR). The IMR would not be a suitable measurement to use, as many deaths occur in children over the age of 1 year. Statistics are not available for all countries and, where they are, may not be entirely reliable as countries do not all have a registration system of births and deaths. A report by UNICEF in 1993 suggests that, overall, the U5MR has halved since 1960, which is encouraging. However, this figure hides important variations; Malawi has a mortality rate of 228 per 1000 that has hardly altered, whereas India has dropped its U5MR by two-thirds to 94 per 1000. Even here there are differences, with the mortality rate in Uttar Pradesh standing at 123 per 1000 and the mortality rate in Kerala standing at 28 per 1000 (UNICEF 1993). As in the United Kingdom, the differences relate to the wealth of individual families. The gap between the rich and the poor in India is even more marked, even though the families may be living in close proximity to each other.

Diarrhoea and malnutrition

Diarrhoea would have been a major cause of death in the United Kingdom 100 years ago. It was not until Victorian times that clean water and adequate sewage disposal became widely available. Even in the 1950s, children commonly died from diarrhoea, as standards of hygiene were often poor and there was little understanding amongst the general population of the spread of infection. There was an emergency team working from St Mary's Paddington that would be sent to homes to rehydrate children before bringing them to hospital. Intravenous or subcutaneous rehydration was the commonest intervention and it was not until the 1980s that oral rehydration therapy (ORT) became more popular. It is now used world-wide and is thought to be saving 1 million lives each year (UNICEF 1992).

Many families in developing countries still do not have access to clean water and it is estimated that 5 million children world-wide still die each year from dehydration. The importance of the diarrhoeal diseases is not just the mortality rate. Each episode of diarrhoea weakens children by compromising their nutrition. Not only are they unlikely to eat whilst they are ill, but they also lose important nutrients in their stools. The policy of giving children clear fluids for several days following an episode will further debilitate them. In this country, where the majority of children are well nourished, this may not be important, but in developing countries it can be a crucial factor in determining future health, as children may average five episodes of diarrhoea per year.

The media coverage of famines in the developing countries has made people aware of the appalling consequences of starvation. Many people do not, however, realise that approximately 1 in every 3 children living in the developing world is chronically malnourished (UNICEF 1993). When children are malnourished they have a reduced resistance to disease and are at risk of dying from the common infectious diseases of childhood and from respiratory infections. These diseases were also the major killers in the United Kingdom 100 years ago.

Tuberculosis

Tuberculosis is another important disease where there is a link between mortality and poverty. In the United Kingdom, the fall in mortality rates was most marked from the middle of the 19th century to the middle of this century. The introduction of chemotherapy and the BCG vaccination in the 1950s had little impact on mortality rates, which were already reduced (McKeown 1976). It was, however, still a relatively common disease and many children were hospitalised for many months with tuberculosis of the bones or respiratory tuberculosis. It was not uncommon for children to be kept in spinal plasters for months whilst they received chemotherapy. One of the causes of the fall in the number of cases seen, has been the introduction of tuberculin testing for cows. Many children were infected with tuberculosis by drinking contaminated milk.

Tuberculosis remains a major problem in the developing countries. Drug-resistant strains are appearing and those whose immune system is damaged by measles or the HIV virus fall victim to the disease. In this country, it remains a disease of poverty. There is an increased incidence amongst Indian, Pakistani and Bangladeshi children. A survey was done in 1978/9 and, due to alarm that the incidence may be increasing, a further survey is currently being undertaken. Rates amongst Asian children born in this country are about half the rates of those who have come to this country through immigration;

however, they remain significantly higher than the rates of the white population (Woodroffe et al 1993). The high rates amongst the Asian children are thought to be due to a number of factors. Some have acquired the disease abroad, either before coming to this country or on a visit to Asia. Some children have acquired the disease from relatives who are recent immigrants. However, many Asian children are living in poor housing and this is also thought to be a contributory factor.

Measles

Measles is one of the most severe infectious diseases of childhood and an interesting one to consider. Measles in a malnourished child is a devastating disease and causes many deaths from diarrhoea and pneumonia. It is estimated that in 1980 measles claimed 2.5 million children's lives world-wide. As many as 5% of the children affected die during the acute attack and a further 5% are likely to die during the following months, as a result of further damage to the immune system and a worsening of their nutritional status (UNICEF 1993). A similar picture would have

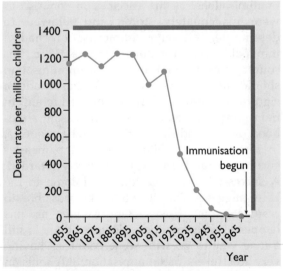

Figure 3.1 Measles: death rates of children under 15, England and Wales. (From McKeown T 1976 The modern rise of population. Reproduced by permission of Edward Arnold (Publishers) Limited.).

been seen in this country in 1900, and by studying the decline of mortality from measles it is evident that the decline had nothing to do with immunisation, but everything to do with the improved standard of living and improved nutritional status of children (see Fig. 3.1).

The influence of immunisation

Immunisation against measles

In the 1980s, the World Health Organization set targets for the reduction of the common infectious diseases and the extended programme of immunisation was launched. As a result, it is estimated that the total number of cases of measles has fallen from about 75 million a year to 25 million. The mortality from measles has fallen to 900 000 (UNICEF 1993). A great deal of time and energy has gone into increasing the uptake of immunisation and in improving the cold chain. (The cold chain refers to the transport of vaccines, ensuring that they are kept at a sufficiently low temperature from the time that they leave the manufacturers until the time that they are administered to the child.) In the past, children may have been given useless immunisations, as the vaccines in some cases were inadequately stored and allowed to deteriorate. Although immunisation had a minimal effect in reducing mortality in this country, this does not mean that immunisation should not be encouraged. It has made a significant contribution to the reduction in morbidity. Measles is a very unpleasant childhood disease and may have disabling sequelae. In rare cases the child may develop measles encephalitis and can be left severely retarded. A successful immunisation programme in the USA suggests that it would be possible to eradicate the disease world-wide, as has happened with smallpox. However there is still a long way to go with some countries having very low levels of immunisation: Afghanistan 29%; Ethiopia 17%; and Chad 21% (UNICEF 1993). The percentage of children immunised against measles in the United Kingdom, has

risen from 46% in 1971 to 89% in 1991. This was boosted by the introduction of the combined measles, mumps and rubella vaccine in 1988. There has been a corresponding reduction in the numbers of notifications of measles.

The effect of the WHO's expanded programme of immunisation in the developing world has been considerable. It is a sad reality that it is easier to launch and implement a programme of this nature than it is to abolish poverty and ensure that the world's children are adequately fed.

Immunisation against other infectious diseases

Other infectious diseases are also of importance. Whooping cough, polio, tetanus and diphtheria are all responsible for considerable mortality and morbidity in the developing world and used to be in this country. In 1900, approximately 900 per million children died each year from diphtheria. With the improvement in living conditions and the introduction of antitoxin, this had fallen to approximately 250 per million in 1940 (McKeown 1976). The national immunisation programme in 1942 reduced this further to a figure of 2 cases in 1992 with no deaths. However, there is no cause for complacency. In the former USSR, the disease was almost wiped out by the national immunisation programme of the 1960s. With the break-up of the USSR, the immunisation programme has faltered and diphtheria has now become Russia's most widespread, fatal infectious disease, affecting nearly 5000 people in the first half of 1993 (DoH 1993). With improved travel, it is conceivable that there could be cases seen again in the United Kingdom where 5% of children remain unprotected. In this country, adverse media coverage of the effects of the pertussis vaccine in the 1970s led to a decrease in the rates of immunisation. The general public required a lot of encouragement to take their children to the clinics.

It is possible for children to be immunised against a growing number of diseases. The introduction of the *Haemophilus influenzae* vaccine (Hib) in October 1992 is already having an impact on the numbers of cases of haemophilus meningitis. The immunisation is estimated to have reduced the incidence by 70%. There has also been a reduction in the number of children admitted with epiglottitis, although this was a less common condition. There are now vaccines available for meningococcal meningitis, which remains a significant cause of childhood illness, with some fatal cases. Unfortunately the vaccine is not effective against strain B of *Neisseria meningitidis*, which is the commonest strain in the United Kingdom, and it is therefore usually only made available to those who are travelling to countries with a high incidence of disease caused by other strains.

CAUSES OF MORTALITY TODAY

The mortality rate for children of all ages has continued to decline in this country, with some quite marked falls even since 1970 (see Fig. 3.2).

The causes of mortality and morbidity today are best considered under specific age groups.

Neonatal deaths

Neonatal deaths are deaths occurring during the first 28 days of life.

The highest numbers of deaths in children occur during the neonatal period and the main causes are prematurity, congenital abnormalities or respiratory disease. Of these, congenital abnormalities are the most important. One in every 20 live babies is born with an abnormality and 50% of these are classified as major abnormalities (see Ch. 20). There is still a class gradient for mortality rate from abnormalities, with a higher rate in children born to mothers from Social Class V than for children born to mothers from Social Class I (OPCS 1988). This is

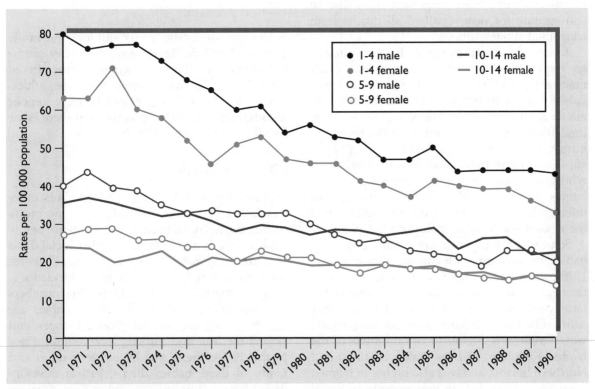

Figure 3.2 Childhood mortality rates by sex and age, 1970–1990, England and Wales. (Source: 1990 Mortality statistics: childhood, HMSO 1992)

particularly true for the neural tube defects and may be a result of a poorer diet during pregnancy, leading to low levels of folic acid.

Congenital abnormalities

Congenital heart disease accounts for approximately half of all major abnormalities— 8 in every 1000 live births are likely to have a heart defect. It was only in the early 1960s that heart surgery became possible. Prior to this, few children with major defects survived. With the development of the heart–lung bypass and the use of hypothermia, surgeons were able to stop the heart whilst surgery was carried out. Initially the failure rate was high. Ventilators and machines that had been developed for adults were found to be unsuitable for babies and children. Surgical procedures and supportive care following surgery have improved and the majority of heart defects can now be treated. However, deaths from congenital heart disease still account for nearly half of all deaths from congenital abnormalities.

Technological improvements have resulted in an improved outcome for some of the other major abnormalities. Gastroschisis is one of these. Babies born with this serious abdominal defect are unable to absorb food for some considerable time following surgery. Before the introduction of intravenous alimentation, these children rarely survived. Their nutritional status deteriorated whilst their gut recovered from surgery. The babies were then at risk from intercurrent infections, which were often due to breakdown of the wound as a result of their poor nutrition.

Screening programmes are resulting in fewer babies being born with abnormalities. In the 1970s, it became common practice to screen for the neural tube defects. Women with an affected fetus could be offered a termination. Statistics showed that the incidence of neural tube defects was significantly higher in certain areas of the United Kingdom, such as Wales, Scotland and Northern Ireland, and was also higher in women from Social Class V than in women from Social Class I. This led to research into diet during pregnancy and the role of folic acid in preventing neural tube defects. The incidence of neural tube defects in 1990 was only 25% of the incidence in 1986 (Woodroffe et al 1993).

There has been increasing interest in other factors which affect the developing fetus, one of the most notorious being a drug called thalidomide (Distaval). In the 1960s the drug was prescribed for many women with morning sickness during pregnancy. There was a sudden realisation that there was an increase in babies being born with phocomelia (absent or deformed limbs). For the families involved it was a disaster, but inadvertently some benefits did eventually arise. A national fund was set up under the auspices of Lady Hoare and as a result a great deal of money was raised and utilised to develop prostheses for these children. All children with phocomelia benefited from the increased interest and developments that took place at that time.

Genetic disorders

Screening can also be carried out for some of the genetic disorders. An increasing number can be detected prior to birth and women can be offered termination. For many people this raises ethical dilemmas and it is preferable to offer genetic counselling prior to the pregnancy if there is the likelihood of an affected baby.

Prematurity and low birth weight

Prematurity and low birth weight are other significant causes of mortality and morbidity during the neonatal period. The incidence of low birth weight is higher for mothers in Social Class V, accounting for 68 per 1000 births, than for mothers in Social Class I, where the incidence is 47 per 1000 (OPCS 1992). Increasing numbers of preterm and low birth weight babies are surviving due to technological advances and skilled medical and nursing intervention. Prior to the 1960s, there was little intervention and many of these babies died. Medical developments have led to increasing numbers of babies surviving. However, during the 1960s it was realised that many of these babies were subsequently found to be blind. The practice of giving high oxygen concentrations to immature infants was found to be causing a condition known as retrolental fibroplasia. Since then, babies requiring oxygen have had their oxygen saturations carefully monitored in order to prevent this complication arising.

In the early 1970s, it was rare for an infant of less than 28 weeks' gestation to survive. Nowadays, some babies of 23 weeks' gestation are surviving. Previously rare or unheard of complications have resulted. In the 1980s, it was realised that many of these very immature infants had had an intraventricular bleed. The more immature the infant, the more likely it was that intraventricular bleeding would occur. However, it was not until it was possible to do scans on the babies, that the true incidence became apparent. It is now possible to grade these haemorrhages and give some indication of the future outlook for the baby. Another complication due to the survival of these very immature infants is bronchopulmonary dysplasia (BPD). Infants are often surviving with severe lung damage and requiring long-term oxygenation. These infants may now be discharged into the community with their supplies of oxygen and with back-up from paediatric or neonatal nurses (see Ch. 20).

There has been much discussion on the long-term outlook for these very immature infants. One survey done in the Mersey region between 1967 and 1984, found that 9% of very low birth weight babies (babies weighing less than 1500 g) have cerebral palsy. However, most infants who develop cerebral palsy weigh more than 2500 g, and the overall incidence has not increased but remains between 1.5 and 2 per 1000 live births (Woodroffe et al 1993). A further study assessed the outcome of very low birth weight babies at the age of 8 years. The study was small: 51 children, who had weighed less than 1250 g at birth, were assessed at school and a significant number were found to have problems in reading, spelling and arithmetic (Marlow et al 1993).

The ethics of using scarce resources on more and more immature infants continue to be debated. However, babies who in the past would have been damaged by hypoxia, hypoglycaemia or other problems are surviving intact as a result of the advances in medical and nursing care.

Infant deaths

The infant mortality rate in the United Kingdom has continued to fall and currently stands at 7.4 per 1000 live births. This figure hides some important variations. The mortality rates are higher in inner city areas and amongst socially deprived families. In 1988–1990, the infant mortality rate in rural Huntingdon was 4.7 and in central Birmingham 14.0 per thousand (OPCS 1991b). The rates are much higher for the children of unskilled and semi-skilled workers. The IMR for Social Class I is currently 6 per thousand, whilst for Social Class V, it is 10 per thousand (OPCS 1992). The mortality rate is higher for boys than it is for girls, as is the case for all age groups.

Sudden infant death syndrome

The commonest cause of death between the ages of 1 month and 1 year is sudden infant death syndrome (SIDS). An increasing number of deaths were notified as due to SIDS until the peak in 1988. Most of these deaths occur during the winter months and the greatest number of deaths is recorded in infants between the ages of 1 and 4 months. More boys than girls are affected. The increasing incidence was attributed to several factors. As fewer babies died from other causes, SIDS was more commonly identified as the cause of death on the registration certificate. It also became practice in the United Kingdom for babies to be nursed in the prone position. This was felt to be safer than laying them on their backs, which was considered as putting them at risk from the aspiration of vomit. At the end of the 1980s, research from New Zealand, which had a particularly high rate of SIDS, and studies of the incidence of SIDS in countries where babies were not nursed prone, suggested that the positioning of babies was a contributory factor. Another factor was the overheating of babies as a result of an increase in the number of houses with central heating, the introduction of duvets and the stress placed on keeping babies warm. In 1991, the Department of Health launched the 'Back to Sleep' campaign. Mothers were advised to place their babies on their backs to sleep and also to ensure that they were not overheated. Other advice included the promotion of breast-feeding and the in-advisability of smoking. Both of these factors had also been shown to have an effect. The campaign appears to have been very effective. Between January and June 1992, there was a fall of 46% in the number of deaths (OPCS 1993). However, SIDS still accounts for the deaths of many babies and, for the families involved, each death is a tragedy. As research continues, there should be a steady decrease in the numbers of deaths, as more is learnt about their causes.

Childhood deaths

Accidents

After the age of 1 year, the commonest cause of death in children and adolescents is accidents. They are also a significant cause of morbidity. About 700 children die each year and a further 2 000 000 (one child in every five) attends an accident and emergency department; 200 000 spend at least one night in hospital (Levene 1992). The type of accident suffered by the child is linked to his or her developmental stage. Young children are more likely to suffer accidents within the home; older children are at risk in the wider environment. Accidents to child pedestrians are the main cause of death. The high rates of accidents to children are sometimes attributed to their lack of concentration or irresponsible behaviour. James Thompson (1991), in *The Facts about Child Pedestrian Accidents*, suggests that there are a number of factors involved. Children are small and therefore they have a limited vision of the road, and are also less likely to be seen by other road users. The

road is also proportionately wider to a small child. Children are also less skilled at judging both speed and distance. They are also easily distracted and may act impetuously, for instance in running after a ball. Adults often overestimate the child's ability and skill. A study of children under the age of 5 who were killed in traffic accidents found that over 50% were un-accompanied by an adult at the time of death. Accidents on the roads are significantly higher in Social Class V than in Social Class I. Children between the ages of 1 and 14 from Social Class V have a death rate from injuries nearly four times higher than in children from Social Class I. The more deprived child may only have the street available as a play area and may also be less well supervised.

The other common types of accidents affecting children are burns and scalds, poisoning and falls. Toddlers are at particular risk from scalds and, in house fires, it is often the young children who are killed. They are dependent on adults to rescue them and are often trapped in their rooms. Publicity is being given to the advisability of fixing smoke alarms in houses, which would alert the household. Most children who die in fires, die from the inhalation of smoke or toxic fumes. Child-proof medicine bottles have led to a decrease in the numbers of children who ingest medicines, but medicines remain the most significant cause of death from poisoning. The Government has recognised accidents as a major cause of mortality and morbidity and in *The Health of the Nation* (DoH 1992) has set the targets of reducing deaths in the under-15s by at least one-third by the year 2005.

Cancer

Cancer remains a significant cause of childhood mortality and morbidity. The incidence in childhood is highest between the ages of 1 and 4 and lowest between the ages of 5 and 9. Leukaemia remains the most common of child-hood cancers but has shown the greatest response to treatment. Children who were

Activity 3.1

Visit your accident and emergency department and ask the staff about the numbers of children they see daily who have been injured. Try to find out the types of injury, the ages of the children and how each injury occurred. Do you think these accidents could have been prevented?

diagnosed with acute lymphoblastic leukaemia in the 1950s had a life expectancy of about 6 months. Children who were diagnosed between 1971 and 1973 had a 37% chance of being alive 5 years later. This 5-year survival rate has now risen to about 70% (Woodroffe et al 1993). Survival from most other types of childhood cancer has also improved, but the increased survival is not without significant psychological cost to both the child and the family. Treatments have many unpleasant side effects. The child may require many episodes of hospitalisation, though with the introduction of paediatric community nursing teams in many parts of the country, increasing numbers of children are being cared for at home. Siblings of affected children may suffer from jealousy at the attention given to the affected child (see Ch. 24).

Although there has been much research into the causes of cancers and leukaemia, the only confirmed link is that with radiation. Over the last two decades, leukaemia clusters have been identified near to nuclear installations and links have been made to the occupation of fathers in the nuclear industry. Currently the link remains unproved, with conflicting results from research studies. There has also been a suggestion that there is a link between a high electromagnetic field and high levels of childhood cancer. Researchers are also investigating the role of infectious agents in the development of leukaemia. One puzzling fact is that leukaemia in childhood appears to be four times more common in wealthy countries than in poor ones.

CHRONIC ILLNESS

Children's wards in the mid-1950s were very different from the wards today. Many children were admitted with diseases that are now rarely seen. Rheumatic fever, glomerular nephritis and scarlet fever were common childhood diseases. Improved living conditions, the availability of antibiotics and the decreased virulence of some organisms seem to be the main reasons for the fewer cases. Children stayed in hospital for much longer periods and the throughput was much less. However, there remains a core of children with chronic illness or disability, whose needs are not always being met. The report on health services for school-age children by the British Paediatric Association (1993) found that 9.6% of children under the age of 15 have an illness chronically affecting their functional capacity.

Cystic fibrosis

Of the chronic diseases affecting children, cystic fibrosis remains one of the most important. It is the commonest serious genetic disorder amongst Caucasians—1 in 20 of the population carries the defective gene. As it is a recessive disorder, both parents must be carriers if the child is to present with the disease. The gene responsible for the disorder was discovered in the late 1980s and it is now theoretically possible to screen all women of reproductive age. If a woman was found to be carrying the gene responsible, her partner could also be screened. If this became national policy, the incidence of cystic fibrosis, which currently stands at 1 in 2000, would be reduced. With modern treatment, the life expectancy of these children has increased significantly. In the 1950s few of them would have survived into their teens. Now, many survive into adulthood and they have formed their own branch of the cystic fibrosis association. Babies born with cystic fibrosis in the 1990s have a life expectancy of about 40 years, although they may require considerable medical intervention during this time. It is common practice to give these children intravenous antibiotics early on during an infection, to minimise the pulmonary damage. In some areas this will require hospitalisation, in others, where there is a paediatric community nursing service, parents may learn to give the intravenous drugs themselves, with support from the paediatric nurse. Some children have benefited from heart/lung transplants, but the numbers are small and the long-term results need to be evaluated. Transplants are unlikely to become common practice but will be reserved for those children with the most severe lung damage. They are not a cure and the future may lie in genetic engineering.

Other genetic disorders

With increasing numbers of children from ethnic minorities being born and living in Britain, other genetic disorders are being seen more frequently. Sickle cell disease is a severe genetic disorder affecting the Afro-Caribbean population. It is particularly common amongst people of West African origin. Thalassaemia is a common disorder affecting people from the Mediterranean and Asian countries.

Asthma

There are other chronic disorders that are being seen more frequently in children. The incidence of asthma appears to have increased, with 1 in every 7 children now suffering. There has been considerable debate as to whether there is an actual increase, or whether the apparent increase is due to better diagnosis. A study done by Ninan & Russell in 1992 found that there had been an increase from 10.4% of the child population in 1964 to 19.8% of the population in 1989. Other authors suggest that the increase is due to improved diagnosis which has led to the inclusion of children who previously would have been diagnosed as having wheezy bronchitis. Children's wards have all reported increasing numbers of admissions due to asthma; an estimated doubling since the mid-1970s.

The role of the house dust mite as an allergen is now accepted. Warner & Price (1978) found that 80% of asthmatic children were sensitive to the house dust mite. The house dust mite thrives in an environment which has a temperature of 25°C and a relative humidity of 80%. With increasing numbers of houses having central heating and double glazing, and more families being able to afford carpets on the floor, the house dust mite is likely to be found in large numbers, especially in beds and bedrooms. Over 50% of asthmatic children are found to be sensitive to animal dander. Cats and dogs are particularly important and over 50% of homes now have one or other of these pets.

Another factor that has been studied is the effect of parental smoking on the child with asthma. There has been increasing interest in the effect of passive smoking on the health of the population in general, and several studies have also been done looking specifically at the child with asthma. A study by Magnusson in 1986 found that maternal smoking during pregnancy increased the risk of the infant developing allergic disease. Parents of an asthmatic child are advised not to smoke in their child's presence, and if they can cut down their consumption of cigarettes, the incidence of wheezy attacks in the child is found to decrease.

Air pollution is another area that is currently attracting interest. The role of car exhaust fumes is under consideration, with several studies suggesting that increased levels of nitrogen dioxide and sulphur dioxide, and low levels of ozone may well cause children to wheeze. In the 1960s, severe smog in London and other large British cities caused serious respiratory illness in all age groups, with many deaths. This led to the introduction of the Clean Air Act 1968, which concentrated on the emissions from industry and led to a decrease in the amount of pollutants discharged into the atmosphere. Since that time, there has been a major increase in road traffic and an increase in pollution from this source. There has been concern that the death rate from asthma has increased, as well as the frequency. In the 1960s, there was an increased mortality rate due to the overuse of isoprenaline inhalers.

Since that time, the mortality rate for children has decreased but there has been an increase in deaths amongst those aged 15–19 years (Anderson & Strachan 1991).

Activity 3.2

Consider the number of children who are being admitted to your wards with asthma. Try to discover what the parents think causes the attacks and how disruptive it is proving to be to a child's life. Talk to the permanent staff and find out whether there has been an increase or decrease in admissions of children with asthma. At what time of year are admissions most likely to occur and do the staff have any thoughts about the reasons for this?

Diabetes mellitus

Another chronic disease of childhood which is increasing is diabetes mellitus. In 1988, there were 19 000 children under the age of 20 in the United Kingdom with diabetes mellitus. 3200 new cases are diagnosed each year. A survey by Nabarro in 1988 showed that the incidence in children aged between 10 and 11 years was 10 cases per 100 000 population in 1956; this had risen to 60 cases per 100 000 in 1968 and 130 cases per 100 000 in 1980. The reason for this increase is unclear. The onset of diabetes often appears in clusters, and virus infections are thought to precipitate the onset in children who have a genetic predisposition to the disease. British children have a high intake of refined sugars and this may be a factor. The incidence of diabetes is low in countries where the intake of refined sugars is low and the intake of fibre is high. Nabarro's study also showed that the increase in diabetes is most marked in the higher social classes. No cause has been discovered for this difference.

OBESITY

Overall, British families are more affluent than they were in 1900 or in 1950 and therefore the diseases of affluence are becoming more significant. Increasing numbers of children are found to be overweight or obese. This pattern is a cause for concern, as obesity makes a significant contribution to ill health in later life. Obesity in childhood often leads to obesity in adulthood and the 'Health of the Nation' target is to reduce the proportion of men and women aged 16–64 who are obese, by at least 25% and 33% respectively, by 2005 (to no more than 6% of men and 8% of women).

Even during childhood, obesity can cause problems, with overweight babies presenting with bronchiolitis and school-age children with Perthes' disease. Blood pressure is also likely to be raised, which may have later detrimental effects. Overweight children do not always eat more than their slimmer peers, but they often take significantly less exercise. They may be teased in school and are therefore less likely to take part in physical activity for which they have a poor tolerance.

Diet

Increasing attention is being paid to the diet of children, which is often less than optimal. A new term has crept into the vocabulary, that of 'grazing'. Family lifestyles have altered over the past 20 years, with increasing numbers of working mothers. Fast foods have become more popular as people have less time to prepare food, and microwave ovens offer a quick solution to the 'instant' meal. Some children rarely sit down to a family meal but gather food at intervals; hence the term 'grazing'. School meals used to be an important factor in providing at least one healthy meal per day for children. However, the 1980 Education Act abolished nutritional standards for school meals and also the need for schools to provide meals. Since then, increasing numbers of children take packed lunches to school or rely on the tuck shop. Some parents will go to great lengths to ensure that the packed lunch is a healthy one. Others are not so particular, and children will often swap items from their lunch boxes with each other. A programme on television, considered a small research study which appeared to show that the diets of children were significantly low in some of the important minerals and vitamins. The programme went on to suggest that by giving vitamin supplements, the ability of children to concentrate and their intellectual ability could be improved. There was a sudden increase in the sales of vitamins following the programme, but since then the results of the study have been questioned.

However, there is increasing concern that children are having a relatively poor diet, which is too high in saturated fats and refined sugars and too low in minerals, vitamins and fibre. Together with the fact that many children take little or no exercise, the increase in overweight children is to be expected. Dietary habits laid down in childhood will influence the diet of the adult and the 'Health of the Nation' target is to reduce the average percentage of food energy derived from total fat by at least 12% by the year 2005 (to no more than 35% of total food energy).

In some areas, school nurses are making an impact on the eating habits of children. They have taken the initiative in meeting with school teachers and discussing the meals provided in school canteens. This has resulted in healthier meals being offered in some instances. There have also been initiatives taken by school nurses in persuading the school tuck shop to stock fewer snacks with high fat and sugar content and to promote the sale of healthier foods.

Activity

The activity of children appears to be decreasing with the greater use of the motor car. In the past, many children would have walked or cycled to school. This is now relatively uncommon. School buses collect many children; parents take others by car. Roads are much busier than they used to be and many villages do not have adequate footpaths or pavements. There is also a great deal of media coverage of abducted or assaulted children. Although these cases are uncommon, the publicity they receive makes many parents fearful of allowing their children to walk to school on their own.

Organised games at school are less common than they used to be and sometimes are arranged for evenings or weekends, so that children can avoid them completely. The television at home has become a convenient way of entertaining children on their return from school, so there may be little incentive for them to take any exercise. Video and computer games are other favourite leisure activities that require no physical activity.

The osteoporosis society has expressed concern over the combined poor diet of children and lack of physical activity. As bone tissue is laid down in childhood and requires a good intake of calcium and vitamin D and stressing from exercise, the society is predicting an increase in the incidence of osteoporosis, when today's children reach old age. Boys take more exercise than girls and therefore the incidence of osteoporosis in women may rise even higher than it is at present.

DENTAL HEALTH

In spite of the high sugar intake of some children, the incidence of dental caries is falling, thanks to the fluoridation of water. Many water companies add fluoride to the water supplies, but it is still not country-wide due to public opposition. Fluoride is also added to many brands of toothpaste, so there is no reason why dental caries should not be almost eliminated. However, a significant number of 5-year-olds are still reporting with dental caries. The routine brushing of teeth is not encouraged in all households and

Activity 3.3

When you are with a group of schoolchildren, try to decide how many of them are overweight. Ask some of the children about their diets, what their favourite foods are and what they have eaten and drunk over the past 24 hours. Also ask them what they do when they get home from school and whether they walk to school or go on the bus or by car. Find out how often they take exercise in a week, what form this exercise takes and how long they spend on it.

children have to be taught good oral hygiene and correct methods of brushing. The 'grazing' of sugary foods and drinks is particularly harmful. The high level of sugar in canned and boxed fruit drinks is not widely appreciated. A 250 ml carton of Five Alive fruit drink contains the equivalent of 10–12 lumps of sugar. Other makes have equally high levels with a 250 ml carton of Ribena containing the equivalent of 15 lumps (Lang 1992). Many parents are totally unaware of this fact and may buy these drinks for their children with excellent intentions. The energy level is quoted on the side of the carton or can, but few will appreciate the significance. It is relatively difficult to find a carton or can of fruit juice with a low energy value.

HIV AND AIDS

The first cases of AIDS in children were seen in this country in the mid-1980s. The first children in this country to become infected with the HIV virus were those with haemophilia. The United Kingdom did not produce enough blood products to be self-sufficient and used to buy factor VIII, which is used to treat haemophiliacs during a bleed, from the USA. In this country, blood donors give their blood without being financially rewarded. In the USA, blood donors are paid. In some instances, drug addicts who were short of money, sold their blood, and they were amongst the first to be infected with the HIV virus. Haemophiliacs who were given factor VIII were particularly at risk, as factor VIII was made from pooled plasma. There was therefore an increased risk of blood becoming contaminated. Blood products are now subjected to much tighter control and are heat treated to destroy the virus. More recently, babies have been born to HIV-positive mothers. The babies are often HIV-positive at birth, and initially it was predicted that they would all develop full-blown AIDS. Fortunately, that has not proved to be the case. Many of the children who are HIV-positive at birth will seroconvert at a later stage and will test negative. By July 1992, a total of 403 children under the age of 15 had been

diagnosed as HIV-positive and of these 47 had died. Sadly, this number is likely to increase (Woodroffe et al 1993).

SOCIAL FACTORS

Physical well-being is not the only component of health. Social well-being is also important. Research carried out by the National Children's Bureau (Kumar 1992) showed that the number of children living in poverty has risen from 1.4 million in 1979 to 3.9 million in 1991. Poverty is always relative and, compared to children in the developing countries, these children would not be counted poor. However, the definition of poverty in the United Kingdom is; 'families with incomes below 50% of the average'.

There are many reasons for this increase in poverty. Since 1979 there have been two major recessions leading to mass unemployment. Unemployment tends to affect the unskilled and semiskilled first, and these are the families who are least likely to be able to move to other areas in search of work or have any resources to tide them over bad times. The latest recession has also hit the white collar workforce and high unemployment in areas with normally full employment is a new phenomenon. More women now form part of the workforce and many of them have low-paid and part-time jobs. Some of these women are the only wage earner in the family, either because their partners are unemployed or because they are single parents. The number of dependent children living with single parents has increased rapidly from 1 million in 1971 to 1.9 million in 1989 (Haskey 1991).

Children living in poverty are likely to have increased mortality and morbidity rates but are often also socially deprived. They live in the worst housing, with less access to safe play areas and in a less-stimulating environment. The incidence of smoking and substance abuse is also higher, although teenagers who had been offered drugs were slightly more likely to have come from the higher socio-economic groups. The 'Health of the Nation' target is to reduce the prevalence of 11- to 15-year-olds who

Activity 3.4

Discuss with your friends the concept of poverty. What are the factors that make you think that a child is living in poverty and what effect is this having on that child's health and welfare? Find out how many children on the ward are living with single parents. Do you consider that all of these children are living in poverty?

smoke, by at least 33% by 1994 (to less than 6%). Most adult smokers start during their teenage years and currently 27% of girls and 26% of boys in the fifth year of secondary school, are smokers (BPA 1993).

Deprivation can have long-term consequences. The children may develop a low self-esteem and the lack of social facilities may lead to unsocial behaviour. As they grow into adolescents, many will realise that job opportunities are not good and a sense of frustration may lead to an increased incidence of criminality.

Poverty also affects the mental well-being of children and the recent figures published by the Mental Health Foundation are disturbing. They estimate that 2 million children are likely to be suffering from emotional problems (MHF 1995). This accounts for almost a quarter of all children who attend GP surgeries. Even more disturbing is the fact that only a small percentage of them are likely to be identified as having a problem. Suicide and attempted suicide in children is rare but appears to be rising in adolescents. True figures are difficult to obtain as often the coroner will give a verdict of accidental death in order to spare the parents further anguish. Behaviour problems, depression and anorexia are other common mental health problems seen in children and adolescents. These will be discussed in more depth in Chapter 23.

CONCLUSION

In conclusion, the last 100 years have seen major changes in mortality rates and morbidity in children. Initially, the improved standard of living and nutrition accounted for the greatest changes. Latterly, the technological advances and improved medical and nursing care have had some effect. Some of the diseases that are seen today are the diseases of affluence; however, poverty still has a part to play. There are increased mortality rates for all ages in the lower socioeconomic groups and, for many diseases, there is increased morbidity.

REFERENCES

Anderson H R, Strachan D P 1991 Asthma mortality in England and Wales 1979–1989. British Medical Journal 337: 1357

British Paediatric Association 1993 Health services for school age children. Consultation Report of the Joint Working Party. British Medical Association, London

Clean Air Act 1968 HMSO, London

Department of Health 1992 The health of the nation: a strategy for health in England. HMSO, London

Department of Health 1993 Diphtheria in the former USSR. HMSO, London

Education Act 1980 HMSO, London

Haskey J 1991 Estimated numbers and demographic characteristics of one-parent families in Great Britain. OPCS Population Trends 63: 22–25

Kumar V 1992 Poverty and inequality in the UK: the effects on children. National Children's Bureau, London

Lang T 1992 Food policy and public health. Public Health 106: 91–125

Levene S 1992 Preventing accidental injuries to children. Paediatric Nursing 4(9): 12–14

McKeown T 1976 The modern rise of population. Edward Arnold, Kent

Magnusson C G M 1986 Maternal smoking influences cord serum IgE and IgD levels and increases the risk for subsequent infant allergy. Journal of Allergy and Clinical Immunology 78: 898–904

Marlow N, Roberts L, Cooke R 1993 Outcome at eight years for children with birth weights of 1250 g or less. Archives of Disease in Childhood 68(3): 286–290

Mental Health Foundation 1995 Mental health and the young. Mental Health Foundation, London

Nabarro J D N 1988 Diabetes in the United Kingdom: some facts and figures. Diabetic Medicine 5: 816–822

Ninan T, Russell G 1992 Respiratory symptoms and atopy in Aberdeen schoolchildren: evidence from two surveys 25 years apart. British Medical Journal 304: 873–875

Office of Population Censuses and Surveys 1988 Childhood mortality. DS8. HMSO, London

Office of Population Censuses and Surveys 1989 Mortality statistics: surveillance (time trends). DH1/19. HMSO, London

Office of Population Censuses and Surveys 1990 Mortality statistics: perinatal and infant. HMSO, London

Office of Population Censuses and Surveys 1991a Mortality statistics: cause. DH2/17. HMSO, London

Office of Population Censuses and Surveys 1991b Mortality statistics: perinatal and infant. DH3 91/2. HMSO, London

Office of Population Censuses and Surveys 1992 Mortality statistics: perinatal and infant: birthweight. DH3/24. HMSO, London

Office of Population Censuses and Surveys 1993 Sudden infant deaths: 1988–1992. DH3 93/2. HMSO, London

Thompson J 1991 The facts about child pedestrian accidents. Cassell Educational, London

United Nations Children's Fund 1992 The state of the world's children. UNICEF, New York

United Nations Children's Fund 1993 Progress of nations. UNICEF, New York

Warner J O, Price J F 1978 House dust mite sensitivity in childhood asthma. Archives of Disease in Childhood 53: 710–713

Woodroffe C, Glickman M, Barker M, Power C 1993 Children, teenagers and health. The key data. Open University Press, Buckingham

World Health Organization 1958 Charter. WHO, Geneva

FURTHER READING

British Paediatric Association 1993 Health services for school age children. Consultation Report of the Joint Working Party. British Medical Association, London

Child Accident Prevention Trust 1989 Basic principles of child accident prevention. CAPT, London

Department of Health 1992 The health of the nation: a strategy for health in England. HMSO, London

Foundation for the Study of Infant Death 1991 Reduce the risk of cot death. Foundation for the Study of Infant Death, London

Health Education Authority 1992 Today's young adults. 16–19 year olds look at diet, alcohol, smoking, drugs and sexual behaviour. HEA, London

Health Education Authority 1992 Tomorrow's young adults. 9–15 year olds look at alcohol, drugs, exercise and smoking. HEA, London

Levene S 1992 Play it safe: the complete guide to child accident prevention. BBC Books, London

Putland S 1993 Off to a poor start. Nursing Times 89(44): 46–49

Woodroffe C, Glickman M, Barker M, Power C 1993 Children, teenagers and health. The key data. Open University Press, Buckingham

USEFUL ADDRESSES

Child Accident Prevention Trust
4th Floor
Clerk's Court
18–20 Farringdon Lane
London EC1R 3AU

National Children's Bureau
8 Wakeley Street
London EC1V 7QE

Royal Society for Prevention of Accidents
Cannon House
The Priory
Queensway
Birmingham B4 6BS

4

Sociology and social policy

Penny Reid   Jean Neave

This chapter introduces the student to different concepts of the family and childhood and examines the effects of social policy on the provision of services for children.

The chapter aims to:

- discuss the varying sociological perspectives on the family, and changing family structure, family breakdown and size of families

- highlight the concept of the changing role of women within the family, looking at mothering, delayed mothering, young mothers and the relationship with social class and working patterns

- examine 'childhood' through the ages, exploring the ways in which it has evolved and the influence of the family on socialisation, the role of education and the growing influence of the media

- discuss services for children with reference to health, education, social services and their remit for children, and the effect of the 1989 Children Act on services

- discuss the voluntary sector in relation to its growing role as a result of changes being implemented by Government.

FAMILY AND MARRIAGE IN THE UNITED KINGDOM

The term 'family' is likely to hold different meanings for different people and is unlikely to conform to any stereotypical image, although certain general characteristics apply to the population as a whole.

Monogamy is established in the law and the majority of the population follow this course, although recent trends in marriage patterns suggest rather a serial monogamy where we can have more than one spouse in sequence over a period of time. British marriage is based on the notion of romantic love. Couples are expected to develop long-lasting ties of affection based on attraction and compatibility with each other. The emphasis on personal satisfaction may have raised expectations that cannot be met, which could be one factor involved in the rising divorce rate.

Generally speaking, the British family is nuclear, consisting of two parents (though due to the rising divorce rate there are a growing number of single-parent families) living in a household with their children. The Second World War disrupted marriage and family life. The divorce rate in 1947 was 10 times higher than it had been in previous years and, although the rate subsequently dropped, it rose sharply again in the early 1960s. The passing of the Legal Aid Act in 1949 opened the possibility of divorce to many who, because of the expense, had never previously been able to consider it. There was, however, no decline in the popularity of marriage; three-quarters of those who had divorced remarried.

A brief baby 'boom' occurred in the immediate post-war period, with the birth rate (numbers of live births per thousand adults in any one year) reaching a peak of 20.7 in 1947. Thereafter, the birth rate levelled off and has since remained quite stable.

Single-parent households have become increasingly common. The vast majority are headed by women, since the wife usually obtains custody of the children following a divorce. The term 'single-parent family' covers several kinds of families with quite different backgrounds and histories. For instance, it could describe:

- a family which was functioning well until the death of one of the adults
- a family headed by a mother who has never married, and who has always raised her child alone
- a family whose single-parent status is the result of a dissolved marriage—these families form the largest single-parent group.

There are 1.3 million single-parent households in Britain today, and the number is expected to increase at five times the rate of two-parent families between now and the end of this decade. Such households constitute one in five of all families with dependent children. On average they are amongst the poorest groups in contemporary society (Bradshaw 1989). This may well be because women find it impossible to work and pay for child care, so they have to rely on the state benefit system. Benefits are set at such a level that they often act as a disincentive to work; the mother may find that if she earns too much she will lose benefits and thus make herself economically worse off. Most lone mothers remain stuck in a poverty trap where child care is both unobtainable and unaffordable, and part-time work would constitute a net loss in income; even full-time employment would need to be very well paid to make a direct difference to this. Housing is another issue where the single parent is disadvantaged and one-parent families are more likely than any other group of families to experience homelessness through marriage break-up or eviction because of pregnancy.

Many lone parents, whether they have been

Activity 4.1

Think about the different family structures you have encountered. What proportion of them fall into the category of single-parent families? Can you identify ways in which these families have been socially disadvantaged, or is society becoming more accepting of their situation?

married or not, still face societal disapproval as well as economic insecurity. However, earlier more judgemental terms such as 'deserted wives', 'fatherless families' and 'broken homes' are tending to disappear.

Differing perspectives on the family

The Marxist perspective

Marxists regard the nuclear family as a particular feature of capitalist society, preserving the class-based nature of that society and fulfilling the needs of capitalism. They believe that nuclear families encourage and reproduce hierarchical, inegalitarian relationships, acting as a safety valve to dampen down discontent so that it is robbed of revolutionary content. In providing a place where children can be safely conceived, born and reared, the family is providing tomorrow's labour force. At the same time, by offering a centre for relaxation, recreation, refreshment and rest, the family helps to ensure that the current labour force is returned to work each day with their capacity to work renewed and strengthened. Children are taught the necessity of work and the basic forms of work discipline (punctuality, obedience) in the context of the family, though supplemented by the school. Adults are kept working in boring jobs by the expectation that 'good' husbands/ mothers/parents must do their utmost to earn enough to buy their families and themselves certain comforts and advantages.

The privatisation of family life is also seen as contributing to the survival of capitalist society. On the one hand, small and fairly self-sufficient family units offer an enormous market for the sale of domestic goods, which is encouraged by advertising. On the other hand, the privatisation of the family acts as a barrier to the development of strong, organised and collective opposition to the status quo. It undermines class conscious-ness by emphasising one's loyalty to the family.

Finally, according to some Marxists, the family quells rebellious spirits in two other ways. First, through socialisation of children and through day-to-day relationships, people are inculcated with patterns of obedience and power; thus patriarchal relationships outside the family, or the habit of submission to the 'boss', have a foundation in family life. Second, to the extent that family life is warm and satisfying, it can help to sustain unfair and unfree structures outside the family, by offering an escape from these and a chance for recuperation.

Therefore, in Marxist tradition, although the family is seen as relatively strong, this strength is seen as detrimental to the development of the individual and of society. The family helps to preserve the unsatisfactory and constraining patterns of capitalism, and therefore prevents the emergence of better, more enriching ways of life. The irony is that the less fulfilling work and life in the public sphere are, the more desperately people cling to their one potential source of satisfaction, the family.

The Functionalist perspective

Functionalists stress the importance of inte-gration and harmony between the parts of society. Parsons (1951) argues that the isolated nuclear family is best adapted to the needs of an industrial society, giving as it does a degree of flexibility and ease of movement so that family members are able to be geographically mobile in order to seek work. Individual family members are not tied down by the demands of their kin, but are able to take their specialised skills where they are in most demand.

They regard the functions of the family as its most important aspect. George Murdock (1949) considered the four basic functions of the family to be the sexual, the reproductive, the socialising and the economic. Although these functions are constantly evolving, he considered them to be overwhelming.

Sex and reproduction according to the func-tionalist view take place best within marriage and a nuclear family, providing the best oppor-tunity for socially controlled expression of the sex drive and the necessary institutional stability for the reproduction and nurture of children. The latter requires considerable time and effort and, ideally, should be a part of the role of the people who produced the child.

The family's role in laying down the basis of culture through socialisation is universally stressed by functionalists.

The basic function of the family is to provide food and shelter for its members. In pre-industrial societies, many families produced much of what they consumed. Now individuals work for wages, but the family remains an important unit of consumption of industrially produced goods.

Functionalists tend to assume a 'fit' between the nuclear family and society as a whole, even though they may concede that it may be internally under stress. Arguably, they are over-influenced by the harmony explicit in the organic analogy in making this assumption.

Marriage in Britain today

The term 'family' conjures up a picture of mother, father and 2.4 children; yet this vision accounts for only 5% of families living in Britain today as the average number of children is now 1.8.

Getting married is still popular. By the age of 49, 95% of women will have married as will 91% of men. The actual numbers of marriages in 1984, the latest year for which figures are available, was 349 000, an increase of 5000 over 1983.

First-time marriage remains low when considered over a period of decades. The figures reached a peak in 1970, fell by one-third in 1976, levelled off until 1980, and are now beginning to rise again. Remarriages, by contrast, were two-thirds higher in 1984 than in 1970. Marriages in which one or both partners had previously been married now form 35% of all marriages, largely because of increases in remarriages among people who are divorced.

Both sexes are marrying at a later age and are choosing to have fewer children; 50% of couples are tending to live together before getting married.

Following the Matrimony and Family Proceedings Act 1984, the number of divorces has increased dramatically; the rate of 12 divorces per 1000 marriages means that one in three new marriages will end in divorce. Marriage breakdown causes great stress to the children involved. Their emotional and security needs, which under normal circumstances are met by both parents, are apt to be set aside as the parents resolve their differences, when paradoxically the children need more reassurance (Randall 1989). One of the consequences of rising divorce is an increase in the numbers of one-parent families. There are now an estimated 1.3 million such families in Britain, which means that:

- one in every eight families is headed by a lone parent
- 1.5 million children live in one-parent families
- 20% of all dependent children live with a lone mother compared with 1% who live with a lone father.

The fact that most lone parents are women is a reflection of the increase in the numbers of single and divorced mothers and the fact that divorced mothers usually get custody of the children. In general, a one-parent family will be financially worse off than a two-parent family. In 1983, only 39% of single parents received the major part of their income from paid employment, compared with 92% of two-parent families. The opportunities for lone parents to take paid work, full or part-time, are limited by the age of children, the availability of child care facilities and attitudes of employers (Bradshaw 1989).

One-parent families are more likely than others to rely on state benefits (Payne 1991). In 1981, nearly half of all one-parent families had an income 20% below that of two-parent families. Thus, an 'underclass' of children in poverty, with poorer educational and life chances, is emerging (Halsey 1993).

Partly because of later marriages and fewer children, women now spend a greater proportion of their lives at work. Most married women work full time until the birth of their first child and are likely to return quickly to work.

The demographic evidence suggests that

families are still important as a social institution. An increasing number of adults will live with their partner before marriage, and two-thirds of marriages will survive until the death of one partner. Therefore, the vast majority of children will grow up living with both natural parents. But a significant and growing number of children will be affected by the divorce of their parents and spend some part of their childhood in step-parent or one-parent families. However, the average child in a two-parent family does better in health, personality and in educational attainment than the child in the care of one parent (Halsey 1993). The dominant type of family unit for those with dependent children remains the nuclear family, and the typical experience of most people is to have been raised in such families, even if they now live alone.

Men and women get different things from the family, both good and bad, often at the same time. Circumstances change, family situations alter, children grow up and parents age. How we experience families, what we want and what we actually get from our family cannot simply be explained by the internal dynamics of family life and interpersonal relationships. The family exists within a wider social, political and economic environment which creates, structures and constrains the individual opportunities and choices available to those within it.

Familial ideology in our society asserts that the co-resident nuclear family is a universal and desirable way to live, and that the prevailing sexual division of labour, in which the woman is a housewife and mother and primarily located within the private world of the family and the man is the wage earner and breadwinner located in the public world of work, is universal and normatively desirable. There is clearly material basis to this ideology; in capitalist societies production does take place outside the home and does make it difficult for a woman not to be dependent on a man. So the family itself is both the ideological site in which gender differences are constructed and creates the material relations in which men and women are differently engaged in waged labour.

The dominance of this ideology in our society therefore leads us to expect that we will live our lives in the family; it is the starting point from which we judge alternative ways of living. Those who are excluded from the family can be massively disadvantaged individually and socially (for example single people, children in care). Those who choose alternative lifestyles will have to struggle and constantly justify themselves, for ideals of family relationships have become enshrined in our legal, social, religious and economic systems, which in turn reinforce the ideology and penalise or ostracise those who transgress it. Thus there are real pressures on people to conform, to lead their lives according to acceptable norms and practices. These pressures partly explain the appeal of the family.

Familial ideology is constantly being reinforced by wider arrangements and organisation in society (e.g. Government, and housing policy) and is embedded and shaped in other non-familial institutions such as welfare and public health provision.

The main role of the family in child rearing is socialisation, this being the process by which individuals learn the culture of their society. By responding to the approval and disapproval of their parents and by copying their example, children learn the language and many of the basic behaviour patterns of society.

Most of the influence of the family at this initial stage during the socialisation process is unintended and takes place informally as a product of social interaction between people in extremely close physical proximity to one another. Although the family has an important influence in infancy other agents of socialisation also contribute as the child gets older. For example friends and playmates can have a significant socialising influence. This agency, called the peer group, is probably the first means by which children encounter ideas and ways of behaving that are different from those at home. Clearly, it is important that children are exposed to these influences early on in order for them to develop fully their confidence and personality.

THE HISTORY OF CHILDHOOD

The Greeks, it appears, did not pay too much attention to childhood as a specific category. Indeed, the words 'child' and 'youth' seemed only to mark out the broad sweep of time between infancy and old age. They did, however, believe passionately in education. Youth was seen as a legitimate time for intervention and training. The Romans followed this thinking and even developed some notions of childhood which we can guess at from pictorial records on vases and pottery. Europe's descent into the dark and middle ages after the collapse of the Roman empire has been claimed to be particularly relevant to childhood, notably the disappearance of education and literacy. Aries (1962) also tries to demonstrate that in medieval times childhood was of no consequence. He uses as evidence the fact that no records were kept of childhood or age.

Prior to the Industrial Revolution (1750–1850), Britain was predominantly an agricultural society and the family structure and relationships were different from our present type. The social structure consisted mainly of two social classes: the aristocracy and the labouring poor (agricultural workers and those involved in cottage industries such as weaving). The merchant and professional classes who were to become the middle classes of the future industrial society were a small minority. Aristocratic families prided themselves on not having to work for a living—their wealth was based on the ownership of large estates. They monopolised positions of power throughout the country.

Harry Hendrick (1994) writes that from the late 17th century a new attitude towards children began to manifest itself. Points of view on childhood were polarised between children being seen as the originators of original sin and therefore subject to harsh and often cruel treatment, countered by the more benign influence of the humanists, who believed in the child's capacity for good and the moral neutrality of a child's impulses. Here was an optimism which acted as a corrective against the more dour Protestantism.

Nevertheless, the 18th century social construction of childhood emerged fragmented and ambiguous, torn as it was between the notion of 'innocence' and a pessimism born of evangelical and political anxieties. Hendrick talks of the portrayal of childhood in the literature of the time, where the romantics constructed a particular childhood, narrowly confined to an elite, as a literary and educational theme in order to combat much of the century's materialism and rationalism, or what Mill described as 'the revolt of the human mind against the philosophy of the eighteenth century'. The Romantics turned to childhood because they were in search of a new awareness and psychological insights. All in all this was a search which helped to assign a new importance to childhood, and one that saw the condition as optimistic and life-enhancing. At the most basic level, therefore, this construction related to the contest for a particular kind of society—for a particular set of beliefs—which was to stand between 18th century rationalism and 19th century industrialism.

The 19th century discussion on the meaning of childhood in an industrialising and urbanising nation was very much the work of evangelicals who produced their own agenda for reform, largely through publicly promoting a domestic ideal which emphasised home, family, duty and respect.

Three views of childhood through history are to be found in the literature:

- the factory child
- the delinquent child
- the school child.

The factory child

This is probably one of the best known of all historical stories: the struggle to rescue 'little children' from long hours and cruel conditions in factories, mines, and workshops. The early Factory Acts prohibited children under the age of 9 from employment in a variety of mills. There was nothing new about children working in the Industrial Revolution, for it had long been established that they should contribute to the family economy. By the early 19th century they were widely employed in textiles, dress, mining, agriculture, domestic service, docks and navigation, metals, and machinery and tools. However, it was their work in textile mills, mines and as chimney sweeps which most dramatically captured the imagination of reformers and philanthropists who campaigned against this form of exploitation.

The delinquent child

The 19th century saw a number of Acts passed regarding youthful offenders which were important for four reasons. First, they provided the initial recognition in legislative terms of juvenile delinquency as a separate category. Children coming before the courts were seen as beings with their own special characteristics, and not always responsible for their actions, rather than as small adults. Second, they introduced 'care and protection' features, which referred to potentially delinquent children; and, third, they established reformatory schools with the intention of 'treating' and 'reclaiming' delinquents, rather than merely punishing them. Fourth, the cumulative effects of these changes was to extend 'childhood' beyond the customary first 7 years. Accordingly, the legislation defined children as 'different'; reinforced the view that they were not 'free' agents; drew attention to the child–parent relationship, with the latter expected to exercise control and discipline; and emphasised the danger of those in need of 'care and protection' becoming delinquents—neglect and delinquency were seen to stand side by side. One of the most important consequences of the Acts was the perception of working-class children as 'precocious' sexually and otherwise. The Acts were intended to 'save' such children who had a detailed knowledge of 'the adult world and its pleasures'. Clearly, the intention was to make working-class children conform to the reformers' middle-class notion of what constituted childhood—a constitution characterised by dependency.

In order to understand the significance of developments in the concept of juvenile delinquency, it has to be remembered that the movement to create the beginnings of a separate order of juvenile justice emerged from three sources: the debate on child labour, the economic and political upheavals of the 1830s and 1840s, and the increasing popularity of the school as a means of class control.

Here was a turning-point in the history of age-relations, second only in significance to compulsory mass schooling. For under construction was a carefully defined 'nature', which also posed a return to an earlier mythical condition of childhood. The clue to the success of the reformers lay in the 'care and protection' clauses of the Acts. These took the concept of the Romantic child as it was being popularised by 19th century literature and, with the help of religious conviction produced an image of the 'innocent' child, who needed to have the protection, guidance, discipline and love of a family. Given the widespread criticisms of working-class family life, in particular that of the poor, in their failure to conform to middle-class standards, the reformatory schools were seen as providing a replacement for these 'inadequate' families.

The school child

Children had received a schoolroom education through state and voluntary provision since the early 19th century. However, the Elementary Education Act of 1870 made possible free and compulsory education, which came with the Acts of 1876 and 1880, although it was not free for the majority of elementary school children until 1891.

The immediate impact of compulsory schooling was to prohibit wage-labour by children of school age. Since only a small minority of young children were so employed, those most affected were older children aged 10 and over. However, schooling affected not only wage-earning children, but also those who were unpaid domestic workers in their own homes. Whatever the 'educational' benefits, in prohibiting full-time wage-labour, schooling probably reduced older children's sense of their own value, especially those who were conscious of the significance of their contribution to the family economy, and may therefore, have prevented them from maintaining their sense of individual worth.

In terms of the developing emergence of the child, compulsory schooling made its impact in four significant respects:

• Education, though not in itself new to working-class children, served to emphasise their ignorance; school was the place where 'knowledge' could be 'learnt'. The working-class cultural knowledge that children possessed was deemed to be both useless and harmful in that it encouraged precocious behaviour.
• The allegedly precocious behaviour of working class children—not least the ability many of them had apparently to survive independently of their parents—was taken to be evidence of their moral weakness and, therefore, they could only be made 'innocent' again by being made incapable of such 'adult' behaviour.
• Children were compelled by law to submit themselves to the discipline of the school whose teachers were given the legal right to subject them to corporal punishment. This was a conspicuous example of how, in the process of emerging, the child's body helped to define its status insofar as it could be legally assaulted by virtue of its age.
• Education was a decisive point in separating and segregating the child from adult society; the child's proper place in the school (middle-class children had long been kept separate from adults through nurseries, nannies and boarding schools); the adult's proper place, the workplace and, for women, the home.

The role of schooling in the universalisation of childhood was one that subjected children to overtly political agendas which have nothing to do with their welfare.

The 20th century has seen the reinforcement of childhood as a dependent state, with adults in control, though there is a growing lobby to improve the civil rights of children, which may

Activity 4.2

Can you think of any ways in which children's rights and status have been improved during this century?

go some way towards destroying this notion of dependency.

As pointed out by Halsey (1993), 'The quality of childhood is highly varied because although the twentieth century is the single "century of the child" it is still more the century of the individual which also means a flight from parenthood'.

THE CHANGING ROLE OF WOMEN

This century has seen a dramatic rise in the level of participation of married women in the labour market. At the time of the 1931 census, 10% of married women were employed; by 1987 the proportion had risen to 60%. Virtually all of this increase was in part-time employment.

Currently the position seems to be that each successive group of new mothers returns to the labour market more quickly than the one before. The numbers of children, but more particularly the age of the youngest child, tend to be the constraints. Yet 46% of mothers with children aged 3–4 years are working (35% part time, 11% full time) as are 30% of mothers with children aged 0–2 years (19% part time, 11% full time).

Employment patterns of mothers are still substantially different from those of fathers. Nevertheless, increasingly in recent years—and it may be more so in the late 1990s—the employment patterns of women have become more like those of men. However, many mothers with dependent children are still likely to be working part time, either through choice or because of the lack of adequate child care provision.

These trends have led to a rise in the number of 'dual worker' families; both partners are now working in over half of families (52% of married couples with children). For couples with one child the figure is 53%, falling to 41% for couples with three children. Where the youngest child is under 5, about one-third (33%) of partners are both working. Married mothers are more likely than lone mothers to be in employment; 52% of married women with children of all ages were working in 1984/86 compared with 42% of lone mothers. Again, the age of the children is important; lone mothers with children under 5 were less likely to be working than other mothers—18% were working (9% part time and 9% full time). Lone mothers with older children worked in 53% of cases (31% part time and 22% full time) (Wicks 1990).

SERVICES AVAILABLE TO CHILDREN

In the first part of the chapter the great changes that have taken place in the family and family relationships have been discussed. In this part of the chapter the three main services available to children, health, education, and social services, will be described and the social policy framework within which they have evolved will be discussed. However, it is important to appreciate that there has always been an historical reluctance in British society to become involved in what is seen as being the 'private' sphere of the family, and there is a lack of common philosophy about what should be provided for children and by whom. Provision for the care of children has tended to respond to political and economic factors rather than to be developed within a comprehensive framework (Pugh 1988).

However, the Audit Commission in their report *Seen but not heard*, published in 1994, found that children's services still often fail to help those in need. It criticised the providers of community health services and social services for their poor focus, with much of the £2 billion the services cost wasted on families the commission considered did not need support. Education authorities were criticised also, for allowing up to 40% of children in residential care not to attend school. The Audit Commission recommended that the Government should impose a statutory obligation on social service departments, and that health and education

authorities publish joint strategic plans to help children in need.

They recommend investment in the creation of family centres which would provide a range of services for children and families in need. These services would be offered by statutory services and voluntary groups working in partnership. Costs for new initiatives could be found in part by moving spending away from residential care. The Audit Commission also recommended that local authorities move funding away from child abuse work, and requested that the Government clarify guidance on risk management of child abuse.

Increasingly, however, government policy has emphasised the responsibilities of families to care for their dependants, although the number of children living within traditional family structures has declined. There has been a shift away from services provided by the State and stress placed on the rights of individuals to find suitable provision within the free market and voluntary sectors. However, because of the increasing vulnerability and fragility of the traditional family, the number of families living on state benefits has continued to rise, which has placed additional pressures on the services that are provided for children.

The National Health Service

Nursing services for children are discussed in greater detail in Chapter 5, but the social policy framework within which child health policy has developed will be outlined here and an overview given of the services available for children in the National Health Service.

Primary health services

The National Health Service (NHS) is the most universally used service by children and adolescents. The principle underlying the NHS, created by the NHS Act 1948, is that health services should be free at the point of delivery. All children and their families are entitled to be registered with a general practitioner, who provides medical care at his or her practice premises or at the patients' homes, and has responsibility for referral to hospital-based consultants for more specialist care. In England and Wales, it is a legal requirement under the Births and Deaths Registration Act 1874 to register a birth before the child is 6 weeks old. At this time, a child's parents are given a card to enable the child to be registered under the care of a general practitioner. Newborn babies are discharged from the care of midwives to a health visitor who is a registered nurse with a post-registration quali-fication in health visiting. Health visitors now work predominantly in primary health care teams with general practitioners, district nurses, practice nurses and school nurses. It is envisaged in the report *New World, New Opportunities* (NHSME 1993) that all health visitors should be general practice based, but there is also a need for health visitors to have a locality, or neighbourhood, as not all children are registered with general practitioners, e.g. homeless families, highly mobile families, and these are often children who may be most at risk (see Ch. 28).

The health visitor's role with children is essentially one based on disease prevention and health education. She is responsible, with the child's parents and other members of the primary health care team, for ensuring that a child's development is carefully monitored and, if there are any concerns about a child's well-being and development, that these are referred for appropriate help. She normally continues to maintain her role with the family until the child enters full-time education. The greater involve-ment of primary health care teams in the health surveillance of all children was recommended in a comprehensive report on child health services published in 1976 under the chairmanship of Professor Donald Court (DHSS 1976) after a 3-year review of the provision made for health services for children. The enquiry was initiated because of a growing recognition that children have specific needs and that a healthy childhood is vitally important in ensuring optimum health in adult life. The Court Report recommended that there should be a more integrated child

health service based on the integration of acute and preventive health services linked with supporting hospital and consultant care. It recommended that the ability of parents to bring up their children in the best possible way should be reinforced. The service should provide acces-sible skilled help to all children and be oriented towards prevention. There should be extra paediatric training for general practitioners, and health visitors should be involved in curative as well as preventive work with children. All chil-dren should be offered a programme of health surveillance, which the Court Committee envis-aged would take place within primary care. Specialist district handicap teams should be set up, based in district hospitals, which would provide assessment and help to children who were chronically sick or had handicaps, and give advice and support to parents.

Although the Court Report was not debated in the House of Commons, the Government accepted its overall philosophy, but made only three recommendations:

- Child development teams were to be set up.
- A children's committee was to be established to advise the Government on the coordination and development of health and social services in relation to children and their families.
- Hospital-based paediatric services were to be extended into the community (Rogers 1984).

Since the Court Report, there has been a growth in multidisciplinary child development teams, community paediatrics as a discipline has developed steadily and general practitioners are much more involved in preventive aspects of care (Kurtz & Tomlinson 1991).

Hospital services

The Platt Report (MoH 1959) laid the foundations for child- and adolescent-centred hospital services. The special committee under the chairmanship of Sir Harry Platt had been appointed in 1956 by the Central Health Services Council following pressure from a wide range of professional and voluntary organisations. They were requested to make a special study of the arrangements in hospitals for the welfare of ill children. In their report, they stated that the guiding principle for the care of children in hospitals was that they should be subjected to the least possible disturbance of the routines to which they were formerly accustomed (Rogers 1984).

They made 55 important recommendations for change. These included:

- Children should not be admitted to hospital if it can possibly be avoided.
- Children and adolescents should not be nursed on adult wards.
- A children's physician should have a general concern for the care of all children in hospital.
- Mothers should be admitted with their children, especially if the child is under 5 and during the first few days in hospital.
- Children must be visited frequently to preserve the continuity of their lives.
- Parents should be allowed to visit whenever they can and to help as much as possible with the care of the child.
- The training of doctors and nurses should include a greater understanding of the emotional and social needs of children and their families (Belson 1993, p. 197).

The Ministry of Health accepted the Platt Committee's recommendations, particularly those calling for an end to nursing children on adult wards, and the unrestricted visiting of children in hospital. However, Rogers (1984) maintains that progress to implement the changes would have been much slower without the involvement of the National Association for the Welfare of Children in Hospital. This pressure group, now called Action for Sick Children, was formed in 1961 to ensure that the Platt Report's recommendations were implemented and to give advice and support to parents about becoming more involved in their children's care in hospital. Professionals also joined the group, and Action for Sick Children has given credit to the work of sick children's nurses for the

improvement of care given to sick children in hospitals (Belson 1993).

The Court Report, *Fit for the Future* (DHSS 1976), re-affirmed the principles of the Platt Report, that all children should be nursed in children's wards and cared for by nurses with specialist knowledge of their needs. However, the Court Report commented that 17 years after the Platt Report children's wards were still often staffed without the benefit of trained children's nurses and there was patchy provision of such nurses in charge of children's outpatient departments. As previously stated, they recommended that hospital care should be centralised in district general hospitals and consultant paediatrician and hospital-based specialists should provide an accessible service to all children and continuing support for the primary health care teams in their district (see Ch. 21).

Although, since the publication of the Platt Report in 1959, there has been a steady improvement in the care of sick children in hospitals, the lengths of children's stays in hospital are shorter and more paediatric home care teams are available, the standard of care and staffing remains variable. In their 1992 survey of hospital services for children, the Audit Commission (1993) found that there was still a lack of provision of accommodation for parents. Although the Audit Commission found that registered sick children's nurses were present on wards, many wards during the day were staffed with only one RSCN and at night the situation was even worse. The needs of adolescents for separate provision were frequently still not met and there was a lack of specialised paediatric medical and nursing care in accident and emergency departments in district general hospitals.

Action for Sick Children has now embarked on a campaign to ensure that their quality standards and Department of Health guidelines will be used by all health authorities in developing contract specifications for children's services. They continue to give credit for the improvement in services for sick children to sick children's nurses, whether they work on children's wards or are involved in management or education (Belson 1993).

Child care

Britain has a low level of publicly funded child care, compared to most other countries in the European Union. This can be partly explained by a deeply held belief that full-time motherhood in a child's early years is in the best interests of the child and also by a reluctance of government to become too involved in the private sphere of the family. However, in the Second World War, when women with young children were needed to work in order to help the war effort, the number of local authority day nurseries expanded rapidly. At the end of the war, the number of day nurseries was drastically reduced and it was expected that women with children would revert to the status of 'full-time mothers'. An example of this expectation can be seen in the special provisions made for married women in the National Insurance Act 1946.

Because of the great changes that have taken place in British society and in families, which have been discussed earlier in the chapter, many more women with young children are working than was envisaged in post-war Britain. Pressure for child care has grown steadily and, although the number of places has increased, demand outstrips supply. The biggest growth has been in the private sector as government policy has been to promote this sector in preference to local authority provision. Between 1966 and 1991 the number of places in day nurseries, playgroups and with registered child minders grew from 128 000 to 899 000; this rise was primarily due to the growth of playgroups in the voluntary sector. The number of children attending nursery schools has also risen; in 1966 only 15% of children aged 3 and 4 years attended pre-school facilities, whereas in 1991 over half of all children under 5 years went to nursery school (CSO 1993). However, national statistics do not reveal the differences between education authorities and they do not indicate whether children are attending nursery school full time or part time. Mothers requiring full-time care for their children, in order to work, face many problems, and pressure groups like Working for Child Care

have lobbied for improvements to the poor provision of good quality care available. Day nursery places, for example, are available to fewer than 2% of children under 5, whereas the proportion of mothers with children under 5 who are working full time is 11% (Utting 1991).

Recently the Government has responded to pressure for better child care provision, which on average costs working mothers a quarter of their salary. The Government also wants to encourage parents who are reliant on state benefits to obtain work, as the number of lone-parent families dependent on state benefits has risen. In the 1990 Budget, tax concessions were introduced for workplace nurseries, but there are still only a small number of these. This is partly due to the recession and also because employers would like further tax concessions, comparable to those offered in some other European countries (Garrett 1993). The Child Support Act 1991 also encourages mothers to work, as, for example, the maintenance element has been disregarded on some means-tested benefits (Edwards 1993).

In October 1994, the Child Care Allowance was introduced. The purpose behind this is to help low-paid families continue to work and also to encourage parents who are not working to obtain work. Child care costs of £40 per week are offset against earnings for children under 11 years. Parents eligible for the benefit are those who claim family credit, disability working allowance, housing benefit or council tax benefit; lone parents must be working 16 hours a week, and married couples must both be working full time. However, there is no extra allowance for additional children and the average costs for full-time child care range from £60–70 per child (Lakhani 1994).

It would appear that although there have been some developments to assist with child care costs, there is not the same commitment by government policy for child care provision to be extended to match that provided in other countries in the European Union. In Denmark, for example, 44% of children attend nurseries and full-time day care centres from birth until they are 2 years old. Between the ages of 3 and 6 years,

87% go to kindergarten and pre-school centres (Griffin & Young 1993). In the United Kingdom the emphasis, as has been indicated, is on the growth of private and voluntary provision.

Social services

Local authorities are responsible for the provision of personal social services to children and their families. Social service departments are involved in a wide range of responsibilities and the provision of services to a number of vulnerable groups, including not only children but other care groups such as the elderly and people with disabilities. Their work may involve advising about benefits, welfare rights, group work, community work or intensive case work. The principles behind these services are not only to give help and support, but also to help clients gain insight into their problems. Their areas of responsibility have grown rapidly but Hill (1988) maintains that this growth is perceived with some anxiety by society since most of the activities of social services departments were formerly carried out within the family or community. As discussed earlier in the chapter, concerns about the welfare of children and their families reflect societal values and divisions about how much the State should intervene in the private sphere of the family. However, children are seen by society to be a priority group because of their vulnerability and their need for care and protection. It is recognised that families play a vital role in the nurture and socialisation of children, and care of families who need support is regarded as vital in trying to reduce the long-term problems that may be caused by family breakdown, which has increased in frequency.

Social services departments work within tight budgetary limits imposed by the Government and help can only be concentrated on those who suffer the most disadvantages. Legislation regarding the care of children is provided by the Children Act 1989, which was implemented in 1991 and reflects some of the changes which have occurred in society's attitudes to children, the changing nature of the family and concern about the need to provide a more unified body of legislation. The Children Act was enacted, therefore, to provide a single and consistent statement on the care, upbringing, and protection of children, based on the belief that children are generally best looked after within the family, with both parents playing a full part.

The Act uses the phrase 'parental responsibility' to define the duties, rights and authority which parents have in respect of their child. Reflecting the changes in family structure, unmarried fathers have easier rights to parental responsibility. The welfare of children is seen to be the paramount consideration when reaching any decision about their upbringing, and children's wishes must be taken into account. Local authorities, under the Children Act, are given a new duty to promote the upbringing of children in need by their families and to give support to their families. This should reduce the need for children to be in care or to be brought before the courts. It is also the duty of the local authority to return children they have looked after to their families, unless it is against those children's interests. When local authorities are looking after children, they must ensure that these children have contact with their parents (DoH 1989).

Packman (1993) considers that, although 'partnership' was not a term used in the Act, it is a concept which encapsulates the spirit of the legislation. The responsibilities of the family and the State are seen as complementary and not confrontational. Moreover, within the legislation there is a move towards preventive and support services and away from a reactive stance to a more proactive stance.

Educational services

Compulsory full-time education commences at the age of 5 years for children in Great Britain and at the age of 4 years in Northern Ireland. The provision of compulsory, free elementary education was introduced after a series of Education Acts in 1870, 1880 and 1891. However, it was not until the Education Act 1944 that universal free secondary education became available to all pupils in the state system. The school leaving age was raised to 16 years in 1972/73. The age at which full-time education starts in the United Kingdom is younger in comparison with other western countries, where the more usual age is 6 years. A strong private sector is also a feature of the British education system; in 1991 an average of 7% of all pupils attended private (independent) schools. This percentage is greater than in 1976, for example, when it was an average of 5%. The percentage also increases with the age of pupils, and in 1991 20% of boys and 15% of girls aged 16 and over were in independent schools (Central Statistical Office 1993).

Primary education is usually provided in infant schools for children aged between 5 and 7 years and junior schools for pupils between the ages of 7 and 11 years, although in Scotland primary education is provided for 7 years in a single primary school. Primary schools are normally quite small; the majority cater for around 100–200 children from the surrounding area. However, competition for the 'popular schools' can be very intense and parents then have to be highly motivated and have knowledge of how the education system operates to obtain their first choice of school. There can be a wide disparity between the best primary and other schools.

This disparity was highlighted in the Plowden Report (Central Advisory Council for Education 1967), which made a detailed analysis of the situation that existed then and important recommendations for raising the level of the 'poor schools' to those of the best. Their analysis had revealed that children from poor homes in socially deprived areas were more often attending primary schools with poor resources, large classes and a high staff turnover. The Plowden Report recommended a national policy of 'positive discrimination' and some efforts were made to implement the recommendations by creating educational priority area schools which received extra funding (Brown & Payne 1990). However, education cannot by itself overcome deep-seated inequalities between children in different areas and between different social classes.

Secondary education is provided for children between the ages of 11 and 19 years and has been the subject of much political debate and controversy and parental dissatisfaction. Following the 1944 Education Act, a tripartite system was developed based on grammar, technical and secondary modern schools. Following an examination at 11 years, children were selected for grammar or technical schools and the remainder went to secondary modern schools, where they often received an inferior education. Gradually, doubts arose and evidence became available of the unfairness of the selection process and the psychological damage to children who were not successful. The system also failed to make good sense of the talents of young people. In the 1960s, arguments in favour of comprehensive schooling prevailed and by 1991 over 90% of pupils of secondary school age were educated in comprehensive schools (Central Statistical Office 1993). However, the arguments in favour of selection still have much support, especially within the Conservative Party.

There have been major changes in England in the provision of state education in the primary and secondary sectors following the Education Reform Act 1988. This act introduced and advocated the local management of schools—each school now has control of its own budget and the school governors decide how the budget is spent. The local education authority is responsible for the allocation of money to schools within its area and provides services such as the inspectorate of schools, provision for the assessment of children with special educational needs and training for school governors. The school governing body now has responsibility for the pay of teachers, within agreed scales, and discipline and health and safety.

The Education Act 1988 had already changed the composition of school governing bodies, as part of the Government's strategy to give parents and the local community more say in how their schools were run and thus devolve power from local education authorities. Also, under the

Education Reform Act 1988, schools could apply for grant-maintained status and receive grants directly from the Department of Education. The governing body would then be responsible for overall control of the school. A ballot of parents has to be taken first. In May 1994, 1504 ballots had been conducted and 75.2% were in favour of grant-maintained status; 590 primary schools and 914 secondary schools had participated. Grant-maintained schools are now run by the Funding Agency for Schools (FAS) and, where more than 75% of secondary schools have opted out of local education authority control, the FAS has assumed responsibility for all the schools in the local authority area. Some grant-maintained schools have obtained permission to select pupils according to their academic ability (Kingston 1994).

The 1988 Education Reform Act also introduced the National Curriculum for all schools and a set of core and foundation subjects which all schools in England, Northern Ireland and Wales must teach. The core subjects are mathematics, English, and science, and the foundation subjects are history, geography, technology, music, art, physical education and a modern foreign language. Since 1989, pupils have to be tested at the ages of 7, 11, 14 and 16 by national tests.

Education for children with special needs

Education for children with special needs covers a wide spectrum of needs, including those of highly gifted children and children with dyslexia, language problems, or hearing and visual impairment. It is vitally important that children's needs are individually assessed and met if each child is to achieve his or her full potential. The framework for the education of children with special needs was radically changed following the publication of the Warnock Report in 1978 (DES 1978). The report was produced following the first committee of enquiry to review the educational provision for all handicapped children in Great Britain under the chairmanship of Mary Warnock. Although the Education (Handicapped Children) Act 1970

had ensured that all handicapped children received an education, however severe their problems, this had usually been based on the medical 'category' of their physical or mental handicap, rather than on their educational needs. The Warnock Report, however, recommended that children should no longer be viewed in terms of two distinct groups, i.e. handicapped or non-handicapped, but in terms of their individual educational needs. Special education should be seen as part of the continuum of educational provision available (Rogers 1984).

The Warnock Report recommended, as the Court Report 1976 had also proposed, that there should be a programme of health surveillance for all children and that children who might in the future have special educational needs should be identified as early as possible, so that extra help could be offered to them before compulsory education began at 5 years. It was recommended that a named person, usually the health visitor, should be available to give support and help to parents, the district handicap team should assess the child's progress and the local education authorities should be notified, in advance, of children who might need special education. When a child started school, the named person should normally become the head teacher and the child's progress should be reviewed every year.

A statement should be drawn up by a multi-professional team which would profile the child's needs, the recommendations for special help and how these are to be met. Parents should be fully involved as partners but they also would be able to appeal against the Local Education Authority's decision that their child was in need of special education and also against a decision that their child was not. Education should take place as much as possible in mainstream schools. The Warnock Committee estimated that there would be about 2% of children who would require statements of special need, and about 18% of children would be likely to be in need of special educational provision at some time in their school life.

Most of the recommendations of the Warnock Report were incorporated into the 1981 Education

Act, which came into effect in England and Wales in April 1983. However, local education authorities were not given the necessary resources to fund the Act. Since the Act was implemented, delays have appeared in the system and many parents have become dissatisfied with the way the Act was being implemented. Moreover, although it was envisaged that only 2% of children would need statements, some parents have found that the only way that their child can receive special education provision is to request a statement. The Audit Commission in *Getting in on the Act* (1992) criticised the special education available. The 1993 Education Act seeks to streamline the process and to make it faster and easier for children to have statements. A code of practice on special educational needs came into effect in September 1994. Parental choice and specialist support for children and teachers are central themes of the code of practice.

It was envisaged that the number of those with severe problems would gradually fall, but more children are surviving because of advances in medicine and technology. Latest figures reveal that 2.5% of children have had statements. In 1993, 179 132 school-age children in England received statements, which was 37 500 more than predicted. However, local authorities are identifying children's needs earlier. Integration of children into ordinary schools has also grown and 28 local authorities now have less than 1% of their pupils in special schools. The highest percentages of children in special schools, over 3%, are to be found in Wandsworth and Lambeth, two London boroughs. It was estimated that the cost of special educational provision would rise to £320 million in 1995 and local education authorities are concerned about these increasing costs, and greater expectations from parents and schools (MacLeod 1994; see also Ch. 21).

The Warnock Report did not consider the needs of children who are gifted; however, the 1980 Education Act made provision for means-tested assisted places in independent schools for clever children. The number of places available has been expanded recently from 235 000 to 350 000. City technology colleges have also been set up in inner city areas; these colleges operate independently of local education authorities and will also 'cream off' talented pupils from the state sector (Moran & Jones 1991).

School nurse service

The first school nurse services were established at the end of the last century and grew rapidly when, in 1907, local education authorities had to provide medical examinations for children in elementary schools. They were also obliged to make arrangements for medical treatment. There was much evidence at the beginning of the century that young people were in poor health. The examination of recruits for the Boer War had revealed that 40–60% of young men were too medically unfit to join the army (Owen 1968). Therefore, in the early days of the school nurse service, school nurses were principally involved in the treatment of physical handicaps resulting from malnutrition and infections, in order that school children could benefit from their education.

Today, the primary role of school nurses is still to assist school children to fulfil their educational potential and to derive maximum benefit from their school education. However, the way they carry out their role has changed, because of the changing nature of children's needs and health care. They are responsible for health surveillance and immunisation of the children within their schools, and for the early detection of health and psychological problems and for appropriate help and referral. Their work has become much more complex and they have an important role in child protection, health promotion, health education and achieving the 'Health of the Nation' targets (DoH 1992). They may also be attached to special schools and are much more involved with other members of the primary health care team.

However, the expansion of the school health service, recommended in the 1976 Court Report, has not taken place. The report advocated that there should be one school nurse per 2500 school-age population. Despite a rise in the school-age population, school nurse numbers have not increased; in 1992 there were 2440 school nurses compared with 2450 in 1988 (Cohen 1994), and there was a fall in the ratio of school nurses to pupils aged 5–14 years of 5.3% in 1991.

This part of the chapter has described the development of the three major services for children, but much more coordination is required between them to achieve a more effective child policy.

CONCLUSION

In this chapter the sociological perspectives on the family have been described and the rapid changes occurring within the family have been discussed. These changes have occurred so quickly that frequently the services required as a result of the changes have not been in place or have been slow to respond. It has been shown that the vulnerability of some children has increased and that the number of lone-parent families dependent on benefits has risen. However, the particular needs of children and their families received recognition in 1994 by the appointment of a Minister of the Family and, as a result, it is hoped that a more comprehensive policy for families will emerge.

REFERENCES

Aries P 1962 Translated by Baldwick R 1973 Centuries of childhood. Penguin, London

Audit Commission 1992 Getting in on the Act. HMSO, London

Audit Commission 1993 Children first. HMSO, London

Audit Commission 1994 Seen but not heard. HMSO, London

Belson P 1993 Children in hospital. Children and Society 7(2): 196–210

Bradshaw J 1989 Lone parents: policy in the doldrums. Occasional Paper No. 9, Family Policy Studies Unit, London

Brown M, Payne S 1990 Introduction to social administration in Britain. Unwin Hyman, London

Central Advisory Council for Education (England) 1967 Children and their primary schools: the Plowden report. HMSO, London

Central Statistical Office 1993 Social trends 23. HMSO, London

Child Support Act 1991 HMSO, London

Children Act 1989 HMSO, London

Cohen P 1994 Immunisation campaign spotlights school nurses. Health Visitor 67(9): 285

Department of Education and Science (DES) 1978 Special educational needs: the Warnock Report. HMSO, London

Department of Health (DoH) 1989 An introduction to the Children Act. HMSO, London

Department of Health (DoH) 1992 The health of the nation: a strategy for health in England. Cm 1986. HMSO, London

Department of Health and Social Security (DHSS) 1976 Fit for the future: report of the Committee on Child Health Services. (Court Report) HMSO, London

Education (Handicapped Children) Act 1970 HMSO, London

Education Act 1944 HMSO, London

Education Act 1980 HMSO, London

Education Act 1981 HMSO, London

Education Act 1988 HMSO, London

Education Act 1993 HMSO, London

Education Reform Act 1988 HMSO, London

Edwards R 1993 Give children a break. The Observer 8 Aug: 18–19

Garrett A 1993 Give child care a break. The Observer 8 Aug: 23

Griffin, Young 1993 Mum's the word for confusion. The Guardian 22 Oct: 18–19

Hale R, Loveland M, Owen G The principles and practice of health visiting. Pergamon Press, Oxford

Halsey A H 1993 Changes in the family. Children and Society 7(2): 125–136

Hendrick H 1994 Child welfare: England 1872–1989. Routledge, London

Hill M 1988 Understanding social policy. Basil Blackwell, Oxford

Kingston P 1994 The ballot of Britain. Guardian Education 24 May: 2–3

Kurtz Z, Tomlinson J 1991 How do we value our children today, as reflected by children's health, health care and policy? Children and Society 5(3): 207–224

Lakhani B 1994 Child care allowance: an incentive to work? Health Visitor 67(9 Sept): 1994

Legal Aid Act 1949 HMSO, London

MacLeod D 1994 Family stress causing pupil problems. The Guardian 22 Sept: 9

Matrimony and Family Proceedings Act 1984 HMSO, London

Ministry of Health (MoH) 1959 The report of the Committee on the Welfare of Children in Hospital. (Platt Report) HMSO, London

Moran M, Jones B 1991 Economic policy. In: Jones B (ed) Politics UK. Wheatsheaf, Hemel Hempstead

Murdock G P 1949 Social structure. Macmillan, New York

National Health Service Management Executive (NHSME) 1993 New world, new opportunities. HMSO, London

National Insurance Act 1946 HMSO, London

NHS Act 1948 HMSO, London

Packman J 1993 From prevention to partnership: child welfare services across three decades. Children and Society 7(2): 183–195

Parsons T 1951 The social system. The Free Press, New York

Payne S 1991 Women, health and poverty. Wheatsheaf, London

Pugh G 1988 Services for under fives: developing a co-ordinated approach. National Children's Bureau, London

Randall P E 1989 Marital breakdown and young children. Midwife, Health Visitor and Community Nurse 25(9)

Rogers R 1984 Crowther to Warnock, 2nd edn. Heinemann Educational Books, London

Utting D 1991 Family policy bulletin March 1991. Family Policy Studies Centre, London

Wicks M 1990 The Family Policy Studies Centre. Joseph Rowntree Memorial Trust, York

FURTHER READING

Central Advisory Council for Education (England) 1967 Children and the primary schools: the Plowden Report. HMSO, London

Department of Health 1989 An introduction to the Children Act. HMSO, London

Hendrick H 1994 Child welfare: England 1872–1989. Routledge, London

MacLeod D 1994 Family stress causing pupil problems. The Guardian 22 Sept: 9

National Health Service Management Executive (NHSME) 1993 New world, new opportunities. HMSO, London

Pugh G 1988 Services for under fives: developing a co-ordinated approach. National Children's Bureau, London

Wicks M 1990 The Family Policy Studies Centre. Joseph Rowntree Memorial Trust, York

2

Nursing: fundamental principles

The children's nurse works with families to ensure that nursing care is adapted to meet the needs of the individual child, taking account of the family situation, the social context and the health needs. Nursing is influenced by legislation, by changes in provision of health care and by technological advances. Children's nurses need to be able to adapt their practice to take account of developments as they occur.

5

Development of paediatric nursing

Esther Parker

This chapter aims to:
- **examine some of the social changes which necessitated the specialised care of children**
- **describe some of the leading influences in the development of specialised children's nursing**
- **look at some of the most influential legislation concerned with children's nursing**
- **examine how the development of Project 2000 has affected the specialist children's nurse.**

It is the real test of a nurse whether she can nurse a sick infant.

Nightingale 1859

Paediatric nursing and the training of paediatric nurses have undergone many changes throughout their history. They have continued to adapt and develop to meet the needs of their various patients. These have varied as the pattern of childhood diseases has changed and the provision of health care altered. There are 15 million children and teenagers under 19 years old making up one-quarter of the population of the United Kingdom. Children under 15 years of age make up approximately one-fifth of the population of the United Kingdom and Europe. By contrast, this age group forms one-third of the world's population, while in some East African countries it rises to one-half (Woodroffe et al 1993). The incidence of chronic illness in children in the UK has more than doubled between 1972 and 1991, with one-fifth of all children aged 16–19 stating that they have a long-standing illness (OPCS 1991).

Paediatric nurses, therefore, have a large potential client group, many of whom, because of advances in care and medicine, are living longer, healthier lives. Major medical advances in treatment have extended life expectancy of those children with many now reaching adulthood.

Rather than solely considering the 'patient' in isolation, the aim of paediatric nursing is to promote and provide family-centred care, recognising and respecting the needs of the child within the context of the whole family and adjusting care accordingly. The skills and knowledge of paediatric nurses sometimes appear to be undervalued, especially by those who are not directly involved with child care provision. The qualification has at times been seen as an optional extra instead of a necessary requirement for those nursing children. This has been despite many government reports that have said that children should be cared for by a nurse who is qualified to care for children (MoH 1959, DoH 1991, Audit Commission 1993). Changes in attitude have occurred since the Clothier Report (DoH 1994), which emphasised how important it is for children to be nursed by children's trained nurses. The report additionally upheld the requirement for a minimum of two such nurses to be on duty per shift, per 24 hours, on each children's ward (Audit Commission 1993).

HISTORICAL PERSPECTIVE

Throughout the ages children have always been cared for by their elders. This could have been a member of the family, the extended family, a nanny or hired nurse or, when they were very young, a 'wet' nurse (Burr 1989, Saunders 1982). Many babies died during birth, and if they survived, childhood was hard. Mortality during infancy and childhood was high due to the exposure to numerous diseases, insufficient nourishment and general poor living conditions. Until the turn of the last century women had many children in the hope that some would survive to adulthood. This was to provide an heir or an additional pair of hands to support the family. Queen Anne produced 17 children for

instance, only one of whom survived infancy. Children were frequently treated as miniature adults or drudges; they were often vital to the family and its survival, as breadwinners or as minders for younger siblings.

There was little medical treatment. What there was often consisted of purging and bleeding with leeches. This tended to have the effect of killing rather than curing. Some religious orders did provide medical, herbal or nursing care for those who required it. Institutions and hospitals gradually evolved, but these mainly treated adults. Care was given by anyone who could be employed; previous patients or people from the domestic servant class. Sisters and matrons came from higher classes. They might have been widows whose circumstances were reduced, or people who had 'lived in a respectable rank of life' (Abel-Smith 1960).

The first facility that offered any relief for sick children was a dispensary opened by Dr Armstrong in 1769. He had produced the only English-language book of the time that dealt with diseases of children. His clinics gave advice and medicine to children 'of the industrious poor' up to the age of 10 or 12. These children were treated only as outpatients. He argued that it would not be convenient for the mothers, that mothers and nurses would not agree with each other, and 'if you take a sick child away from the parents, you break its heart immediately' (Miles 1986). More dispensaries opened in London and the provinces but they were not used as teaching and training establishments nor did they provide any nursing care.

Almost half of the people who died annually in London in the 1840s were children under 10. In 1843, there were 2363 patients in London hospitals. Only 26 of them were children under 10 (Saunders 1982).

At around this time, Dr Charles West, another London physician, had been running a clinic at Red Lion Square. His experiences taught him that outpatient treatments were not adequate to cope with the problems of children. General uncleanliness, malnutrition and poverty increased the dangers of infection to the child, the family and the immediate neighbourhood. The parents worked all day, while older children, often only 7 or 8 years old, were nursing the ill child. He felt these considerations should outweigh the psychological traumas of separation.

Training for children's nurses

Whilst working in the clinic, Dr West had made copious notes. These he put together to publish a book on the diseases of children. It was the sale of this book that helped him raise the finance required for the Hospital for Sick Children, Great Ormond Street, which opened on 14 February 1852. One of his aims for the new hospital was for it to be 'employed as a school for the education and training of women in the special duties of children's nursing'. By achieving this aim, he provided the beginning of the education and training for sick children's nurses (Miles 1986).

Several other specialist children's hospitals opened in London and major cities across the United Kingdom during the next decade. These were voluntary hospitals, relying on public subscriptions raised by campaigns frequently initiated by local physicians and surgeons.

Nursing must have been very demanding in those early days. Children were admitted to the care of the nursing and medical staff on arrival at hospital with little or no parental involvement. Off-duty time for nurses was limited to 2 hours daily, with 1½ days off per month. Annual leave was 3 weeks per year. Pay in children's hospitals was not as high as that in general hospitals, but nurses could commence training at the age of 21 instead of 23 or 24. Lectures were given by the medical staff, who were also consulted about all new nursing staff appointments. Meanwhile, demonstrations of bandaging and other such practical skills were given by the sisters. Perhaps surprisingly, considering the times, the sisters' role also included instructing new doctors and house officers. In 1897 a nurse probationer noted: 'there were some stray lectures given, some rather antiquated medical books and a dummy upon which to practice bandaging. The taking of temperatures, pulse and ordinary tests

for urine being strictly the work of medical students' (Seymour 1961). The matron's role was administrative. She was not necessarily a nurse, neither was she involved in supervising nurses or nursing duties (Abel-Smith 1960).

Miss Catherine Wood

In 1888, Miss Wood, the Lady Superintendent of Nurses at the Great Ormond Street Hospital, wrote the words that must set the yardstick for children's nursing: '... that sick children's nurses require special training.'

She advocated many ideas, some of which may be seen as recent or present-day innovations. They were open visiting, the importance of careful and accurate observations, patient allocation and the necessity of play and learning for the children. Patients, she wrote, should be allocated to a nurse, who was then responsible for the entire care. The nurse should accompany the sister and the doctor in order to give information on the child's state and progress. Catherine Wood felt that children would not get better as quickly if they had frequent changes of nurses. One nurse would get to know the child's individual likes and dislikes. In order for the nurse to be able to care for her charges properly, the ward would have to be organised in such a way as to facilitate this (Wood 1888).

Could this have been the earliest documentation of primary nursing?

In the same article she wrote:

The same regularity and order cannot be maintained among the children as among the adults. Order and discipline there must be, or the children will not be happy; but the ward that is tidied up to perfection, in which the little ones look like well drilled soldiers, when the lack of liberty is absent, and nothing is out of place, is hardly suggestive of the happy heart of a child. Toys and games share as much a part of the treatment as physic, and the ceaseless chatter and careless distribution of the toys are surely consistent with a well-ordered children's ward.

Wood 1888

Despite her support for open visiting, children admitted to hospital continued to be

Activity 5.1

It was only relatively recently that open visiting and resident parents became the norm.

Speak to somebody who was admitted to hospital as a child when it was not possible for parents to stay:

1. What are the strongest memories?
2. Has it affected their feelings about hospitals now?
3. Would they have preferred to have one of their parents with them?
4. Were there any 'substitute mothers' available on the ward?
5. Did it seem right or wrong not to have a parent with them?

completely 'surrendered' to the care of the medical and nursing staff. Visiting generally consisted of 2–3 hours twice a week. It was even more limited for children who were admitted with an infectious condition or disease, when the isolated child was cared for by white-gowned nurses. Parents were only permitted a short visit if the child's name was on the danger list.

Mrs Ethel Fenwick

The general public, at this time, would have had difficulty in judging the professional competence of any nurse. Training for nurses was very variable in amount and standard. Towards the end of the 1800s there were moves to establish some form of professional register. Nurses who discredited the profession could then be removed from it. Many nurses wanted a register that recorded only those who were fit to practice. They also pressed for some form of central body to be set up, with general examinations which would act as a recognisable standard. Ethel Mason had started nursing at the Children's Hospital in Nottingham. She subsequently went on to become Matron at St Bartholomew's Hospital before marrying Dr Bedford Fenwick in 1887. Her time then became devoted to organising the nursing profession. She did much to encourage recruitment from higher social classes, partly by encouraging educational and financial requirements in order to enter

training. With her husband, she worked to promote nurses' registration, advocating a 3-year initial training.

They were involved in establishing the British Nurses' Association and the International Council of Nurses (ICN). Speaking at the Congress of the ICN in 1901, she made a call for university facilities for nurses (Seymour 1961), something that has only recently become a reality for many nurses.

Legislation for nurse registration

It was not until 1919 that the Nurses' Registration Act finally achieved royal assent and become law. The Act required a register to be set up consisting of a general part for nurses who satisfied the conditions for that part, and four supplementary parts. These were for registered male nurses, those caring for patients with mental diseases, sick children's nurses and a part for 'others' (Burnard & Chapman 1990). Sick children's nursing was included after much lobbying and a great deal of support by eminent paediatricians. The Register was opened in 1921 and the General Nursing Council (GNC) elected. Individual hospitals were recognised as training schools and could issue their own certificates on completion of a course (Checkland & Lamb 1982). An early effect of registration was that the lack of children's trained nurses was identified (Miles 1986).

Post-war changes

The two world wars affected nursing and nurse training. Many of the people who were given a basic introductory nursing course, followed by what was often extensive experience, felt that they should be able to register without undertaking further training. This resulted in a change in the law, allowing a roll to be established to record the status of assistant nurses. During the Second World War, a committee was established to examine the post-war nursing and educational needs. Their report, in 1947, advocated tackling wastage and giving full student status to student nurses; it called for training institutions rather than hospitals to provide education.

The report also recommended a training that had an 18-month common element followed by 18 months of specialist area activity, and adequate, appropriately trained teaching staff (Pyne 1982).

The need for specialist parts of the Register was reviewed as the committee felt they could be converted to post-registration qualifications registrable with the GNC. In the end, however, the committee recognised the specialist skills of the sick children's nurse and the mental nurse, and the independent registers were maintained (Miles 1986).

Effects of hospitalisation on children identified

It was around this time that Bowlby, for the World Health Organization, and Robertson, for the Tavistock Institute of Human Relationships, started their individual research studies. They both showed the damaging effects on children of separation from their mothers and families. These works were the catalyst for many of the changes that have occurred within the care of hospitalised children. As a direct result, the Platt Report (MoH 1959) was commissioned and its findings, together with a showing of Robertson's film on television, saw the beginnings of the National Association for the Welfare of Children in Hospital (NAWCH) in 1961. This organisation was later renamed Action for Sick Children.

Whilst some of the recommendations were slowly implemented, particularly open visiting for families and the availability of facilities for resident parents, both the Court Report (DHSS 1976) and more recent Audit Commission Report (1993) continued to identify the need for children to be admitted to hospital only when they could not be cared for at home and to be cared for by children's trained nurses within facilities dedicated to the care of children.

Paediatric community services

For those managers who had had the foresight and inspiration to set up paediatric community

services, this recommendation must have been uplifting. Rotherham, Yorkshire, set up a service in 1948, followed by Birmingham and Paddington, London, in 1954 (Gillet 1954, Semellie 1956, Lightwood 1956). By the 1970s, five schemes were in existence, growing to 28 general care schemes by the late 1980s.

The Court Report (DHSS 1976) recommended that community services should be expanded for all children, while existing services should work towards improved coordination. The Royal College of Nursing, in their directory of paediatric community services, recorded 74 general services throughout the country, with a further 58 specialist services (Whiting 1994). These included services such as those supporting children with cancers or cystic fibrosis and neonatal babies. As more conditions are treated and children survive longer, the children and their parents need more care and support. Children are being discharged from hospital whilst receiving on-going treatment and, therefore, require nursing care at home or in school settings. The role of the paediatric community nurse is becoming more diverse, and at the same time more specialised.

Updating and post-registration education is increasingly important for these nurses. It is still uncommon to find a post-registration course that addresses the needs of the child in the community and, as a consequence, nurses are often having to undertake a general district nursing course to progress in a career in community nursing.

Activity 5.2

Speak to the community paediatric nurses in your area:

1. What is their basic qualification—RSCN or RN (Part 15)?
2. Do they have post-registration qualifications?
3. Does having completed a Project 2000 course affect the need for post-registration qualification?
4. Should it?

General hospitals

Within the children's wards, student nurses became an important element of the workforce in many district general hospitals, while they gained experience of the welfare of children and the care of sick children (Glasper & Ireland 1988). This experience was identified as being one element required by the European Community in order for the general training to meet agreed requirements.

Rye (1982) highlighted a conflict between the patients' needs for the nursing care and the needs of the nurse in training, causing significant manpower problems. Student nurses, who were part of the workforce, had to gain experience in a limited number of children's wards. This raised issues regarding supervision of the students, due to the large numbers of them having to be placed in a limited number of children's wards. It meant that inexperienced and often young nurses, with a limited knowledge of children, were providing care for the sick child.

Towards the end of the 1950s, pressures on paediatric nurses increased with hospital managers demanding dual qualifications in order for paediatric nurses to be promoted. In response, combined courses were introduced. These enabled the qualifying nurse to achieve both RGN and RSCN in 4 years. In England, this led to the 3-year RSCN course being withdrawn in the early 1970s and the post-registration RSCN becoming more available.

CHANGES IN NURSE PREPARATION—PROJECT 2000 IMPLEMENTED

A review of the preparation and training of nurses led in 1989 to the commencement in England of the first Project 2000 diploma courses (UKCC 1986). This was a 3-year course that had an 18-month common foundation course, followed by a branch that was client specific. The branches available were, care of the Adult, care of the Mentally Ill, care of the Mentally Handicapped and care of the Child. A staged implementation of Project 2000 courses throughout the United Kingdom began. In England, colleges changed their pre-registration courses to the new format as funding became available.

Wales, Northern Ireland and Scotland introduced Project 2000 between 1991 and 1992, choosing to go for a single implementation phase in their respective countries.

At the same time as Project 2000 was commenced, there was a rationalisation of colleges of nursing, with many of them amalgamating to form more viable centres of education. This allowed them to offer a wider range of opportunities for both pre-and post-registration courses and clinical experience. As a result, more colleges were able to offer the Children's Branch. Project 2000 courses also forged closer links with higher education, being validated by the appropriate national board in conjunction with an institute of higher education (Robertson 1990). This meant that, on completion, the nurse gained both nurse registration and a higher education diploma. These courses also had a high emphasis on nursing in the community with the diplomates achieving a qualification which enabled them to nurse in the community or the hospital setting (UKCC 1986).

This was an important development as there was a greater shift to care taking place in the community. Children were being admitted less routinely and the period of hospitalisation was increasingly reduced. The use of day care and day surgery has been promoted and expanded so that children are not separated from their parents and families longer than necessary.

As the number of paediatric community teams increases, more treatments and monitoring of conditions are carried out within the home, decreasing the need for hospitalisation. There is also a greater emphasis on family involvement in care, with parents being taught to give long-term treatment at home to chronically ill children who would otherwise need to be admitted to hospital.

.3

Think a   pe of care that can be provided at
home b   ith the support of community nurses.
    Spe   families who are routinely involved in
the spe   sing care of their children at home:

1. Hov   el when the child has to be admitted?
2. Do   t they wish to 'give up' their responsi-
   biliti   rses?
3. Do   if they are expected to do so?
4. Do   full part in planning the inpatient care
   for   do they feel awkward about doing so?

Generic or specialist?

The format of pre-registration education is constantly being monitored and discussed to ensure that the courses continue to meet the needs of the students and their future clients. Changes that have taken place due to the introduction of Project 2000, diploma level education and the effects of implementing the findings of various government reports, have done much for the nursing of children. Practitioners have responded to the diploma students by looking to their own professional updating and striving to ensure that they are adequately prepared as mentor/assessors.

However, specialisation at a pre-registration level has meant that the Child Branch diplomate can not automatically achieve reciprocal registration in many overseas countries. This, together with a questioning of the possible role of the RN (Part 15) in units such as accident and emergency departments or intensive care units, has led to discussions regarding the equity among the various branches (Parker & Coulson 1995). The rationale of specialist training as opposed to a generic education followed by a future specialisation to a particular client group has been raised again, especially when comparisons are being made with nurse education in other countries (Boxall 1989, Campbell 1994/5, Powell 1995). No doubt this debate will continue whilst the evaluations of Project 2000 are collated and the career progression of its diplomates is monitored.

POST-REGISTRATION EDUCATION

With the implementation of PREP in April 1995 by the UKCC to ensure that all nurses undertake regular updating in practice and education, colleges have been reviewing their post-registration courses to ensure that they meet the needs of a diverse nursing profession. Nurses wishing to become specialists or advanced practitioners need to undertake studies to first degree or master's level in order to achieve registration within these categories. There are challenges and opportunities available for paediatric nurses, regardless of their work situation, and it will be up to the individual to use them within his/her own professional development.

Formal study days or courses are not the only way to achieve the requirements of PREP. Visits can be made to units so that services or facilities can be compared or evaluated, leading perhaps to a change or expansion of current services or an introduction of new ones. A study of a clinical condition or interest through a review of current literature may be undertaken. This could extend one's knowledge and allow an evaluation or comparison of current research and practice. Any of these activities are then recorded as part of the practitioner's professional portfolio.

Reflective practice

Reflective practice is something that is now being positively encouraged for all nurses. The professional development as a statutory requirement for re-registration (UKCC 1994) has been designed to allow each nurse time for professional updating. As part of this, the nurse must produce a portfolio which will provide a record of what activities she/he has undertaken. An essential element of the portfolio will be a summary of an event or learning activity together with an account of how that learning will affect or influence future practice.

Reflective practice, the ability to reflect on previous actions during their practice, is a concept that has been around for many years. Schon

(1983) explored the use of this technical and rational process as a way of learning and developing skills. He has since talked about it having a relationship with the development of expertise by the practitioner. The individuals, by reflecting on their performance, adjust and enhance their skills in order to progress from being the able practitioner to the competent one. By using reflective practice, nurses could move along the continuum identified by Benner (1984), from novice to expert. It should be a thoughtful and conscious process. Those who did not utilise it would be likely to nurse by rote, stuck in the ritual and routine of day-to-day practice.

Many nurses and students think that they regularly undertake reflective practice as they informally gather to mull over the day's events. They feel that they talk the situation through and rationalise their handling of the scenario. They may be reflecting on their practice, but they are not normally undertaking a rigorous, objective analysis of the situation and their feelings, and identifying alternative ways to handle a similar situation in the future.

It is possible to reflect as an individual, using a reflective journal and allowing time to go back over experiences. It is also useful to share experiences, in order to help each other to consider good and caring practice. Both Burnard (1991, 1993) and Darbyshire (1993) emphasise the importance of setting up such a group appropriately.

For effective reflection, sufficient time must be allowed. The group must be structured with a clear idea of why they are meeting. The number in the group is important; Burnard (1993) advocates about 10 as being the optimum. In practice this may be difficult, as in the ward situation, for instance, there would rarely be 10 members of staff available at one time. Perhaps a senior member of staff could be used to take the reflective thoughts from one group to another to initiate a discussion if that were thought appropriate. This may be particularly useful in the case of unusual occurrences which several members of staff wish to discuss—perhaps a child with an eating disorder or one who has recently been diagnosed as having a terminal illness.

The group must provide a safe and non-judgemental setting in order to allow all the individuals to participate. How the group is then conducted is up to the individuals and the facilitator. The facilitator may be nominated on a sessional basis or may be someone from outside the work area. It does not need to be the most senior member of staff who is chosen, but perhaps one who has experience of the situation under discussion. He/she has an important role to play, by not allowing the group to degenerate into a dirty washing or moaning session. The facilitator should declare at the outset the expected length of the meeting and set, or ask for, some objectives of the session. He/she should ensure that all staff have an equal opportunity to contribute, and allow this to happen.

The structure of the group meetings may vary—perhaps members would each like to identify one episode of care that they feel they carried out well, which they can relate to the group. Alternatively the group may wish to explore just one or two situations in depth. It is important that if this format is followed all members of the group have the opportunity to contribute, and also present situations to future meetings.

There are a number of stages which make up the reflective process and these are shown in Figure 5.1.

Stage 1: Experiencing

The particular event is focused on and described, giving as much relevant detail as possible in order to set the scene. In early experiences of sharing, positive episodes of care should be identified. As the group becomes more comfortable and supportive, difficult or awkward situations may well be discussed.

Stage 2: Reflection

After the scene setting, the raconteur reflects on the situation giving more detail, including evidence to support what is being said. This may be observations of feelings, thoughts, experiences and physical signs such as sweaty palms

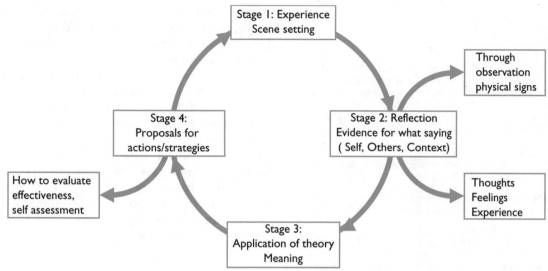

Figure 5.1 The reflective cycle.

or shaky hands. Information should include all those present and involved in the experience, including self and others, and be put into the context of the situation. Finally, all the elements are drawn together. The reflective group may help during this phase by asking questions to clarify or help explore further. The facilitator must ensure that the main focus of the scenario is maintained.

Stage 3: Application of theory

The third stage is the application of knowledge, theory and relevant practice. This gives sense or meaning to the situation. It should draw on the whole group's experiences and knowledge, with everyone contributing.

Stage 4: Proposals and strategies

The final stage looks at future practice and decides how to handle or anticipate similar situations. It may be that new policies, procedures or standards need to be developed as a result of the reflection. An evaluation strategy, formal or informal, must be included to ensure that the action taken is effective or show whether there is a need for further refinement or flexibility.

When a written account is needed as part of a journal or as a written assessment, then further elements should be included. Firstly, an overall review of the reflective process; whether, for example, it was difficult or easy, or whether there were any blind spots or blanks—this is the self-assessment part of the process and, secondly, a reference list which details the literature drawn upon during the analysis.

The situation considered in Activity 5.4 may be a seemingly simple one which we encounter many times in a day. Through reflection, however, we can see just how complex it is and how easily it could go wrong. When you know what you are trying to say and the people with whom you are communicating appear to have heard and understood, it is easy to overlook the fact that they could either have misunderstood you or have been so preoccupied that they did not even hear. This is frequently the case when parents are extremely worried about their child or have just been given bad news.

You could try another situation that went well and try to reflect with a friend. Perhaps then you

Activity 5.4

It is not easy to start meaningful reflection without help or experience. Choose a situation that you encounter frequently such as talking to parents. Now focus on one particular situation when you really felt you related to them well. Using Figure 5.1 follow the cycle round and just note down for yourself a few key words for each stage.

Example

Stage 1. Setting the scene: ward situation (main ward or cubicle), community (child's home):

- Why were you talking to them?
- Were you interrupted and, if so, by whom?

Stage 2. What made you think it went well?
Think about ease of communication, nonverbal expressions such as smiles, eye contact, touching, body language. Think of yourself, the parents and the situation you were in.

- Did you understand them and do you think they understood what you were saying?
- Did the environment help you?

It is easier to have contact when you are both on the same level and, conversely, more difficult when one is sitting and one is standing.

- How did you feel at the time?
- How do you think the parents felt?
- What makes you come to that conclusion?

Stage 3. Application of theory and knowledge:

- What communication theory did you utilise, intentionally or otherwise?
- Did you draw on past experience?
- Were you using the theory you had learnt on your course, or on a study day, to give information?
- Were you perhaps using developmental theory to help you discuss how the child was coping?

Stage 4. How would you approach the same or a similar situation in the future?

- Would you use the same setting; would you position yourself differently?
- Could you ensure that there would be no interruptions?
- How would you evaluate, formally or informally?
- How would you test the knowledge given?

could look at an experience where you felt that you did not handle the situation particularly well. In Stages 3 and 4 identify what you could have done by drawing on appropriate theory and then set yourself some aims that will enable you to approach a similar situation in a different way. Remember—how are you going to evaluate?

Reflective practice is, of course, not confined to those nurses who work with children, but the special needs of children and their families can be very stressful. The many reports referred to in this chapter highlight just how important it is that children are treated differently when they come into contact with the health services. Children's nurses have a responsibility to ensure that children have access to the right sort of care. There is plenty of evidence, and guidance, to support them in striving to provide the appropriate specialist service.

REFERENCES

Abel-Smith B 1960 A history of the nursing profession. Heinemann, London

Audit Commission 1993 Children first: a study of hospital services. HMSO, London

Benner 1984 From novice to expert: excellence and power in clinical nursing practice. Addison Wesley, California

Boxall L 1989 Nurse education in the USA and the UK. Paediatric Nursing (Dec): 20–21

Burnard P 1991 Improving through reflection. Journal of District Nursing 9(11): 10–12

Burnard P 1993 Guidelines for reflection. Journal of Community Nursing 7(7): 26–28

Burnard P, Chapman C 1990 Nurse education—the way forward. Scutari Press, London

Burr S 1989 Aspects of paediatric nursing (development of children's nursing in Britain). Senior Nurse 9(3): 16–18

Campbell S 1994/5 New light on an old debate? Child Health 2(4): 136

Chapman C 1982 Degrees in nursing. In: Allan P, Jolley M (eds) Nursing, midwifery and health visiting since 1900. Faber & Faber, London

Checkland O, Lamb M 1982 Health care as social history: the Glasgow case. Aberdeen University Press, Aberdeen

Darbyshire P 1993 In the hall of mirrors. Nursing Times 89(49): 26–29

Department of Health (DoH) 1991 Welfare of children and young people in hospital. HMSO, London

Department of Health (DoH) 1994 The Clothier Report. HMSO, London

Department of Health and Social Security (DHSS) 1976 Fit for the future: report of the Committee on Child Health Services. (Court Report) HMSO, London

Gillet J 1954 Domiciliary treatment of children. The Practitioner 172: 281

Glasper A, Ireland L 1988 A special kind of learner (the paediatric nursing module in RGN education). Senior Nurse 8(4): 13–14

Lightwood R 1956 The home care of sick children. The Practitioner 177: 10–14

Miles 1986 The emergence of sick children's nursing. Parts 1 & 2. Nurse Education Today 6(2): 82–87; 6(3) 133–138

Ministry of Health (MoH) 1959 The welfare of children in hospital. Report of the Committee on Child Health Services. (Platt Report) HMSO, London

Nightingale F 1859 Notes on nursing: what it is and what it is not. Republished 1974, Blackie, Glasgow

Office of Population Censuses and Surveys (OPCS) 1991 General household survey. HMSO, London

Parker E, Coulson J 1995 Equity or discrimination? Paediatric Nursing 7(1): 10–12

Powell C 1995 Should we go Dutch? Child Health 2(5): 182–185

Pyne R 1982 The general nursing councils. In: Allen P, Jolley M (eds) Nursing, midwifery and health visiting since 1900. Faber & Faber, London

Robertson L 1990 The challenge of Project 2000 (development of the Common Foundation Programme and the implications for paediatric nursing). Paediatric Nursing (Feb): 6–8

Rye D 1982 Prospective: post-1980. In: Allen P, Jolley M (eds) Nursing, midwifery and health visiting since 1900. Faber & Faber, London

Saunders D 1982 Sick children's nursing. In: Allen P, Jolley M (eds) Nursing, midwifery and health visiting since 1900. Faber & Faber, London

Schon D 1983 The reflective practitioner: how professionals think in action. Temple Smith, London

Semellie J M 1956 Domiciliary nursing service for infants and children. British Medical Journal 5: 256

Seymour L 1961 A general history of nursing. Faber & Faber, London

United Kingdom Central Council for Nursing, Midwifery and Health Visiting (UKCC) 1986 Project 2000: a new preparation for practice. UKCC, London

United Kingdom Central Council for Nursing, Midwifery and Health Visiting (UKCC) 1994 The Council's standards for education and practice following registration. UKCC, London

United Kingdom Central Council for Nursing, Midwifery and Health Visiting (UKCC) 1995 PREP and you. UKCC, London

Whiting M 1994 Meeting needs: RSCNs in the community (training needs of community paediatric nurses). Paediatric nursing 6(1): 9–11

Wood 1888 Training of nurses for sick children. Nursing Record 36: 507–510

Woodroffe C, Glickman M, Barker M, Power C 1993 Children, teenagers and health, the key data. Open University Press, Buckingham

FURTHER READING

Baly M 1980 Nursing and social change, 2nd edn. Heinemann Medical, London

Beattie J 1990 The future of paediatric nursing. Nursing 4(16) 29–31

Boxall L 1989 Nurse education in the USA and the UK. Paediatric Nursing (Dec): 20–21

English National Board for Nursing, Midwifery and Health Visiting 1990 A new structure for professional development. ENB, London

Fradd E 1992 The evolution of the RSCN. Journal of Clinical Nursing 1: 309–314

Laurent C 1990 Building for the future. The case for paediatric nurses. Nursing Times 86(10): 70–72

6

Professional role of the children's nurse

Linda McQuaid

In this chapter the student examines the factors which affect the way that nurses function. The chapter will then consider the ways in which the role of the nurse has changed, is changing and will change in the future.

The chapter:
- **looks at legislation governing the Health Service and nurse training**
- **explores the influences of different theories of care delivery**
- **investigates the ways in which care can be documented**
- **supports the notion that nurses are at the forefront of change.**

INTRODUCTION

The 'professional' role of the nurse conjures up many pictures and it is worth considering the notion in its broadest context before examining the issues in more detail. Is it, for instance, to do with appearance? One only has to remember the countless discussions in the nursing and national press when any mention is made of a change to the uniform, such as the abolition of the frilly cap. There are apparently large numbers of otherwise intelligent people who are convinced that the nurse is 'real' only if she is wearing a traditional uniform with a cap. There is often no recognition of the fact that the nurse may be male.

The real concept of the professional role of the nurse is far more to do with her/his performance. There are many influences on nurses today and the acronym used by marketing managers sums them up nicely:

P   Political
E   Economic
S   Social
T   Technological

Political influences

The recent changes in the politics of the Health Service have had many effects on nursing. The general management review reported by Sir Roy Griffiths in 1983 reduced the power of senior nurses and gave many of them advisory responsibilities only. In the next few years we saw the introduction of Project 2000 and the reorganisation of the Health Service.

Economic influences

It may have been the desire of the Conservative party to make the Health Service more efficient but the effects of the recession of the late 80s have certainly complicated the issue. There is simply less money to satisfy an ever-increasing demand for health provision and nurses are by necessity becoming ever more aware of this. Skill-mix reviews have reduced the numbers of qualified nurses and in many cases downgraded the posts that remain.

Social influences

Social pressures such as the large decrease in the numbers of available recruits for nurse training and then the very real possibility of unemployment at the end of the training period are linked with the economic factors described above. In addition, the increasing age of the population means that there will be more people needing care, which is likely to be delivered by a smaller pool of qualified nurses.

Technological influences

The use of technology, both in terms of the equipment used to deliver and monitor patient care, and in the increasing use of computers, has changed the working day. Student nurses used to spend time counting the 'drops' required to deliver an intravenous infusion at a certain rate but now a machine can (almost) be relied upon to do it for us. Ward-based computer systems can be used for care-planning, rostering and budgeting.

On a larger scale, hospital information systems are used to monitor contracts and so balance income and expenditure in a manner that was unheard of in the public sector only a few years ago. Patient information may be available at ward level, increasing accuracy and saving time. This may include the results of laboratory tests as well as the biographic details of patients and the history of their previous admissions to the hospital.

THE CODE OF PROFESSIONAL CONDUCT

'The Code of Professional Conduct', as stated by the United Kingdom Central Council (UKCC) in 1983 and updated in 1992, acts as a guide to professional behaviour for all registered nurses, midwives and health visitors. The clauses of the Code were examined in detail by Cynthia Gilling (1992) and the updated version appears in Box 6.1.

The Scope of Professional Practice, issued by the UKCC in 1992, enlarges on the Code and gives guidance and direction about the extension of the role of the nurse, midwife and health visitor. The Council accepts that it is constantly being asked to change and to consider new practices, but wishes to ensure that any such alterations remain subject to guidelines. It remains implicit that a nurse should not be asked to carry out a procedure for which she/he has not been trained, but Point 3 of the document, 'Education for Professional Practice', recognises that some of this training can be given in the pre-registration curriculum.

Box 6.1 UKCC Code of Professional Conduct (UKCC 1992a)

As a registered nurse, midwife or health visitor, you are personally accountable for your practice, and in the exercise of your professional accountability, must:

1. Act always in such a manner as to promote and safeguard the interests and well-being of patients and clients;
2. Ensure that no action or omission on your part, or within your sphere of responsibility, is detrimental to the interests, condition or safety of patients and clients;
3. Maintain and improve your professional knowledge and competence;
4. Acknowledge any limitations in your knowledge and competence and decline any duties or responsibilities unless able to perform them in a safe and skilled manner;
5. Work in an open and cooperative manner with patients, clients and their families, foster their independence and recognise and respect their involvement in the planning and delivery of care;
6. Work in a collaborative and cooperative manner with health care professionals and others involved in providing care, and recognise and respect their particular contributions within the care team;
7. Recognise and respect the uniqueness and dignity of each patient and client, and respond to their need for care, irrespective of their ethnic origin, religious beliefs, personal attributes, the nature of their health problems or any other factor;
8. Report to an appropriate person or authority, at the earliest possible time, any conscientious objection which may be relevant to your professional practice;
9. Avoid any abuse of your privileged relationship with patients and clients and of the privileged access allowed to their person, property, residence or workplace;
10. Protect all confidential information concerning patients and clients obtained in the course of professional practice and make disclosures only with consent, where required by the order of a court or where you can justify disclosure in the wider public interest;
11. Report to an appropriate person or authority, having regard to the physical, psychological and social effects on patients and clients, any circumstances in the environment of care which could jeopardise standards of practice;
12. Report to an appropriate person or authority any circumstances in which safe and appropriate care for patients cannot be provided;
13. Report to an appropriate person or authority where it appears that the health or safety of colleagues is at risk, as such circumstances may compromise standards of practice and care;
14. Assist professional colleagues, in the context of your own knowledge, experience and sphere of responsibility, to develop their professional competence, and assist others in the care team, including informal carers, to contribute safely and to a degree appropriate to their roles;
15. Refuse any gift, favour or hospitality from patients and clients currently in your care which might be interpreted as seeking to influence preferential consideration; and
16. Ensure that your registration status is not used in the promotion of commercial products or services, declare any financial or other interests in relevant organisations providing such goods or services and ensure that your professional judgement is not influenced by any commercial considerations.

The administration of intravenous drugs, for example, for so long a so-called 'extended role', is being included in the last study block for some final-year student nurses. This is rightly recognising it as a natural extension to the teaching of administration of all other medicines and can only enhance the nurse's role as a total provider of care.

CHANGES TO THE TRADITIONAL ROLE OF THE NURSE

The last few years have seen many changes to the traditional picture of the 'bedside' nurse—not all of them are improvements. It is essential, however, for the truly professional nurse to take the opportunities which are being offered and see them in a positive way rather than as a threat.

Project 2000

The introduction of Project 2000 nurse training was announced by John Moore, then Secretary of State for Health, during a turbulent time for the Health Service. Towards the end of 1987 there had been increasing publicity about lengthening waiting lists and ward closures, but the event which drew the largest comments was the cancellation of paediatric cardiac surgery in Birmingham due to staff shortages. A national strike was called and, quite suddenly, Margaret Thatcher announced that she intended to hold a review of the Health Service. This announcement was completely unexpected and came as a great surprise to everybody. The result of this review was the White Paper 'Working for Patients' (DoH 1989).

John Moore's announcement about Project 2000 was therefore yet another change from the old-style Health Service. There had been many discussions about the way nurses were trained and there were three major issues:

1. Student nurses were expected to contribute to the delivery of care almost from their first days on the ward. This level of contribution varied between wards and specialities; it could be simply the relatively small amount that was provided by first-year student nurses or the much greater contribution of some final ward students who acted as junior staff nurses. This was not only difficult for them, but it also meant that enormous demands were placed on the trained staff on the ward. Supervision of students was inconsistent and could vary from day to day and ward to ward. Some trained staff were also very reluctant to 'teach' students as there was a belief that the only form of teaching that was acceptable had to be in the ward office during the 'handover' period.
2. Even quite small hospitals had nurse training schools linked to them and nurse training was not linked to higher education establishments. There was a two-tier system of training leading to either registration or enrolment with the General Nursing Council (UKCC after 1983). A large emphasis was placed on the attainment of practical skills, particularly for enrolled nurses undergoing the shorter 2-year training. For the nurse aiming for registration, the training tended to follow a 'medical model' method of teaching disease processes. Nurses were not necessarily taught to think or question but rather to 'do'.
3. The training took place almost exclusively in the hospital setting, with very little emphasis on community care. The focus was definitely on the sick patient, with only lip service being paid to the contribution of any agency other than the hospital.

Project 2000 was seen as the solution to these problems, with an academic training given to nurses who had student status and were not expected to be part of the workforce. Changing

Table 6.1 The United Kingdom population age structure: 2010. (Source: King's Fund Acute Services Initiative: reproduced from Bryant 1991 by kind permission of The King's Fund.)

Age group	Change
20–24	- 600 000
30–34	- 1 100 000
35–59	- 700 000
60–64	+ 600 000
65–79	+ 100 000
80 +	+ 600 000

Activity 6.1

Think about the definition of 'supernumerary' and how it affects you:

1. What is your understanding of supernumerary status?
2. To what extent have you found it to be understood by ward staff?
3. Do you think that it is the best way to learn?

patterns of demography identified a twofold problem; there would be a shortfall in the numbers of young people wishing to enter nurse training and a rise in the number of people who would require care (see Table 6.1).

A smaller, but more highly qualified, number of nurses would address this problem. The students would be granted supernumerary status and the use of this one word has generated many discussions.

The actual interpretation of the status of 'supernumerary' varies from area to area. When Project 2000 nurses started their training, with a consequent decline in the numbers of traditional students, money was allocated to budgets to allow for replacement staff. Paediatric areas often received very little of this extra money because it was (wrongly) assumed that students had always been supernumerary in specialist areas. This put additional pressure on the trained staff, who were already struggling to cope with shrinking budgets.

What has Project 2000 achieved for the children's nurse?

For many years, it has been recognised that the optimum care for the child in hospital should only be provided by the 'appropriately trained staff, fully aware of the physical and emotional needs of each age group' (NAWCH 1984). It has never been easy to achieve this due to the limited number of places available for training. The would-be children's nurse could either opt for the combined RGN/RSCN training, or qualify first as an RGN and then undertake post-registration RSCN training. This inevitably meant that the most junior staff nurses were not qualified as children's nurses but gaining experience prior to RSCN training.

Project 2000 has worked to both the advantage and disadvantage of children's nursing. The philosophy of the training, that one is trained for the precise Branch in which one wishes to work, is a good one. It means that at the end of the training period there is a supply of highly trained nurses who have received a training directed towards the care of the child. It does not, however, address the needs of the inevitable oversupply of nurses who qualified prior to the introduction of Project 2000 and now find themselves as RGNs with a shrinking number of RSCN courses to join. For some, the solution may be to join a Project 2000 course at the beginning of the Child Branch element. This route has been approved by the ENB, provided the course is of at least 1 year's duration. The successful student at the end of this course receives a Diploma in Child Health and can be entered in Part 15 of the Register.

This brings inevitable problems at ward level for the newly qualified RN who may find him/herself in the position of being challenged by the more senior staff nurses who, although they have experience at working on the ward, do not hold a formal qualification. The team structure of the ward should be designed in such a way that there is a balance of qualifications and experience on each team.

Reduction in junior doctors' hours

The recent legislation (DoH 1991a) aimed at reducing the hours worked by junior doctors has put further pressure on nurses. There has been a gradual shift in the type of procedure that once was performed only by the doctor but has now been absorbed into the nursing role. At one time, for instance, only doctors could record blood pressures but nobody would dream of suggesting that a nurse should call a doctor for this task. The administration of intravenous drugs has become a real problem in some areas. A nurse is required to be trained and certificated to carry out this role but cannot always carry this 'qualification' to another hospital. Surveys of medical staff have identified procedures which they feel could be better carried out by nursing staff. These include venepuncture, intravenous injections, suturing, application and removal of plaster casts, changing of tracheostomy and nasogastric tubes and ECG recording (Hunter 1991). Many of these are of course already being performed by nurses as part of their everyday role, but doctors may still feel that the ultimate responsibility is theirs.

It should not be a case of dividing the work and assessing who should carry out the job on the basis of some outdated definition of what the nursing role is. It is far more important for the nurse to grasp the opportunity to expand the area of responsibility. For children who have to come into contact with the Health Service in whatever capacity, the number of contacts they have with different professionals should be kept at a minimum. It is astonishing how many parents cannot stay with their children while they undergo procedures such as venepuncture because they themselves are terrified. How did they all become so frightened of hospitals? Is it because they themselves had bad experiences as children in hospital when visiting was restricted and the very special needs of the hospitalised child were not so well known?

There is a great temptation for the 'extended role' argument to be used and to expect many of the more mundane jobs currently being carried out by medical staff to be delegated to nurses. This principle should be resisted at all costs, but only by using reasoned arguments. Trevor Clay, in his book, *Nurses, Power and Politics* (1987), refers to the Green Paper on Health Care of 1986 and the question that was posed at the time: 'Are we realising the full potential of nurses?' He stated that we were not, for professional and economic reasons, but was also concerned that nurses would be used merely to 'fill the gaps left by doctors'.

At the time he wrote his book, he bemoaned the fact that all patients 'belonged' to doctors who prescribed and directed their care. He made reference to the rise and importance of primary nursing and, in the years since the book appeared, there have been endless debates and arguments about whether it 'works' or not.

Primary nursing—does it affect the professionalism of the nurse?

The four elements of primary nursing have been described as accountability, autonomy, coordination and comprehensiveness (Bowman & Carter 1990, Coe-Legg et al 1990). These factors combine to make the primary nurse responsible for planning the care of the individual child and family for 24 hours a day, during the entire episode of care. The nurse is obviously not expected to be on duty for all of those 24 hours, and so careful communication and coordination of care from one shift to the other is an inherent part of the planning process. It is a clear move away from the notion of nurses following the instructions of other professionals and means that nurses have professional responsibility in their own right.

It has been difficult at times for nurses to grasp the true meaning of accountability simply because for so long it was possible to pass responsibility on to the 'nurse in charge'. The UKCC Code of Professional Conduct makes it clear in its first sentence that all nurses are accountable, i.e. responsible, for their own actions and must be able to justify taking them. The Patients' Charter (DoH 1991b) made it

Activity 6.2

Think about the 'named nurse' concept and how it may be used when caring for children and their families:

1. Are there any specific issues unique to paediatrics which may affect the effectiveness of the 'named nurse' concept?
2. How can these be addressed?
3. What is the role of the ward sister?

quite clear that there should be 'a named nurse, midwife or health visitor responsible for each patient'. At the time of its introduction, it was wrongly thought to be Government acceptance and approval of the concept of primary nursing. In fact, the concept of the 'named nurse' is open to abuse and, at its extreme, can be interpreted as merely the admitting nurse entering her/his name on the patient documentation. Rather than just pay lip service to the notion, it is far better for the professional nurse to grasp the opportunity to increase personal responsibility and thus job satisfaction.

Each individual ward or area will choose to implement its own version of primary nursing, and indeed it should be tailored to the needs of the type of children seen on the ward. A surgical ward with a very short length of stay and a low readmission rate obviously functions in a way that is entirely different from an oncology ward in a specialist children's hospital. Regardless of this factor, there is now a great opportunity for nurses to explore areas previously closed to them and become more rounded professionals.

The fundamental needs of children and their families whenever they come into contact with any aspect of the Health Service are irrefutable. They need continuity of care, good communication and respect. They should be treated by professionals who can absorb legislation and regulations aimed at the population as a whole, and then adapt them for children. Primary nursing, or the requirement to have a named nurse, is no exception. The way this concept is practised on each individual children's ward is up to the people working on it. It is infinitely preferable for all the staff to develop their own model which works for them and the children and families in their care, than to attempt to reproduce a standard package which may work perfectly well somewhere else.

SPECIFIC ISSUES TO CONSIDER FOR THE CHILDREN'S NURSE

Caring for children also means caring for their families. Although this is true for every branch of nursing, there are issues which are unique to paediatrics. The nurse is expected to be the patient's advocate, but how easy is this when, for instance, a particular treatment that would help the child is opposed by the parents? This can occur particularly in oncology nursing or perhaps when nursing the child with anorexia nervosa. There can be instances when the parents are insisting that the diagnosis is not disclosed to the child but the nurse is sure that the child knows that the illness is terminal. At the root of this is often the fact that the parents are denying the diagnosis to themselves and are having difficulty in accepting it. The nurse is often in the position of mediating between the doctor and the family, and this can be very stressful. These issues are discussed in more detail in Chapters 7 and 24.

THE NURSE'S ROLE IN THE DIRECT CARE PROCESS

A critical element of the professional role of the nurse is to ensure that as much time as possible is spent in the direct care of the child. The best way to do this is to ensure that the time of trained and qualified nurses is being used appropriately. If, as discussed in the introduction to this chapter, we face a time where we have fewer, more highly qualified nurses we must ensure that we use them properly. Professor Roger Dyson examined the question of the changing profile of the workforce and observed that all of the different professions involved in

the Health Service had their own structure of hierarchies (Dyson 1991). It had always been assumed that these boundaries could not be crossed, and they were in fact jealously guarded. He identified that what was needed was a new approach to the skill mix of staff in all areas, including nurses involved in the direct care-giving process.

Project 2000 will result in, among other benefits, an increase in the quality of care through the use of planned interventions. For this to be possible, there must be available a support structure of other staff. This is not just in the hospital setting, but also in the community where there has been a rise in the numbers of unqualified staff delivering care in the patients' homes.

The logical next step from reviewing the mix of staff in a given area is to examine the areas of responsibility. The strict demarcation lines between the professions are being broken down with nurses especially absorbing more into their roles than once was expected. The traditional role of the nurse had very definite boundaries and any embellishments were encompassed by the general heading of 'the extended role'. In order to extend the role, one had to undergo some sort of additional training, be tested and observed actually carrying out the procedure and then awarded a certificate, which was a proof of competence. This concept is shifting, partly in response to the factors already discussed that will result in a reduction in numbers of nurses. It is also because we are creating a profession much more used to questioning practice and seeking ways to improve it. Nurses are quite rightly no longer content to defer to others to finish a job they may have started.

The Scope of Professional Practice (UKCC 1992b) states quite clearly that 'the terms "extended" or "extending" roles … are no longer suitable since they limit, rather than extend, the parameters of practice.' This is a recognition that nurses want to expand their areas of responsibility to enable them to take a more active role in the whole spectrum of care. This will be discussed later when looking at the development of the patient-focused hospital.

STANDARD SETTING

The formal setting of standards is a well-established procedure allowing practice at ward level to be regularly evaluated. The writing of standards can be an unnecessarily complicated process and should be simplified so that all staff can understand the aims of the standard statement. The standard should have three elements:

• the statement
• the main issues concerned with the statement
• a foolproof method of auditing.

The last element is essential; if the process of audit is made as simple as possible, it will be performed. By stating clearly what the audit criteria are, the nurse knows that every audit will be carried out in the same way.

This uncomplicated approach can be used at ward level, at unit level and at hospital level. It will work equally well in a community setting or even in a field not connected with health care. Box 6.2 is an example of a standard, written in conjunction with a policy document, for the administration of medicines.

Standards are written by the whole team concerned with the delivery of care. They should not be seen as another piece of paperwork which nurses have devised for their exclusive use, but rather as a tool for the benefit of everybody. The increasingly businesslike environment of the Health Service has led to purchasers writing quality demands into contracts. In order to satisfy these, and demonstrate that they are being met, written standards can be used. Many of these quality specifications are written around the demands of the Patients' Charter and will specify for instance the timescales that should be followed when a patient is referred to the outpatient clinic. This will include length of time between referral letter and appointment, length of waiting time in the clinic and length of time between the appointment and the report being sent to the general practitioner.

It may seem that these are issues over which the nurse has very little control, but the reality

---

Box 6.2   Nursing standard—administration of medicines

Standard statement: All members of the nursing staff will administer medicines in accordance with the policy 'Administration, Control and Storage of Drugs'.

Criteria
1. All wards/departments will have the current policy available and staff will be conversant with it.
2. All staff will receive practical instruction as required by the policy.
3. All patients will be wearing identification bands.
4. Controlled medicine cupboard keys will be separate from other keys.
5. Medicines will be stored in locked cupboards/trolleys/refrigerators.

Audit criteria
1. Is the policy visible?

    Yes   [   ]   If yes, ask staff to show you the policy.
    No   [   ]   If no, ask why not.

Please state . . . .

2. Have all staff received instruction? (Ask all staff.)

    Yes   [   ]
    No   [   ]

3. Are all patients wearing identification bands? (Check all the patients.)

    Yes   [   ]
    No   [   ]

4. Are the keys separated? (Ask to see the keys.)

    Yes   [   ]
    No   [   ] .

5. Is the trolley locked and immobilised?

    Yes   [   ]
    No   [   ]   If no, ask why not.

Please state . . . . : . . . .

6. Are the cupboards locked? (Ask to see the cupboards and refrigerator.)

    Yes   [   ]
    No   [   ]   If no, ask why not.

Please state . . . .

is different. Resource management and the directorate structure has shifted management responsibilities. Prior to 1991 and the Health Service reforms, senior nurses had responsibility for nurse management only and did not have any input into the running of some of the peripheral services that are so important to good patient care. One of the positive benefits of the reforms has been the opportunity that it has given for the total management of the entire service to be under the control of one person. Titles vary in different organisations, and in themselves are not important, but the senior manager takes on far more than pure nursing management. It is important that this Directorate or Service or Speciality Manager is a nurse to ensure that basic principles of good care are not sacrificed for financial reasons.

In paediatrics there is a real danger of the service being marginalised if directorates merge. Some organisations have for instance a 'women and children's' directorate which may be led by a midwife. This ensures that the midwives have a supervisor, a statutory requirement of the UKCC, but does nothing to address the problem of the management of children's nurses. The Audit Commission made the point in their 1993 report, *Children First*, when they said: 'There should be a senior children's nurse above ward sister level to provide the focus for implementing consistent policies for the care of children in all parts of the hospital'.

Importance of the role of senior children's nurse

There must be an advocate for children's rights within every organisation. In this way, it is to be hoped that no major decisions would be taken without considering how to ensure that the needs of the child are met. In the community, for instance, the paediatric community nursing service is a vital, but small, part of the whole district nursing team. If these nurses are not recognised for their specialist knowledge, but absorbed into the general community nursing

services, the children may ultimately suffer. These nurses should be part of a total paediatric service, liaising with colleagues in the school nursing service and health visiting as well as those in the hospital.

The Audit Commission accepted that the ward manager on the children's ward should not be expected to take the responsibility for issues concerning children either elsewhere in the hospital or in the community. This place should be taken by a more senior nurse who has the managerial role within the directorate. These global issues may include acting as the professional head of children's nursing as well as monitoring contracts and taking financial control.

NURSING MODELS

From the introduction of the Activities of Living model described by Roper, Logan & Tierney in 1980, there has been a substantial amount of work carried out looking at nursing models. These are discussed in more detail in Chapter 8. The usefulness of a model depends very much on the individual nurse's interpretation of it and there have been many criticisms about, among other things, the sheer length of time involved in completing the documentation.

This can be a real issue in paediatrics when the length of stay is so short. There is a danger that people feel they have to write 'something' and the content of what is actually written may not always be relevant. In addition, the depth of questioning which would be needed for a child who is admitted with pallor, weight loss and bruising is simply not required for a child who has been admitted for routine day case surgery.

This has led inevitably to standard care plans which could be customised for each child. These are particularly useful on a regular operation day when perhaps five children are admitted for adenotonsillectomy. There is a natural extension to this though, and that is looking at the total expected care of these children and not just the expected form-filling.

INCREASING PRESSURES IN CARE DELIVERY—A SOLUTION?

If the many pressures discussed are put together, it is clear that a radical rethink of the way in which care is delivered is needed. We have fewer staff, who may be more highly trained but are expected to expand their position as never before. Finance for the National Health Service may be increasing but it will never be enough to meet demand. Increasing technical expertise will raise expectations and the changing demography illustrated in Table 6.1 places additional upward pressure on finite resources.

A further element is the introduction of competition among the providers of health care. The Patients' Charter (DoH 1991b) has made patients more aware of their rights and more ready to demand them. If they have a bad experience in hospital, they will quite rightly complain and may even resort to legal action to claim compensation for substandard care. In the event of a return visit being necessary, they are likely to ask their general practitioner to send them to another hospital. This is not as easy as it sounds, particularly in more rural areas, but in London and other big cities, where there is said to be an oversupply of hospitals, this has had the effect of forcing hospitals to examine the way in which they look after patients.

One way of realigning care to make better use of resources and improve the experience of the patient is by the introduction of the patient-focused hospital.

The patient-focused hospital

It was Booz, Allen & Hamilton (BAH) who first described the patient-focused hospital concept in 1988 when they published a paper titled *Operational Restructuring—a Recipe for Success* (Lathrop & Crauff 1988). They examined the traditional methods of delivery of patient care and found that hospitals are generally organised around the staff rather than the patient. All professionals involved in the care of the patient had their own boundaries which could not be

---

Box 6.3   Booz Allen Hamilton: patient-focused care

1. The organisation must be decompartmentalised to ensure that staff resources are both patient-focused and better utilised.
2. 'Jobs' on these operating units must be structured to emphasise the greatest possible continuity of care to the patients. Some unit members, including nursing staff, will be cross-trained to perform procedures outside their 'primary area and expertise'.
3. The operating approach must stress responsiveness, substantially improving the quality of care and services provided to patients.
4. The operational construct must emphasise accountability.

---

crossed. Often this meant that the patient would be waiting an unnecessarily long time for the next stage in the process. An example of this could be the patient whose routine postoperative mobilisation would have to wait until a Monday rather than happen on a Saturday because only emergency physiotherapy is available at the weekend.

BAH devised four steps which were required to reorganise the traditional patterns of work and therefore provide a higher quality of health care: these are listed in Box 6.3.

Several hospitals have chosen to investigate and subsequently implement the patient-focused model of care. The key objectives of the project in one of these hospitals—to improve patient and staff satisfaction, deliver predictable, prompt and effective care, and provide an informed choice—are basic principles of good care.

The model chosen by one of these sites, Central Middlesex NHS Trust in North West London, was designed to provide an innovative method of health care and had four major principles (see Box 6.4).

The principles are as relevant in paediatrics as any other speciality and have been shown to increase the professional standing of the nurse.

Initially a project team must be formed to implement such a radical change in the delivery of care, and this may comprise staff already employed in the hospital or those recruited from outside. Because of the uniqueness of paediatrics,

> **Box 6.4 Central Middlesex: patient-focused care (Morgan 1993, Fuchter & Garside 1992)**
>
> 1. All care to be on the 'patient-focused' model and managed by multiskilled, multidisciplinary care teams led by an appropriately trained registered nurse. This model has large training implications and also implies changes in roles and the breaking down or 'blurring' of traditional professional barriers, with nurses taking on a wider range of responsibilities.
> 2. Patient care will be organised and managed according to protocols which are developed by staff from all disciplines to encourage ownership and ensure that the protocol becomes a working tool.
> 3. The emphasis will be on ambulatory care with a minimal use of inpatient beds.
> 4. An integrated information system must support management and clinical changes. This will result in a reduction of documentation and eventually a 'paperless' system.

it is important that the children's services are well represented on this type of team. Ill children, regardless of their diagnosis, should be on the children's ward and the senior paediatric nurse is able to coordinate care for all specialities.

Getting started

Enthusiasm and commitment are essential to the success of any project and this one will be no different. It involves such a drastic rethink of established practice that each member of the team has to be convinced that it will work. There must be a clear leader, capable of devising deadlines and ensuring that the members stick to them.

One of the first elements of the project should be to carry out an analysis of just how care is being delivered. The simplest way of doing this is to carry out a work flow study. This involves examining the work of all members of the team, preferably by a group of impartial observers. There are several ways of doing this but one of the simplest is as follows:

1. Draw up a list of tasks carried out by the staff on the ward. These should include both direct and indirect patient care as well as those tasks which are 'non-nursing'. There should also be a space to document 'non-productive' time. Not all of the entries in this category should be assumed to be time-wasting—for instance three nurses in an outpatient clinic may be assessed to be doing nothing simply because the doctors have been delayed and the clinic does not start on time. Supplementary notes in this type of case can be useful later when the data are analysed.

2. A team of observers should be assigned to the ward or area on a given day, and each one should be assigned several members of staff to observe. Every 5 minutes, a note should be made of what each person is doing.

3. Analysis of the data can be used to show percentage of time, by grade, spent on direct and indirect care, documentation and communication. This latter is important as it is vital to see how the various members of the team share information and transmit it to each other.

When the data have been examined, they should then be fed back to all of the staff who were involved in the study. There may have been initial resentment, and the method of feedback should be informal in order to allay these fears. There will undoubtedly be many issues thrown up for discussion as some interesting facts and figures will be brought to light.

Work flow studies which have been carried out at various sites have shown that there is very little difference between adult and children's wards as far as the percentage of direct patient care is concerned. The amount seemed to be fairly standard at around 39%. Communication is often higher in paediatrics than in the adult

> **Activity 6.3**
>
> Consider the different ways in which you work and how much of your day is spent in giving 'hands-on' care:
>
> 1. What percentage of the total time spent on the ward do you expect to be devoted to direct patient care?
> 2. What percentage of the total time spent on the ward do you expect to be devoted to documentation?
> 3. Do you think that the amount varies significantly amongst different groups of patients?

wards, both with the families and with the various disciplines in the ward team. The amount of time spent on documentation has been found to be around 14% and has led to attempts to reduce it.

DOCUMENTATION AND RECORD KEEPING

The importance of record keeping, and the implications of inaccurate documentation are crucial elements of the nurse's role. For many years, nursing records were kept in a 'Kardex'. Each patient had a page, and essentials of care were noted in the record, usually by the sister or at least the nurse in charge. Indeed, to be in possession of the Kardex was as good as delivering a message that one was 'in charge of the ward'. Some wards had an additional page for each record which was where instructions for the following shift were noted. These would be filled in by the most senior nurse on the shift and would often be duplications of either the main nursing notes or the entries in the medical notes.

The advent of the nursing process brought, among its benefits, a large increase in paperwork. Nurses began to plan care and to take note of many extra details. Patients were encouraged to take part and, in the case of children, their parents became more actively involved. Nursing models began to be developed which documented care assigned solely to the parent, and the pile of paperwork grew.

Linked with some of the patient-focused hospital projects was a desire to reduce the levels of documentation by the development of a unitary record. This addresses the issue of not only the number of times a patient was asked the same question, but also the number of times the answer was noted down.

Nurses are often acknowledged by doctors as being accurate recorders of information, particularly of events which occur on the ward. The treatment of this kind of information is addressed later. For the time being, let us consider the routine documentation of admission details. On arrival in the accident and emergency department for example, the mother is asked the child's name, address, date of birth, general practitioner, etc. The triage nurse may repeat some of these questions, the A&E doctor asks them again and then may request the opinion of the paediatrician. Some more repetition is inevitable and then the child is sent to the ward for admission. It is almost certain that at least the name, address, date of birth and general practitioner are requested, and documented, again. All of this takes time and is completely unnecessary if only the information transfer is dealt with properly.

A particular issue in the care of the child in hospital is simply the sheer number of professionals who may visit the children's ward in one day. In a general hospital there may be only one or two wards devoted to children, with all consultants 'sharing' the beds. The recommendations of the 1993 Audit Commission report *Children First* look at this problem. In the report it is clearly stated that paediatric surgery should be carried out only by those with expertise. The obvious way to address this is for only one or two surgeons to be responsible for routine surgery, including orchidopexy, circumcision and hernia repair. Nevertheless, even with a limited number of designated surgeons, there remain several other professionals involved in the care of the child, all of whom have slightly different ways of working and documenting that work. The common link among all these teams is the nurse. Although the unitary record is being developed for widespread use, when the issue of many and multidisciplinary professionals involved with children is considered, it can be seen that its use is of real benefit in paediatrics. The introduction, development and evaluation of projects such as these should be nurse-led. This is not because the nurse should necessarily lead the team but because he or she is at the centre of it. For the children's nurse working on a children's ward in a general hospital this responsibility is more keenly felt. The nurse must be the child's advocate in an atmosphere geared towards the care of the adult. It is for the nurse to set the standard and the unitary record is a good starting point.

Development of the unitary record

The UKCC has issued guidance on the subject of documentation—*Standards for Records and Record Keeping* (1993). This document enlarges on the purpose, importance and standards for records. It covers ethical aspects, the recording of decisions on resuscitation and the legal status. Section 37, 'Shared Records', examines the question of the 'shared' record and 'recognises the advantage'. It makes the point, however, that there must be 'a broadly agreed local protocol' and 'where relevant preparatory work has been undertaken' with 'each practitioner's contribution ... seen as of equal importance.'

It is not just nurses and doctors who look after children in hospital—what about physiotherapists, dietitians, occupational therapists, etc.? Each of these groups can record their own findings and not share the information. Nurses form the largest group of professionals involved in patient care and are well placed to see the whole picture.

A group should be formed with representatives of all the professionals who document aspects of the child's care. All of these groups are invited to list information that they consider to be essential. Duplication can then be eradicated and a core is left which should be acceptable to all. It may be possible for instance to take out information which is held on the hospital information system if there are ward terminals which all staff are familiar with. The view may be taken that if the information is stored electronically, the patient or parent has already been asked for it and so should not be asked again. It should be remembered, however, that children often have more than one hospital admission and it is essential that all computer-held data is correct. Each hospital will have its own way of dealing with this—perhaps the computer screen should be displayed to the parents with an invitation for them to view it and thus validate it.

Having developed the unitary record and had the drafts accepted by all users, the pilot study can begin. It is advisable to opt for a short pilot time and a rapid evaluation. In this way, any problems can be addressed quickly and opposition dealt with before it threatens to be permanent.

Figure 6.1 is an extract from the document produced using the procedure described above. It was part of the first booklet developed for children having day care surgery, although further refinements have since taken place.

The multidisciplinary care plan

The day-to-day reporting of a child's care is not carried out in a standard manner. Each hospital often devises its own system which is tailor-made to its own requirements. Within the confines of the ward, this is probably satisfactory but is subject to a great deal of 'human error'. The record of care is a legal document and could be produced in a court of law years after most of its contributors have left the ward. Often the handwriting is illegible and, even if it can be read, the signature gives no clue to the identity of the writer.

An agency nurse, perhaps working in several different hospitals simultaneously, cannot be expected to be completely at ease with all the different methods of working and record keeping. The development of care protocols, either within the patient-focused concept or as a stand-alone project can help with this problem.

A care protocol is a set of clear activities which are agreed by the entire team concerned with the care of the child. Looked at in isolation, a protocol can appear to be merely a list of tasks which actually detract from the professionalism of the team. It is only by the scrupulous way it is designed and managed that it is possible to answer this argument with any clarity.

Given that many of the children on the ward are not under the direct care of the paediatrician, but are patients of the general or orthopaedic surgeon, the urologist, the haematologist, etc. there are many people to be convinced of the effectiveness of the protocol. In fact, as McNicol (1992) pointed out, we have had protocols for many years in the care of patients requiring chemotherapy for leukaemias.

Paediatric day case multidisciplinary assessment

PATIENT'S NAME: ....

Date: .... Time: ....

Accompanied by: .... Next of kin notified?   Yes/No

Health visitor: .... Telephone number: ....

Address: ....

This section must be completed for the under-fives
School/Nursery/Childminder

Name: .... Telephone number: ....

Address: ....

Ethnic origin: .... Language spoken: ....

Religion: .... Baptised: ....

Family details
Draw family tree, including names and occupations of parents

Daytime contact telephone numbers: ....

Evening contact telephone numbers: ....

PAST MEDICAL HISTORY:

Born at: .... Weight: .... Gestation: ....

Complications of pregnancy: ....

Neonatal problems: ....

Past infections (insert date)

Measles: .... Mumps: .... Pertussis: .... Chickenpox: ....

Others: ....

Immunisations (insert date)

DTP/Polio:

1: .... 2: .... 3: .... Pre-school: ....

MMR: .... BCG: ....

© Central Middlesex Hospital NHS Trust 1995

Figure 6.1 (A) Extract from day care document. (Reproduced with kind permission from Central Middlesex Hospital NHS Trust.)

Day care procedures

To be completed by the Doctor or Consultant in the Outpatient Department

SELECTION OF PATIENTS

Patients need to be screened for their suitability for day surgery at the time of their initial consultation. They should be screened for:

Medical fitness, including any necessary routine investigations;
Provision of postoperative care at home;
Suitability of home circumstances (e.g. availability and accessibility of a telephone);
Distance of travel after procedure;
Access to suitable means of transport and escort home.

NB for local anaesthesia, all of the above may not be applicable.

OUTPATIENT CLINIC ASSESSSMENT FORM

Date of assessment: ....
Diagnosis: ....
Planned procedure:
Anaesthesia proposed: (please tick)   General/regional block   Local infiltration

Doctor's signature: .... Print name: ....

FOR GENERAL ANAESTHESIA/REGIONAL BLOCK PATIENTS ONLY

Does your son/daughter have; or has he/she ever had
Rheumatic fever   Yes/No
Fits   Yes/No
Cough regularly   Yes/No
Asthma   Yes/No
Bronchitis   Yes/No

Is there anything else you think the Surgeon or Anaesthetist should know?

Figure 6.1   (B) Day care procedures. (Reproduced with kind permission from Central Middlesex Hospital NHS Trust.)

From idea to implementation

Assuming that the entire team are in agreement about the usefulness and effectiveness of a protocol, the stage from idea to implementation can take several months. Although the input of every member of the team is essential, it is the nurse who will be taking the responsibility for the day-to-day care of the child and actually *managing* the protocol. It is now that there can be seen a true shift of the professional role. It is suggested that the first protocol to write should be one for a condition that is seen frequently on the ward and has a short expected length of stay. The reasons for this are:

- It is likely to be familiar to all members of the team.
- It is likely to be uncomplicated.
- It is likely that audit data from using the protocol will quickly become available.

Types of conditions which fall into this category are probably surgical—an adenotonsillectomy or circumcision for instance. This means liaison with surgeons as well as all the other members of the team, but although this may sound unnecessarily complicated for a new project, it need not be so.

The team members should be given a short presentation on the benefits of the patient-focused approach, preferably from one of the project members. This is not about convincing doctors, but rather about reassuring the whole team that care will be delivered in a structured way.

Assuming that the subject under discussion is adenotonsillectomy, who should be on the list of invitees?

- Nurses—trained, untrained and students
- Consultant surgeon and his registrar/SHO/HO
- Pharmacist
- Anaesthetist
- Dietitian
- Paediatrician
- Ward clerk
- Anaesthetic/recovery nurse
- Play leader.

This is just a start—the list should consist of anybody who potentially comes in contact with the child during his stay.

Each person is then invited to consider his or her own contribution to the child's care and at this point it often becomes clear that more than one person thinks that they are doing the same thing and that different people think that different things should happen in different ways.

It is not practical for this full list of people to be involved in the entire process and so a smaller project team should be composed of key members. These people will compile the documentation and then present it to the original group for comments and subsequent agreement.

No one person is right or wrong, but an agreement has to be reached eventually. There should then be a list or a flow diagram of the agreed steps that the child takes during the episode of care. These then have to be chronicled in such a way that is clear and easy to read.

If procedures on the ward are documented separately as Standards of Care and adhered to, there is the potential for further saving on repetitive recording. If for instance there is a standard for the 'routine admission to the ward' which includes steps such as:

- Show child and family around the ward
- Introduce children in adjacent beds
- Give ward telephone numbers etc.

there is no need for the multidisciplinary care plan to state anything other than: 'Routine admission as per Standard Statement No. x'.

This document then becomes the standard multidisciplinary care plan for all professionals involved in the care. It is not written in tablets of stone, but is merely an expectation of what will happen in an uncomplicated episode. There is space for any variations to be noted and these are picked up as part of the audit process.

Management of the protocol

The protocol is managed by the nurse who has taken responsibility for the care of the child. This may be the named nurse or the primary nurse or

Multidisciplinary gastroenteritis protocol

	Date of admission .... Time	Sign
Assessment	1. Dr assessment-dehydration assessed at .... 2. Nursing assessment 3. Stool chart and fluid balance chart	....
Investigations	Minimum requirements Stools for bacteriology: 1 [] 2 [] 3 [] Refer to computer system-menu 'Gastroenteritis(Child)' State which blood tests have been ordered	....
Treatments/ procedures	Calculate deficit .... ml Calculate maintenance .... ml % dehydration x body weight (kg) 1000 1st 10 kg 150 ml/kg 100 10–20 kg 100 ml/kg 20+ kg 50 ml/kg FLUID REPLACEMENT = Oral [ ] IV [ ] If i.v. in situ-c/o i.v. and mouth care	....
Drugs/IVI's	THIS IS NOT A PRESCRIPTION Hourly fluid intake = Deficit + maintenance/24 REASSESS REGULARLY Await sodium result and then: If low/normal Replace deficit and maintenance with 4% Dextrose, 0.18% Saline over 24 hours If high Replace deficit as 1/2 Normal Saline over (>150 mmol/l) 24-48 hours If shocked or Normal Saline and 4% albumin at 10 ml/kg over 10 >15% minutes. This is minimum and to be repeated if dehydrated shock persists	....
Mobility	Nurse in side room with enteric precautions	....
Diet	If <10% dehydrated Offer breast milk if breast-fed otherwise Dextrolyte	....
Psychological support	1. Care plan discussed and explained to by: .... 2. Parent education:	....
Discharge planning	Home when tolerating oral fluid, vomiting settled and diarrhoea decreased enough for family to feel confident to manage child at home	....
Additional information	If notifiable disease and/or suspected food poisoning, inform Consultant in Communicable Disease Control in Borough of child's residence	....
Care leader	a.m. p.m.	....

© Central Middlesex Hospital NHS Trust 1995

Figure 6.2   Multidisciplinary gastroenteritis protocol. (Reproduced with kind permission from Central Middlesex Hospital NHS Trust.)

somebody acting under their guidance. The terms 'named' and 'primary' may not be used and, in the example protocol shown in Figure 6.2, this role is held by the 'care leader'. This person ensures that care is given as stated on the protocol although does not necessarily give it personally. She/he may be supervising the care being given by a student or a health care assistant or a more junior RN. The important fact is the recognition that care is directed by the person who is managing the protocol and who signs the document. This signature is the statement that care has taken place and, by signing next to the instruction, the action is deemed to have occurred.

Full signature or initials?

The UKCC have published clarification of this issue in *Standards for Records and Record Keeping* (1993). Point 15 of this document states:

> In hospitals or other institutions providing care, a local index record of signatures should be held. Where initials are regarded as acceptable for any purpose, these should also feature in the index, together with the full name in printed form.

It is likely that a pre-printed protocol will only have space for initials, due to the large amount of information that the protocols contain. If this is the case, a complete record of initials should be kept in a 'signatures book'. This should include any temporary or agency staff so that, in the event of any future query about the care given to a particular child, it will be easy to trace the writer.

AUDIT

Medical audit has been carried out for many years but often not shared with other disciplines. As a logical step from a multidisciplinary care plan or protocol, there exists a simple way to carry out multidisciplinary audit. In this way, all of the group involved in the care-giving process are able to evaluate current practice and discuss ways to improve it.

When the date of implementation is decided upon, the next important event to be agreed is the date for the first audit. As stated, there is opportunity for the protocol to be supplemented with free text if care should vary for any reason from the expected path. This may be for any number of reasons, but the recording of the change, and the reason why it occurred should be added to the record. At all times remember that it is a legal document and, in the event of any actions being questioned in the future, the rationale for taking those actions must be clear.

Such variances could be that a planned test or X-ray did not take place as expected. To state it in these terms would not be very helpful, but to say why it was delayed may help to improve the next child's care. Perhaps the planned blood test could not happen because the doctor was delayed in theatre. Suppose out of 20 protocols examined at the end of the pilot period a large percentage had a blood test delayed because the doctor was unavailable. The obvious answer would be for somebody else to take the blood. This would eliminate the delay and improve the total care.

Specific audit forms which deal with the protocol can also be designed and an example is shown in Figure 6.3. When the initial meetings are set up to discuss the text of the protocol, it is not uncommon to find that each consultant has a different perception of how the child is treated. In order to establish exactly how care proceeds, a form can be used alongside the protocol. This will request certain information to be documented which can then be analysed when sufficient data are collected. In the case of the example shown in Figure 6.3 the following were included:

- Who assessed the level of dehydration? What was it?
- Was rehydration oral or intravenous?

Agreed definitions of 5%, 10% and 15% dehydration will aid the doctor or nurse in assessing the precise level. This can then be used to back up both the protocol and the audit forms.

MULTISKILLING THE CARE TEAM

As mentioned earlier, multiskilling is not, and should not be seen as, a way for the nurse to

---

Gastroenteritis audit

Audit completed by Consultant: ....   Named nurse: ....

Date of admission: ....   Date of discharge: ....

Off or return to protocol: please give dates and reason
....
....

Co-morbidity: ....

Dehydration assessment: % by: ....

Method of rehydration—please circle: i.v. oral

If i.v. state indication: ....

Please record all other protocol variations below

DATE	VARIATION	CODE OF VARIATION	ACTION TAKEN

© Central Middlesex Hospital NHS Trust 1995

Figure 6.3   Gastroenteritis audit. (Reproduced with kind permission from Central Middlesex Hospital NHS Trust.)

---

relieve the doctor of some of the more tedious tasks. It is the way that multiskilling is approached that will enhance the professional role of the nurse. What is actually better for the child and the nurse:

- the nurse having to apologise for the doctor's delay and being unable to do anything about it, or
- the nurse completing the process of admission by moving smoothly from the administrative

element to the total nursing care including the recording of baseline observations and performing routine preoperative venepuncture?

There are, however, several roles that can be readily taken on by nurses to enhance their professional standing. This will help to iron out some of the anomalies which can exist if one type of nurse is trained to take on an 'extended' role and one is not. As already mentioned, the UKCC would prefer that practice 'will continue to be shaped by developments in care and treatment, and by other events that influence it' (UKCC 1992b).

The concept of multiskilling should not be assumed to be something that only nurses do but should include all members of the team. A health care assistant for instance should not have the role limited to nursing but should rather be part of the whole team. During the course of a day, many people other than doctors and nurses affect the care of the child. Surely, if the number of contacts were reduced, we would be helping to create a more friendly environment for children and their families.

The list will include as a minimum the porter, postman, phlebotomist, ward clerk, domestic assistant, etc. It may seem that these are all quite separate roles with clearly defined boundaries, but is this the best way to function? The notion of the multiskilled worker is as important to the patient-focused process as the elements of reorganising documentation and designing protocols. Having drawn up a list of people, the next step should be to look at the tasks they perform and how best they can be combined. You then

Activity 6.4

Think about whether all the care that the child in hospital receives should be given by a registered nurse.

1. How many different people come into contact with the child during the length of stay, however briefly?
2. Could any of the functions be amalgamated?
3. Is there a minimum level of competency you would want from a support worker?

have the basis for a job description, designed by you for your ward or area, which best fits your needs. For ease of training there should be a core of responsibilities that would be common to all areas, which are then customised to fit the needs of the child.

For example, the basic skills may include:

• Transport service. This could include taking patients to theatre, but it need only include children who have had a premedication. Others may walk to theatre or ride a bicycle. It is not only patients who have to be transported but also specimens, post, meal trolleys, etc. Currently hospitals often have different porters for different transport functions, but there is no necessity for this.
• Domestic duties. This may include all the cleaning activities as well as serving meals where appropriate.
• Ward maintenance. Small tasks that ordinarily require the input of another department and several forms to be completed in triplicate should be taken on by the support worker. This could be changing light bulbs or small repairs to non-specialised equipment etc.

The management of these staff should fall under the direct responsibility of the ward/unit manager. This will allow for a training programme to be tailored to fit identified needs. It also means that objectives can be set which relate specifically to the role which is required.

The training period should not be a long one as most of the practical training will be gained through observation in the work area. It should consist of such general principles as the background to the 'new' NHS and the specific role of the support worker. Regardless of the type of work which will be expected the core training should encompass:

• health and safety
• lifting and handling
• bedmaking and basic housekeeping
• CPR training—not necessarily to train how to resuscitate but the importance of rapid actions.

Activity 6.5

Consider the following questions that relate to the training of support workers:

1. What are the specific tasks in your ward/area which could be undertaken by a support worker?
2. Which skills are essential to perform these tasks?
3. Which skills would help the support worker to understand the role more clearly?

This can then be supplemented by additional modules as identified by the manager in the area—a support worker in a health centre will not have the same role as one in an operating theatre.

The role in the team should be made clear and then, depending on the type of area and its expectations, there should be a few sessions of training on the specific elements. This may include stock maintenance, customer care, infant feeding, administration of outpatient clinics, assisting with patient hygiene, etc. The important part is that with the support of a training department, who will ensure that competencies are identified and certificated, the trained nurse is able to plan care knowing that there is an effective, properly trained backup.

The ways that have been described in this chapter of accepting the necessity for change and in some cases driving it, will work to the benefit of the professional nurse. It is only by understanding that these challenges are not a problem, but an opportunity, that the role of the children's nurse will survive in a strengthened form.

REFERENCES

Audit Commission 1993 Children first. HMSO, London
Bowman G, Carter E 1990 Making sense of primary nursing. Nursing Times 86(27): 39–41
Bryant J 1991 Nursing manpower options—the future. Paper presented at conference: How many nurses do you need? organised by Mercia Publications, London. University of Keele, Staffs
Clay T, in association with Dunn A, Stewart N 1987 Nurses, power and politics. Heinemann Nursing, London

Coe-Legg J, Morgan H, Hanmer V 1990 First things first. Nursing Times 86(36): 609
Department of Health (DoH) 1989 Working for patients. HMSO, London
Department of Health (DoH) 1991a The new deal. DoH, London
Department of Health (DoH) 1991b The Patients' Charter. HMSO, London
Dyson R 1991 Changing labour utilisation in NHS Trusts. University of Keele Centre for Health Planning and Management
Fuchter E, Garside P 1992 Patient-focusing Central Middlesex. The Health Summary 9: 9
Gilling C 1992 The professional role of the nurse. In: Kenworthy N, Snowley G, Gilling C (eds) Common foundation studies in nursing. Churchill Livingstone, Edinburgh
Hunter S 1991 Nurses and junior doctors. Paper presented at conference: How many nurses do you need? organised by Mercia Publications, London. University of Keele, Staffs
Lathrop P, Crauff K 1988 Operational restructuring—a recipe for success. Booz, Allen & Hamilton, London
McNicol M 1992 Achieving quality improvement by structured patient management. Quality in Health Care 1 (Suppl.): S40–S41
Morgan G 1993 The implications of patient focused care. Nursing Standard 7: 52
National Association for the Welfare of Children in Hospital (NAWCH) 1984 Charter for children in hospital. NAWCH, London
Roper N, Logan W W, Tierney A J 1980 The elements of nursing. Churchill Livingstone, Edinburgh
United Kingdom Central Council for Nursing, Midwifery and Health Visiting (UKCC) 1992a Code of professional conduct for the nurse, midwife and health visitor, 3rd edn. UKCC, London
United Kingdom Central Council for Nursing, Midwifery and Health Visiting (UKCC) 1992b The scope of professional practice. UKCC, London
United Kingdom Central Council for Nursing, Midwifery and Health Visiting (UKCC) 1993 Standards for records and record keeping. UKCC, London

FURTHER READING

Alderson P 1990 Choosing for children: parents' consent to surgery. Oxford University Press, Oxford
Alderson P 1993 Children's consent to surgery. Open University Press, Milton Keynes
Bishop J 1988 Monitoring the quality of paediatric nursing. University of Birmingham Health Services Management Centre, Birmingham
Buchanan D, Huczynski A 1991 Organisational behaviour, 2nd edn. Prentice Hall, New York
Child J 1988 Organisation, a guide to problems and practice. Paul Harper, London
Clay T, in association with Dunn A, Stewart N 1987 Nurses, power and politics. Heinemann Nursing, London
Drucker P 1994 Management—tasks, responsibilities and practice. Butterworth-Heinemann, Oxford

Ellis J, Hartley C 1984 Nursing in today's world. Lippincott, Philadephia

Mawhinney J 1993 Speech to RCN Congress, 17. 5. 93. Unpublished

Nightingale F 1859 Notes on nursing. London. Facsimile published by J B Lippincott, Philadelphia

Royal College of Nursing 1993 Buying paediatric community nursing. RCN, London

Salvage J 1985 The politics of nursing. Heinemann Nursing, London

Wright S 1989 Changing nursing practice. Edward Arnold, London

7

Morals and ethics in children's nursing

Jean Beattie   Dympna O'Grady

This chapter will provide students with the opportunity to build on and combine their knowledge of ethics and legal issues gained during their common foundation course and assist them in applying this knowledge when caring for children.

The chapter aims to:
- **consider some ethical and legal issues related to children**
- **provide the opportunity for reflection on personal experiences**
- **stimulate comparisons with examples from observations made during clinical practice**
- **assist the individual in coming to terms with ethical issues encountered in both institutional and community settings**
- **enhance the student's knowledge of legal matters related to children**
- **assist the student to appreciate the importance of valuing each individual, and the beliefs and value systems of different people**
- **encourage the student to consider those issues which may not have clear-cut answers.**

INTRODUCTION

This chapter is intended to provide an introduction to the ethical and legal issues encountered in caring for children. Examples and scenarios are included to enable you to consider ethical and legal issues related to children; these are based on experiences of nurses working in the field of child care. Not all examples relate to a child with an illness, as there are instances where any child may confide in those caring for them or seek advice about matters which could have ethical and legal consequences. Where examples or scenarios are given, you might like to compare these with examples from your own experiences, reflecting on how situations were addressed and how you personally felt about the outcomes.

Throughout the chapter there are activities for you to carry out *before* you read the supporting text. The purpose of these is to enable you to identify your thoughts and opinions about a given set of circumstances before those ideas are affected by the chapter material.

Remember that ethical ideas, like nursing, are dynamic, constantly being reviewed and changing as society develops and changes. Ethics as a science arises out of the discipline of philosophy, which indicates that the topics under review can be approached from a variety of angles. Issues are often contentious and open to debate, and you may like to discuss some of the material with your colleagues to enable you to measure/compare your ideas with theirs. Many of the scenarios and examples do not have a right or wrong answer; perhaps the important issue is that the question was asked and considered in the light of the particular circumstances. The other thing to remember is that ethics and law are closely interrelated in that each informs the other. This is why the two issues are addressed together in this chapter.

SOME ETHICAL THEORIES

Immanuel Kant the philosopher who lived from 1724–1804 postulated that all human beings are capable of good or moral will and it is this that separates us from other species. He argued that because of this capacity all human beings should be able to be given absolute respect and should not be treated as a means to an end in themselves. The idea of being a means to an end is bound up with notions of consequentialism and deontology.

Consequentialism

Consequentialism—the commonest form of which is utilitarianism—can be related to the ideas of such philosophers as John Stuart Mill (1806–1873) and Thomas Hobbes (1588–1679), who wrote from a hedonist or pleasure-seeking point of view. In simplistic terms, they subscribed to the idea that the aim should be to do the greatest good for the greatest number of people. The basis of this argument was that, by so doing, most people would benefit and therefore society would be happier. Not only were they concerned with the notion of greatest good, but they firmly believed that the consequences or outcomes were more important than the means by which the outcomes were reached. If the consequence or outcome could be measured as beneficial, then how that outcome was reached was unimportant. In other words, the ends justified the means.

Deontology

By contrast, deontology, which comes from the Greek word meaning duty, is concerned with the importance of the individual as an individual. Whilst the notion of doing the greatest good for the greatest number has merit, the deontologists—Immanuel Kant (1724–1804) for example—would argue that it should not be achieved at cost to the individual. Additionally, those who support the rights of the individual also support the idea that how a consequence is achieved is just as important as the consequence itself. In other words, the ends do not justify the means but must be considered very carefully.

These ideas, which form the opposite ends of a continuum, can be illustrated in medicine—especially at a time when there are limited resources and those concerned with health care delivery are being asked to account for their actions.

Example: children with different medical needs

In the United Kingdom there are many children with ear, nose and throat problems, who require relatively minor surgery to remove or reduce the misery caused by constant earache, sore throat and reduced hearing capacity, which in turn affects social interaction and educational progress.

There are also children with conditions such as congenital abnormalities, organ failure and severe life-threatening disease processes, who require major surgery and/or costly long-term medication. An example here might be major heart surgery.

From the utilitarian/consequentialist standpoint it could be argued that meeting the needs of the first group would produce the greatest good for the greatest number as the cost could be far below treating one child from the second group. The outcome or end would be that more children could be treated, thereby doing the greatest good for the greatest number of children. The end or outcome would justify ignoring the means (disregarding the needs of the second group of children) by which it was obtained.

The deontological argument would run counter to this in that, as each human being is an end in him- or herself and the means are as important as the end, the needs of both groups of children should be considered. This means that equal consideration should be given to the needs of the children who fall into the second group, despite the fact that the cost of their treatment far outweighs the cost per child in the first group. This leads us on to notions of justice and equality.

Activity 7.1

The words 'justice and equality' bring to mind ideas about fairness and sharing equally. It is often said that all people should be treated equally as this would be the fairest thing to do.

Stop and think about this and write down whether you think this is a good idea or not and why you think as you do.

JUSTICE AND EQUALITY

At first glance, the idea of treating everyone the same seems to be a good one until we remember that no two people are the same and therefore it may be neither fair nor appropriate to treat everyone in the same way.

Perhaps we should reflect on what Aristotle saw justice to be. In essence he suggested that:

- like should be treated as like
- different cases should be treated differently

In other words we should look at the individuals concerned, assess the needs of each of them and, within whatever resources we have, address those needs rather than treating all people equally.

Example: when equitable treatment is inappropriate

Peter and his brothers and sisters were all treated equally at home. Frequently there was nothing prepared for meals and the children often had no clean clothes to wear. Neither parent spent much time with the children, who basically cared for themselves. With the exception of Peter, all the other children were growing and developing well and appeared happy and thriving. Peter, however, was adversely affected; he was an unhappy and withdrawn little boy whose growth and development were adversely affected by his environment.

He was taken into care and subsequently went to live with his grandparents where he thrived well, thus indicating that his needs were 'different' from those of his brothers and sisters. Whilst he and his siblings had been treated in the same way, to treat Peter the same (equally) was clearly inappropriate, and the Aristotelian concept of treating different cases differently can be seen to be the fair and appropriate course to adopt.

The United Nations Convention on the Rights of the Child

A United Nations convention is binding on those countries that agree to ratify it and there are procedures in place for monitoring a country's

Box 7.1   **The rights of the child (UN 1989)**

Definition of a child: all persons under 18 years, unless by law majority is attained at an earlier age.

All rights apply to all children. Every child has the right to:

- have a name and be granted a nationality
- live with parents unless this is deemed incompatible with the child's best interests
- express opinions and have them taken into account
- information
- freedom of thought, conscience and religion
- expect freedom from neglect and abuse
- education, with primary education being free and compulsory
- the highest level of health care possible
- enjoy and practice his or her own culture, language and religion
- leisure, play and participation in cultural and aesthetic activities
- protection under the law and to have respect of the human rights under the due process of law.

The State has an obligation towards:

- the abolition of harmful traditional practices
- the protection of children from exploitation as a labour force
- the protection of children from drug abuse and sexual exploitation
- ensuring respect for humanitarian law as it applies to children.

All children who become refugees or who are handicapped in any way have the right to special protection, special care and education to enable their independence.

Activity 7.2

Jane, an intelligent 13-year-old is currently receiving treatment which necessitates rigid control of her fluid intake. She is always thirsty and therefore reluctant to follow the instructions given to her. Because she is refusing to comply with the prescribed regime she is being cared for in an isolation cubicle away from the adolescent unit where she would prefer to be. There are no facilities in the cubicle and Jane is only allowed to leave the cubicle when accompanied by a member of the nursing staff. Jane is only allowed to drink at set times when fluids are brought to her. Jane's parents support the medical and nursing staff in this course of action.

How do you feel about the above scenario? Jot down your opinions about Jane's treatment.

Who should decide the form of treatment Jane should receive? What role does Jane have?

compliance with the articles that have been agreed.

The UN Convention on the Rights of the Child acknowledges that, on an international basis, children have distinct and particular rights (Box 7.1). It has taken 30 years for the UN General Assembly to pass the Convention unanimously; it was adopted by the General Assembly on 20 November 1989 and entered into force on 2 September 1990.

The right to refuse treatment

Before reading further, consider the scenario in Activity 7.2 and the questions that follow it.

Traditionally, decisions regarding treatment

have fallen within the medical domain. Doctors as professionals are considered to have the knowledge and skills to make informed judgements about what is in the best interest of the patient. Formal consent is not usually required unless the intervention is of a surgical nature as, just by being present, the patient is presumed to be consenting. This is based on the existing right of patients to be given 'a clear explanation of any treatment proposed, including any risk and any alternatives' (DoH 1991a) before they decide whether or not to accept the proposed treatment.

However, these assumptions have not usually applied to children. Prior to 1986, individuals under 16 years of age were deemed to be legally incompetent to give consent to medical treatment. Parents were required to give consent, except in emergency/life-threatening situations. Following the 1985 'Gillick' decision (*Gillick* v. *Wisbech and West Norfolk AHA revised* 1985b; see Box 7.2), autonomy and confidentiality were given to those under 16 years who sought contraceptive advice and treatment and were judged by the doctor to be of sufficient understanding and intelligence. Since then, this notion has been broadened and 'Gillick competent' is now a term used to describe anyone under the age of 16 years who is of sufficient understanding and intelligence to give consent to medical treatment.

To return to the example of Jane in Activity 7.2, if she is considered to be 'Gillick competent', it follows that she should be considered competent to make decisions about treatment regimes. However, in this case, because Jane appears to be non-compliant, the issue is not one of consent, but of her right to refuse. Bearing in mind that the doctor in charge is the person who decides Jane's competence, it is very easy to ignore her wishes if they are not seen to be in accord with those of the doctors, particularly when her parents are willing to give their consent to the treatment. The question here is whether Jane's wishes should be taken into consideration, as they would be if she were an adult, and alternative means sought to overcome her reluctance to comply with the prescribed treatment without resorting to the punitive measures described in the scenario.

AUTONOMY

The ethical and legal issues raised regarding the autonomy of children are ones which nurses need to address, particularly in the light of the Children Act 1989, the United Nations Convention on the Rights of the Child (1989), to which this country is a signatory, and the guidance given by the Government publication entitled *Welfare of Children and Young People in Hospital* (DoH 1991b).

Contrary to popular belief the Children Act 1989 does not give automatic right to consent to or refuse treatment to those under 16 years of age. There is very little in the Act which deals specifically with matters of medical treatment. Where it is covered, the issue is only addressed in relation to those children who are in family placements or under supervision orders.

Whilst the underlying philosophy of the Act could be said to accept the right of those under 16 to exercise autonomy in relation to medical treatment, the lack of clear instructions has meant that this issue is open to a variety of interpretations.

The term 'autonomy' is derived from the Greek —*autos* (self) and *nomos* (rule or governance). It

---

Box 7.2   Gillick in a nutshell

Mrs Gillick took issue with Wisbech and West Norfolk Area Health Authority over its circulation of a notice raised by the then Department of Health and Social Security (DHSS) which stated that, whilst it was desirable to consult the parents of a person under 16 years of age who was seeking contraceptive help and advice, the relationship between the patient (a minor) and the doctor was confidential and therefore the doctor should be able to protect the young person's right to privacy where he thought it was in the young person's (minor's) best interest.

The thrust of Mrs Gillick's argument centred on two issues:

1. If a man has sexual intercourse with a female under 16 years of age, this is a criminal offence (Sexual Offences Act 1956). Therefore the notice put out by the DHSS that contraceptive advice and treatment might be provided by the doctor without parental knowledge and consent was also unlawful. The doctor, in giving such advice and treatment, was encouraging illegal acts or was an accessory to illegal acts.

2. The giving of medical treatment to minors without parental permission was 'inconsistent with the rights of parents and their ability to properly and effectively discharge their duties supervising the moral welfare of their children' (Mr Justice Woolf, *Gillick v. Wisbech and West Norfolk AHA* 1984).

In the Crown Court (*Gillick v Wisbech and West Norfolk AHA* 1984) Mrs Gillick lost her case; at Appeal Court (*Gillick v. Wisbech and West Norfolk AHA revised* 1985a) the decision was reversed; but it was reinstated by the Law Lords (*Gillick v. Wisbech and West Norfolk AHA revised* 1985b). Both Lord Scarman and Lord Justice Frazer adopted the view that once a child has 'attained sufficient maturity and understanding, he has the full capacity to enter into legal relationships without the consent of his parents' and in such circumstances parental rights yielded to those of the child concerned.

---

is used to refer to such issues as liberty, rights and freedom of choice and therefore encompasses a diversity of thoughts and ideals. The autonomous person is one who is capable of acting within a freely self-chosen and informed manner. This autonomy arises from the capacity to obtain relevant information, reflect on that information and then take rational, considered decisions and actions based on that information. Additionally, the autonomous individual has the capacity to amend all the foregoing phases in order to adapt to changing circumstances.

Activity 7.3

List those individuals who you consider to be autonomous.
   Now list those individuals who you consider are not autonomous.

When does a person achieve autonomy?

Autonomy is frequently perceived as an all-or-nothing state and no consideration is given to the level of capabilities and competencies needed for the issue on which a decision is required. Legally, individuals over the age of 18 years are considered to be fully autonomous in law unless it can be proved otherwise. By contrast, those under the age of 18 years have to prove that they have sufficient intelligence and understanding in order to be considered competent and therefore autonomous. In relation to consent to medical treatment, of course, the cut-off age of consent is 16 years in England and Wales (Family Law Reform Act 1969) and 14 years in Scotland, whilst there is potential for younger individuals who are considered to be 'Gillick competent' to be involved in making decisions about their own treatment.

The measure of autonomy appears to rely heavily on chronological age rather than the attainment of the ability to make an informed choice. However, this ability is dependent on the individual's rate of development and the experiences to which she or he has been exposed, not simply on achieving a particular birthday (see Ch. 1).

Individuals under the age of 16 years are not generally considered to have reached sufficient maturity to make informed decisions, despite the work of psychologists such as Piaget & Inhelder (1958), Weithorn & Campbell (1982), Kohlberg (1986), Nicholson (1986) and many others, which clearly indicates that children from 11 years onwards may have, and can frequently demonstrate, the capability and capacity to make informed decisions. Interestingly, this research also indicates that some so-called competent adults may never reach this stage of development and maturity, and that their decision-making skills may be questionable.

This brings us back to the difficulties raised when autonomy is considered to be an all-or-nothing state. Perhaps the autonomy of individuals under 16 years of age would be more readily identifiable if it were remembered that decisions are not people but *actions* applied to a range of situations which may vary in severity and complexity. For example, nowhere near as much thought is required to make decisions about having two stitches inserted in a small clean superficial wound on your arm as would be needed for a decision about major surgery which may affect you for the rest of your life.

Perhaps we should not be so surprised at the assumptions made about the capacity of someone under 16 years old to make rational decisions about treatment when we remember that the notion of informed consent is a relatively new concept for adults requiring medical intervention.

Another reason often given for excluding young people from making decisions is that, particularly where their opinion is in conflict with that of their parents and/or the doctor, the 'adults' take over on the grounds that they know what is best and will therefore act in the young person's best interests. This reflects the belief held by some that it is important to make decisions on behalf of children in order to protect them from the harsh realities of life and to preserve the state of childhood.

This attitude of knowing what is best for children by both the medical profession and parents has been reflected in the judicial system. The practice of law is based on comparisons to similar cases which have been brought to court (such as the Gillick ruling). Cases brought to court since the enactment of the Children Act 1989 will have a bearing on the amount of autonomy afforded to children. Many decisions regarding the need for medical treatment are made every day and carried out professionally and efficiently. Occasionally situations arise which are the exception rather than the rule and issues of autonomy and ethics, in relation to individual freedom, are raised. This is usually brought about when there is disagreement between one or more of the parties concerned and it is in these cases that the courts become involved. Precedents set by these cases then set the scene in similar situations. (See the case of Re W below for an example.)

The Children Act 1989 does not address what happens when there is a difference of opinion between the child and those with parental responsibility. Parental responsibility is defined in the Act as: 'all rights, duties, powers, responsibilities and authority which by law a parent of a child has in relation to the child'.

The Children Act 1989 relies on what has become known as the Welfare Check List (see Box 7.3). This, and the statement in the Act 'that the child's welfare shall be the court's paramount consideration' should ensure that the child's voice is heard in all areas where there is an element of choice involving children's lives. This provision in the Children Act 1989, together with the fact that those over the age of 16 years have the right in law to consent to medical treatment, and those under the age of 16 years but 'Gillick competent' can also consent to medical treatment, would seem to increase autonomy for children. The trend of increasing autonomy has not been borne out by recent judgements, which have added a new dimension to the issue of consent, that of the right to refuse treatment.

The case of Re W

The case of Re W (1992) concerned a 16-year-old girl in the care of the local authority, who was refusing consent to medical treatment for anorexia nervosa. As a 16-year-old, she had the right to consent to medical treatment under the Family Law Reform Act 1969. Although it is not possible to have all the details of the case, it appears that the issue was her refusal to be removed from the adolescent unit where she was staying to a specialist hospital. This may have been an attempt at control over her own life or

---

Box 7.3 Welfare Check List

The Welfare Check List contained in Section 1 (3) of The Children Act 1989 has been welcomed by many as an innovation which will provide the courts with a useful yardstick for decisions about what is best for the child. Although the courts are directed to have regard to the check list in certain proceedings, the principles contained in the list can be considered in all proceedings involving children. It is the first time that courts have been directed to have regard to the child's own wishes, which is a significant advance for childhood autonomy. In practice, the list is being used to provide a systematic approach to decisions concerning children. It requires the following factors to be taken into account when decisions are made:

a. the ascertainable wishes and feelings of the child concerned (considered in the light of his age and understanding)
b. his physical and emotional needs
c. the likely effect on him of any changes in his circumstances
d. his age, sex, background and any characteristics of his which the court considers relevant
e. any harm which he has suffered or is at risk of suffering
f. how capable each of his parents, and any other person in relation to whom the court considers the question to be relevant, is of meeting his needs
g. the range of powers available to the court under this Act in the proceedings in question.

---

equally a manipulative ploy. Nevertheless, negotiations could have included the option of staying at the adolescent unit if she would agree to follow treatment. Anorexia is not concerned with food; essentially it is an attempt by sufferers to gain control over their own bodies. In making the decision, the court focused on the physical need to ensure W did not starve and ordered her removal to the specialist hospital. A satisfactory outcome may have been achieved by allowing W to stay where she was, thereby solving both problems—the need to follow treatment and the need for her to have control. In the end W did agree to the treatment but ultimately lost control over her life, perhaps the most important aspect for her at that particular time.

Box 7.4 summarises the law as it now stands in relation to the right of children to consent to or refuse treatment.

Box 7.4   The law as it stands

Family Law Reform Act 1969
The Act lowered the legal age of maturity from 21 to 18 and gave those aged between 16 and 18 the right to consent as if of full age.

Gillick v. Wisbech Area Health Authority 1985
Parental rights gave way to the child's right to make his or her own decisions when deemed of sufficient understanding and intelligence, regardless of age.

United Nations Convention on the Rights of the Child 1989
Particularly article 12 which gave the child the right to freedom of expression and ideas which includes the receiving and giving of information and the right to express his or her views.

The Children Act 1989
The wishes and feelings of the child must be ascertained and given due consideration when making a decision in respect of that child.

Cases brought to court
Precedents set by cases since the Gillick judgement have in effect given anyone who has parental responsibility for the child the right to give consent to the doctor for medical treatment even when a child of over 16 years of age has refused. The court also has inherent jurisdiction which can give consent for medical treatment.

The role of the nurse when the wishes of the adult and child conflict

Consider now the questions raised by the scenario outlined in Activity 7.4.

Legally, if doctors decide that a child such as Anne is not of sufficient understanding and intelligence to give consent to treatment, they are at liberty to act on the consent given by the parents. In situations where it would be necessary to physically restrain a child who is refusing treatment, particularly when refusal is not life-threatening, the nurse acting as the advocate is in an ideal position to negotiate with all parties involved, the child, parents and medical staff, to agree an alternative. In this case then the nurse may need to support the parents in accepting a treatment to which they did not originally agree, if a satisfactory alternative can be found. If an alternative cannot be agreed and the original treatment is still prescribed, the nurse may be

Activity 7.4

The doctor has prescribed a rectal enema for Anne, a 9-year-old girl who is complaining of abdominal pain. Anne is refusing to allow this but her parents agree with the doctor. You are asked to assist another nurse in the administration of the enema.

What would you do in this situation? Are there any alternatives? If so, is it a nurse's responsibility to pursue alternatives?

able to discuss this with the child and provide an explanation appropriate to that child of the proposed treatment and its rationale. By involving the child in decisions, such as choosing the time and place of treatment and the person who will carry it out, an agreement may be reached whereby the treatment is carried out with the child having some control over the situation (autonomy). It may be that the child will still not consent to the treatment and the nurse may wish to support the child in this decision. Where a trusting relationship has developed between nurse and child, it can be a difficult and painful experience for them both in those instances where the nurse has to go against the wishes of the child (or indeed to go against the wishes of the parents and medical staff). However, the nurse must remember that it is his or her duty to act always in the best interests of the child.

The notion of acting in the child's best interest is based on the assumption that, were the young person of sufficient maturity, he or she would make the same decision as that made on his or her behalf.

It is very difficult for a child faced with this sort of situation to go against the wishes of adults. Therefore it is sometimes the case that young people who do not want to participate in a prescribed course of treatment or investigation frequently agree because this is the easiest option when the adults believe that they are acting in the child's best interest.

Douglas 1992 states that 'overcoming a refusal means having to interfere with a person's autonomy both intellectually and bodily'. Therefore the assault is both physical and mental. However, it must be remembered when conflict arises that the adults concerned are acting in a way which they *believe* to be in the child's best interest. There is, however, a need to question whether adults will always make a decision which *is* in the individual child's best interest.

THE PRINCIPLE OF 'BEST INTEREST': SOME CONSIDERATIONS

Consider first the principle of best interest as it applies to the situation described in Activity 7.5.

In the scenario there are three parties to whom the best interest principle could be applied. Firstly there is Samuel, the recipient child, for whom it can be clearly demonstrated that his best interests would be served by receiving a bone marrow transplant which could improve not only his life chances but also the quality of his life. Secondly there is Daniel, the donor child. Is it in Daniel's best interest to submit him to a general anaesthetic and a surgical procedure, with all the possible complications that may ensue? Suppose that the transplant fails and Samuel dies; the feeling of failure on the part of Daniel could hardly be said to be in his best interest. Thirdly, there are the parents, whose best interests might be served by the knowledge that Samuel has been given every possible chance of survival.

There is of course always the possibility that Daniel may not wish to participate in such a procedure. He then can be subjected to pressure from all those adults (and even Samuel) who consider that it is his duty to participate.

Activity 7.5

There are two children in a family. One of the children, Samuel, requires a bone marrow transplant, but even if he is given a transplant his prognosis is poor. The only suitable donor that can be found is his brother Daniel.

Who in your opinion should take priority when applying the best interest principle in this example?

Now suppose that Daniel is handicapped and has little understanding of the situation. Does this make any difference to your opinion of the priority you give when applying the best interest principle? Is Daniel, in some way, less worthy of consideration because of his handicap? Would you make different decisions depending on the type of his handicap? If he is mentally handicapped, is he is less worthy of consideration than a child who is physically handicapped and mentally normal?

There are no easy answers to such dilemmas, but in such a situation there is perhaps a case for appointing an independent individual such as a guardian ad litem to protect the best interests of the donor child. A guardian ad litem is a person appointed by the courts to act in another individual's best interest where there may be a conflict of interests as in the scenario above. Since the Children Act 1989, the notion of appointing a guardian ad litem has been extended, and such a person may be appointed to ensure that the child's best interests are protected at a case conference, for example. A guardian ad litem has to act in the individual's best interest. This may not always be what the individual might want. Whilst this goes a long way in protecting the interests of the individual child, it must be remembered that the outcome may still be in conflict with what the child might wish. For example, if Daniel (not handicapped) did wish to donate bone marrow to Samuel, the guardian ad litem might recommend that this course of action should not be followed because it was not perceived to be in Daniel's best interest to subject him to all the procedures involved, particularly as a successful outcome for Samuel could not be guaranteed.

Children's nurses are continually confronted by ethical issues, and one of the most difficult areas is the birth of a baby either prematurely or with severe congenital abnormalities. Consider the scenario presented in Activity 7.6.

It is difficult to apply the best interest principle to Simon, as the outcome is unknown. Even if he survives severely handicapped, it may not be right to assume that it would have been in his

Activity 7.6

Simon is born at 23 weeks' gestation, weighting only 530 g. His chances of survival are very slim and, even if he does survive, he may well be left with severe handicaps. He may die quite quickly, in spite of all efforts to save him. He may, however, develop one complication after another. If he is on life support, someone may need to take the decision whether this should be continued or switched off. These decisions are normally discussed with the parents and nursing staff, but the doctor presenting the case may weight the arguments according to his own beliefs.

If the parents have been trying to have a child for several years and the mother has had several miscarriages, does this alter the way in which the case is considered? Or, if the mother has got four children already, all of whom have been taken into care?

Discuss this scenario with your friends, applying the principle of best interest to both Simon and his parents.

best interest had he died. If he survives severely handicapped, however, it might not be in his parents' best interest.

Family-centred care—in the child's best interest?

The concept of family-centred care is a developing and dynamic approach to the nursing care of children. The consensus that the family is the best place for the growing and developing child is true for most children and this is encouraged by a family-centred approach to the nursing care of children.

Children's wards should all have a written philosophy, and indeed Action for Sick Children (originally the National Association for the Welfare of Children in Hospital) has issued a *Charter for Children in Hospital* (NAWCH 1984) and the Royal College of Nursing (1992) has issued a *Philosophy of Care* for sick children, both of which endorse the importance of family-centred care. If the concept is taken seriously by both nurses and management, quality assurance measurement of nursing care can include measuring the amount of involvement the family has in the care of their child. Whilst fully endorsing the philosophy of a family-centred approach, nurses

involved in the care of children need to be able to distinguish between the best interest for individual children and the best interest of the family as a whole when the two interests are not the same.

Compulsory treatment is never satisfactory because of the stress and distress such a course of action engenders. Children are best cared for in an holistic and family-centred environment. Dissent from any party, be it the child, parents or professionals will always cause conflict and disrupt relationships. This disruption is to the detriment of the child. The best course of action is always a negotiated settlement, with the child's welfare as the paramount consideration.

CONCLUSION

Children, in common with all other groups, have the right to expect consideration of their special needs. This does not, or should not, mean that they have less rights than anyone else. Nursing and medical staff need to examine their practice in regard to giving information, requesting consent and giving the option of refusal when caring for children. Where a child requires medical treatment, it is the child who is the client, not those with parental responsibility or even the courts. It is a requirement of professionals that they act in such a way as to safeguard the interests of their clients (UKCC 1992; see Box 7.5). If professionals working with children genuinely support the right of the competent child to have autonomy over his or her own body, they must approach the issue of consent to and refusal of medical treatment from the child's perspective. Those children who do not fall within the 'competent' child domain also have rights. It must never be forgotten that children are unique individuals who are entitled to their own ideas and opinions. Even where those ideas and opinions have to be overridden for sound medical reasons, respect should be accorded to the child's right to hold them. Perhaps one of the most important aspects of nursing care is to ensure that children do know that they are respected and unique individuals and that their opinions and ideas will be listened to and valued by those caring for them.

> **Box 7.5   Extracts from the Code of Professional Conduct (UKCC 1992)**
>
> Each registered nurse, midwife and health visitor shall act, at all times, in such a manner as to:
>
> - safeguard and promote the interests of individual patients and clients;
> - serve the interests of society;
> - justify public trust and confidence and
> - uphold and enhance the good standing and reputation of the professions.
>
> As a registered nurse, midwife or health visitor you are personally accountable for your practice and, in the exercise of your professional accountability, must:
>
> 1. act always in such a manner as to promote and safeguard the interests and well-being of patients and clients;
> 2. ensure that no action or omission on your part, or within your sphere of responsibility, is detrimental to the interests, condition or safety of patients and clients;
>   ...
> 5. work in an open and co-operative manner with patients, clients and their families, foster their independence and recognise and respect their involvement in the planning and delivery of care;
>   ....

REFERENCES

Children Act 1989 HMSO, London

Department of Health (DoH) 1991a The Patients' Charter. HMSO, London

Department of Health (DoH) 1991b Welfare of children and young people in hospital. HMSO, London

Douglas G 1992 The retreat from Gillick. The Modern Law Review 55 (July): 569–576

Family Law Reform Act 1969 HMSO, London

Gillick v. *Wisbech and West Norfolk Area Health Authority* [1984] All ER 635

Gillick v. *Wisbech and West Norfolk Area Health Authority* revised [1985a] 1 All ER 533 CP

Gillick v. *Wisbech and West Norfolk Area Health Authority* revised [1985b] 1 All ER 402 HZ

Kohlberg L 1986 Moral stages and moralization, the cognitive developmental approach. In: Lickona T (ed) Moral development and behaviour theory : research and social issues. Holt, Rinehart & Winston, New York, pp 31–53

National Association for the Welfare of Children in Hospital (NAWCH) 1984 Charter for children in hospital. NAWCH, London

Nicholson R (ed) 1986 Medical research with children: ethics law and practice. Oxford University Press, Oxford

Piaget J, Inhelder B 1958 The growth of logical thinking from childhood to adolescence. Routledge & Kegan Paul, London

Re W [1992] 4 All ER 672

Royal College of Nursing (RCN) 1992 Philosophy of care. Scutari, London

Sexual Offences Act 1956 HMSO, London

United Kingdom Central Council for Nursing, Midwifery and Health Visiting (UKCC) 1992 Code of professional conduct, 3rd edn. UKCC, London

United Nations (UN) 1989 Convention on the rights of the child. UN, New York

Wiethorn L A, Campbell S B 1982 The competency of children and adolescents to make informed treatment decisions. Child Development 53: 1589–1598

FURTHER READING

Alderson P 1990 Choosing for children: parents' consent to surgery. Oxford University Press, Oxford

Alderson P 1992 In the genes or in the stars? Children's competence to consent. Journal of Medical Ethics 18: 119–124

Alderson P 1993 Children's consent to surgery. Open University Press, Milton Keynes

Bainham A 1990 Children the new law. The Children Act 1989. Family Law, London

Beauchamp T, Childress J 1989 Principles of biomedical ethics, 3rd edn. Oxford University Press, New York

Booth B 1994 'A giving Act?' Nursing Times 90(8)

British Medical Association 1993 Medical ethics today: its practice and philosophy. BMJ Publishing Group, London, ch 3

Brykczynska G (ed) 1989 Ethics in paediatric nursing. Chapman & Hall, London

Buchanan A, Brock D 1989 Deciding for others: the ethics of surrogate decision making. Cambridge University Press, Cambridge, ch 5

Day A T 1993 Consent and the teenager. Maternal and Child Health (May): 139–142

Dickenson D 1993 Suffer the children. Nursing Standard 7(35): 50–52

Franklin P 1994 Straight talking. Nursing Times 90(8): 33–34

Gilman C 1993 The dilemma of parental choice. New Law Journal 20 Aug: 1219–1220

Hendrick J 1993 Child care law for health professionals. Radcliffe Medical Press, Oxford

Korgaonkar G, Tribe D 1993 Children and consent to medical treatment. Family Law 2(7): 383–384

Peace G 1994 Sensitive choices. Nursing Times 90(8): 35–36

Pithers D 1994 Acting fair. Nursing Times 90(8): 32

Shelly P 1993 Attitude to teenagers in hospital: why they need to change. Professional Care of the Mother and Child (Oct): 248–249

8

Concepts of individualised care

Sue Price

In working through the contents of this chapter the student is introduced to the concept of individualised care.

The chapter aims to:
- outline the needs of children
- outline developments in nursing which contribute to the delivery of individualised care
- describe the nursing process and the ways in which children and their parents can be involved in their own assessment and the planning of care
- discuss the use of nursing models with children and their families
- describe different methods of organising nursing work and the impact that they have on the ability to deliver individualised care.

KNOWING THE INDIVIDUAL

The needs of children

A belief that children are individuals with specific needs is the first step towards the development of individualised care. Over the last 30–40 years our attention has been drawn to these 'special needs' (DoH 1991) of children. Nurses have been encouraged to provide care for the child 'as a whole' (DoH 1991) rather than just the medical problem.

A major influence in changing attitudes towards the care of children in the 1950s was the work of John Bowlby and later James Robertson on the effects of separating children from their families. They, among others, presented evidence to the Committee on the Welfare of Children in Hospital. The result of the Committee's deliberations, the Platt Report, was published in 1959 and started a change in the way that children were cared for in hospital.

The Platt Report put forward important recommendations in relation to preparing children for admission to hospital and changes in the arrangements for parental visiting of children. It stated that children admitted to hospital were to be helped to maintain their normal routines as much as possible, taking into account the need for medical treatment. In particular the Committee emphasised the need to consider the child as an individual with emotional, educational and physical needs.

Since the publication of the Platt Report (MoH 1959), the belief that children have needs that are individual has continued to be developed through the publication of government reports and recommendations about the provision of health services. In 1976, the report *Fit for the Future*, the Court Report (DHSS 1976), expanded the list of children's needs by adding psychological and social needs to those proposed by the Platt Report. More recently, government guidelines for the provision of a 'good quality service for children' (DoH 1991) have clearly indicated a belief that children have both emotional and physical needs.

The belief that children's needs are special (DoH 1991) and require specially trained nurses to enable them to be met has meant that the United Kingdom has continued to maintain a separate register for children's nurses (Glasper 1993). Such nurses should be able to identify the 'physical, psychological, social and spiritual needs of the patient' (HMSO 1989).

Although various reports and recommendations may express the needs of children in slightly different terms, there is overall agreement that children have needs that are individual to themselves (Table 8.1). Essential to the meeting of these needs is the provision of individualised care for the 'child as a whole' (DoH

Table 8.1 The needs of children (adapted from Price 1994)

Need	Identified as special (✓) by		
	MoH (1959)	HMSO (1976)	HMSO (1989)
Physical	✓	✓	✓
Psychological		✓	✓
Social		✓	✓
Emotional	✓	✓	
Physiological			
Intellectual			
Educational	✓	✓	
Spiritual			✓

1991), as well as care in which the child and the family are central.

The nursing process

The nursing process is the 'core and essence' of nursing (Yura & Walsh 1988). It enables nurses to use a 'systematic' approach to the gathering of information about individual children and their families. The cyclical nature of the nursing process enables nurses to constantly review the nursing care that is planned to ensure that it continues to meet the identified needs.

Assessment

Assessment is the first stage of the nursing process. Roper et al (1990) prefer to use the term 'assessing' for this phase to indicate that this should be an ongoing activity. Information about the child and family can be gathered in a number of ways. Nurses may use questioning, observation, examination or measurement. For Roper et al, the involvement of the patient wherever possible is seen as a prerequisite for success.

When caring for children and their families, a sound knowledge of child development will enable the nurse to ensure that the correct people are involved in the assessment. Depending upon the age of the child, these could be the family, or the child and family, with the nurse. For the adolescent it may be essential, in order to complete a full assessment, that privacy is ensured during the gathering of some assessment information.

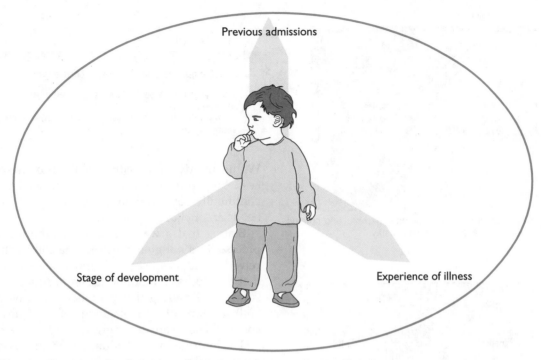

Figure 8.1   The experiences that may influence how a child responds to hospital

In order to get to know each child, nurses have to deploy a variety of skills and have a thorough knowledge of the wide range of children's needs. This requires knowledge of the normal needs of children as well as understanding of the effect that illness, previous hospitalisation or family experience may have upon those needs (Fig. 8.1).

Planning

An effective assessment will enable the nurse to determine the 'plan of action' (Yura & Walsh 1988) for the child and family. Such a plan should establish priorities of care for the child and family.

There have been increasing moves to involve parents in the care of their child during hospital admission. It is not enough, however, to simply state that this is so. In a study by Dearmun, over half of the nurses on the ward acknowledged that they 'sometimes discussed the care plan with parents' (Dearmun 1992). However, throughout the study it became evident that parent participation in the activities of caring was variable.

For successful parental involvement in care to take place, it is necessary for them to be involved in the assessment and the planning of care. During a stay in hospital, parents may be able to become increasingly involved in the care of their child (Fig. 8.2). A plan of care for children should also clarify which actions will be carried out by the nurse, the family or when appropriate the child. The family may wish to change their level of involvement in care, as also may the child (Fig. 8.3). In such situations there should be a clear statement about how responsibilities for nursing actions can be devolved or resumed by nurses.

Activity 8.1

Using the headings in Figure 8.1, describe how the different influences have affected some of the children that you have cared for.

Hospital stay

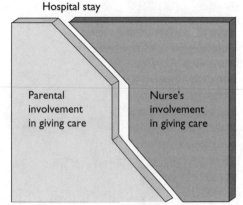

Figure 8.2 Diagram of the change in parental and nursing involvement in care during a hospital stay.

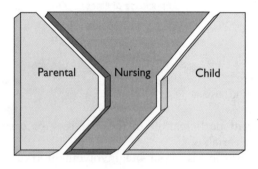

Hospital stay

Figure 8.3 Diagram to illustrate how involvement in care may change between parents, nurse and child.

Positive action has to be taken to ensure that parents have the opportunity to be fully involved in all aspects of care. Such an action could be the involvement of the nursing team in the development of standards of care. The standard would reflect the beliefs of the team and make a clear statement to others about the role of the parents in the assessment and planning process. The creation of such a standard would also require the team to monitor how well it was being achieved. In this way the degree to which parents are being involved can be more easily monitored.

Statements about the outcomes of particular aspects of care should be clear, so that there is an understanding of the goals that have been set.

Activity 8.2

Look at the nursing care plans of the children you care for:

1. Can you see clearly how the parents are to be involved in care?
2. How might the parents' involvement in care be made more explicit?

Within the dynamic nature of the nursing process, both priorities and goals will need to be continually reviewed to ensure that children's needs are met appropriately.

Stating that a ward or unit uses the nursing process does not guarantee that the child will receive individualised care. Simply acknowledging that a child has an individual set of needs is not sufficient. Ensuring that parents are involved in both assessment and planning will not always ensure that the care that is given is individualised.

The information that is gained through assessment requires comparison with knowledge of what is usual or to be expected. Such a comparison will enable those planning the care to determine areas where nursing activity may be required. It will also ensure that needs which are apparently being met appropriately will continue to be monitored. Action can then be taken if there are changes in the child's situation.

NURSING MODELS

All nurses will have their own private beliefs about the purpose of their nursing care. However, nurses are seldom made to clarify their beliefs to the other members of the care team. Such a situation may result in children and their families being cared for

Activity 8.3

Look at the care plans of two children of different ages, admitted to hospital for similar reasons:

1. How do the plans of care differ?
2. Are the child's particular developmental needs reflected in the care plan?

by nurses with different approaches to nursing. This has the potential to lead to confusion for the child and family. The adoption of a common set of beliefs will help to reduce such confusion.

Nursing models provide such a set of beliefs against which the child's assessment can be compared. They provide a philosophical framework which can guide the way in which the child is assessed, care is planned and goals are set. Models provide a set of beliefs about nursing that should be explicit and can therefore be adopted by a group of nurses on a particular ward or unit. Nursing models should contain statements about the four main concepts:

- the person
- health
- the environment
- nursing.

Choosing the most suitable model for the ward or unit will enhance the care that is planned and implemented.

Analysing nursing models

Nursing models can be seen as 'images of nursing' (Fawcett 1989). By putting forward such statements and sets of beliefs about nursing and its purpose, the authors provide others with a framework which can be used to guide practice. The formal, widely published nursing models are usually devoted to the care of the adult. Such models will require careful reading and possibly adaptation by those who are caring for children and their families.

The use of a framework to analyse a nursing model means that each of the different concepts within the model are examined. Statements can be made that clarify the meaning of the individual concept and how it links to the others. The assumptions made by the author of the model should also be made clear. In this way the potential users of a model can compare their beliefs with of those of the author.

Both Fawcett (1989) and Aggleton & Chalmers

Table 8.2	Comparison of major concepts from three models of nursing		
	Roper et al (Roper et al 1990)	Orem (Orem 1991)	Roy (Roy & Andrews 1991)
Nursing	'Nursing is viewed as helping patients to prevent, alleviate or solve or cope with problems (actual or potential) related to the activities of living'	Nursing is a helping service: • acting or doing for another • guiding another • supporting another • providing an environment that promotes person development • teaching another	'The science and practice of promoting adaptation for the purpose of affecting health positively'
The nursing process	Four stages: • Assessing • Planning • Implementing • Evaluating	Three stages: • Diagnosis and prescription • Designing and planning • Provision of care	Six stages: • Assessment—of behaviour in the adaptive modes • Identification of the stimuli that have influenced behaviour • Nursing diagnosis • Setting goals • Intervention • Evaluation
Health	'... health can be conceptualised as a dynamic process with many facets'	Accepts the WHO definition of health	'The state and process of being and becoming an integrated and whole person'

(1986) provide a list of similar questions to be asked when analysing models of nursing. The purpose of analysis is to 'clarify the content of the conceptual model' (Fawcett 1989). In the process of clarification it is then possible to see how the different concepts fit together.

A thorough analysis should mean that the four main concepts of the model are fully understood. There should be statements about the person and the environment. There should also be definitions of nursing and health and an explanation of the nursing process as used by the model (Table 8.2). Following an analysis, the nursing team should be able to see the relationship between the four concepts.

Analysis of a conceptual model is not sufficient. Before adopting a model into practice, its credibility should also be examined. This process of evaluation requires judgements to be made about the model. Fawcett (1989) details many of the questions that she believes should be asked.

While analysing nursing models to determine which would be the best for a particular area of practice, the changes which have occurred in their development should become clear. Over a period of years, the main ideas in the model should be seen to be changing. They should evolve, taking into account changing practices and developing knowledge.

For a model to be useful in practice it must, amongst many other things, suit the society into which it is to be introduced. Nurses caring for children should care for both the physical and psychological needs of children. A model of nursing which has an emphasis on only one of these areas of need may not be appropriate for use with children.

Nursing models should be 'comprehensive enough to provide direction for research, practice, education and administration' (Fawcett 1989). Fawcett states that the assumptions upon which a model is based should be clear. Roper et al (1990), for example, have clear statements of their assumptions. Providing these in an explicit way makes it more easy for practitioners to assess the model's potential for use.

When choosing a model of care, those who are going to use the model should feel comfortable with its central beliefs. For example a nursing model may make very specific statements about the goal of nursing which are very different from the beliefs of the majority of the staff. In such a situation there would be conflict between the different sets of beliefs. Such conflict could lead to an inconsistent approach to the children and their families, leaving them confused and uncertain.

Choosing a nursing model

There are a number of ways in which a nurse's knowledge of nursing models and their application to the care of children and their families can be developed. If the most appropriate model is to be chosen, this ought to be a careful process that uses as many resources as are available.

Ideally, there should be at least one member of the team who is knowledgeable about nursing models and can act as the agent of change (Wright 1985). As part of the process of change, this person may encourage team members to develop a philosophy for the area in which they work. This would clarify the feelings and beliefs about nursing children and their families that are central to that area.

A number of different resources are available to help in the process of choosing a model that best reflects the philosophy of the nursing team. It may be appropriate to start with summaries of different models that provide a brief outline of the concepts of the model (e.g. Aggleton & Chalmers 1986). If such outlines seem to fit with the expressed philosophy of the team, then more detailed information should be sought (e.g. Andrews & Roy 1986).

There may also be examples in the literature describing how others have attempted to scale down a model to suit children (e.g. Cheetam 1988, Stephenson 1987). Such sources may also be able to point out some of the problems that can arise when attempting to change practice.

The final choice should be made when there is a full understanding of the model as a whole. This may take some time to achieve. There may be the feeling that most of the model

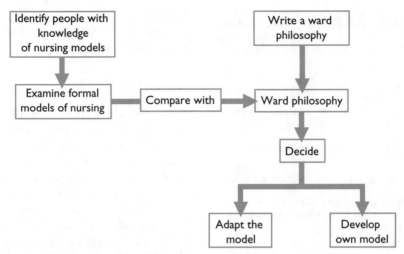

Figure 8.4 Choosing an appropriate nursing model.

is appropriate. It is important to note that any decisions about adapting the model are based on a solid understanding of the whole of the model. To gain this understanding, the definitive text of the model should be utilised (e.g. Orem 1991).

It may, however, seem more appropriate for the ward team to develop a model of care that is specific to their own situation. To do this the team of nurses have to establish a clear statement of their beliefs about nursing children and their families (Fig. 8.4).

Alternatively, nurses may wish to follow the example of Clark & Bishop (1988) in mixing aspects of different models. As Wilding et al (1988) demonstrate, it is then possible to design a model to suit a very specialist group of children and their families. Casey (1988) describes how this process was carried out in a specialist children's hospital.

Casey's Partnership model (Casey 1988, Casey & Mobbs 1988) relates the concepts to children's nursing (see Box 8.1). The concept of the person is divided into the child and the family, thus recognising the importance of the family to the child. Casey (1988) does not provide a 'list of needs to be assessed' as children can potentially be nursed in a large variety of different settings, each of which has a particular set of priorities.

GIVING INDIVIDUALISED CARE

Belief in children as individuals with specific needs, combined with the adoption of a philosophy or model of care, is not sufficient to ensure individualised care. Such beliefs have to be combined with a system of organising nursing work that enhances their effectiveness. The organisation of work and a clear understanding of who is responsible for nursing decisions will ensure that children and their families become the central focus of nursing.

Decision making

When caring for children in hospital, decisions about their nursing care can be made at a variety of different levels. There are major decisions about the overall plan of care and the best way that it can be implemented. There are more minor decisions that relate to day-to-day care.

Activity 8.4

Find the philosophy of care that has been adopted by the ward you are working on. How is this reflected in the way nursing care is planned?

Box 8.1   Concepts of the Partnership model (Casey 1988)

The person

The child

- Growing, developing
- Needs: 'protection, sustenance, stimulation, love'
- Capable of some independent activity, e.g. breathing, sleeping
- Moves from dependence to independence

The family

- Meets the child's activities that are dependent on others
- Includes parents and significant others
- Factors that affect the family's ability to care are the concern of the nurse

Environment

- A child can be affected by 'ethnic, social, psychological or physical' influences on its environment

Health

- A healthy child should be able to reach full potential
- Growth and development are influenced by ill health
- Health and ill health are part of a continuum

Nursing

- Family care—the care the child would normally receive—usually given by parents (nurse will give this care if family cannot)
- Nursing care—care that is needed as a result of the need for treatment—given by nurses, or parents with advice, help and support from nurses

The way in which the ward is organised can have a great influence on how many different nurses are involved in decision making. The greater the number of nurses involved with a particular child the less chance there is that there will be continuity and consistency in decision making.

To ensure continuity and consistency, two main factors should be taken into consideration. The method of organising nursing work should facilitate the use of a small number of nurses for each patient (HMSO 1992). It should also allow for the nurse who is deciding the care to have maximum contact with the child and his or her family.

Organising the care

There are a number of different ways in which the organisation of nursing work can be planned. Some are more effective than others in enhancing both decision making and the giving of individualised care.

Task allocation

In task allocation, nurses are allocated tasks that they carry out for a large group of patients. A particular nurse may, for example, be responsible for doing all of the dressings on a particular shift. Patients therefore come into contact with a potentially large group of nurses.

Hawthorn's study, *Nurse—I want my Mummy!*, published in 1974, looked at nine children's wards, eight of which were using task allocation. The data for the study had been collected about 10 years after the publication of the Platt Report. Despite the recommendation that children should be nursed using case assignment, only one children's ward in London was found to be using this method. Some of the children who had spent up to 1 week in hospital on task allocation wards had had contact with 15 different nurses.

In times of crisis, task allocation may be the only way of ensuring adequate nursing with limited staff numbers (Roper et al 1990). However, it does not enhance either continuity of decision making or maximise the contact between a small group of nurses and the child and his or her family.

Team nursing

On wards where team nursing is the chosen method of organising the delivery of care, the nursing staff are divided into small groups with responsibility for a specific group of patients (Roper et al 1990). Ideally the team leader is responsible for the planning of the care required by the allocated group of patients. Team nursing has the potential to allow the differing skills of the team members to be used in the best possible way (Hegavary 1982). Team nursing is one way to implement child-centred individualised care.

For team nursing to be effective as a mechanism

to improve the continuity of individualised care, a number of factors must be considered. If the members of the team are constantly being changed, there will be little chance for continuity of care. The duty rota will need to be looked at in a different way to take into account the maintenance of stable 'subgroups' of nurses (Audit Commission 1993).

There is one other important aspect of organisation to be taken into account in ensuring that team nursing enhances the opportunity to provide individualised care. On many wards, as their level of dependency reduces, children are moved to different areas of the ward. The team of nurses should, therefore, be allocated to a specific group of children and their families, rather than a specific area of the ward.

Patient allocation

In 1959, the Platt Report (MoH 1959) recommended that children should be cared for by the method of case assignment. This was seen as a way of increasing children's sense of security when they were in hospital. By reducing the number of different carers, children would experience less emotional stress. This form of organising nursing is now more usually called patient allocation.

In patient allocation, nurses are given specific patients for whom they will care. This can be achieved by a nurse being allocated a group of patients (Marks-Maran 1978) or working as an individual within a group of nurses, who have an allocation of patients. Nurses are specifically responsible for the care of their allocated patients. Patients may be allocated on a day-to-day basis, for a few days consecutively, for the length of their stay (Marks-Maran 1978) or for a set period, for example 2 weeks (Wright 1985).

If patient allocation is the preferred method of organising nursing work, then effective communication between the individual nurses caring for the same child is essential. Such communication should ensure that the care that the child and family receive is consistent. The level to which the family is involved in care can then be maintained

and any information or teaching has the same message, thereby reducing the risks of confusion.

Brown (1989), in her study of individualised care, compared the care given on a children's ward where the sister employed patient allocation, with a ward using task allocation. She concluded that the nature of the interaction between the nurses and children on the patient allocation ward acknowledged the children as 'unique individuals'. As might be expected, the nature of the interaction on the task allocation ward related much more to the completion of the task rather than interaction with the child. Although this was only a small study, it distinguishes some of the potential differences between these two different methods of organising the giving of nursing care.

Primary nursing

Primary nursing is seen as a method of organising nursing work that provides the best opportunities for consistent decision making and the individualising of patient care.

Primary nursing is a system for delivering nursing service that consists of four design elements:

1. 'allocation and acceptance of individual responsibility for decision-making to one individual'
2. 'assignments of daily care by case method'
3. 'direct person-to-person communication'
4. 'one person operationally responsible for the quality of care administered to patients on a unit twenty-four hours a day, seven days a week' (Manthey 1980, p. 31).

 Activity 8.5

When you are on the ward, look through the care plans of the children you are caring for:

1. How long have the children been in hospital?
2. How many different nurses have been involved in implementing their care?

Working in a primary nursing unit creates changes for the nurse. The primary nurse has involvement with children and their families from admission until discharge. There are specific associate nurses allocated, who are involved in the planning of care and are able to use their own professional judgement when caring for the child.

Such a system of organising nursing work will enable more individualised care to be given. There can be greater consistency in preparation of children for stressful situations. Teaching plans before discharge home can be better coordinated if a particular group of nurses are involved and cooperating in a definite plan of care.

In 1988, Fradd described the process of changing to primary nursing on a children's unit. Such a change had the effect of changing the way in which the whole ward was organised. The introduction of primary nursing means that the ward sister can no longer be the one who is consulted about every aspect of a child's care. The responsibility for the quality of a child's care is specifically placed on a small group of nurses.

SUMMARY

Children have very individual needs which change as they pass through the different stages of physical growth and cognitive development. In trying to meet these needs nurses have to get to know the individual. This process of assessment forms the first stage of the nursing process, a 'systematic approach' to planning care.

The care given by the whole team of nurses involved with specific children and their families can be enhanced by the adoption of a common set of beliefs. A carefully chosen model of nursing, or a model created by the caring team can provide such a set of beliefs.

Activity 8.6

Plot a chart to illustrate the effect that being nursed on a ward using primary nursing may have on the number of nurses who come into contact with a child.

The organisation of the ward to reduce the number of nurses interacting with different children and their families enhances the effect of both the nursing process and the use of a nursing model.

When all three components come together in the same place then the result will be individualised care.

REFERENCES

Aggleton P, Chalmers H 1989 Neuman's systems model. Nursing Times 85(51): 27–29

Andrews H, Roy C 1986 The essentials of the Roy Adaptation model. Appleton-Century-Crofts, Norwalk CT

Audit Commission 1993 Children first: a study of hospital service. HMSO, London

Bowlby J 1965 Child care and the growth of love. Pelican, Harmondsworth

Brown R A 1989 Individualised care: the role of the ward sister. Scutari Press, Middlesex

Casey A 1988 A partnership with child and family. Senior Nurse 8(4): 8–9

Casey A, Mobbs S 1988 Partnership in practice. Nursing Times 84(44): 67–68

Cheetam T 1988 Model care in the surgical ward. Senior Nurse 8(4): 10–12

Clark J, Bishop J 1988 Model making. Nursing Times 84 (27): 37–40

Dearmun A 1992 Perceptions of parental participation. Paediatric Nursing 4(7): 6–9

Department of Health (DoH) 1991 Welfare of children and young people in hospital. HMSO, London

Department of Health and Social Security (DHSS) 1976 Fit for the future: report of the Committee on Child Health Services. (Court Report) HMSO, London

Fawcett J 1989 Analysis and evaluation of conceptual models of nursing. F A Davis, Philadelphia

Fradd E 1988 Achieving new roles. Nursing Times 84 (50): 39–41

Glasper A 1993 Back to the future. Child Health 1(3): 93–96

Hawthorn P 1974 Nurse—I want my Mummy! Royal College of Nursing, London

Hegavary S T 1982 The change to primary nursing. C V Mosby, St. Louis

HMSO 1989 Statutory Instrument No 1456 The Nurses, Midwives and Health Visitors (Registered Fever Nurses Amendment Rules and Training Amendment Rules) Approval Order 1989. HMSO, London

HMSO 1992 Making time for patients: a handbook for ward sisters. HMSO, London

Kershaw B, Salvage J (eds) 1986 Models for nursing. John Wiley, Chichester

Manthey M 1980 The practice of primary nursing. Blackwell, Boston

Marks-Maran D 1978 Patient allocation v. task allocation in relation to the nursing process. Nursing Times 74: 413–416

Ministry of Health (MoH) 1959 The report of the Committee on the Welfare of Children in Hospital. (Platt Report) HMSO, London

Muller D J, Harris P J, Wattley L, Taylor J D 1992 Nursing children: psychology, research and practice, 2nd edn. Chapman & Hall, London

Orem D 1991 Nursing concepts of practice, 4th edn. Mosby, St Louis

Price S 1994 The special needs of children. Journal of Advanced Nursing 20: 227–232

Robertson J 1970 Young children in hospital, 2nd edn. Tavistock, London

Roper N, Logan W W, Tierney A J 1990 The elements of nursing, 3rd edn. Churchill Livingstone, Edinburgh

Roy C, Andrews H A 1991 The Roy Adaptation model: the definitive statement. Appleton & Lange, Norwalk CT

Royal College of Nursing (RCN) 1990 Standards of care for paediatric nursing. Scutari Projects, Middlesex

Stephenson P 1987 Models for action. Nursing Times 83(29): 62–63

Walsh M 1990 From model to care plan. In: Salvage J, Kershaw B (eds) 1990 Models for nursing 2. Scutari Press, London

Wilding C, Wells M, Wilson J 1988 A model for family care. Nursing Times 84(15): 38–41

Wright S 1985 Special assignment. Nursing Times (28 Aug): 36–37

Yura H, Walsh M B 1988 The nursing process, 5th edn. Appleton & Lange, Norwalk CT

FURTHER READING

Aggleton P, Chalmers H 1990 Model future. Nursing Times 86(3): 41–43

Aggleton P, Chalmers H 1986 Nursing models and the nursing process. Macmillan Education, London

Binnie A 1987 Structural changes. Nursing Times 83(39): 36–37

Chavasse J M 1987 A comparison of three models of nursing. Nurse Education Today 7: 177–186

de la Cuesta C 1983 The nursing process: from development to implementation. Journal of Advanced Nursing 8: 365–371

Giovannetti P 1986 Evaluation of primary nursing. Annual Review of Nursing Research 4: 127–151

Hale C A 1988 Innovations in nursing care. Royal College of Nursing, London

Henderson V 1982 The nursing process—is the title right? Journal of Advanced Nursing 7: 103–109

McKenna H 1990 Which model? Nursing Times 86(25): 50–52

Malby R 1988 All you need is thought. Nursing Times 84(51): 46–48

Newton C 1991 The Roper–Logan–Tierney model in action. Macmillan, Basingstoke

Pearson A 1988 Primary nursing. Croom Helm, London

Pearson A, Vaughan B 1986 Nursing models for practice. Heinemann Nursing, London

Roper N, Logan W W, Tierney A J 1981 Learning to use the process of nursing. Churchill Livingstone, Edinburgh

Royal College of Nursing (RCN) 1990 Standards of care for paediatric nursing. Scutari Projects, Middlesex

Salvage J, Kershaw B 1990 Models for nursing 2. Scutari Press, London

Sutcliffe E 1990 Reviewing the nursing process. Senior Nurse 10(9): 9–13

Wilding C, Wells M, Wilson J 1988 A model for family care. Nursing Times 84(15): 38–41

Wright S 1990 My patient—my nurse. Scutari Press, London

Wright S 1990 Organisational issues of nursing models. Surgical Nurse 3(3): 22–26

9

General concepts in child care

Philippa Smith

In this chapter the student is introduced to a variety of general concepts that are pertinent to nursing children. It is hoped that, at the end of this chapter, the student will appreciate the importance of the child being nursed by an appropriately trained nurse and will be able to define the major differences between adult and paediatric nurses.

The chapter includes:
- the concept of family-centred care
- the effect of hospitalisation on the child and the family
- the importance of preparation of children and their parents for hospitalisation and surgery
- information on preoperative and postoperative care
- pain control
- the importance of play in hospital
- the uses of play during hospitalisation.

FAMILY-CENTRED CARE

The principle of making a child's stay in hospital as untraumatic as possible originates from the concept of family-centred care. This concept is a well-used but poorly defined idea which forms the basis for paediatric nursing. The main theme is that all care is based around the needs of the children and their families. Brunner & Suddarth (1981) define family-centred care as 'providing an opportunity to care for hospitalised children under nursing supervision, the goal being to maintain or strengthen the roles and ties of the family with the hospitalised child in order to promote normality of the family unit.' This may mean that the nurse becomes more of a teacher and assessor, an enabler rather than a doer (Stower 1992). This can be quite threatening for the nurse and is a move away from the traditional role, but it is of greater benefit to the child and his family, for all of whom the nurse is caring.

An important aspect of partnership in care is that, once it has been decided who is going to fulfil what aspects of nursing care, the decision is documented, otherwise things can get forgotten and care can be missed. This can be incorporated into care plans, and more units are redesigning their care plans to give space for the parents to sign to say what they are happy, confident and competent to take on. Casey's Partnership model (see Ch. 8) is especially for use within paediatrics, since it incorporates the concepts of family-centred care and partnership in care. The actual taking on of nursing skills by parents is not the only way that family-centred care can work. Some parents may not feel able to take on more responsibilities, or it may be that the child does not want his parents to become nurses. Robbins (1991, p. 36) suggested that they 'may simply be present as a reassuring and familiar figure, to give their child a sense of security in a strange environment, to play and support him through his stay', and this still comes within the concept of family-centred care.

In the past, when parental involvement was unheard of and visiting was once a week, the negative effects of hospitalisation were immense. One just has to look at the work of Bowlby (1965) and Robertson (1970) on separation anxiety to see evidence of this.

Much research has been done in this area and many theories have been suggested. As long ago as 1959, the Platt Committee looked at how children were being treated in hospital and advised admission of children with their mothers and unrestricted visiting (MoH 1959). The Platt Report stated that the new approach to

Activity 9.1

To what extent are parents involved in their children's care on the ward on which you work? How would you improve their level of involvement, or, if it is already good, how would you ensure that the level is maintained? What are important facts to remember in partnership in care?

the care of children should be based on mutual understanding between hospital staff and parents. This, of course, is still true today and is what family-centred care is aiming towards and, it is hoped, achieving.

There are, however, still staff who see parental involvement as a nuisance or as meaning the need for very little nursing input. There is a happy medium, which more units are managing to achieve with careful writing of philosophies and partnership with parents from the beginning. For this kind of philosophy to work, it is imperative that all staff interpret family-centred care in the same way and that parents have a good understanding of the concept.

It is important to remember that the family is a system in which no member exists alone. Action for Sick Children have done a lot of work for the rights of the child in hospital and, together with the Children Act 1989 and the Audit Commission Report (1992), they help to ensure that children receive the most appropriate care while they are in hospital. From a very practical point of view, a nurse dealing with an upset child, who has just been subjected to a very traumatic invasive procedure, will welcome parental involvement, because the parents are the only people who have a chance of settling a hysterical child.

THE EFFECTS OF HOSPITALISATION

The effects of hospitalisation will vary with age, but all age groups can show regression, 'the act of returning, going back' (Collins English Dictionary 1987, p. 444). In this case it means that children will go back to doing things that they

Activity 9.2

The parent of a 4-year-old child is very worried because the child has started to wet the bed again since coming into hospital. What reasons would you give and how would you reassure the parent?

did at a younger age. It is most visible in toddlers who may start wetting the bed after being dry at night, or only drinking from a bottle when they have been using a cup. It also happens to teenagers who will want their parents to stay when they are usually very independent or will have a temper tantrum over something fairly minor. It is children's way of showing that they are psychologically upset. Usually they will revert back to normal on discharge; sometimes regression may persist for a while after discharge but disappear when normality has been achieved.

It is important to allow children to take a familiar comforter and keep it with them at all times whilst in a strange environment like hospital. However old and disgusting you or their parents think it is, the child loves it and will receive a lot of comfort and reassurance from it.

Parents need support

Parents in hospital need support; it is a time of increased stress to them regardless of why their child is there. Be it an emergency admission, a booked admission for elective surgery or one of many hospitalisations for a chronic problem, the need for support will still be the same. It is important to remember that, as a nurse, you see many of the procedures that the children are admitted for every day and know that they are very routine, common and carry almost no risks;

Activity 9.3

How would you encourage an extremely worried and anxious parent to take some much-needed time-out?

parents do not and, even if they did, it is totally different when it is their child. They may feel guilty, that the reason their child is sick is somehow their fault. They may feel guilt if they do not stay with their child, or guilt for the other children who are left at home if they do stay at the hospital.

In hospital, they may feel that they have been made redundant as parents and end up feeling useless, that they have nothing to offer the child, or they may feel pressurised into taking on roles that they do not feel happy or confident with, simply because the staff expect it of them. This is where partnership in care should come into its own. The nurse and the parents should sit down and discuss what each person's role is, and the parents should feel free at any time to have their role reviewed, either because they feel able to take on more or because they need time-out to get themselves together or simply to have a rest.

Parents may not be able to comprehend what is happening and why, so the nurse must be sufficiently perceptive to recognise this situation and be there with explanations at the appropriate times. Parents often feel very alone, their partner may have gone home to care for the other children and they are left feeling frightened and redundant. If the child is suffering from a serious illness, the parents may feel that they must be strong for the child, yet not have come to terms with the diagnosis or their own feelings about it. This puts a lot of pressure on a parent. They may have to make decisions about things and, if that causes their child to suffer, they may well wonder whether they have made the right choice. If hospitalisation is prolonged, they may feel fed up and angry with the system and the whole situation and feel helpless and trapped. There are often financial worries which increase as the hospitalisation goes on.

It is important for the nurse to be aware of the actual or potential problems of parents, as it will probably be the nurse who bears the brunt of this pent-up anger. It is the nurse's role to help the whole family to accept the hospital experience as a positive one, although this can be understandably difficult at times. The nurse must:

- give support when necessary and back off at times
- give information, not only about the child's illness but practical information about where parents can leave their car, how a social worker can help them if they need one and where the canteen is
- remember that parents will not necessarily be able to take in a lot of information in one go so positive reinforcement and repetition is crucial
- help parents to tackle one problem at a time, using a problem-solving approach to come up with a coping strategy that includes the family as a whole—parents, siblings, grandparents and the extended family (Robbins 1991)
- stress the importance of parents having time together, alone and with the sick child's siblings—grandparents and friends are usually willing surrogate parents for an afternoon.

Including siblings is crucial; if they know what is going on they will feel part of it and less left out. If they understand or at least feel included, they may not feel as resentful about not seeing as much of their parents as their sick sibling (Bendor 1990). They may also not feel guilty, as siblings of sick children often do, thinking that the whole thing is their fault because of something they did, said or even thought (Taylor 1980). Sometimes they are understandably jealous of the sick child because, from their perspective, the sick child is getting spoilt with toys and attention whilst they are getting nothing (Kramer & Moore 1983). If they are included right from the beginning, they will have a better understanding.

As their nurse, you want to encourage parents to maintain as normal a routine as possible both at home and hospital, although that can take some imagination and work from both sides. You are there as much for the family as for the sick child. The parents' feelings will affect the sick child. If the parents are very upset and anxious, this will be passed on to the child; if the parents are relaxed as a result of being aware of what is happening and why, the child will be also. Do not force the parents to do anything that they are not happy with, and sometimes offer to do things that they normally do at home as they may feel like a break and their child being in hospital provides the perfect opportunity to have one. Just be there to offer support, encouragement, an ear to listen, a shoulder to cry on and friendship. Nights are often the time when relationships are built up with parents as they feel that you have more time and they are not keeping you from doing other things.

Support groups

Many intensive areas will have support groups for parents, run either by staff or by the parents themselves. These are usually very good, and some parents find it very useful to be with people who understand what they are feeling and going through, as they find that very few of their friend or relatives do. Parents will also support each other on a much more informal basis in the kitchen or in the smoking area and this is just as useful as a formal support group. It is important to remember that you cannot and should not try to force parents to attend these groups; you will usually find that they will go when they are ready.

More places now are starting to organise support groups for the siblings of children with serious conditions and these seem to be proving very worthwhile (Stone 1993).

PREPARING CHILDREN FOR ADMISSION TO HOSPITAL

A hospital admission is an anxiety-provoking experience for anybody. For a child who has limited or no past experience, or has preconceived ideas derived from the media or bad experiences, e.g. a grandparent who died in hospital or a 'helpful' friend who has already been in hospital, it can be even more frightening, especially for those experiencing emergency admissions. A lot of work has been done with adults, proving that providing information about an impending admission or procedure decreases anxiety and worry. Visintainer & Wolfer (1975) have proved that the same thing is true in children. Information increases their cooperation and decreases upset behaviour, resulting in less anxiety.

Unfortunately, pre-admission programmes are still not the norm in British hospitals, but are growing in favour thanks to the Department of Health endorsing the concept that modern child health care needs integration between hospital and community. A pre-admission programme is just this and would provide information to meet the social, emotional, psychological and spiritual needs of the whole family (Kiely 1989, Glasper et al 1989), although Acharya (1992) found that too much information increased anxiety levels.

This preparation could start at home if the parents were sent information that told them what to expect—unfortunately many parents do not mention a forthcoming hospitalisation to the child, as they do not know what to expect or what to tell their child and they themselves are very anxious about the situation (Acharya 1992). Jolly (1981) recommends that primary health care workers—GPs and health visitors—have a role in preparing children for hospitalisation, but this does not seem to work.

School-based education programmes

Elkins & Roberts (1983) have advocated that school-based education programmes are useful and that all children should participate routinely, giving all school-age children some idea of what to expect. This could be done in two ways:

- an organised hospital tour—McGarvey (1983) reported that a programme for pre-schoolers

Activity 9.4

What would you say to a parent whose child was coming into hospital for an operation, about the importance of telling the child that this was where he was going? How would you cope if you felt very strongly that the child needed to know, but the parent thought not?

to experience what happens in hospitals was well received by children, teachers and parents
- setting up a 'play hospital' at school, encouraging children to play with real hospital equipment in both free and structured play.

Both of these ideas could be organised and worked through with school nurses and teachers, with parental involvement, and could produce the basis for a whole term's topic work, at the same time as familiarising the children with the hospital situation. This would be beneficial to all children, as emergency admission is a possibility for any child.

When the time of admission is known

Children coming in as booked admissions should be easier to prepare because the reason for the admission and its time are already established. An increasing number of hospitals are practising day care surgery for routine operations. For children, this is a definite advantage (Campbell et al 1988) and it has the added benefit of being a cheaper option for hospitals, something that is important nowadays. Children who are having day care procedures need just as much preparation as those who will be hospitalised for a longer time, but as there is less time it will often be missed or reduced to the bare minimum.

Children can have 'funny' ideas as to why they have come into hospital. They may, for example, regard it is a punishment for being naughty or because their parents do not want them any more, so it is very important for staff to give parents enough information to enable them to start preparing their child before admission. It is important that everybody involved knows what the child has been told, and what the child has been told should be exactly what happens. Children will trust and believe what they have been told and, if what happens is different, they will lose their trust in whoever told them, which can make life very difficult for all involved and is very unfair on the child.

Pre-admission programmes

A preoperative admission programme may well be beneficial for children who are being admitted for booked procedures. This would include:

- information being sent to the parents well in advance of the admission
- an invitation to the unit to have a look around
- the chance to meet some of the staff including the play therapists, who have a very important role, and the theatre staff.

Parents should have what is expected of them explained and the ward philosophy should also be discussed. There should be a chance for asking questions, and parents should be given useful information such as sleeping arrangements, facilities available and what they need to bring for themselves and their child. Like their children, they need to be shown around and to see things such as the bathroom, pay phone, school room, playroom, shop, canteen, smoking area, parents' room and nursing office.

The children should also have what is going to happen explained to them and be given a chance to ask questions or voice any worries that they may have. They should have the opportunity to play with equipment that will be used on them. It is also important for them to have something to take home that will promote discussion between them and their parents. The parents may also find it useful to have the information that they have been given written down to take away. The time between the visit and the admission should not be so long that they may forget things, but should be long enough to allow them a few days to assimilate the information and have the chance to ask questions.

On admission, there should be reiteration of information and an opportunity for questions. It is also a good idea to try to find out how much the parents and child understand, allowing the nurse to know what areas need to be repeated in more detail. Many places that are introducing pre-admission visits use questionnaires to audit the usefulness of the visit and reveal any areas that need further attention.

PREPARATION FOR SURGERY

A day case is a child who has been seen as an outpatient and whose condition is considered suitable for day case surgery. This will depend on the type of operation, how far away from the hospital the family live and whether there are any other health problems. In the outpatients' department, the surgeon will give a full explanation of what the operation entails and, when happy, the parent will sign the consent form. The child will be examined and any blood tests that are needed will be done. This is a perfect opportunity for preparation of the child and the family, which should begin months before day surgery (Norris 1992). It is very important to prepare both family and child for a stressful event, as one will affect the other (Crocker 1980).

Parents should receive adequate information through the post about when to start fasting their child and why they are doing it. This should be worked out for each child individually and there should not be a blanket time for all children, e.g. 12 midnight. It will depend on what time the child is going to theatre, morning or afternoon, and how old the child is. A baby need only be fasted for 4 hours, whilst an older child should be fasted for 6 hours preoperatively.

Admission

On admission, the child will be re-oriented to the ward and the nurse should go through the plan for the day, ensuring that both child and parents are aware of what their roles are and are happy with them. A good first impression is imperative as there is only a short time in which to gain the family's trust. Baseline observations of temperature, pulse, respirations and blood pressure should be recorded along with weight and height. A name band should be put on the child and his bed and gown (if necessary) shown to him. At this point, he should be allowed to go to the playroom or do whatever he wants, although it is a good idea to put a sticker on him saying that he cannot have anything to eat or drink to stop other parents feeding him when he says he is hungry. The admitting nurse should then inform the surgeon's team and the anaesthetist that the child is on the ward, and check the notes for the consent form and blood results.

The role of the parents

Action for Sick Children have written a policy, *Just for the Day* (Thornes 1984), offering guidelines for day care surgery. They have also written a policy for the emotional care of children who are going to have surgery (Action for Sick Children 1990b), and any area that admits children for surgical procedures should strive to comply with their suggestions. One of their beliefs is that a child needs the support of his parents on the day of operation and that they should be able to accompany the child from the ward to the anaesthetic room and be with the child until he is asleep. This has been met with mixed reactions from those involved, and many studies have been done to test the hypothesis that children benefit from parental presence in the anaesthetic room. On reviewing the literature, the general consensus was that with adequate preparation and counselling about their role, what to do and when to leave, parental presence was beneficial and made the induction of anaesthesia a calm procedure for the child. It sometimes produced anxiety in the parents but, even then, most parents said that they were pleased to have been there and would repeat the exercise if necessary (Glasper 1988, Coulson 1988). Turner (1989) found little difference between the children whose parents were present and those whose parents were not. The ultimate decision is made by the anaesthetist, and reasons that anaesthetists gave for not allowing parents to be present included the worry that a parent would faint and become an extra patient and that parents were an infection risk.

Premedication and induction

The anaesthetist will decide on the most appropriate premedication, although this is often just a personal preference (Redford 1990). With the increasing number of day cases that are being done, no premedication is given, so methods of getting to theatre that produce less anxiety can be used; tricycles and bikes make the journey to theatre different and fun. The anaesthetist will also decide the method of induction that is most suitable, ideally in consultation with the parents. If a needle is necessary the anaesthetist should ensure that EMLA (a local anaesthetic) is prescribed on the drug chart, and ward staff should ensure that it is applied and has time to work properly. If it does not work, the child will lose faith in the cream and will not want it again. The need for the use of intramuscular injections has now gone, and very few children will have them as a premedication. The argument for using them is usually that the analgesic content will carry the child through the postoperative pain, although it could be argued that it would be kinder to give the injection straight after the operation, while the child is still anaesthetised (Colliss 1990). Whatever premedication a child has, once it has been taken the child should be encouraged to be quiet and relaxed to get the optimum effect from it.

During the operation, the surgeon should ensure that as many painful procedures are performed as necessary, for example the insertion of peripheral cannulae, giving of intramuscular analgesia and even minor things like the removal of old plasters which take seconds to do and can prevent a lot of upset and discomfort for the child. 'Dressings, drains and catheters should be adequately fixed because the awake,

Activity 9.5

What action could you take if an anaesthetist had promised a child and her mother that no needles would be used until the child was asleep using gas, and that old plasters would be removed whilst asleep. In the anaesthetic room no attempt is made to give the child gas, a cannula is inserted without EMLA cream and mother and child are very upset. How would you cope? Who would you be the advocate for?

disorientated child can remove all attachments in record time if given the opportunity' (Colliss 1990, p. 16).

PAIN CONTROL

Pain relief is another area that involves anaesthetists and surgeons. Contrary to the belief that babies and children do not feel pain like adults do, 'pain is what the patient says it is' (McCaffery 1969; cited by McCaffery & Beebe 1986) regardless of whether the patient is an adult, a child, or a baby whose only way of communicating is by crying. For major surgical procedures, there are now subcutaneous or intravenous infusion pumps that can deliver either nurse- or patient-controlled analgesia (PCA). These pumps give a background continuous infusion of analgesic with the opportunity for the child to instigate a bolus dose when necessary. It is quite possible for children of adequate cognitive ability to use these pumps as long as they understand what they must do, when they must do it and what the effect is. Children must be encouraged to give themselves a bolus as soon as they start to hurt, by pushing the handset. The pumps have a lock-out system, so it is impossible for children to give themselves too much analgesia. The pumps are carefully set by nurse specialists or anaesthetists and closed with a key, making accidentally changing the rate impossible. The pump will tell you how many times the child has tried to give himself a bolus and how many of these were good tries, which aids in evaluating his pain control. There is no set age at which a child can use one of these pumps and children must be assessed individually. Children must also understand that the pump will make them hurt less and not make them completely free of pain. 'A PCA pump is a valuable option for carefully assessed patients, but both medical and nursing staff must be aware of the potential problems and limitations to get the most from them' (Llewellyn 1993, p. 13). This is just one way of decreasing the amount of intramuscular injections a child will need to have, the fear of which will force a child

to lie about the degree of pain he is in (Burr 1993). There are many oral analgesics that can be given to children as soon as they are able to swallow. Children will not become addicted to opiates through their use after surgery, so adequate pain relief should and must be given to all children.

In the past there has been an under-treatment of children's pain, mainly due to the difficulty involved in assessing and measuring the pain that a child is in (Goldman & Lloyd Thomas 1991) and this has lead to the use of pain assessment charts. The chart that is used must be appropriate to the child's age, and the child must understand what it does. Pain assessment charts may not be useful to all children, but are still worth trying. Some staff may need encouragement to use them. Examples of pain assessment charts include the 'Oucher' by Beyer (1984) and Eland's Colour Chart (Foster et al 1989). When looking at a child's degree of pain, it is important to include the parents, as they know their child best and they know how their child likes to be comforted (Dearmun 1993).

There are methods other than pharmacological ones that can be used as pain relief. These include distraction therapy, positioning and hypnotherapy; often a combination of these methods gives the best results.

POSTOPERATIVE CARE

Practical aspects of postoperative care include explaining things age-appropriately to children and their parents so that they have some ideas of what to expect. They should be told, for example:

Activity 9.6

In what ways, other than verbally, could you assess the amount of pain that a child is in, and how well the pain is controlled? What else, and what other methods could you use?

- that the child may vomit
- that it is routine to record observations of pulse and respirations frequently on return to the ward
- that the child may well sleep for the remainder of the day.

For day case surgery the discharge will have been discussed with the parents at the outpatient appointment, but it is important to reiterate this information—that the child must be fully awake, have eaten, drunk, passed urine and not be in excessive pain. The parents must be happy to take the child home, have information about analgesia, a number to ring in an emergency, an appointment for when the child will be next seen, an idea about how long the child needs to take off school and information about removal of sutures or dressings. Areas that are lucky enough to have a paediatric community nurse team may have a policy that the nurse will visit all day cases the next day to check that everything is all right.

Discharge planning should start from admission, from both the health professionals' and parents' points of view. Parents should be given as much information, help and practical advice as they need to ensure that the discharge goes smoothly (Norris 1992).

THE IMPORTANCE OF PLAY

It is said that play is the work of a child (Foster et al 1989); it contributes to and is an expression of development. As children play, social, cognitive, physical and emotional skills are learnt and perfected. Children start to play at a very early age and this continues in various shapes and forms until adulthood. Through the medium of play 'children learn what no-one can teach them' (Goldensen & Hartley 1963; cited by Foster et al 1989, p. 663).

Uses of play to the hospitalised child

There are many ways in which play is important to children in hospital and useful to the nurses

caring for them. As soon as children are put into a strange environment their anxiety levels will rise. A good way of relaxing children is with toys and games, as they are safe things that children consider themselves to be experts with. Vessey & Mahon (1990) talk about two different types of play:

- normative play
- therapeutic play.

Normative play. All children use normative play. This is something that is spontaneous and pleasurable, child led and voluntary with no extrinsic goals. This play is very important to hospitalised children and their siblings as it maintains some normality in an otherwise abnormal and strange situation.

Therapeutic play. This is different in its design and intent. It is guided by professionals who have goals that the play is going to achieve, the main one being to 'facilitate the emotional and physical well-being of hospitalised children' (Vessey & Mahon 1990, p. 328).

Through both types of play, specialists can tell a lot about how children feel about what is happening to them. Through play, a child may show fear of an upcoming procedure or a sibling may show guilt about hospitalisation, a lack of trust, anger or fear. Vessey & Mahon (1990) talk of three types of therapeutic play:

- emotional outlet play
- instructional play
- physiologically enhancing play.

Emotional outlet play

Children will turn to play for emotional release when they are unable to cope with the situation that they find themselves in. Emotional outlet play is initiated to facilitate this. Children are encouraged to re-enact events with the ability to be in control of the situation and to resolve the problems they were faced with. This type of play is often used to diagnose child abuse and the use of anatomically correct dolls has made this of greater benefit. It can also be used to help hospitalised children come to terms with a new physical disability, but needs to be done in a safe, non-threatening environment. Specialists can help children express their fantasies and anxieties through play, but it will take time and perseverance for children to build up enough trust in an individual to do so. Therefore this type of play cannot be rushed and must be taken at the child's own pace.

Instructional play

The second type of therapeutic play that Vessey & Mahon discuss is instructional play. This is the preparation for forthcoming procedures through play. Smallwood (1988) discusses the preparation of children for surgery through play and includes the use of real equipment in a safe and non-threatening environment where they can participate as much or as little as they like. He suggests the use of disposable equipment for children to keep to promote further discussion at home.

Instructional play can also be used to clarify information that children have already got. A method often used involves puppets which the children can work, and often the puppets will have their own fears and anxieties about the forthcoming procedures. Oncology wards will often have teddy bears with Hickman lines or dolls with no hair.

It is important in this type of play to show children that some things will be reversible. An example is a board game used to teach children about cancer. It introduces a child, either a boy or girl, who has had to come into hospital, and goes into detail about the blood cells and what their

jobs are, for example the white blood cells are the soldiers, and what happens to them when they are attacked by the 'baddie' cells. The child will need to have medicine through a drip and by mouth and in the end will lose his hair, feel ill and the doctors may have to do nasty things to him to make him better, but in the end the little boy's hair will grow back and he will be well again. It is surprising how many children do not mind losing their hair as long as they know that it will grow back when they are better. This kind of game will explain to children what is happening and can be as personalised as they or the parents wish it to be. It will introduce some new and strange words to them, but will also reassure them that although things may be horrible at that moment, in time things will be all right. This gives the children the chance to ask questions if they wish to and have fun at the same time. The information given through this game can be as much or as little as the play specialist wishes and is usually discussed with the parents first. The game can be returned to at each stage of treatment. It can also be made age appropriate which is an important factor in all therapeutic play.

Physiologically enhancing play

Physiologically enhancing play is play that is used to get children to do exercises or actions that are necessary to improve their condition but that they will not do when asked. A good example of this would be a child who has a chest infection and needs to be encouraged to do deep breathing exercises. If children are asked to breathe in deeply 10 times every hour, it is unlikely they would do so simply because they had been asked to, even if they understood the request and were able to comply with it. Deep breathing exercises can, however, become a part of play. Blowing bubbles or paint blowing will both enhance deep breathing and the child will be having fun at the same time, so the exercise does not become a task. The activities that are encouraged should be to treat a specific pathological condition and be age appropriate (Vessey & Mahon 1990).

Activity 9.7

In what ways could you begin to work with an extremely needle-phobic child, who you know will need a lot of injections in the near future? What other professionals could you involve?

Play, both normalising and therapeutic should be used in all anxiety-provoking areas, including the GP's surgery, dentist's surgery and clinics. It reduces tension, keeps children busy and occupied and allows the professional to see them at play, a medium through which a lot can be told. Throughout all types of play, children need the acceptance of an important adult. A parent or significant other can help to promote the child's development by encouraging participation in a variety of activities and should be encouraged to recognise the child's individuality.

I hope that this chapter has given you an insight into a number of subjects that are of utmost importance to a children's nurse, making it obvious why a child has the right to a specifically trained nurse. I hope it has emphasised the differences between adults and children in hospital and provided information about the nurse's role in caring for both the child and the family. It is important to remember, as stated by Casey (1988), that the child and the family are interlinked and you will never get one without the other.

With a little bit of forward planning and insight, a child's experience of hospital can be trouble-free, non-anxiety-producing and non-threatening and will result in no long-term psychological or physical ill effects. You must remember that these children are the parents of the future. If they have no bad memories of their time in hospital, they will pass on only positive impressions to their children. As Redford (1990, p. 12) states, 'if the child needs further hospitalisation and comes back without fear then we know we got it right the first time.'

REFERENCES

Acharya S 1992 Assessing the need for pre-admission visits. Paediatric Nursing 4(9): 20–23

Action for Sick Children 1990a Charter number two. HMSO, London

Action For Sick Children 1990b Emotional preparation for surgery. Nursing Standard 4(32): 4

Audit Commission Report 1992 HMSO, London

Bendor S 1990 Anxiety and isolation in siblings of pediatric cancer patient. Social Work in Health Care 14(3): 17–33

Beyer J 1984 The Oucher: a user's manual and technical report. The Hospital Play Equipment Company, Evanston Ill

Bowlby J 1965 Child care and growth of love. Pelican, Harmondsworth

Brunner L, Suddarth D S 1981, Lippincott manual of paediatric nursing. HarperCollins, London

Burr S 1993 Myths in practice in managing pain in children. Nursing Standard Supplement 7(25): 4

Campbell I et al 1988 Psychological effects of day case surgery, compared with inpatient surgery. Archives of Disease in Childhood 63: 415–417

Campbell P et al 1993 Keeping it in the family. Child Health 1(1): 17–20

Casey A 1988 A partnership with child and family. Senior Nurse 8(4): 8–9

Children Act 1989 HMSO, London

Collins 1987 Collins English dictionary. Collins, London, p 444

Colliss V 1990 Pre and post-operative management. Paediatric Nursing 2(15): 12–13

Coulson D 1988 A proper place for parents. Nursing Times 84(19): 26–28

Crocker E 1980 Reactions of children to health care encounters. In: Robinson G, Clarke H (eds) The hospital care of children. Oxford University Press, New York

Dearmun A 1993 Towards a partnership in pain management. Paediatric Nursing 5(5): 8–10

Eiser C et al 1989 Preparing children for hospital; a school based intervention. Professional Nurse 4(6): 297–299

Elkins R, Roberts M 1983 Psychological preparation for paediatric hospitalisation. Clinical Psychological Review 3: 275–295

Foster R et al 1989 Family centred nursing care of children. Saunders, Philadelphia, pp 868–877

Glasper A 1988 Parents in the anaesthetic room: a blessing or a curse. Professional Nurse 3(4): 112–115

Glasper A et al 1989 Preparing children for admission. Paediatric Nursing 1(5): 18–20

Goldman A, Lloyd Thomas A 1991 Pain management in children. British Medical Bulletin 47(3): 676–689

Jolly M 1981 The other side of paediatrics—a guide to the everyday care of sick children. Macmillan, London

Kiely T 1989 Preparing children for admission to hospital. Nursing 3(33): 42–44

Kramer R, Moore I 1983 Meeting the special needs of healthy siblings. Cancer Nursing 6(3): 213–217

Llewellyn N 1993 The use of PCA for paediatric post-operative pain management. Paediatric Nursing 5(5): 12–15

McCaffery M, Beebe A 1986 Pain: clinical manual for nursing practice. Mosby, St Louis, p 7

McGarvey M 1983 Preschool hospital tours. Children's Health Care 13: 31–36

Ministry of Health (MoH) 1959 The welfare of children in hospital. Report of the Committee on Child Health Services. (Platt Report) HMSO, London

Norris E 1992 Making the day bearable. Paediatric Nursing 4(3): 21–23

Redford P 1990 Physical and emotional care. Paediatric Nursing 2(5): 12–13

Robbins M 1991 Sharing the care. Nursing Times 87(8): 36–38

Robertson J 1970 Young children in hospital, 2nd edn. Tavistock, London

Robinson G, Clarke H 1980 Reactions of children to health care encounters. Hospital care of children. Oxford University Press, Oxford

Smallwood S 1988 Preparing children for surgery. AORN Journal 47(1): 177–185

Stone F 1993 Lending an ear to the unheard. Child Health 1(2): 54–58

Stower S 1992 Partnership in caring. Journal of Clinical Nursing 1: 67–72

Taylor S 1980 Siblings need a plan of care too. Pediatric Nursing 6(6): 9–13

Thornes R 1984 Just for the day. Caring for children in the Health Service. Action for Sick Children (formerly NAWCH), London

Turner L 1989 Creating the right atmosphere. Nursing Times 85(32): 34–35

Vessey J, Mahon 1990 Therapeutic play and the hospitalised child. Journal of Pediatric Nursing 5(5): 328–333

Visintainer M, Wolfer J 1975 Psychological preparation for surgical paediatric patients. The effects on children's and parents' stress responses and adjustment. Paediatrics 56(2): 187–202

FURTHER READING

Eiser C et al 1984 Children's perceptions of hospital. British Journal of Nursing Studies 21(1): 45–50

Fradd E 1987 A child alone. Nursing Times 83(42): 16–17

McClowry S 1988 A review of literature pertaining to psycho-social responses of school age children. Journal of Pediatric Nursing 3(5): 296–299

Marriner J 1988 A children's tour. Nursing Times 8(40): 39–40

3 Nursing: principles and skills for practice

The child is physiologically immature and therefore has different physiological needs to that of an adult. This section aims to illustrate some of these differences and to discuss the changes that take place during childhood. These differences will affect the way in which the infant and the child is affected by ill health. Children's nurses need to develop special skills to enable them to meet the needs of the sick child.

10

The circulatory system

Sue Davies   Linda McQuaid

The aim of this chapter is to:
- describe the changes from the fetal circulatory system to that of the infant
- describe the main cardiac abnormalities that may compromise a child's cardiovascular system, their effects and the treatments required
- consider the effects upon the family of a child with cardiac disease and the care the family will require
- describe the basic principles of cardiovascular health assessment outlining some of the more detailed investigations
- outline some of the haematological problems affecting children
- identify key nursing issues when using intravenous therapy, having looked at the reasons why it may be necessary.

CHANGES IN THE CIRCULATION AT BIRTH

In the fetus, blood is relatively well oxygenated due to several factors:

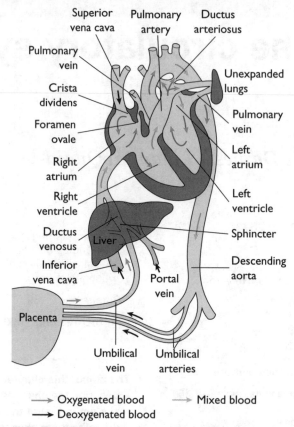

Figure 10.1   The fetal circulation. Arrows indicate the direction of blood flow.
(Reproduced from Kelnar & Harvey 1988 by kind permission.)

- the ability of fetal haemoglobin to carry more oxygen than maternal haemoglobin does
- a high haemoglobin count of 18–20 g/100 ml
- a high erythrocyte count.

Fetal blood passes from the placenta through the umbilical vein (Fig. 10.1). This vessel is unusual in that it is one of the few veins in the body carrying oxygenated blood. From here it passes through the ductus venosus and then the inferior vena cava to the right atrium. Most of this blood goes through the foramen ovale to the left atrium because, in the fetus, the pressure in the right side of the heart is higher than in the left side.

From the left atrium, the blood passes into the left ventricle where it is pumped into the ascending aorta. The superior vena cava receives blood from the fetal head, neck and coronary sinuses. This empties into the right atrium, passes through the tricuspid valve and out through the pulmonary artery. As the fetal lung is not expanded, there is a high pulmonary resistance due to the constricted arteries. A small amount of blood will pass to the pulmonary vessels but most will pass across the ductus arteriosus into the aorta. Blood will flow back to the placenta from the descending aorta via the two umbilical arteries.

At birth the most significant change occurs when the first breath expands the lungs and the pulmonary vascular resistance falls. The placental blood flow will be lost and there will be an increase in the systemic vascular resistance. The pressure will now be higher in the left atrium than in the right atrium, causing the foramen ovale to close (Fig. 10.2). The rise in oxygen

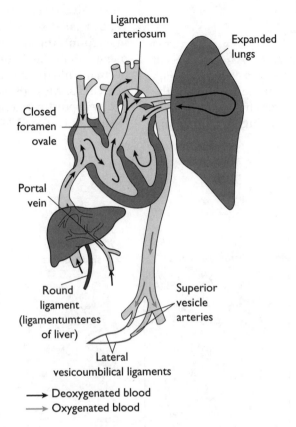

Ligamentum
arteriosum

Expanded
lungs

Closed
foramen
ovale

Portal
vein

Round
ligament
(ligamentumteres
of liver)

Superior
vesicle
arteries

Lateral
vesicoumbilical ligaments

⟶ Deoxygenated blood
⟶ Oxygenated blood

Figure 10.2   The circulation at birth. Arrows indicate the direction of blood flow. (Reproduced from Kelnar & Harvey 1988 by kind permission.)

saturation, as respiration is established, will cause the closure of the ductus arteriosus. As the umbilical vessels are cut, the ductus venosus loses its blood flow and will close, eventually forming a ligament.

These are not all immediate occurrences and a premature baby for instance may have a persistent patent ductus arteriosus for several weeks following birth (see Ch. 20).

CONGENITAL HEART DEFECTS

The majority of cardiac disease in children is due to a congenital defect and the clinical consequences of that defect. Approximately eight children in every 1000 will have a congenital heart defect (Jordan & Scott 1989) but only four of the eight children will require treatment—either cardiac surgery or invasive cardiac catheterisation techniques, for example septostomy.

If cardiac disease or abnormality is confirmed, or either is strongly suspected, the child should be referred to a paediatric cardiac unit for further assessment and management.

Congenital heart defects can be divided into acyanotic defects (pink babies) and cyanotic defects (blue babies). A right-to-left shunt causes central cyanosis, as some blood passes from the right to the left of the heart without perfusing the alveoli so that there is deoxygenated blood in the systemic circulation. In a left-to-right shunt, blood passes back from the left to the right of the heart during one circulatory phase.

Left-to-right shunt

Ventricular septal defect (VSD)

This is the most common defect. A hole is present in the septum between the two ventricles (Fig. 10.3A), shunting blood from the left side of the heart to the right and increasing blood flow to the lungs. At birth, there is higher pulmonary artery resistance and consequent higher right ventricular pressure and so there is often minimal shunt through the defect initially. This means that the baby's heart usually sounds normal until pressure in the right side of the heart falls. Most (80%) of VSDs close normally and without treatment before the age of 8 years (Kelnar & Harvey 1988).

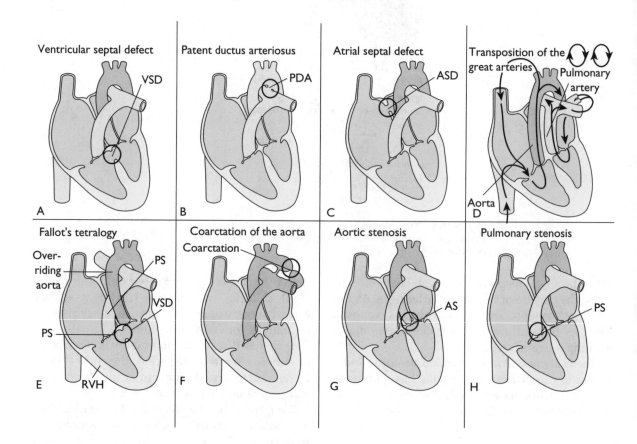

Figure 10.3   Congenital heart defects. Key: AS = aortic stenosis; ASD = atrial septal defect; PDA = patent ductus arteriosus; PS = pulmonary stenosis; RVH = right ventricular hypertrophy; TGA = transposition of the great arteries; VSD = ventricular septal defect.

Patent ductus arteriosus (PDA)

In this defect, the ductus arteriosus fails to close following birth (Fig. 10.3B). Blood flow reverses and flows through the duct from the aorta to the pulmonary artery increasing blood flow to the lungs. Babies with rubella syndrome often have a PDA in conjunction with a septal defect. The premature baby will often have a persistent PDA, although closure is usually spontaneous. See also Chapter 20.

Atrial septal defect (ASD)

As in VSD there is a hole present in the septum, but this time between the two atria (Fig. 10.3C). This causes blood to flow from the left side of the heart to the right, increasing flow to the lungs. There are two types of ASD—ostium primum, which is the more serious, and ostium secundum, which is the higher defect, i.e. an opening in the upper part of the atrial septum. The more serious defect is at the lower part of the septum and is found in conjunction with mitral valve abnormalities.

Right-to-left shunt

Transposition of the great arteries

This is a condition requiring urgent treatment to save the baby's life. The aorta and pulmonary artery are transposed and arise from the wrong ventricle, i.e. the aorta arises from the right - ventricle and the pulmonary artery from the left (Fig. 10.3D). There are therefore two separate circulations; blood is returning from the left side of the heart to the lungs and from the right side of the heart to the body. Initially, after birth, there is mixing of blood between the pulmonary and systemic circulations, through the patent ductus arteriosus and foramen ovale. As the ductus closes, generally within the first 24 hours of life, the baby becomes progressively cyanosed.

Fallot's tetralogy

There are four abnormalities (Fig. 10.3E):

- ventricular septal defect
- overriding aorta
- pulmonary stenosis—see 'Obstructive lesions' below
- right ventricular hypertrophy.

The child may have marked cyanosis if:

- the aorta overrides the VSD to a great extent, when deoxygenated blood will be drawn into the aorta and enter the systemic circulation, and/or
- the pulmonary stenosis is severe, leading to a greatly diminished blood flow to the lungs.

Obstructive lesions

Coarctation of the aorta

The aorta is narrowed (Fig. 10.3F) and there is diminished blood flow to the lower half of the body.

Aortic stenosis

The aortic valve is narrowed (Fig. 10.3G) and there is diminished blood flow through the valve into the aorta. The left ventricle becomes hypertrophied as it pumps against the resistance. There may be pulmonary congestion.

Pulmonary stenosis

The pulmonary valve leaflets are thickened (Fig. 10.3H) and there is diminished blood flow to the lungs. This may result in cyanosis, although luckily both this and aortic stenosis rarely produce heart failure in the newborn period.

SIGNS OF HEART DISEASE IN THE NEWBORN

A full cardiovascular assessment is indicated if one or more of the following signs are present:

1. tachypnoea—above 60 breaths/minute
2. cyanosis
3. tachycardia—above 160 beats/minute

4. dyspnoea
5. difficulty with feeds
6. grunting
7. abnormal heart sounds—'murmurs'
8. increased weight gain in spite of poor feeding.

If it is suspected that the child has a heart defect, investigations will be needed to help reach a diagnosis. As with any potentially serious condition, the parents will be devastated and the nurse will often be needed to repeat and reinforce the information that they have been given by somebody else.

ASSESSMENT OF THE CARDIOVASCULAR SYSTEM

The child whose cardiovascular system is being assessed should be quiet and rested. If he is struggling and upset, or has been exercising, the recording may not truly reflect the child's condition.

It is not always easy to gain the cooperation of some younger children and, as with any unfamiliar technique, as much time as necessary should be spent explaining the procedures to the children and their families. Small children will often prefer to sit on their mothers' laps, but the mothers' fears must be allayed for this to be really helpful. Allow the children to handle any equipment and demonstrate it on their toys. If, despite all this, the child is still very distressed, it may be necessary to withdraw for a while and return later.

Assessment of a child's cardiovascular system involves a combination of observation and measurement of the following indicators of the child's condition.

Colour

This should be uniform across the body; the mucous membranes, palms of hands and soles of feet should be pink. If the circulation is compromised, the child may be mottled with pale palms and soles. The mucous membranes, especially the lips and tongue, are the best place to check for signs of cyanosis because of their vascularity.

The child may be cyanosed constantly or intermittently, perhaps on exertion such as feeding in a baby or exercise in an older child. Continual assessments of colour change over time are crucial.

Perfusion of the extremities

The child's hands and feet should be warm with brisk capillary refill. If the circulation is compromised and perfusion of the extremities poor, the hands and feet will be cold to the touch with delayed capillary filling. It is important to remember that a low atmospheric temperature may affect the temperature of the child's hands and feet.

Pulse

When measuring the pulse rate, count for 1 minute, noting the regularity of the pulse as well as its strength. Sites at which the pulse rate can be measured are shown in Figure 10.4. Normal heart rates for children are given in Table 10.1.

Babies

It is very difficult to feel the radial pulse in either a newborn or an older baby due to the small size of the blood vessels. Babies may also have chubby wrists, which again makes identification of the radial pulse difficult. Sites at which the pulse is more easily felt are the carotid and femoral and it may be helpful to practice feeling

Table 10.1 Normal heart rates in children (adapted from Adamson & Hill 1984)

Age	Beats per minute
Birth	110–150
Infants	100–140
1–5 years	80–120
5–15 years	70–100

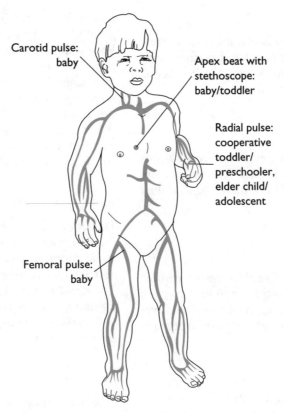

Figure 10.4 Sites for measuring the pulse rate.

the latter when changing a baby's nappy. In general, however, it is probably easiest and less disturbing to listen to the baby's heartbeat with a stethoscope—listening to the apical impulse of the heart. This is heard by placing the stethoscope on the left side of the child's chest, just below the nipple, and counting the beats for 1 minute.

It is possible to listen through a vest or thin clothing so as not to disturb the baby too much. If care is taken, it can be done when the baby is asleep.

Toddlers and pre-school-age children

If the child is cooperative, it may be possible to feel a radial pulse, but toddlers also have a desire to wriggle and twist their hands, making an accurate recording impossible. Again, it may be easier for child and nurse to count the toddler's apex beat by listening through a stethoscope.

School-age children and adolescents

With careful explanation, cooperation should be possible in both age groups and a radial pulse can be taken.

Respiration

When observing a respiratory pattern, again count for 1 minute when the child is at rest. Note the rise and fall of the chest, the rate and depth of respiration plus any irregularities of breathing pattern, grunting, sternal retraction or nasal flaring.

Babies

The respirations are probably most accurately recorded by lightly placing a hand on the baby's chest to feel the chest movement. This technique may also be applied to toddlers.

Older children

This age group should have their respirations observed whilst the pulse and temperature are being taken so that they are unaware that they are being watched.

Oxygen saturation

If there is any suspicion of cyanosis or cardiac disease, the child should have an oxygen saturation recording made. The method of carrying this out is covered more fully in Chapter 11.

Blood pressure

This may be measured manually using a mercury sphygmomanometer or electronically using a device such as a 'Dinamap'. It is likely to be easier, quicker and more accurate to use an electronic device to take the blood pressure of babies and young children, due to the difficulty in hearing the younger child's pulse using an auscultatory method with the mercury sphygmomanometer.

Selecting the correct size of cuff

When taking a blood pressure using either device, it is crucial to select the correct size of blood pressure cuff. Failure to do so will result in inaccurate measurements. When considering the cuff size, it is the bladder within the cuff that is important not the overall size of the material cuff. It is important to ensure that the inflatable bladder is able to encircle the limb that is being used for the blood pressure measurement (Frohlich et al 1988). If the bladder does not encircle the limb, the measurement will be falsely high, and if the bladder overlaps itself greatly, the measurement will be falsely low. Wrong measurement may then lead to inappropriate treatments. Some cuffs with Velcro fastenings have range markings to assist with selecting the correct cuff size. If the overlap of the cuff occurs within the two range lines then the correct size has been selected and if not the cuff is either too large or too small. This sort of cuff is mainly found with the electronic devices.

Reassuring the child before the measurement

The child should be relaxed and cooperative. Explain what is to happen in simple terms that are appropriate to the child's developmental age and let him handle the equipment to be used. The child should be warned that the cuff will tighten round his arm, and told that keeping still will make the measurement easier to do and so over more quickly.

Measurement of the blood pressure

Mercury sphygmomanometer. Using a stethoscope in the antecubital fossa, the systolic pressure value should be recorded at the start of the first Korotkoff sound—the clear tapping sound. The diastolic pressure should be recorded in children up to 12 years of age at the fourth Korotkoff sound—the low-pitched muffled sound. Children over the age of 12 years have the diastolic pressure recorded at the disappearance of all sound—the fifth Korotkoff sound (Whaley & Wong 1991).

If no sounds can be heard with a stethoscope, a systolic recording only can be taken by palpating the pulse as the cuff is deflated—the value is recorded as the point at which the pulse reappears. Alternatively, a small Doppler instrument may be applied to the pulse point; the systolic value is recorded as the point at which the pulse became inaudible (Weller 1978).

Electronic method. Devices such as 'Dinamaps' are commonly available on children's wards and are especially useful for frequent blood pressure recordings. If using an electronic

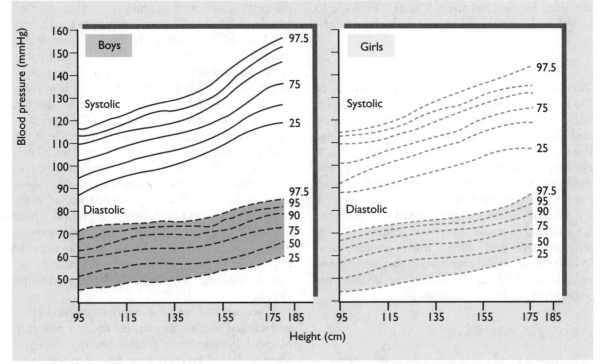

Figure 10.5 The relation of blood pressure to height in children. Figures are percentages of boys and girls. (Reproduced from de Swiet et al 1989 by kind permission.)

device, the child can be involved more readily by asking him to press the start button on the machine. Some children requiring regular blood pressure monitoring become quite adept at helping to carry out their own measurements.

Graphs of normal paediatric blood pressure values are given in Figure 10.5.

INVESTIGATIONS

Electrocardiography

An electrocardiogram (ECG) can be difficult to assess in the newborn period because of the rapid changes that are taking place. Nevertheless, information can be gained about the rate and rhythm patterns as well as looking for myocardial damage or hypertrophy. Although the test is non-invasive and does not hurt, a baby may be distressed simply by being held and, again, much reassurance for the parents will be necessary. Older children should have the test

explained to them by the nurse and/or hospital play specialist in language and style appropriate to their developmental age. For instance, if they understand the concepts of electrical power, they can be told that it is a test that will record the electrical activity of the heart. They should be given time to look at the ECG machine and handle the leads if they wish. It may be beneficial to reassure them that the test will be completed quickly if they can lie as still as possible. Certificates or stickers proclaiming achievements such as 'I lay still for my ECG' are often useful incentives.

Radiography

X-ray examination of the chest is carried out to determine the size and position of the heart and, once again, a full explanation for both the child and the family is essential. The procedure is difficult in the newborn, but radiographs can be very useful when they show a large heart which can then aid the diagnosis. It is also possible to establish the number of vessels in the lung fields.

Echocardiography

This uses sound waves to build up an image of the heart in the same way that ultrasonography scans the unborn child. It is highly sophisticated and gives accurate images of the heart, enabling the skilled operator to see any abnormalities. It can be performed using a mobile machine by the mother's bedside or in the special care nursery, thus avoiding moving the baby to another department. Older children need to be asked to lie still and warned about the coldness of the jelly on their chests, but as this is another non-invasive test, careful preparation usually leads to compliance. Light oral sedation can be used for very young children and babies.

CARE OF THE FAMILY

Whenever a family is told that there is something wrong with their child they will be devastated. When a cardiac abnormality is suspected or confirmed, however, the seriousness of the situation often appears even greater.

As with any abnormality or chronic illness, they are likely to react with feelings of grief as they mourn the loss of their 'normal' child and the 'normal' family life they had planned to enjoy (Johns 1971). Initially, intense sorrow, shock and anger are likely to be the most commonly exhibited emotions. Parents, especially mothers, may feel guilty that they have caused the heart abnormality as they search for meaning and a reason for their tragedy (Camaroff & Maguire 1981).

A nurse working in a general paediatric ward referring such a child, or a community nurse attending a family waiting for assessment of their child will witness the family's distress and can be an invaluable support at a difficult time. For the most part, it is possible to reassure the family, as the vast majority of children with congenital heart disease can be offered treatment bringing life-long health and fitness. For a

minority, a series of operations may be needed but the child can ultimately expect to lead a normal life with minimal limitations on exercise and lifestyle. For a very small minority, treatment is either not possible or carries a very high risk of mortality or morbidity. It is therefore best for a specialist paediatric cardiac centre to discuss fully with the parents the diagnosis and prognosis of their child's condition, as they will be in the best position to advise of the options. They should also have access to appropriate educational material for the parents and be able to put families in contact with specialist social work support and local family support groups. These are run by parents who have first-hand experience of congenital heart disease and can provide friendship and support to newly diagnosed families struggling to come to terms with the situation.

If you are caring for a newly diagnosed child and family in the community or in a referring hospital, the paediatric cardiac unit that the child attends should be more than happy to send you information on the child's heart condition and the effects this may have upon the child.

HEART FAILURE

Some children suffering from congenital heart problems will develop heart failure. This occurs when the heart fails to pump enough blood round the body to meet metabolic demands

Activity 10.1

Peter is a 3-month-old baby who has recently been diagnosed as having a ventricular septal defect. He is awaiting admission to hospital for further investigations with a view to possible surgery. He is feeding poorly although his weight gain is being maintained with calorie supplements in his bottle feeds. His parents are in their early 20s and Peter is their first child. They feel confused and distressed about their son's condition and have no local family support.

As Peter's community nurse, what sort of practical advice and support could you offer the family? What other agencies could be asked for help?

(Jordan & Scott 1989). It is most common in the first 3 months of life, although not all congenital heart problems lead to heart failure.

The child may have some or all of the following:

- tachycardia, above 180 beats/minute for a baby and above 150 beats/minute in an older child
- breathlessness, perhaps on exertion—this is best demonstrated in babies who cannot complete feeds or take much longer than normal to do so
- sweating due to the increased metabolic rate—the child's hair and pillow may be soaked in sweat
- failure to thrive
- weight gain despite poor dietary intake—this indicates fluid retention and is the reason why children in cardiac failure are weighed daily in hospital.

Main principles of treatment

- The improvement of cardiac function through drug administration and careful monitoring of the response. Three main groups of drugs are used:
    —inotropes, e.g. digoxin
    —diuretics, e.g. frusemide
    —vasodilators, e.g. captopril.

Activity 10.2

Joanne is a 1-month-old baby who has a large ventricular septal defect, which has led her to suffer from heart failure. This has been controlled with diuretic therapy. Joanne was failing to thrive and still requires nasogastric feeds to maintain an adequate weight gain. The feeds are in bolus form during the day and by continuous pump feed overnight. It is felt, however, that Joanne is now well enough to go home and her parents are keen for her to do so. There is one other child in the family, Luke aged 2 years. Joanne's mother does not intend to return to work.

As Joanne's primary nurse, consider what sort of training and education programme Joanne's parents will need before they can take her home. Also, consider what support and resources Joanne and her family require once Joanne is discharged from hospital to her home?

- The reduction of respiratory stress with correct positioning and comfort.
- The maintenance of adequate fluid and nutritional intake, bearing in mind that there may be a need for supplemental feeding (Torbet 1994).
- The support of both the child and the family with encouragement and teaching of the parents to participate in their child's care. If parents have been very involved in the care of the child at home, they should not be expected to 'surrender' that care as soon as there is a need for admission. Partnership models of care recognise that the parents should have as big a part in care planning as they wish.

BLOOD DISORDERS

As blood passes through the lungs, the red blood cells absorb oxygen and transport it to the body. For this process to be as efficient as possible, the proportion of red cells to total blood volume must be correct.

If the proportion is too low, insufficient oxygen is carried and if the proportion is too high, the blood becomes too thick, slowing the flow through the tissues.

The most common of the red blood cell disorders, the anaemias, are found when the proportion of red cells in the blood is too low or when the concentration of haemoglobin in the red cells is too low.

Iron deficiency anaemia (see Ch. 12)

Often found in the child who has a history of poor intake of foods containing iron, iron deficiency anaemia may also be seen in those children who have fatty stools, steatorrhoea, which may need further investigation. If the stools are negative when tested for occult blood, a dietary assessment followed by advice on a balanced diet in conjunction with oral iron therapy should produce an improvement. As these children may otherwise be well, prolonged hospital admission is not necessary, but instead the input of the community paediatric nurses will be invaluable. The child who does not readily eat well will be far less inclined to do so away from home and so should be discharged as soon as possible.

Sickle cell anaemia

This is the most common inherited blood disorder with at least 150 babies with sickle cell disease born per year in England alone (Brozovic & Davies 1987). It is most commonly found in people of Afro-Caribbean or West African origin but can also be seen in those from the Middle East, Asia and around the Mediterranean.

This is a recessively inherited disorder. If both parents carry a recessive gene that codes for structurally abnormal haemoglobin, their off-spring have a one in four chance of receiving a copy of the gene from each parent (the homozy-gous condition) and therefore inheriting the dis-ease. Those with only one copy of the gene (the heterozygous condition) have sickle cell trait, which is usually asymptomatic unless the carrier is subjected to severe hypoxia (e.g. at high alti-tudes).

The first manifestations of sickle cell anaemia may appear soon after birth, perhaps by 3 months, and it is the first 3 years of life which carry the highest risk of death. The prognosis is improving, however, and life expectancy is in-creasing, with some patients surviving into their fifth, sixth and seventh decades.

The first signs in a young child may be bacte-rial infection and it is infection by a pneumococ-cus which can cause death in childhood from meningitis, septicaemia, pneumonia or peritoni-tis. It is not known precisely why patients with sickle cell disease are more likely to suffer from such serious infections but the spleen, which has an important role in fighting infection, is dam-aged by sickle cell disease. Repeated infections cause the spleen to atrophy and so as the child becomes older splenomegaly is less common.

The most common symptom of sickle cell dis-ease is the crisis caused by occlusion of the vein when the abnormally (sickle) shaped cells clump together. This is a crisis and is a reaction to a low-ered oxygen saturation which occurs when there is dehydration. This crisis causes severe pain which may follow infection, dehydration, stress, exercise or may simply occur without any warn-ing. Treatment is symptomatic and includes antibiotics, hydration to counter the effects of a slowed circulation and possible renal impair-ment, warmth, and analgesia.

Thalassaemia

Again, this illness is inherited from both parents, and the gene from one alone will give rise to a trait which could result in full disease in the patient's offspring. It is most commonly found among Mediterranean and Asian races and is divided into alpha and beta types. The latter is the more common and the homozygous (in-herited from both parents) form is characterised by severe anaemia which can be treated to a certain extent by repeated blood transfusions. Unfortunately, this causes iron overload and tissue damage and infusion of desferrioxamine at night helps to restore the iron balance. This symptomatic treatment is, unfortunately, denied to many children suffering from the condition in developing countries.

It is possible to offer antenatal diagnosis with the option of termination for parents who wish to consider further pregnancies but such deci-sions are not easily made.

In heterozygous (inherited from one parent) beta thalassaemia, there is mild anaemia which may be confused with that caused by iron deficiency.

Bruising disorders

It is not unusual for a child to develop spontaneous bruising as a symptom in isolation. This may occur with or without an associated anaemia.

Henoch–Schoenlein purpura (HSP)

The child has a normal platelet count and papules on the skin develop into a haemorrhagic rash. The bleeding is a result of increased permeability of the capillary walls leading to 'leakage' of blood and bruising. Admission to hospital will be needed if the child has abdominal pain, haematuria or arthritis. Nursing care will include effective analgesia and observation of the urine for frank haematuria which could be a sign of glomerulonephritis. Intussusception can be a serious complication.

Idiopathic thrombocytopenic purpura (ITP)

This often follows an infection or drug therapy and differs from HSP in that, although there is also a purpura with bruising, this time the platelet count is very low. As the presenting symptoms may be similar to those of leukaemia, a bone marrow aspiration may be carried out to ascertain the precise diagnosis. The parents will need a great deal of support over this difficult time when they will have been told that their child possibly has a life-threatening disease.

For most children the purpura will disappear within 3 months, although if symptoms remain, other treatments such as steroid therapy or very occasionally splenectomy may be necessary.

Acute leukaemia

A child presenting with symptoms which are indicative of leukaemia should have an urgent bone marrow aspiration to confirm the diagnosis. Chapter 24 should be consulted for details of treatment, prognosis and implications for nursing care.

Bleeding disorders

Haemophilia

As already stated, children bruise very easily and most bruises are due to nothing more sinister than normal activity. Some, however, may require a closer examination, perhaps if bleeding is prolonged after injury or dental extraction. Haemophilia, which is caused by low levels of factor VIII, affects only males but is carried by the female, with each male child having a 50% chance of being affected. Affected children, like those suffering from other chronic blood disorders such as sickle cell anaemia or thalassaemia, used to require frequent hospital admissions which were disruptive to school and social life. It is important therefore to ensure that each admission is as well planned as possible and the nurse who is trained and competent at venepuncture and cannulation will be invaluable in this process. Nowadays, many children are cared for at home, and their parents taught to administer the factor VIII as required. The community paediatric nurse is an important support.

Other bleeding disorders include Christmas disease where there is a factor IX deficiency and Von Willebrand's disease where there is a vascular defect; both present problems to nurses that are similar to those of haemophilia.

INTRAVENOUS THERAPY

For many of the conditions described above, intravenous fluids may be required when the child is unable to take sufficient fluid by the orogastric route.

Dehydration occurs more rapidly in children than in adults, which will compromise the child's cardiovascular system because of low circulating blood volume. It will also give rise to electrolyte imbalance which could lead to cardiac arrhythmias. If possible, fluid should be given by nasogastric tube, but this is not feasible in children who are more seriously ill and so an intravenous infusion will be required to maintain fluid and electrolyte balance.

A child may need intravenous fluids if there is:

- inability to feed—coma, serious illness, dyspnoea, trauma to face or neck, congenital abnormality of the mouth or oesophagus
- severe vomiting—if the child also has diarrhoea, fluid requirement rises and dehydration is rapid.

Setting up an intravenous infusion

Depending on local policy and the skills of the staff involved, the cannula may be inserted by the nurse. Explanation and support for the child and family before, during and after the procedure are vital whether the nurse is cannulating or somebody else is. If time permits, the hospital play specialist may be involved in the preparation.

Local anaesthetic cream such as EMLA should be applied to the preferred site around 1 hour before the infusion is sited to minimise the pain (Farrington 1993). It will also minimise recollection of the procedure if it needs to be repeated. There may not be time for this if the child is unwell. Entonox therapy can be helpful for older children as an anaesthetic while the cannula is inserted.

The fluid should be prescribed before cannula insertion so that time is not wasted. It should be in the correct administration set which is compatible with any pump which is to be used. An inaccurate infusion may be the result of an incompatible pump. It is not recommended to administer intravenous fluids to babies and small children without pumps, due to the difficulty in accurately regulating extremely small flows. Older children and adolescents may not have a pump, however, but administration sets with a burette must be used to prevent over-infusion.

Short-term peripheral infusion—insertion of the cannula

Such an infusion is given via a cannula sited in a peripheral vein which in babies could be in the scalp, hand, arm or foot. In older children the site is more likely to be in the back of the hand or the antecubital fossa. Even with good preparation, the procedure may be traumatic and should be carried out in an area away from other children to ensure privacy and prevent upsetting others. All the equipment should be ready to ensure that the procedure is as quick and efficient as possible.

When the cannula has been inserted and checked for patency, it should be secured with tape and bandages, and then splinted if possible to prevent it becoming dislodged.

Peripheral infusions are also used for the administration of intravenous drug therapy,

especially antibiotics. Local policies should be consulted with regard to such administration.

Care of the infusion

Regular observations are necessary during an infusion:

- *General condition.* Take the pulse and respiratory rates regularly.
- *Fluid balance.* Record the amount infused every hour together with the output. Over-infusion can overload the circulatory system causing tachycardia and tachypnoea, perhaps with a moist cough. Babies and small children are most at risk of this because of their low circulating blood volumes.
- *Cannula site.* This should also be checked hourly for signs of infection or extravasation (leakage) which can cause swelling and at worst a necrotic area requiring skin grafting. This is especially important when using infusion pumps, although most modern pumps have pressure sensors with alarms which alert staff when extra pumping pressures are needed, indicating that the cannula may be dislodged.

Peripheral lines can be used, though it is not recommended, to infuse total parenteral nutrition (TPN). This is used for patients who, over a protracted period of time, are unable to take nutrition via the alimentary tract. If a cannula delivering TPN becomes dislodged and the fluid flows into the tissues, the likely result is a necrotic area, and for this reason a central line is usually used.

Central venous line

The fine catheter is inserted into a large vein, usually the jugular, subclavian or femoral. The catheters are larger and longer than peripheral cannulae and less likely to become dislodged. The maintenance of cleanliness and avoidance of infection around the site are of paramount importance and, in babies and small children with a femoral line, this can be difficult due to their wearing nappies. Nappies should be changed promptly and the area kept scrupulously clean.

Central vein catheters often contain two or three lumens allowing two or three different infusions to run at the same time, each into its own lumen. This allows the infusion of fluids and drugs which would otherwise be incompatible. TPN always has its own lumen, as it is rich in nutrients and therefore runs a higher risk of infection.

Long-term venous access

Children requiring long-term venous access are best served by a surgically implanted device (Hollis 1992). This will include those needing long-term drug therapy for malignancy (Sepion 1990) or cystic fibrosis (Sidey 1989). There are also a small number of children who require long-term TPN.

The use of long-term access allows children to have drug or TPN therapy at home as their parents can be taught how to care for the devices. There are two main types:

• Hickman or Broviac line. The Hickman line is silicone, radio-opaque and usually inserted surgically into the subclavian vein. It is tunnelled under the skin and a Dacron cuff lies inside the entry site, helping to anchor the catheter. As part of the catheter lies outside the body, there is a risk of damage, infection or haemorrhage. It is, however, easy to use in the home situation as soon as the family have been taught how to use and care for the line.
• Totally implantable device—Port-a-Cath, Cordis Miniport, PAS Port. These are inserted surgically into the jugular or subclavian veins, with the injection port in the ipsilateral pectoral area, or the cubital vein with the port in the forearm. As the system is under the skin, it is protected from damage and may give less of a problem with body image than having a Hickman line. Again, the families can manage at home when they have been given adequate instruction on how to use the implanted port.

Both of these systems mean that children requiring long-term intravenous therapy do not require either repeated venepuncture or prolonged hospital admissions.

This last point summarises once again the overriding objective of the care of the sick child—that where possible, he and his family should be given the help to care for him at home if that is what they wish.

REFERENCES

Adamson E F St J, Hill D 1984 Nursing sick children. Churchill Livingstone, Edinburgh
Brozovic M, Davies S C 1987 Management of sickle cell disease. Postgraduate Medical Journal 63: 605–609
Camaroff J, Maguire P 1981 Ambiguity and the search for meaning: childhood leukaemia in the modern clinical context. Social Science and Medicine 15B: 115–123
de Swiet M, Dillon M J, Littler W, O'Brien E, Padfield P L, Petrie J C 1989 Measurement of blood pressure in children. British Medical Journal 299: 497
Farrington E 1993 Paediatric drug information—Lidocaine 2.4%/Philocaine 2.5% EMLA cream. Paediatric Nursing 19(5): 484–486
Frohlich E et al 1988 Recommendations for human blood pressure determination by sphygmomanometers. Circulation 77: 501A
Hollis R 1992 Central venous access in children. Paediatric Nursing (July): 18–21
Hull D, Johnston D 1989 Essential paediatrics. Churchill Livingstone, Edinburgh
Johns N 1971 Family reactions to the birth of a child with a congenital abnormality. The Medical Journal of Australia 1(5): 277–282
Jordan S C, Scott O 1989 Heart disease in paediatrics, 3rd edn. Butterworths, London
Kelnar J H, Harvey D 1988 The sick newborn baby, 2nd edn. Baillière Tindall, London
Midence K, Elander J 1994 Sickle cell disease—a psychosocial approach. Radcliffe Medical Press, Oxford
Sepion B 1990 Intravenous care for children. Paediatric Nursing 2(3): 14–16
Sidey A 1989 Intravenous home care. Paediatric Nursing (May): 14–15
Torbet S 1994 Nutritional aspects of failure to thrive. Paediatric Nursing 6(5): 25–28
Weller B F 1978 The Lippincott manual of paediatric nursing, 2nd edn. Harper & Row, London
Whaley L F, Wong D L 1991 Essentials of paediatric nursing, 4th edn. C V Mosby, St Louis

FURTHER READING

Hazinski M F 1992 Cardiovascular disorders. In: Hazinski M F (ed) Nursing care of the critically ill child, 2nd edn. CV Mosby, London

Jordan S C, Scott O 1989 Heart disease in paediatrics, 3rd edn. Butterworths, London

Meadows S R, Smithells R W 1991 Lecture notes in paediatrics, 6th edn. Blackwell, London

Monro J L, Shore G 1989 A colour atlas of cardiac surgery—congenital heart disease. Wolfe Medical, London

Muller D, Harris P J, Wattley L, Taylor J D 1992 Nursing children, 2nd edn. Chapman & Hall, London

Park M K, Guntheroth W G 1992 How to read paediatric ECGs. C V Mosby, St Louis

Pritchard A P, David J A (eds) 1988 The Royal Marsden Hospital manual of clinical nursing procedures, 2nd edn. Harper & Row, London

Rees P G, Tunstill A M, Pope T, Kinnear D, Rees S 1989 Heart children: a practical handbook for parents. Heart Line Association, Bedfordshire

Whaley L F, Wong D L 1991 Essentials of paediatric nursing, 4th edn. C V Mosby, St Louis, ch 34

11

The respiratory system

Kevin Woodhams   Joanne Trussler   Edwina Wooler

In working through this chapter, the student is
introduced to the normal functioning of the
respiratory system. Major alteration in respiratory
function will be discussed.

The chapter aims to:
- outline the structure and function of the
respiratory system
- review the value of careful history taking and
the application of this skill to aid diagnosis and
subsequent management of the common
respiratory problems of childhood
- discuss the different treatments available to
children according to their needs and condition
and identify those that are most appropriate to
each age group
- discuss the effects of respiratory illness on the
family and the need for support and education
during admission and after discharge.

To understand deficits in respiratory function, it
is important to have a basic understanding of
anatomy and physiology. Figures 11.1 and 11.2
will help to identify and describe the structural
features of the upper and lower respiratory tract.

The principal function of the lung is to perform gaseous exchange. Air inspired into the
lungs is carried via the airways to the alveoli
where oxygen is taken up by pulmonary capillary blood and carbon dioxide is released from
the venous blood. This process is affected by
the volume and distribution of air in the lungs.

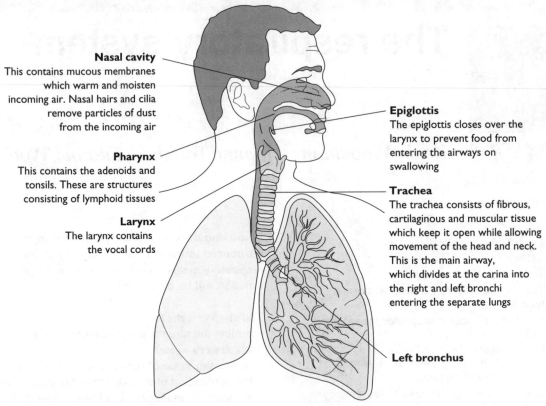

Nasal cavity
This contains mucous membranes which warm and moisten incoming air. Nasal hairs and cilia remove particles of dust from the incoming air

Pharynx
This contains the adenoids and tonsils. These are structures consisting of lymphoid tissues

Larynx
The larynx contains the vocal cords

Epiglottis
The epiglottis closes over the larynx to prevent food from entering the airways on swallowing

Trachea
The trachea consists of fibrous, cartilaginous and muscular tissue which keep it open while allowing movement of the head and neck. This is the main airway, which divides at the carina into the right and left bronchi entering the separate lungs

Left bronchus

Figure 11.1   The upper respiratory tract.

A proportion of each inspired breath remains in the conducting airways where there is no significant exchange of oxygen (O_2) and carbon dioxide (CO_2). This is known as the residual volume. Normal gas exchange depends on O_2 and CO_2 being present in the alveoli in the correct proportions.

It is the amount of CO_2 in the blood that stimulates the respiratory centre in the brain to alter the rate of contraction of the respiratory muscles. In the adult patient with a chronic respiratory illness such as bronchitis, it is the low oxygen concentration which becomes the primary trigger for respiration.

The respiratory tract is lined with a mucous membrane constructed of ciliated epithelial cells. Mucous secretions trap inhaled particles (dust etc.) and the hair-like cilia propel secretions up and out of the airways, ensuring that they do not pool in the respiratory tract.

Breathing

Inspiration is active; the diaphragm contracts and lowers, intercostal muscles contract and the chest cavity expands causing a drop in the air pressure in the alveoli, which draws air into the lungs.

Expiration is a passive mechanism; the diaphragm relaxes and rises, intercostal muscles relax and the chest cavity becomes smaller, forcing air out of the lungs.

Normal breathing patterns

The shape and size of the thorax changes during each respiration. On inspiration, the thorax enlarges as the ribs move upwards and outwards as a result of contraction of the intercostal muscles. The diaphragm moves downwards and air is sucked in. On expiration, the thorax returns to its former size and shape

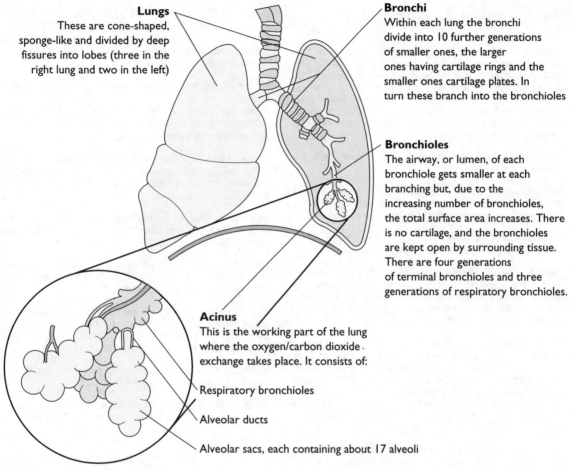

Lungs
These are cone-shaped, sponge-like and divided by deep fissures into lobes (three in the right lung and two in the left)

Bronchi
Within each lung the bronchi divide into 10 further generations of smaller ones, the larger ones having cartilage rings and the smaller ones cartilage plates. In turn these branch into the bronchioles

Bronchioles
The airway, or lumen, of each bronchiole gets smaller at each branching but, due to the increasing number of bronchioles, the total surface area increases. There is no cartilage, and the bronchioles are kept open by surrounding tissue. There are four generations of terminal bronchioles and three generations of respiratory bronchioles.

Acinus
This is the working part of the lung where the oxygen/carbon dioxide exchange takes place. It consists of:

Respiratory bronchioles

Alveolar ducts

Alveolar sacs, each containing about 17 alveoli

Figure 11.2   The lower respiratory tract.

as the diaphragm and intercostal muscles relax.

Infants until the age of 3 months are habitual nose breathers and this will have a significant effect on management of respiratory illness. The respiratory rate in this age group is erratic and may follow no particular pattern.

Normal respiratory rates in infants and children are given in Table 11.1.

Table 11.1	Respiratory rates in children
Age	Respiratory rate (breaths per minute)
Newborn	60
1–12 months	40
1–4 years	32
5–10 years	28
11–14 years	24

Activity 11.1

To understand the effect that asthma can have on normal breathing patterns, take a normal breath in and only release half on expiration. Repeat this several times. How does this feel? What happens to the rib cage and shoulders?

Box 11.1 Terms used in respiratory illness

Apnoea. A term used to denote that respiration has ceased. It is commonly used in relation to infants. The episode can last from a matter of seconds to minutes. The longer an infant is apnoeic the more likely it is that gas exchange will be affected and, subsequently, the oxygen supply to the brain Most apnoeic infants respond to stimulation and often picking them up or gentle movement will 'remind' them to breath.

Auscultation. Examination of the chest with a stethoscope.

Bronchospasm. Sudden spasm of the smooth muscle in the walls of the airway; often associated with inhalation of an allergen such as house dust in the case of asthma.

Consolidation. A state in which areas of the lungs become 'solid' with secretions, as in pneumonia.

Cough. The type of cough with which a child presents may give a strong indication of the diagnosis, and it is rarely sufficient simply to use the term 'cough' on its own. Listed below are the common types of cough which are associated with paediatric respiratory illness.

Paroxysmal cough. This type of cough is characteristic of pertussis (whooping cough) although it may be seen following inhalation of a foreign body. It is characterised by a sudden onset of multiple, forceful and prolonged coughing spasms during expiration, which can last for 20–30 seconds. The characteristic whoop at the end of the coughing episode is caused by the sudden rush of inspiratory breath through the narrowed glottis.

Croupy cough. Acute laryngotracheobronchitis (croup) is a diagnosis in its own right; however, the type of cough associated with the condition is characteristic. The child has a harsh barking cough and inspiratory stridor (see below). This is caused by air being forced past the oedematous upper airways on inspiration.

Productive cough. This type of cough may be indicative of infection in the lower airways and is also associated with conditions such as cystic fibrosis. When sputum is produced, it is important for the nurse to record its colour, amount and consistency.

Nocturnal cough. This is commonly seen in asthma when the child has recurrent symptoms of cough, particularly at night (Barnes & Levy 1984). This one feature alone may be enough to suggest a diagnosis of asthma but further investigation is indicated.

'Wheezy' cough. The baby with bronchiolitis presents with a typical 'wheezy' cough, unlike that which is seen in asthma. This is due to inflammation of the bronchioles in the lower airways. See Wheeze.

Cyanosis. This is a bluish tinge to the skin and mucous membranes caused by imperfect oxygenation of the blood. The lack of oxygen may be due to:

- poor cardiac output due to combined cardiopulmonary failure
- poor gas exchange in the lungs due to acute respiratory illness or chronic lung disease
- obstruction of the child's airway.

Cyanosis can be observed around the mouth (circumoral), in the mucous membranes within the mouth, or generally of the face, arms and legs. Cyanosis always needs to be treated as an emergency.

Dyspnoea. Difficulty in breathing seen in a number of respiratory illnesses including asthma, cystic fibrosis and pneumonia.

Grunting. Short, laboured expiratory breaths or grunts seen in infants with respiratory illness. It is a characteristic of respiratory distress syndrome.

Hyperinflation. Commonly seen in asthma, this is a condition where air is trapped in the alveoli and the sternum bows outwards. It is usually reversible but may be an indication of poor asthma control.

Hypoxia. A decreased amount of oxygen in the tissues caused by poor oxygenation of the blood.

Nasal flaring. In the child with acute respiratory symptoms, such as an exacerbation of asthma, it is possible to

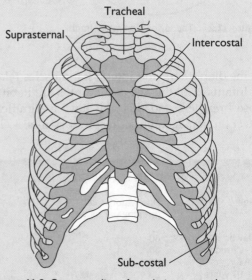

Figure 11.3 Common sites of respiratory recession.

Box 11.1 **continued**

observe the use of the accessory muscles of respiration. Nasal flaring is apparent in these children and is thought to be an attempt to increase the amount of inspired air.

Recession. An indrawing of soft tissues overlying the thorax. It can be described according to the area involved, i.e. intercostal recession—between the ribs (Whaley & Wong 1989) (Fig. 11.3). Recession is a sure sign of increasing respiratory effort and distress, particularly in the infant. It may be present whether the child is awake or asleep; during handling and during periods of activity, recession may become more obvious. Recession may be described as mild, moderate or severe; assessment of the depth of recession relies on clinical judgement (experience). Tachycardia and tachypnoea are commonly associated with recession and these factors will make feeding extremely difficult; this situation is compounded by blocked nostrils.

Secretions. The respiratory tract is lined with a membrane that naturally produces mucus. This prevents drying of the respiratory tract by moistening the inspired air.

Splinting. This describes the way in which a child with respiratory distress will try to increase the amount of inspired air and support the thorax by sitting upright with the elbows supported on a table and the shoulders raised upwards.

Stridor. A harsh sound produced as air is forced through oedematous upper airways. The noise can best be described as being like air being pushed through a narrow tube accompanied by a 'gasping' sound. Stridor can worsen when the child becomes distressed. It may be accompanied by recession and is an indication of acute respiratory illness such as epiglottitis or croup. It can occur during inspiration or expiration.

Tachypnoea. A rapid and often shallow respiratory rate above the normal value.

Tracheal tug. This is another form of recession. See Recession.

Tracheostomy. A surgical opening made into the trachea to maintain respiration in the emergency situation, i.e. inhalation of a foreign body or choking. The operation may be performed electively for congenital abnormalities of the upper airway.

Wheeze. The characteristic whistling sound often heard in the asthmatic child caused by air being forced through narrowed airways during an asthma attack. It may occur during inspiration or expiration. Wheeze is often audible or can be heard by listening to the child's chest with a stethoscope. Recession either subcostal or intercostal may accompany wheezing.

EFFECTS OF RESPIRATORY DISEASE ON NORMAL FUNCTION

An imbalance in gaseous exchange can be caused by the disturbance of either oxygen or carbon dioxide transport. For example in acute laryngo-tracheo bronchitis (croup) there is an obstruction, caused by swelling of the upper airway, that decreases the amount of oxygen which can reach the lungs. In the lower airway, bronchospasm seen in asthma reduces the ability to expire CO_2. When infection is present in the lung, there is disruption of gaseous exchange caused by the accumulation of secretions in affected areas.

A number of terms specific to respiratory illness which may be helpful in establishing a diagnosis are listed in Box 11.1. Definitions of some of the common respiratory illnesses are given in Box 11.2.

THE ROLE OF THE NURSE IN RESPIRATORY ASSESSMENT

The nurse's role in assessment of respiratory status cannot be emphasised enough. Nursing assessment gives vital clues about the child's

Box 11.2 **Some common respiratory illnesses**

Croup. Croup is a disease of the upper airways that is often mild, but can occasionally be severe and life-threatening. It results in inspiratory stridor and a barking cough, and at its most severe is extremely frightening for the child and parent. It is an acute viral infection, usually caused by the para-influenza virus. It resolves spontaneously.

Epiglottitis. Epiglottitis is a severe bacterial infection of the upper respiratory tract caused by the organism *Haemophilus influenzae*. It results in sudden swelling of the epiglottis and should be treated as a medical emergency.

Bronchiolitis. Bronchiolitis is an acute viral infection of the lower airways, usually caused by the respiratory syncytial virus (RSV). It occurs in epidemics in the winter months and affects children in the first 2 years of life.

Pneumonia. Pneumonia is an infection, usually viral but sometimes bacterial, of the terminal airways and air sacs. It results in tachypnoea, respiratory distress, dullness of chest percussion, reduced breath sounds and consolidation shown on chest X-ray.

condition and should be rapid, thorough, on-going and as non-invasive as possible. Keeping these guidelines in mind will ensure that the assessment causes as little stress as possible to both the child and her parents (carers). To avoid confusion, it is essential that the nurse's explanation of the assessment and the reasons for it is kept as simple as possible. The nurse also needs to recognise that the assessment may lead to more formal and possibly invasive methods of investigation.

Before commencing the assessment remember the following points:

• The upper airway in the infant and young child is much narrower than in an adult; there-fore anything that reduces the lumen of the air-way is likely to put the child at risk.
• A child's respiratory tract is shorter compared to that of an adult and this increases the child's susceptibility to infection.
• Infants are obligatory nose breathers until at least 4 weeks of age; therefore blocked nostrils will increase respiratory effort.

It is important when making an assessment to have some knowledge of normal respiratory rates and patterns in infants and children (see p. 173).

The infant's breathing pattern may normally be irregular, with use of the diaphragm more apparent than in older children. Chest wall com-pliance is greater in the infant and does not reach adult values until early adolescence. Hence, dur-ing respiratory illness, signs such as recession and hyperinflation will be more pronounced. External factors such as restrictive clothing or abdominal distension may cause increased respi-ratory embarrassment.

Routine assessment

Following admission, the nurse should make a full assessment of the child's respiratory status. This should include baseline measurements of temperature, pulse and respiration in all cases, and other more specific observations depending on the age and condition of the child.

Temperature

In the child under the age of 6 years, an axillary temperature should be taken; over this age an oral temperature may be taken (Rogers 1992). If the child is pyrexial, this may be an indication of infection; however, small babies may be hypothermic when they have an infection.

Pulse

Take the pulse rate, and note rate and volume. Tachycardia may indicate increased respiratory effort affecting the circulatory system. Where asthma has already been diagnosed, tachycardia may be a side effect of the large amounts of bron-chodilators, e.g. salbutamol or terbutaline, being given to reverse the attack. Small babies with respiratory infections often respond badly to over-handling and this can result in a bradycardia.

Respirations

Record the respiratory rate and observe effort. Note whether the child is using the accessory muscles of respiration. This will be shown by flaring of the nostrils, splinting of the shoulders and recession. Observe also the breathing pattern for regularity of rate, shallow or deep breaths, stridor or wheeze, and whether both sides of the chest wall move equally.

Colour

Observe the child's colour. The hypoxic child may be pale and mottled and the flushed child may be pyrexial. Cyanosis, however, is a life-threatening sign and calls for immediate medical intervention.

Activity 11.2

Record pulse and respiratory rates in children of different ages at rest and after play. Observe the flexibility of the rib cage while doing this.

Hydration

The child may be too breathless to drink and will also be losing fluid through an increased respiratory rate. The child who is pyrexial may also be sweating. Observe the child for reduced tissue turgor, decreased urinary output and dry mouth. Remember that a dry mouth may be a result of mouth breathing and is not always an indication of dehydration.

Sputum

Ask the parents if there has been any sputum produced and, if so, what is its colour and consistency. This is of great importance, particularly in the child with cystic fibrosis. It is, however, common for younger children to be unable to expectorate and they will swallow secretions instead. The parents may then report that the child has vomited and they have noticed mucus in the vomit.

Behaviour

Observe the child and her parents together. The child who is listless or irritable may be hypoxic. Note whether the child responds to her surroundings and her parents; this may help to indicate her level of consciousness. In conditions such as epiglottitis, careful handling by the parents can greatly assist the medical staff in the management of the child. Try to encourage them to stay calm.

Oxygen saturation

Measuring oxygen saturation is now a standard procedure in most paediatric centres. The oxygen saturation monitor, in simple terms, records the amount of oxygen in the circulating blood. The saturation rate should be kept above 92%. The probe may be placed on the child's finger or toe, but care must be taken to position the monitor correctly when recording a reading. In infants, the probe site should be changed every 4–6 hours to prevent burns caused by the sensors.

Investigations and assessments used to establish a diagnosis

Once a history has been taken from the parents, it may be possible for the doctor to make a differential diagnosis, but there are a number of investigations and assessments that may be made to aid in the final diagnosis.

Peak expiratory flow rate (PEFR)

This is the maximum rate at which air can be expelled from the lungs and is measured in litres per minute with a peak flow meter. This is one of the commonest forms of assessment of lung function and can be carried out on most children over the age of 5 years (Milner & Ingram 1970). Children under this age get confused between sucking and blowing and, if inhaled medications are to be used, it is more important to encourage a good inspiratory technique and use clinical judgement to observe lung function. The procedure for using a peak flow meter is given in Box 11.3.

Box 11.3 How to take a reliable measurement of PEFR

- The child should always record the PEFR standing up.
- Ask the child to take a deep breath in, then with the lips sealed round the mouthpiece blow hard into the peak flow meter to give a forced expiration.
- Repeat this three times and record the highest of the readings.
- The expected peak flow can be calculated from a chart, if the child's height is known. It is accepted that the expected peak flow is the highest reading that the child can achieve when well.

Activity 11.3

Borrow a peak flow meter and record your own peak flow rate morning and evening for 1 week. How compliant are you with regular home monitoring?

Spirometry

The simplest form of spirometry uses the Vitalograph machine. The test measures forced vital capacity (FVC) and forced expiratory volume at 1 second (FEV_1). FVC is the total amount of air which can be forcibly expired following full inspiration. FEV_1 is the maximum volume of air that can be forcibly expired in 1 second after full expiration. Computerised spirometry is now available.

Flow volume loops

These tests are a more sophisticated computerised measurement of lung function and can show abnormalities related to obstructive airways disease which cannot be detected using simple spirometry.

Radiography

Traditionally, this has been one of the commonest methods of investigating the lung for infection or other abnormality. In the diagnosis of pneumonia, an X-ray will show the area of consolidation, which will aid the physiotherapist in the clearing of secretions from the chest.

In asthma it is important for an X-ray to taken after diagnosis to confirm that there is no underlying pathology. This is not usually indicated during an acute exacerbation as the X-ray will simply show hyperinflation. It must be remembered that a child should not be exposed to unnecessary radiographic procedures.

Collection of specimens

Sputum. Children from the age of 4–5 years, particularly those with cystic fibrosis, can expectorate with few problems; however, younger children may need assistance from the physiotherapist to obtain an adequate specimen. It is important to ensure that coughed secretions from the lower airways have been produced and not saliva. In infants it may be necessary to use tube suction to obtain a specimen, and this can be traumatic. A physiotherapist or trained nurse should undertake this procedure. Postural drainage or tipping the child over a pillow or wedge may assist in draining secretions to the large airways to allow easier expectoration (Pryor et al 1990).

It is vital, if epiglottitis is suspected, that *no* examination of the nose or throat be made, as this may increase oedema and lead to occlusion of the airway.

Throat swab. A throat swab may be indicated if infection in the throat is suspected. This is carried out by rolling a sterile cotton bud over the tonsillar bed and then sending the swab to the laboratory in transport medium. The procedure often makes smaller children gag, and they need to be restrained briefly whilst the swab is being taken. Once again, this procedure should never be attempted in the child with suspected epiglottitis.

Per-nasal swab. This specimen is usually taken in babies where pertussis (whooping cough) is suspected. It is similar to a throat swab but is obtained by introducing a fine cotton bud attached to thin wire down the baby's nostril into the nasopharynx.

TREATMENTS USED IN THE CARE OF RESPIRATORY ILLNESS

Treatments of diseases of the respiratory tract fall mainly into two categories: physiotherapy and medication.

Physiotherapy

The role of the physiotherapist in treating lung disorders centres on clearing secretions from the child's chest to maintain optimal lung function.

Activity 11.4

Observe a physiotherapist performing postural drainage on a young child and note the difficulty in expectoration. What games might the physiotherapist employ to encourage children to learn the difference between suck and blow?

In the case of the child with cystic fibrosis, this part of management is as important as any drug treatments used. However, it is also important to remember that in some cases physiotherapy is contraindicated; in asthma it may actually increase bronchospasm.

The type of physiotherapy treatment given must be tailored to the condition from which the child is suffering and the child's age. The physiotherapist will advise and educate nursing staff in the delivery of treatment and encourage parents to carry out the procedures at home if this is indicated. The age of the child may determine where treatments will take place. In the case of the small baby, it is often preferable to carry out procedures with the child lying on the lap, whereas the older child will benefit from tipping over pillows etc. to aid drainage of secretions.

Medication

Medications used to treat the respiratory tract are wide ranging and it is not the nurse's role to make decisions on drug therapy. It is, however, important that nurses are able to administer prescribed treatments correctly and teach children and their families about the use of medications.

The most commonly used group of treatments are those which are administered via the inhaled route.

Treatment of asthma

Asthma is a variable condition of the lower respiratory tract, characterised by resistance to flow in the intrapulmonary airways. It is also thought that chronic inflammation is present even when there are no symptoms, although this has not been proved for all types of childhood asthma. Children with asthma experience recurrent cough, wheeze and shortness of breath when they are exposed to certain allergens such as cigarette smoke, house dust mite, pets, pollen, etc. and often during physical activity. Symptoms are often worse at night and with upper respiratory tract infections. Between episodes, many children are completely well. Asthma is the commonest medical condition for which children are admitted to hospital, and inhaled medication provides the quickest relief of symptoms when correctly administered.

The inhaled route is preferred because:

- a smaller dose is required to achieve the same effect as oral medication, because it is delivered direct to its site of action
- the onset of action is quicker, because the drug does not have to be distributed around the body
- there are fewer systemic side effects.

The inhaled route has a few disadvantages related to the technique required to operate the inhaler device. A proportion of the inhaled drug is always swallowed, which will reduce the potential effectiveness of the medication. This is why regular review of inhaler technique by nurses is vitally important.

Inhaled treatments include bronchodilators such as terbutaline and salbutamol and inhaled steroids such as beclomethasone and budesonide. The acute asthma attack is generally treated with nebulised bronchodilator therapy. A nebuliser works by pumping a jet of compressed air or oxygen through a solution of drug. This produces a fine mist which the child inhales through a mouthpiece or mask. This method of administering treatment requires little cooperation from the child. Table 11.2 lists inhalational devices and indicates the suitability of each type for children of different ages.

Oral steroid treatment is also used for the child over the age of 18 months who is experiencing an acute asthma attack. Steroids are potent anti-inflammatory agents and work by reducing mucous secretion and oedema. Concerns have been expressed about the effects of steroid treatment on growth (Speight & Lee 1993, Walthers & Pederson 1990, Wales et al 1991). These concerns may be misplaced fears due to confusion with the effects of corticosteroids and anabolic steroids. It is important that nurses explain fully the use of steroid therapy, as parents may not comply with treatment unless they are fully aware of its effects.

Table 11.2 Inhalation devices suitable for each age group

Device	Age group (years)				Comments
	0–2	2–5	5–10	10+	
Large volume spacer and mask	✓				Nebuhaler/Volumatic, Fisonaire with Laerdal or McCarthy mask
Large volume spacer		✓	✓*	✓*	As above * Spacers indicated for high-dose steroids
Dry powder device			✓	✓	Turbohaler, Spinhaler, Diskhaler, Rotahaler, Accuhaler
Breath-actuated device			✓	✓	Aerolin, Aerobec autohaler, Easi-Breath
Metered-dose inhaler				✓	Ventolin, Becotide, Becloforte, Intal, Bricanyl, Pulmicort
Nebulised therapy	✓	✓	✓	✓	All age groups for treatment

Activity 11.5

List all of the inhaler devices that you are familiar with and think about how you would explain their use to a child. Try to decide which device would be suitable for different age groups, i.e. the under-5s, the school-age child and the adolescent.

Antibiotics

These are substances which have an antibacterial action. A wide variety exist which are specific to different strains of bacteria and should be used with this in mind. However, some have a broad spectrum of activity and can be used where the causative organism is unknown. This does not negate the need for sputum culture wherever this is possible. Antibiotics will have no effect when a virus is the causative organism. As with all paediatric medication, the dose will vary according to the child's age and body weight. Most oral preparations are made to look and taste pleasing to the child but this does not ensure that they will be taken easily.

Only severe infections will require the use of the intravenous route, which is not without its own risks and complications. A child with recurrent respiratory infections, such as occur in cystic fibrosis, may require a long-term venous access device, as repeated venepuncture and cannulation will cause thrombosis and scarring of veins (Sepion 1990). Nebulised antibiotics are sometimes used in patients with cystic fibrosis, especially where the lungs are colonised with pseudomonal infection.

The length of treatment will depend on the severity of the infection and the response of the individual patient. The more prolonged the therapy, the greater the risk of side effects, i.e. diarrhoea, skin rashes and hypersensitivity reactions.

DNAse

Part of the inflammatory process involves the infiltration of the lung tissue with neutrophils. As the infection increases, the neutrophils are destroyed, releasing their own DNA. This material is thick and sticky and increases the viscosity of the lung secretions further. DNAse is an enzyme which, when administered by nebuliser, 'digests' the DNA from the dead neutrophils, thus reducing the viscosity of the secretions and making them easier to expectorate. In trials it was found to improve patients' forced expiratory volume at 1 second (FEV_1) by 15–20% (Dinwiddie 1993).

Mucolytics

These can be administered orally; however, the nebulised route is more commonly used. They act by reducing the tenacity of sputum, so making it easier to expectorate. Their benefit is questionable and it is believed that nebulised normal saline (0.9%) is as effective (Petty 1990).

Oxygen therapy

Oxygen therapy, together with humidification, is used in the treatment of respiratory illness. Oxygen is a drug and, as such, needs to be prescribed by a doctor. However, the need for oxygen therapy is often decided by the nurse, based on assessment of the infant/child. Oxygen is needed to correct cyanosis and hypoxia.

The methods of administering oxygen vary according to the respiratory illness and the age of the child. (For risks associated with oxygen therapy in pre-term infants, see Ch. 20.) It is important if oxygen is being used, that it should be humidified to keep the airway and secretions moist. It can be administered by face mask, nasal prongs or head box. Nasal prongs are often used in preference to a mask which may frighten young children. The head box is a clear perspex box which fits over the child's head and upper body. The box fills with humidified oxygen, but leaves the child visible and accessible. The humidification used may be warmed or cold depending on the illness. It is important that an explanation of why oxygen is needed and how it is to be delivered is given to the parents and the child. It is always preferable to tell parents in advance that treatment may be needed, rather than risk their being made distraught by a sudden decision to start treatment.

If oxygen is being administered, remember that there should be no naked flames or surfaces that could ignite due to friction.

Gene therapy for cystic fibrosis

At the time of writing, gene therapy for cystic fibrosis is still in the trial stages. It involves the introduction of the healthy gene into affected cells, which will then be able to produce the 'normal' cell protein. The protein, cystic fibrosis transmembrane conductance regulator (CFTCR), is believed to control the transport of electrolytes across cell membranes. Where this is faulty, there is dehydration of the epithelial cells lining the respiratory tract and thickening of the secretions it produces (Cuthbert 1993).

Suctioning

This is a technique used when the child is unable to clear secretions naturally from the respiratory tract. Sterile equipment should be used and the principles of asepsis implemented to minimise the risk of cross-infection (Sackner et al 1973). The respiratory tract is lined with delicate structures and care should be taken not to cause trauma to these when administering suction (Young 1984).

Secretions can pool in the mouth, nasopharynx and trachea so suction may be required to any of these areas.

It is important that suction is not prolonged. There are a number of reasons for this:

- the catheter may adhere to the mucosal lining causing trauma
- over-stimulation of the mucosa may cause more secretions to be produced
- laryngospasm, bradycardia and/or cardiac arrhythmias may occur due to stimulation of the nervous supply to the respiratory tract and loss of oxygen.

Suctioning is a frightening and unpleasant procedure which will need to be explained to the child and parents alike. The nurse should be able to assess the effectiveness of suctioning by observing the child's general condition, especially the type and amount of secretions, improved respiratory rate and decreased effort.

Care of the tracheostomy

The child should be nursed near suction and oxygen. There should be a spare tracheostomy tube of the correct size and tracheal dilators by the bedside in case the tube becomes blocked or falls out and needs replacing immediately. Suction catheters of the correct size to clear the lumen of the tube should also be available. Sterile sodium chloride (0.9%) will be required to irrigate the lumen of the tube.

Suction to the tracheostomy will be performed as often as necessary initially, then gradually reduced in frequency as the child learns to cough the secretions out. Because the tracheostomy bypasses the normal defence mechanisms of the upper airway, suction is performed using aseptic technique. Lavage is used to moisten the secretions and make them easier to remove. The danger of secretions drying too much is that the tube may block off completely, putting the child's life in danger.

In order to keep secretions moist and thereby replace the function of the cilia in the upper airway, humidity may be given using oxygen or air postoperatively. This will gradually be reduced and replaced by a 'Swedish nose', which filters expired air from the patient and retains moisture. It fits over the tracheostomy tube and is changed daily. There is no increased resistance during breathing.

It is obviously important to ensure that the infant or child does not introduce any foreign bodies into the tube as this could block the airway. It is also important to prevent fluids entering the tracheostomy. Anyone caring for a child with a tracheostomy should know how to perform suction to the tube and know how to summon help if unsure.

When changing the tracheostomy tube or the tapes that hold it securely in place around the neck, two people should perform the task. This is because children do wriggle, making the procedure hazardous. The tapes are usually changed daily and the tube weekly.

THE PRINCIPLES OF RESUSCITATION

It is uncommon for cardiac arrest to occur in childhood. If it does, it usually follows respiratory arrest and a prolonged period of hypoxia (Kelly 1988). Resuscitation in childhood often follows major events such as suffocation, sudden infant death syndrome, inhalation of foreign body, infectious diseases, respiratory failure, convulsions and, in the infant, hypoglycaemia and hypothermia.

Because the child's metabolic rate is higher than that of an adult, there is an increased demand for oxygen by the body, particularly the brain. Small decreases in the supply of oxygen to the brain affect its function. Hypoxia in children is often characterised by restlessness, crying, 'thrashing about', irritability and anxiety. Eventually the infant/child will become listless and unresponsive.

If hypoxia is present, there is an increase in the heart rate (tachycardia) and in the respiratory rate (tachypnoea). A slow heart rate (bradycardia), below 100 beats per minute, will follow a tachycardia; then there is cessation of breathing (apnoea). It is the nurse's responsibility to recognise these symptoms and know how to initiate resuscitation. Once the nurse has recognised that a respiratory arrest is taking place the following steps should be taken:

1. Call for help; either send someone else to phone or press the emergency buzzer. If the nurse is alone, resuscitation should be started, then help summoned.
2. Remember 'ABC' (airway, breathing, circulation).

Airway. Check that the child's airway is clear; if there is mucus or vomit in the mouth, use suction or a finger to clear it away. Place

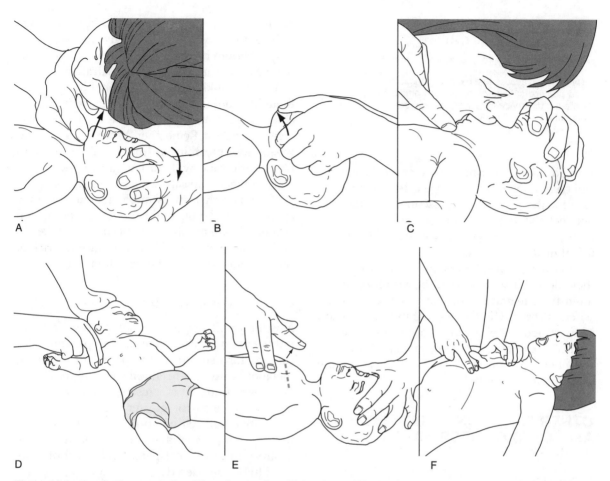

Figure 11.4 Paediatric resuscitation: (A) neck extension; (B) jaw thrust; (C) administering artificial respiration (covering nose and mouth); (D) locating the brachial pulse; (E) positioning fingers for cardiac massage in infant; (F) positioning hand for cardiac massage in the older child.

the child in the supine position and tilt the head backwards (Fig. 11.4A). This will lift the chin, hyperextend the neck and thereby clear the airway.

Breathing. Assess whether the child is breathing by observing the chest wall for movement. Also, listen for breath sounds by placing an ear close the child's nose and mouth. If respiration is absent, resuscitation needs to begin at once. Positioning the child correctly may alone be sufficient to stimulate spontaneous breathing. If this is not the case, mouth-to-mouth resuscitation should be commenced (Fig. 11.4B and C). Alter- natively, a bag and mask may be used for the same purpose. Infants should receive 15–20 breaths per minute, and older children 12–15 breaths per minute. Breaths should not be given too quickly as this often removes carbon dioxide and thereby reduces the response of the higher centres of respiration. Resuscitation should continue until help arrives or the child breathes spontaneously.

Circulation. Check the pulse in the carotid or brachial area (elbow) (Fig. 11.4 D). If the pulse is absent, cardiac compressions may need to take place (Fig. 11.4E and F).

Activity 11.6

Try to obtain access to a paediatric resuscitation dummy and practice cardiac massage and artificial respiration. Note the difference in technique required for adult, child and infant.

In addition to caring for the child during the emergency, the nurse also needs to remember to care for the parents. It is essential that they do not feel themselves to blame for the situation occurring, particularly in the case of sudden infant death syndrome.

Following a respiratory arrest, it is possible that the child will need to be admitted to an intensive care unit and this obviously adds to the parents' stress. The nurse's role in this situation is to support the parents and keep them informed about every stage of management. This will help to reduce anxiety and keep the situation under control.

OTHER FUNCTIONS THAT MAY BE AFFECTED BY RESPIRATORY ILLNESS

Circulation

Where oxygenation is impaired, the heart will attempt to compensate for this. It will beat faster in an effort to deliver the inspired oxygen to the body tissues. Therefore, observation of the apex beat or pulse rate will offer an indication of the child's initial condition and response to treatment. This cannot be used in isolation, however, as other factors, such as anxiety, will also increase the pulse rate.

Hydration

An increase in the respiratory rate will cause an increase in the insensible loss of fluids, since water vapour is lost with every expired breath. This needs to be taken into consideration when planning the child's total care. The encouragement

to drink even small amounts frequently will reduce the possibility of dehydration. Urine output should be observed for deterioration; this will be a clear indication of dehydration.

Where drinking normally cannot be tolerated, thought should be given to administering fluids either via the nasogastric route or as an intravenous infusion. Remember that in younger child where nose breathing is 'the norm' the use of a nasogastric tube will further impair the child's ability to maintain satisfactory oxygenation.

If oxygen therapy is implemented, this may cause further drying of the mouth and nose. Oral and nasal care are therefore needed to make the patient more comfortable and reduce the risk of fungal colonisation and excoriation.

Nutrition/elimination

Nutrition will not be a major concern initially, but the use of nutritious fluids will provide extra calories for use during the period of increased metabolic rate. Where chronic respiratory illness, i.e. cystic fibrosis, is present, there will be a continuous need for greater calorie intake and alternative sources of nutrition in the form of dietary supplements or routes of feeding—gastrostomies or total parenteral nutrition may need to be considered.

With infection and the use of antibiotics, children either expectorate or swallow large amounts of foul-tasting sputum. This can cause a bad taste in the mouth which in turn will reduce the child's desire to eat. The swallowing of sputum can also cause vomiting and a disruption in normal bowel pattern. Stools can become bulky and offensive, and the use of anti-biotics may compound the situation by causing diarrhoea.

Activity 11.7

Find out about dietary supplements that are available and taste a few. How palatable are they? How could you make them more acceptable to the child? Which supplements are available on prescription?

Mobility

Children who are having difficulty breathing will usually not want to be active. Correct positioning will ensure that they are able to use their lungs to full capacity. Where a child has a reversible respiratory problem, e.g. asthma, it is important that treatment is tailored to the child's normal life pattern.

PAIN

Children may suffer pain from repeated coughing. Cough suppression, however, is not thought to be appropriate, as this does not clear the infected mucus from the airways. Analgesia is of course indicated for relief of sore throats, etc. Children often complain of abdominal pain during an acute asthma attack, due to increased use of abdominal muscles and repeated coughing.

THE FAMILY

Whilst difficulty in breathing is distressing for the child, it is also distressing for the parents who feel unable to help their child. Parental anxiety is often relayed to the child, so making the situation worse, particularly in conditions such as epiglottitis where the child should be cared for in a calm atmosphere to avoid a worsening of respiratory status. Adequate explanation of nursing procedures to the family is vital to help alleviate anxiety and encourage them to take an active role in the child's care.

Where an inherited or familial illness is present, e.g. cystic fibrosis or asthma, there may be associated feelings of guilt. Allowing parents time to discuss these feelings will help. Non-judgemental attitudes from both nursing and medical staff are essential.

Health education is indicated where allergy-related problems exist, especially those associated with smoking. Smoking during pregnancy is more harmful than smoking afterwards, and there is now much evidence regarding the harmful effects of smoking on fetal lung growth.

Mothers who smoke during pregnancy have children with a higher incidence of asthma than non-smokers. Children whose mothers smoke, whether before after the child's birth, have worse asthma than those whose mothers do not smoke. There has been a gradual reduction in smoking in the general population, but it is least in young women. The dangers of passive smoking have been well documented and are particularly relevant to children with respiratory disorders (Royal College of Physicians 1992). It is important that nurses are able to help parents who wish to stop smoking by offering advice and appropriate information, and putting them in touch with professional agencies who may be able to help (Barnes & Levy 1984).

Adolescents often bow to peer group pressure over smoking and should be offered support and encouragement from an early age in an effort to discourage them from starting to smoke.

The philosophy of paediatric nursing for many years has included promoting independence within the family. It should be recognised that parents may sometimes be required to include treatments within their normal daily routine long after discharge. Teaching of new skills should be undertaken as soon as parents feel willing and able to learn them. For children with chronic disease, these skills will include physiotherapy and the administration and care of oxygen within the home. The rate at which these skills are taught should be governed by the families themselves.

Liaison with the primary health care team will also be essential in order to identify and resolve any problems which may exist or are likely to occur. Even where children themselves are able to take responsibility for their medication, the parents will need to be aware of correct administration so that they can monitor the children's level of compliance.

Although care should be family-centred, the nurse should be sensitive to the parents' own needs. Where a family have to cope with a chronic illness, an admission to hospital for an acute exacerbation may be greeted as a chance for respite from an otherwise gruelling routine. Part of the nursing admission interview should include discussion and negotiation with the parents regarding the role they want to play.

DEVELOPMENT AND GROWTH

A child learns about life through observation, interaction with others and play. When administering any treatment, the nurse should provide explanations suitable to the child's level of understanding and use play wherever appropriate. Even the language nurses use routinely can be very frightening, and 'magic smoke' sounds far less threatening than a nebuliser. Likening face masks to spacemen and divers may prove successful in administering medication. Where breathing exercises are indicated, e.g. with pneumonia or pneumothorax, the use of blow football or bubble painting is likely to be successful in gaining the child's cooperation; the support of hospital play therapists, where available, is invaluable in implementing such activities.

Poorly controlled respiratory disease can have repercussions on the child in many ways. Poorly controlled asthma can lead to small stature and alteration in the shape of the chest. The inability to participate in sport can further impair these children's ability to be seen as 'normal' by either themselves or their peers, thus perpetuating the stigma asthma sadly still carries. Frequent exacerbations of illness will cause loss of schooling and can lead, in the long term, to poor academic achievement.

SAFETY AND COMFORT

Whilst wishing children to maintain their normal pattern of life as far as possible, their safety needs to be ensured at all times. During the acute phase of their illness, oxygen and suction equipment should be available. When oxygen therapy is in use, friction toys are not advisable due to the high risk of combustion. As mentioned before, parents should be encouraged not to smoke, and this is of increased importance if home oxygen therapy is being used.

CONCLUSION

This chapter can only serve as a brief overview of the nurse's role in the diagnosis and treatment of respiratory illness in children. The disease processes which occur throughout the respiratory tract can rarely be treated in isolation. The multidisciplinary approach to care by an experienced team should always be adopted and it must never be forgotten that the family play an important role within this team. Nurses must be aware of the importance of accurate reporting and recording of observations and information as an aid to diagnosis by medical colleagues.

It is suggested that further reading about the following conditions is required for full understanding of the features and related care of each illness:

- respiratory distress syndrome
- bronchiolitis
- asthma
- pneumonia
- cystic fibrosis
- croup
- epiglottitis.

REFERENCES

American Heart Association 1986 Standards and guidelines for cardiopulmonary resuscitation and emergency cardiac care. Journal of the American Medical Association 255(21): 2956, 2958

Barnes P Levy J 1984 Nocturnal asthma. Royal Society of Medicine International Congress and Symposium Series. Royal Society of Medicine, London

Cuthbert A 1993 The function of the cystic fibrosis gene. Paediatric Respiratory Medicine 1(4): 6–11

Dinwiddie R 1993 New therapies for cystic fibrosis. Paediatric Respiratory Medicine 1(2): 22–25

Kelly S J 1988 Paediatric intensive care nursing. Appleton & Lange, California, pp 103–109

Milner A, Ingram D 1970 Peak expiratory flow rates in children under 5 years of age. Archives of Disease in Childhood 45: 820–823

Petty T 1990 The national mucolytic study. 97: 75–83

Pryor J et al 1990 Effect of chest physiotherapy on oxygen saturation in patients with cystic fibrosis. Thorax 45: 77

Rogers M 1992 Temperature recording in infants and children. Paediatric Nursing (April): 23–26

Royal College of Physicians (RCP) 1992 Smoking and the young. Royal College of Physicians working party report. RCP, London

Sackner M, Landa J et al 1973 Pathogenesis and prevention of tracheobronchial damage with suction procedures. Chest 64: 284–290

Sepion B 1990 Intravenous care for children. Paediatric Nursing 2(3): 14–16

Speight A, Lee D 1993 Under-diagnosis and under-treatment of asthma in childhood. British Medical Journal 286: 1253–1256

Wales J, Barnes N, Swift P 1991 Growth retardation in children on steroids for asthma. Lancet 338: 1535

Walthers O D, Pederson S 1990 Short term linear growth in asthmatic children during treatment with prednisolone. British Medical Journal 301: 145–148

Whaley L F, Wong D L 1989 Nursing care of infants and children, 3rd edn. C V Mosby, St Louis

Young C S 1984 A review of the adverse events and recommended guidelines for airway suction. Physiotherapy 70: 104–108

FURTHER READING

British Thoracic Society 1993 Guidelines on the treatment of asthma. Thorax 48 (Suppl.): S1–S24

Byers C 1989 Managing cystic fibrosis. Paediatric Nursing 1(6): 14–18

Glasper A 1991 Child care—some nursing perspectives. Wolfe Publishing, London

Hinchliff S, Montague S 1991 Physiology for nursing practice. Baillière Tindall, London

Levy S, Barnes G Asthma at your fingertips. Class Publishing, London

Milner A D 1993 Childhood asthma: diagnosis, treatment and management, 2nd edn. Martin Dunitz, London

Taylor C 1993 Nutrition and the child with cystic fibrosis. Paediatric Nursing 5(4): 26–28

Tizzano E F, Buchwald M 1993 Recent advances in cystic fibrosis research. Journal of Paediatrics 122: 985–988

Woodward S 1994 A guide to paediatric resuscitation. Paediatric Nursing 6(2): 16–18

12

Nutrition and the digestive system

Stephanie Moulai   Sally Huband

This chapter introduces the student to the nutrition of children from infancy, through childhood to adolescence. The importance of childhood nutrition and its effect on growth and development will be considered. Common nutritional problems will be discussed.

The chapter aims to:
- discuss the importance of infant feeding and identify factors which may affect this
- review current trends in infant weaning and suggest methods of implementation
- give an overview of child and adolescent nutrition
- discuss the common causes of feeding difficulties in infants and children and methods of management
- discuss the common intolerances and allergies and methods of management
- discuss the common problems of digestion in children.

Children's nutrition is the basis of health during childhood and also influences health in later life. The nurse will need the knowledge to be an adviser and resource to parents so that children are offered the most suitable diet for their age group. Some parents whose children have specific problems will need the additional help of the dietitian. Children have a greater need for calories than adults because of their

Table 12.1 Approximate energy requirements by age group (adapted from Savage-King & Burgess 1992)

Age	Energy requirements (kilocalories per kilogram body weight per 24 hours)
0 +	110
3 +	100
5 +	90
10 +	70

higher metabolic rate and their need to grow (Table 12.1). In addition, their diet needs to be well balanced and adapted to the needs of their age.

INFANT FEEDING

Breast-feeding

It has long been recognised that breast-feeding provides the optimum nutrition for infants. In spite of the publicity given to 'breast is best', the incidence of breast-feeding is not increasing. In 1980, 65% of mothers breast-fed their babies; in 1985, 64% breast-fed; and, in 1990, 63% breast-fed (OPCS 1992). The decision is often taken before the mother visits the antenatal clinic. In one survey, over 80% of women had already decided when they went for a booking clinic; 88.5% of the women who had stated that they wished to breast-feed at this time subsequently did so, and only 1 woman out of 20 who had stated they would bottle-feed subsequently changed her mind (Oxby 1994). Unfortunately, approximately 25% of women who initially breast-feed have ceased to do so after 6 weeks (Martin & White 1988).

Activity 12.1

Ask a group of your female friends whether they would breast-feed their children if they had them. Try to find out what has influenced their decision.

Advantages of breast-feeding

Once well established, breast milk provides complete nutrition for the infant. The first milk to be produced, the colostrum, is a watery yellow substance that is rich in protein and particularly in IgA which will help protect against infection. After the first 2 days, the milk becomes a mixture of colostrum and more mature milk and by the 10th day mature milk is fully established. The mature milk is composed of the foremilk, which is dilute and low in fat, and the hindmilk, which is more concentrated and has a higher fat concentration.

Nutrition:

Protein. The protein content of breast milk is relatively low, constituting 1.1% of the total feed, and most of it is lactalbumen, the whey protein which is easily digested by the infant.

Fat. Fat content is variable. It is usually low at the start of the feed and higher at the end when more of the hindmilk is taken. Breast milk contains an enzyme, lipase, which aids in the digestion of fat. Breast milk also contains the essential long-chain polyunsaturated fats which are important for brain and retinal development.

Carbohydrate. Breast milk is high in lactose, which is important for encouraging the growth of the lactobacillus that maintains the acidic reaction in the gut and inhibits the growth of pathogenic organisms. Lactose is also important for increasing the absorption of calcium and therefore assisting in bone development.

Iron. Full-term babies are born with iron stores in their liver. After birth, there is a rapid breakdown of haemoglobin resulting in further iron stores. These stores should last the baby for the first few months of life. Breast milk is relatively low in iron but what there is, is well absorbed. Lactoferrin, an iron-binding protein present in breast milk, is bacteriostatic and reduces the risk of infection from coliform organisms.

Minerals. The infant's kidneys are unable to deal with a high solute load. Breast milk is low in sodium, calcium, phosphorus and potassium.

Vitamins. It is recommended that vitamin K is administered routinely to all babies at delivery to protect against haemolytic disease of the new-born. Vitamin drops are recommended for all breast-fed infants over the age of 6 months.

Fluoride. The British Dental Association recommends a level of fluoride that cannot be obtained in either breast or formula milk. However, the amount of fluoride in water supplies varies and this has to be taken into account.

Protection against infection. Breast milk contains IgA and IgM. The IgA, which is mainly found in colostrum, protects the intestinal lining from the penetration of intestinal organisms and allergens. There are more lysozymes (bacteriolytic enzymes) in breast milk than in cow's milk.

Babies who are breast-fed are less likely to have gastroenteritis, due to the acidic reaction in the gut, the bacteriostatic effect of lactoferrin and the reduced risk of contamination. There is a reduced risk of otitis media (Duncan et al 1993) and of respiratory infections. There is also less risk of necrotising enterocolitis (NEC) in preterm infants and, as this serious condition has a 20–40% mortality rate, this is a significant factor. The closure of breast milk banks as a result of concern over HIV is estimated to have caused an additional 500 cases of NEC per year (Lucas & Cole 1990).

Additional factors. There has been recent interest in the theory that breast-feeding leads to a higher IQ. Lucas et al (1992) studied a group of infants who had been born preterm and tested them at the age of 18 months and again at 8 years. They found that there was a significant difference between the IQs of babies who had been fed their own mothers' expressed breast milk via a nasogastric tube and those who had been given formula milk. Although the social class, parenting skills and education of the groups studied could be factors, the authors did not feel that this was the explanation.

Breast-feeding is also thought to promote bonding, especially if the baby is put to the breast soon after delivery and this is the current practice in many units. The breast-fed baby appears to have some protection from eczema and there is a reduced incidence amongst families with a history of atopy.

Benefits for the mother. During pregnancy, adipose tissue is laid down in anticipation of breast-feeding. This fat can be mobilised during breast-feeding. The woman who is bottle-feeding may have more difficulty in losing this extra fat. The secretion of oxytocin during breast-feeding encourages the uterus to contract, which is also a benefit. There have been several studies which suggest that breast-feeding protects against breast cancer (United Kingdom National Case-Control Study Group 1993).

Regular and frequent breast-feeding also has a contraceptive effect but is not 100% reliable.

Contraindications to breast-feeding

In the United Kingdom, an HIV-positive mother is advised not to breast-feed, as the infection can pass to the infant via the breast milk. In developing countries, the risk of the baby contracting the virus from breast milk is outweighed by the risks for the infant who is bottle-fed.

Most babies with cleft lip can be breast-fed with encouragement; however, if the baby has a cleft palate, breast-feeding is usually unsuccessful, even with a dental plate, as the baby is unable to form a seal between his mouth and the breast.

If a mother has a chronic illness necessitating drug therapy, the pharmacy will need to be contacted as many drugs are passed into the breast milk. Sometimes safe alternatives can be prescribed.

Factors which can lead to mothers discontinuing breast-feeding

Most of the problems encountered by mothers can be overcome by giving extra support and ensuring that the infant is correctly attached and positioned for feeding.

Pain caused by sore nipples or engorgement. Sore nipples are usually caused by incorrect positioning of the infant, and research has shown that correct positioning is as effective as taking the baby off the breast whilst the nipple heals (Nicholson 1985). The use of creams, sprays, lotions and ointments has no scientific basis and a randomised controlled trial has yet to be carried out (Garcia & Garforth 1985).

Engorgement is due to an increased blood flow to the breasts followed by an over-filling of the breasts with milk. Demand-feeding and correct positioning can help to alleviate this.

Mastitis and breast abscesses.   Mastitis is not always caused by an infection but can be due to milk substances being forced out into the tissues due to an increase in pressure in the alveoli. Infection is usually caused by bacteria entering through a breach in the skin due to cracked or sore nipples. Only if infection is present is antibiotic therapy required; as long as the mother can be monitored closely, there is no need for the baby to stop feeding. If the mother develops a breast abscess, it may require either aspirating or incising. The infant can feed from the affected breast as long as the incision does not make it impossible as this will aid healing (RCM 1991).

Insufficient milk.   The fact that mothers are unable to measure the amount of milk the infant is taking can often lead to anxiety, especially if the baby is fretful. Frequent feeding and correct positioning will usually overcome this problem, as it is uncommon for there to be a real lack of milk if the baby is suckling efficiently. There is little benefit in test weighing; as it is usually inaccurate and the baby is likely to take different amounts at each feed, it needs to be done over a period of time. Test weighing also increases the anxiety of an already worried mother.

Embarrassment and lack of facilities.   Some mothers will give up because they are embarrassed or because they find the attitude of society to people breast-feeding in public unhelpful. There is also a lack of facilities for mothers to

Activity 12.2

Consider how you might present a talk on breast-feeding to a mixed group of 14- to 16-year-olds. What information would you give to help to increase the percentage of breast-fed babies in the future?

breast-feed when they are out and this can lead to social isolation. Some mothers will give up when they return to work. They could be encouraged to continue to breast-feed, even if it is only two breast feeds a day and formula feeds at other times.

Attachment and positioning of the infant

Practical experience is required to enable the nurse to learn how to support the breast-feeding mother and facilitate correct attachment and positioning.

For further information, see RCM (1991).

Frequency and duration of feeds

The baby is the best guide to the number of feeds he requires. Some babies may initially require feeding every 2 hours; others may go for 4–6 hours between feeds. The length of time spent feeding also varies between individual babies, depending on the rate of feeding and the flow of milk. Feeds which regularly last more than 30 minutes may need to be supervised to ensure that the baby is correctly positioned.

Breast-feeding in a paediatric unit.   Children's nurses have a responsibility to ensure that they are knowledgeable and skilful in assisting mothers with breast-feeding. Mothers of babies who are admitted to hospital will need help to continue to breast-feed. They may need to express their milk if the baby is unable to suck. They will also require privacy and support, as anxiety can be a factor in causing mothers to give up.

The preterm infant.   The sucking and swallowing reflex of infants is not fully developed until 32 weeks' gestation; therefore the preterm infant often requires parenteral feeding or feeding by oro- or nasogastric tube initially. Babies are initially nose breathers, so using a nasogastric tube can inhibit the breathing of the small preterm infant; in these cases an orogastric tube will often be used, even though it is less easy to secure. Breast milk is still the best milk for these infants and, if the mother is willing, she can be assisted to express her milk, which is then given to her infant. As the mother may need to continue to express milk for several weeks and this needs to be done 8–12 times in 24 hours, she will need to be well supported. She can be encouraged by the knowledge that she is contributing in a very positive manner to the welfare of her infant (see Chs 11 and 20). Sucking on a blind teat during a tube feed, can improve the weight gain of the infant and this is thought to be due to the release of lingual lipase (RCM 1991).

Bottle-feeding

Mothers who are unwilling or unable to breast-feed should not be made to feel guilty or that they are failing their infants in some manner. They will need information concerning a suitable milk for their baby and the amount that should be offered.

Modified milks and formulae

Following an EEC directive (1991), with which all products had to comply by June 1994, infant milks are based on cow's milk and infant formulae are milks which are not based on cow's milk, e.g. soya formula.

Whey-dominant milks. These are the milks that are made from modified cow's milk and have a whey : casein ratio that is similar to breast milk at 60 : 40. These are most suitable for the youngest babies. Examples of these are Cow & Gate Premium, SMA Gold, Farley's Ostermilk and Milupa Aptamil.

Casein-dominant milks. These milks have the same whey : casein ratio at 20 : 80 as is found in cow's milk. The small baby has difficulty in digesting the casein in these feeds so they are not suitable until the infant is older. Examples of these are Cow & Gate Plus, SMA White, Farley's Ostermilk Two and Milupa Milumil.

Soya formulae. Only babies who are shown to have a cow's milk protein or lactose intoler-ance should be given these milks. They are sometimes encouraged in the belief that the baby who is vomiting or unsettled will fare better with them, but soya, too, is a foreign protein and can cause intolerance. It also has high levels of aluminium and, although there is no evidence that this will cause problems for the healthy infant, these milks should not be used for preterm infants or those with renal disease.

Soya milks also contain high levels of oestrogen, 100 times the amount found in breast milk. Research is currently being carried out in New Zealand to see whether this can cause problems for the young infant. Examples of these milks are Cow & Gate Infasoy, Wyeth Wysoy, Prosobee and Osterby.

Follow-on milks. These milks have come on to the market relatively recently and are designed for the infant over 6 months old. They are not suitable for younger infants, as the protein content and solute load are greater. They are, however, preferable to giving the baby unmodified cow's milk as they have iron and vitamins added to them. They have no advantage over modified infant milks. Examples of these are Cow & Gate Step Up, SMA Progress and Farley's Junior milk.

Cow's milk

Cow's milk is not recommended as the baby's main milk until after the age of 1 year. This is due to the low level of vitamins and iron. There is no reason why babies cannot have some milk on their cereal or with other food, as long as their main milk is either breast milk or an infant milk or formula.

Calculating and timing of babies' feeds

Bottle-fed babies can be demand-fed in the same way as breast-fed babies can. The amount of feed required is based on the baby's weight and varies between 150 and 200 ml per kilogram of body weight per 24 hours. The higher amount of feed is usually only required by the preterm or light for dates infant. The total amount of feed is then divided between the number of feeds per 24 hours, with night feeds being omitted as the baby grows.

Preparation of feeds

Milk is a good growing medium for bacteria so it is important that the feeding utensils are sterilised and the feeds made up with boiled water. Feeds can be made up for 24 hours as long as they can be stored in a refrigerator. Instructions for making up the milks are written on the tins. Scoops are provided with each product. Usually, feeds are made up with 1 scoop to 1 fluid ounce (30 ml) of cooled, boiled water. The powder in the scoop should be levelled off with a knife and not pressed down. It is important that the feeds are made up to the recommended strength and are neither too dilute nor too strong. If the feeds have been kept in a refrigerator they will need to be warmed prior to giving them to the infant. They should not, however, be warmed in a microwave oven, which can produce heat spots that can scald the infant.

Weaning and the weaning diet

Weaning is the gradual introduction of the infant to a mixed diet. It is necessary when milk ceases to provide all the nutrients that the infant requires. It is now recommended that solids are not given before the age of 4 months, but should be offered before 6 months.

 For further information, see DoH (1994).

Weaning is part of the developmental process during which the infant changes from sucking to biting and chewing. These processes help to develop the muscles and movements that will later be necessary for speech. The enzymes required to digest fats and starch are not present in the gut in sufficient quantities until the infant is 3–4 months old, so giving solids before this

time is not recommended. The solid food given is initially puréed and will progress to a consistency that is more lumpy.

First foods

Cereals are usually the first foods offered to the infant, but they should not be wheat-based. The early introduction of wheat-based cereals can lead to an acute onset of coeliac disease in susceptible infants. There is no evidence that delaying the introduction of gluten prevents coeliac disease, as there has been a steady decline in the number of cases amongst children for many years (Stevens et al 1987). However, introducing the infant to gluten-containing cereals after the age of 6 months has led to a later and less acute onset.

Babies tend to be conservative in their tastes and it takes perseverance to introduce the baby to taking solids off the spoon and in introducing new tastes. Tastes are developed during infancy and it is therefore recommended that the food should not contain added salt or sugar. The amount and variety of foods offered should be gradually increased as the intake of milk is reduced. Meat, fish, eggs and all cereals and pulses can be introduced between the ages of 6 and 9 months (DoH 1994). Eggs should be well cooked, until both white and yolk are solid, to destroy the salmonella bacteria, with which some are contaminated (DoH 1993).

Manufactured foods. These may be in jars, tins or dried foods in packets and a wide range is available. They are usually seen as being more expensive than home-puréed foods, but this may not be the case if food is prepared separately for the baby and then only a small amount eaten. The manufactured foods can be given in small quantities and are most useful when families are travelling. However, from the age of about 6–7 months it is probably wise to offer home-produced foods, so that the baby becomes accustomed to a wide range of tastes and textures.

Weaning methods

Solids should be given from a spoon and not added to the bottle. Initially, the baby is likely to spit them out or gag, and perseverance is required. Feeding should be a relaxed time and the mother can choose the meal time at which she first introduces the foods. It is usually preferable to choose a time of day when neither the baby nor the mother is tired. Meal times should not be hurried and there should be the minimum of distractions. Food should not be allowed to become a play medium and mothers may need support to prevent food refusal becoming a manipulative weapon in the hands of even young infants. Often there is a tendency to feed young children too quickly and not allow them the time that an older child would take over the meal. Finger foods can be given from the age of 6–7 months but initially should be those which are softened in the mouth, such as bread or banana. The harder foods, such as a piece of apple or finger of toast, should be delayed until the infant has learnt to chew well. He should be well supervised to prevent choking. From this time he can also be given his own spoon, though this is initially used more as a toy and the infant needs time to develop coordination skills. Drinks can be given from teacher beakers or cups, and bottles should be discouraged after the age of 12 months (DoH 1994).

Nutritional factors concerning the weanling

Milks. Skimmed milks and semi-skimmed milks are not suitable for young children, who still get much of their energy requirements from fat. Fat is particularly important for brain growth, which is at its most rapid from before birth to the age of 2 years. Semi-skimmed milk can be given from the age of 2 years and skimmed milk from the age of 5 years. Goat's and sheep's milks can be given from the age of 1 year, provided that the child's diet contains sufficient iron and vitamin D, which are low in these milks. They should not be given before the age of 1 year. It is important that they conform to the regulations controlling them.

Fruit, herbal drinks and water. There is now a range of drinks on the market for babies. Many of these are relatively high in sugars, but they do have fewer additives than normal fruit squashes. The acidity can cause dental problems later and it has also been questioned whether the herbal extracts may have some pharmacological effect, even though they are dilute (DoH 1994). Water given to young babies should be boiled, until they are 6 months old; after this it can be taken from the mains tap when it is less likely to be contaminated. Some bottled waters are not suitable for young babies because of their high content of solutes, such as nitrate, sodium, fluoride and sulphate (DoH 1994).

Fibre. Fibre is useful in preventing constipation; however, it is bulky and low in calories and the baby has a small stomach and requires a high-energy diet. Fibre also inhibits the absorption of iron. Young children need a balance between sufficient fibre to prevent constipation and an energy-dense diet which will give them the calories they need to grow. Raw bran is not recommended for this age group.

Iron. Full-term infants have sufficient stored iron to last until they are about 4 months of age; after this their diet needs to contain iron to meet their increasing requirements. One of the problems with iron is that the amount present in the food is not a measure of the amount that is absorbed. There are various substances which will hinder the absorption, for example phytic acid from cereals and legumes and tannin from tea. Babies who are breast-fed after 6 months will need additional iron, although if solid food is given at a different time, the amount of iron absorbed from the breast milk is greater (Oski & Landaw 1980). A diet which contains adequate amounts of vitamin C will help in the absorption of iron from the diet. The addition of iron to infant milks and foods is a valuable source for weanlings. In addition, they require meat and lightly cooked fruit and vegetables.

Ethnic minorities

Diets are affected by culture, and Britain is a multicultural and multiracial society. Any advice given concerning diet must take these factors into account. During weaning, some cultures rely mainly on infant formulae or cow's milk for meeting the nutritional needs of the child for too long. This may be because the weaning foods available in this country are unfamiliar or do not conform to the culture. After the age of 6 months, children cannot receive all the nutrients they require to grow from milk only and mothers may need advice on how to prepare food at home which meets the need of the weanling and conforms to their culture. Some communities may continue to bottle-feed until the third year and sugar and honey is often added to these drinks (DoH 1994). Children from these communities have been found to have a higher rate of dental caries, a higher rate of iron deficiency anaemia and to be smaller (DoH 1988). There has also been an increased number of cases of rickets amongst the Asian community, but the reason for this is complex. The formation of vitamin D from exposure to sunlight is reduced in pigmented skins and there are other factors such as late weaning and high fibre content of the diet.

Vegetarian and vegan diets

There is no reason why these diets should not meet the nutritional needs of growing children; however, there are special considerations that need to be borne in mind. Vegans exclude all foods of animal origin and the diet is based on cereals, pulses, vegetables, fruits, nuts and seeds. Human breast milk is acceptable and, if the mother is unable or unwilling to breast-feed, a soya milk can be used. Both diets tend to have a lower energy density, so care needs to be taken during weaning that the child gets sufficient energy from other sources. Other risk areas are the low content of vitamin D in vegan diets in particular, and it is recommended that children should be given a vitamin supplement, such as Abidec, from 6 months to 5 years. Iron may also be a problem and iron deficiency anaemia is particularly common in children on macrobiotic and Rastafarian diets.

PRE-SCHOOL CHILDREN

Pre-school children are still dependent on their carers for when and what they eat, and likes and dislikes are often established during this period. Small children are often resistant to change and it is not sensible to offer them too many choices. 'I don't like it' may be a resistance to trying anything that a child is not accustomed to. Food fads are common and meal times can become a battle with small children refusing or playing with their meals. The guidelines on healthy eating in the COMA and NACNE reports (DHSS 1984, NACNE 1983) are not meant to be applied to this age group. These children still have a high energy requirement and it is important to see that the proportion of sugar in their energy intake is not too high. Payne (1991) found that fruit juices and blackcurrant syrups, which were seen to be healthy, were the main sources of sugar in diets of young children with an exceptionally high sugar intake. This may lead to obesity and also a high sugar intake is related to the development of dental caries. Small children often display erratic eating behaviour, picking at one meal and eating well at another. Some children seem to prefer one particular meal. As long as their energy requirements are met, it is better if they are not forced to eat large portions at each meal, and parents should be encouraged to take a relaxed attitude, looking at the overall pattern and not the behaviour at one specific meal. Between-meals snacks and drinks with a high sugar content may also prevent the child from eating well at meal times. Pre-school children tend to have frequent minor illnesses which will also interfere with their eating. However, they will usually make up for this deficit by increasing their intake once they have recovered.

SCHOOL-AGE CHILDREN

The Education Act of 1980 had a major effect on the provision of school meals. Prior to this time, local education authorities had a statutory obligation to provide meals of a specific nutritional standard at a fixed price. A school meal was meant to provide one-third of the total daily nutritional needs of the child. The 1980 Act abolished these requirements. Now local authorities have to provide a place for children to eat their sandwiches but need only provide meals for those children who are eligible for free school meals, i.e. children from families on income support. This change may have resulted in about 30% of children losing their entitlement. The changes in the benefit system in 1988 meant that, instead of free school meals being provided, some families are now given cash. The problem with this is that the money may not be spent on food (Thomas 1994). A survey commissioned by the DHSS in 1983 (DoH 1989) looked at the effect of the abolition of school meals and found some disturbing facts. A high percentage of children did not have an intake sufficiently high in calcium, iron and vitamin A.

A considerable number of school children do not eat breakfast, so lunch may be the first meal of the day. Children are likely to select familiar foods and those that they like from the school menu, so that even if there is a good menu available, the child may not choose the most nutritional items. Many children take packed lunches to school and these vary in their contents. There is increasing concern over the diet of school children, and schools could make a significant contribution by incorporating teaching on food and nutrition into the school curriculum. However, the theory needs to be matched with children's experience. If eating patterns at home are poor, tuck shops mainly stock sweets, drinks and snacks with a high content of fat and sugar and school meals do not set a good example, the diet of children will remain at risk.

Activity 12.3

Ask a group of school-age children what their favourite foods and drinks are. See if they can remember what they have eaten over a 24-hour period. Also ask them if they know what foods are good for them. See if there is any correlation between what they know and what they have eaten.

ADOLESCENTS

The rapid growth spurt during adolescence means that nutritional requirements are increased. Most girls will have their growth spurt between the ages of 11 and 14 (see App. 3), and during this time there tends to be an increase in body fat with the onset of puberty. Boys have their growth spurt slightly later, between the ages of 13 and 16 (see App. 4), and they increase their lean body mass. On average, boys will grow more than girls and this will affect their energy needs. However, the physical activity of the individual also needs to be taken into account. More boys are involved in strenuous physical activity than girls and this also affects their needs.

Adolescents may also have very erratic eating patterns. They are influenced more by their peers than their parents and may well be trying out new ideas and adopting new principles. They may decide on a vegan or vegetarian diet, or one of the more extreme regimes such as a macrobiotic diet. These have to be taken seriously and the individuals helped to incorporate healthy eating within their chosen diet. They may also be trying out alcohol and spending time in pubs with their friends and there may be a surfeit of snack foods and a lack of a more balanced diet.

Adolescents are also very aware of their body image and girls in particular may develop a fear of obesity. The severe eating disorders of anorexia nervosa and bulimia are more likely to become apparent during the adolescent years and will require psychiatric intervention. (See Ch. 23.)

LOW-INCOME FAMILIES

The diets of families on low incomes have been surveyed on a number of occasions and all surveys have found that a healthy diet is a more expensive one and that families on low incomes are often forced to economise on food. A report by the Central Statistical Office in 1991 found that the highest income groups spent one and a half times as much on food as the low-income families. A report by a charity, The National Children's Home (NCH), in 1991 found that 55% of families on income support said that their children had not had enough to eat during the previous month. Not only is there a lack of food but the food tends to be have a high fat and sugar content. Convenience foods are popular and families are unlikely to experiment with new types of dishes when money is tight. Many families only cook raw food once or twice a week (HEA 1989) and they eat little lean meat, fresh fruit and vegetables, favouring the fish fingers and burgers which are relatively cheap and popular with the children. Cheaper cuts of meat are usually fattier or take longer to cook so use up more fuel. Baked potatoes require considerable cooking, whereas crisps require no preparation. Families in bedsit accommodation have the added disadvantage of shared cooking facilities and often no storage space. Advising families on healthy diets needs to be realistic and must take into account individual circumstances.

CHILDREN IN HOSPITAL

Adequate nutrition is essential for the child who is ill in hospital. During illness, the metabolic rate is increased and calorie consumption is greater. The nurse has a responsibility to monitor the amount of food and fluid taken by the child at meal times. The meals should be served by the nursing staff and preferably eaten at a table with other children. However, young children may be

Activity 12.4

Go with a friend to a supermarket and 'price' a food basket for a family of two adults and two children. One of you can choose a healthy diet, without regard for cost, and the other choose a diet that needs little preparation, appeals to children and is cheap. Compare your prices when you have finished.
    See if you can reduce the price of the healthy eating basket. Is it appealing to children and is it easy to prepare?

distracted by the noise and bustle of a hospital ward and may eat better in a quieter environment. A choice of food is normally offered and should be served at a correct temperature in an organised manner, so that no patient is missed. Appropriately sized cutlery should be used, e.g. small spoon and fork for toddlers. Food should look attractive and where possible should be similar to the food eaten at home. It is usual practice to ask parents and children on admission about their likes and dislikes and any particular practices such as a bottle at bedtime. Sometimes parents will give the answers that they feel the nurse will approve of, e.g. which conform to a healthy diet. Children may give totally different answers. Parents can bring food in from home if they wish and this may tempt children who have a poor appetite because they are unwell, in a strange environment and being offered unfamiliar food. Excessive consumption of sweets and crisps will affect the appetite of children and should be avoided. A survey by Mills et al (1993) found that children were aware of healthy eating, yet whilst in hospital ate more unhealthy food. This may be because sweets and crisps are brought in as 'treats'. Ill children who cannot be tempted to eat can be offered milky or glucose drinks. It is important to keep the fluid intake up, even if the child refuses food. Children who have had anaesthetics can be given water to drink after a few hours. It is advisable to wait until the danger of vomiting is over, but if the child is screaming and very upset, this may not be possible. Children who have had gastrointestinal surgery may need an intravenous infusion and are not allowed anything by mouth until they have been assessed by the doctor. Sips of water are given when allowed and this is gradually increased if there is no vomiting. The child can them have unrestricted fluids, commonly known as 'free fluids'. If these are tolerated, a light diet may be given. This may be toast, cereal or mashed potato and non-greasy fish or meat.

Babies and young children who have undergone major gastrointestinal surgery require total parenteral nutrition (TPN), also known as intravenous feeding. TPN is given directly into a central vein though a catheter (see Ch. 24 for care of central lines).

COMMON NUTRITIONAL PROBLEMS

Posseting

Often when babies are winded, or have completed a feed, they bring up a small amount of milk. It is usually effortless but can cause concern to the parents. Also the baby's clothes tend to smell of stale milk and this is unpleasant.

Treatment is initially observing how the baby feeds. He may be feeding too quickly, may be swallowing excess air, or the size of the hole in the teat may be too big or too small. Some babies need winding more frequently, especially if they are swallowing an excess of air. It is also important to check the quantity of feed being given, as posseting can occur when the baby is being overfed.

Gastro-oesophageal reflux (GOR) also causes posseting and may need further treatment. GOR is caused by the immaturity of the cardiac sphincter of the stomach, which allows milk and gastric secretion to reflux back into the oesophagus. The problem is compounded by the fact that the diet is liquid and the baby is laid flat after a feed. Most babies will improve if they are sat upright after feeding for half an hour and they can also be given a feed thickener (see Box 12.1). This will stop the posseting and prevent oesophagitis from the reflux of gastric acid.

As the baby grows and adopts a more upright position and the food becomes more solid, the problems resolve and the thickeners can be discontinued.

Colic

It is normal for babies to cry (see Ch. 14), particularly in the early weeks. Many babies who cry are diagnosed as having colic, although the rationale for this is unclear. There has been considerable research into both crying and colic in babies and no consensus has yet been reached. Some breast-fed babies seem to be more unsettled if their mothers have eaten a particular food. A small number of babies may be showing signs of cow's milk protein allergy (see p. 207). The majority of cases of crying in babies, however, will not be found to have any particular cause. In the past these babies were given gripe water containing considerable quantities of alcohol. Illingworth found that 'a one month old baby weighing 4 kg, given the upper range of recommended dosage of 5 ml eight times per day, will receive daily as much 90% alcohol per kg as an 80 kg adult gets per kg from almost five tots of whisky' (Illingworth & Timmins 1990). These gripe waters have now been withdrawn, but it is not surprising that they were found to be so effective in settling the baby.

Box 12.1 Examples of feed thickeners

Infant gaviscon. This is easy to use and effective in mild cases; however, it is not a good thickener but it does contain antacid. It must be added to the feed, in the quantities recommended by the manufacturer, immediately before the feed is given. Breast-fed babies can be given the powder mixed with water. The gaviscon reacts with the gastric acid to form a gel, which will prevent the reflux.

Carobel. This is made from carob bean gum and comes in a flaked form, ready to add to warmed feeds. Breast-fed babies can be given this mixed with water prior to the feed; bottle-fed babies have it added to the feed.

Nestargel. This is made from carob bean flour. It requires more preparation and is less often used now that instant thickeners are available.

Instructions for using all thickeners must be followed.

Activity 12.5

Talk to some parents of babies from 0–4 months old and ask them about the crying patterns of their children. Try to find out whether they see this crying as normal or whether they think something is the matter. Find out the time of day/night when the crying is most common.

If parents mention that their baby has colic, try to find out whether there is any difference between the crying of those babies who are said to have colic, and those where it is not mentioned. (Be careful that you do not suggest that the baby does have colic or has anything wrong.)

For further information, see St James-Roberts (1991).

Toddler diarrhoea

This is the term given to a condition in children who present during the toddler years, 6 months to 3 years being the most common, with episodes of diarrhoea, abdominal pain and the passing of undigested food particles in the stools. Mothers report seeing pieces of carrot or undigested peas in the nappies and potties of their children. Typically the children remain well and grow normally and parents should be reassured that the condition is self-limiting and not serious. There does not appear to be one single cause for the condition, rather there are several factors. Taitz & Wardley (1989) suggest that one of the factors may be that the child is now more mobile and more likely to pick up several minor infections. Children in this age group are renowned for putting objects in their mouths. Another factor may be the reduced fat in the weaning diet, as fat slows gastric emptying. Increasing the fibre content of the diet may also contribute to the condition. Only children who are unwell or failing to grow normally need to be investigated.

Constipation

This is a condition in which hard dry stools are passed at infrequent intervals. Many babies appear to strain when passing stools but this does not mean that defaecation is painful or that the baby is constipated. The soiled nappy should be inspected for colour, consistency and amount of stool passed, before passing judgement. Common causes of constipation are either an inadequate fluid intake or over-concentrated feeds. Both of these can be remedied by the nurse giving correct advice. Extra fluid in the form of cooled, boiled water, particularly for the bottle-fed baby, is helpful. In weaned babies, giving

puréed fruits and vegetables may help to solve the problem. Persistent constipation in an infant should be referred to a specialist to exclude Hirschsprung's disease or anal stenosis.

Toddlers who have constipation may require added fibre, which should be introduced gradually. Good sources of fibre are wholemeal bread and whole grain breakfast cereals such as Weetabix, Shreddies and puffed wheat. An adequate fluid intake of between 1200 and 1500 ml per day, dependent on the child's age, is also essential.

School-age children also often present with constipation. Adequate fluids and fibre are also important for this age group. In addition, it is often helpful to ask the family about the level of physical activity taken by the child and also the routine. Some children are very wary of using school toilets and may be 'too busy' to go before leaving for school. The gastrocolic reflex, whereby activity in the stomach triggers activity in the colon, can be made use of by taking the child to the toilet after breakfast and after supper.

Chronic constipation and soiling

Children who have chronic constipation are often referred to the paediatrician because of soiling their underclothes. They may also have abdominal pain and a loss of appetite. On examination, the large bowel is found to be full of faeces and this can be confirmed on an abdominal radiograph. The aim of treatment is to clear the bowel and change the habits of the child.

Medicines used to help clear the bowel include Lactulose, which is an osmotic laxative, and Senna Syrup, which is a stimulant laxative. These are commonly prescribed. Patience and persuasion are the necessary skills for the nurse in encouraging the child to take them.

Activity 12.6

How would you encourage a child who has constipation to take medicine such as 10 ml of Lactulose?

Children can be acutely embarrassed by soiling and may hide soiled clothes in their bedside lockers. The dietary intake, both food and fluid, should be monitored, and a diet high in fibre advised. The child and parents may be seen by the dietitian who can give advice.

Many of the children who present with soiling have disturbed family backgrounds and may need referral to the child guidance clinic or psychiatrist (see Ch. 23).

Stomas

Infants who fail to pass meconium or present with intestinal obstruction in the first few days of life need to be referred to a paediatric surgeon. There are a number of conditions which may result in the infant requiring a stoma to relieve the obstruction in the first instance (Box 12.2).

Most of the infants will have their stomas reversed, once they have had corrective surgery. Corrective surgery is usually delayed until the child is bigger and more able to withstand major surgery.

Following formation of the stoma, it is important to observe the colour of the stoma to ensure that there is a good circulation and no undue bleeding. It is also important to see that the bag fits well and that the skin surrounding the area does not become excoriated. Most infants will have a colostomy but a few may need an ileostomy. Ileostomies may cause more problems, as the faeces are more liquid and it can be difficult to maintain the integrity of the skin. The amount of gut available for absorption may also be reduced and there can be a difficulty in meeting the nutritional needs of the infant.

The parents are likely to need time to come to terms with the fact that their baby has an abnormality. They can be involved in caring for the stoma as soon as possible so that they become competent and confident. Referral to a stoma therapist is often advised. There are a number of bags of suitable sizes available and the families usually adjust quite soon. The nurse can help by emphasising that most stomas in infants are temporary and can be closed when the child has had corrective surgery.

Gastroenteritis

Young children are very vulnerable to infections of the gastrointestinal tract and may present with diarrhoea and vomiting. Viruses are a common cause and include rotavirus and adenovirus. Bacterial infections include salmonella, shigella and campylobacter. The most serious result of vomiting and diarrhoea is dehydration, and young children are particularly prone because of the difference in their fluid balance compared to that of the adult (see Ch. 13).

Signs of dehydration in babies include:

- limpness and lethargy
- sunken anterior fontanelle
- mottled skin, due to poor circulation
- inelastic skin
- decreased urinary output.

Immediate fluid replacement is required.

Mild dehydration (5% or less) can be treated with oral glucose/electrolyte replacement fluids. These are either ready-made solutions (Dextrolyte, Pedilyte) or in sachet form which should be made up according to the instructions. Several flavours are available in this form.

Replacement fluids are given for 24–48 hours and then feeds are gradually reintroduced, using a regrading system. Table 12.2 gives a basic feeding structure which can be modified to suit the needs of an individual infant or child. Regrading depends on the amount of diarrhoea the infant has and the infant's clinical condition. If the baby is breast-fed, breast-feeding can continue with oral rehydration given as a supplement if required.

Box 12.2 **Conditions which require immediate surgical intervention**

- Intestinal atresias
- Imperforate anus
- Hirschsprung's disease
- Meconium ileus (a presentation of cystic fibrosis)

Table 12.2 Regrading system: rehydration fluid only is given initially for first 24 hours

Strength of feed	Volume of feed (ml)	Rehydration fluid (ml)	Milk (ml)
¼	200	150	50
¼	200	150	50
½	200	100	100
½	200	100	100
¾	200	50	150
¾	200	50	150
Full	200	—	200

Toddlers and older children often find the oral glucose/electrolyte solution unpalatable; they can be given very weak fruit juice instead. Toddlers who are hungry and not satisfied by fluids only, may be given a dry rusk or plain biscuit or toast.

The diarrhoea will cease sooner if the baby is given clear fluids, but the weight loss is greater. For babies who are malnourished, it may be preferable to continue their feeds and give supplementary oral rehydration fluid. Studies done using a low-lactose, low-fat formula HN25 have shown that babies given this formula, after they have been rehydrated in the usual way, gain weight faster and have loose stools for a shorter period of time (McClean et al 1990).

Babies with moderate to severe dehydration require intravenous fluid therapy. The type of solution given depends on the patient's blood electrolytes. Sodium chloride and glucose fluids are given when there is a combined water and sodium depletion.

Babies and children who have diarrhoea and vomiting often require admission to the paediatric ward following assessment in the accident and emergency department. The nursing care 10-point plan in Box 12.3 applies to all patients with gastroenteritis and can be used in planning care (see also Ch. 13).

Failure to thrive

This is the term given to children who fail to grow at the normal rate (see Box 12.4).

Nurses should be able to work out the

Box 12.3 Nursing care 10-point plan for the child with gastroenteritis

- Barrier nurse in isolation in a side room with the door closed.
- Place an appropriate sign on the door.
- Wear a disposable apron on entering room and disposable gloves when changing nappies.
- Weigh the patient daily, if a baby.
- An accurate record of fluid intake and output is essential.
- Collect two stool samples. The same sample can be used for different investigations:
  —a sample for virology
  —a sample for microscopy, culture and sensitivity testing.
- Obtain a urine sample for microscopy, culture and sensitivity testing to exclude a urinary tract infection. This is not always possible if the infant's bottom is very sore or if the diarrhoea is severe.
- Nurse the bottom exposed if necessary. Apply a suitable barrier cream, e.g. zinc and castor oil cream or Metanium.
- Dispose of waste inside the room into the correct bag.
- Educate parents and family about hand washing before they leave the room.

expected weight of an infant, once they know the age and birth weight. In addition, all young children should have their weight and height plotted on percentile charts (see Apps 1 and 2). This forms part of the health visitor's remit and should identify the child who is at risk. Parent-held records have been introduced in many areas and are likely to be universal before long. These records provide an invaluable source of information about the progress of the individual child. When estimating expected growth rates it is important to take into account the size of the parents, as small parents are likely to have smaller children than average. There are also racial differences, for example Chinese children tend to be smaller, West African children larger. Adjustments in plotting weights and heights also need to be made if the baby was premature. A baby who is below the 3rd percentile is not necessarily failing to thrive, he may just be a small baby. However, a baby who is born on the 50th percentile and subsequently falls below the 10th percentile, does need to be investigated.

There are many causes of failure to thrive; however, they can usually be grouped according to the main reasons.

- inadequate intake
- persistent vomiting
- malabsorption
- chronic disease.

Inadequate intake

This is the most common cause of failure to thrive and can usually be rectified by giving sensible advice. Unfortunately parents are often subjected to a great deal of conflicting information on how best to feed their children. Professionals, relatives and friends are all eager to pass on advice which is sometimes out of date and incorrect. In the 1960s it was common practice to introduce solids at 6 weeks of age and in some cases even sooner. Diluted evaporated milk was sometimes used to feed babies, in particular preterm infants. Most children came to no harm and mothers of that era may advise their daughters to feed their infants in a similar way.

Breast-fed babies. Breast-fed babies may take longer than bottle-fed babies to regain their birth weight and maintain a steady growth. This is not a cause of concern unless the baby continues to fail to gain weight. The first action should be to check the attachment and positioning of the baby when feeding and increase the number of feeds. In most cases this is all that is necessary. In rare cases, the mother may produce insufficient milk and may need to give supplementary bottle-feeds. This should not, however, be started until all other advice and support has been given.

Bottle-fed infants. A good feeding history needs to be taken, and some overview of the amount of feed the baby is taking and the number of feeds offered per day. In some instances the baby may not be offered sufficient for his needs.

The nurse also needs to check that the mother is making up the milk correctly and not making it too dilute or too strong.

Some babies may have become very difficult feeders. They cry frequently and when offered a feed only take a small amount before falling asleep. Often the mother is exhausted by lack of sleep and a screaming infant. She may also have a significant loss of self-confidence. The rejection of the feed can be interpreted as a rejection of the mothering offered and can cause intense distress. The mother may have tried many different techniques and a variety of formulae or milks. She may state that a certain milk did not suit the baby. There is no evidence that changing the milks will have any benefit, as long as the baby is receiving a suitable one for his age and has no intolerances, and these are uncommon. If the problems cannot be sorted out in the community, a short period in hospital may provide relief for the mother and a chance for the baby to be fed by a nurse. Often the problems will resolve as the baby relaxes and feed time can become a pleasurable time of interaction and not one fraught with anxiety and distress.

If the failure to thrive is diagnosed in a baby whilst being weaned, a history needs to be taken to check that the diet is suitable for the age group; contains sufficient fat and not too high a fibre content. The parents of the older child need to be asked about the intake of sweets or sugary drinks between meals or an excessive intake of snack foods which may inhibit the appetite.

 Activity 12.7

Paul is 6 weeks old and his birth weight was 3.5 kg. How much should he now weigh?

His mother is offering him 100 ml per feed and feeding him five times per 24 hours. Is this sufficient for his needs?

Box 12.5 Other causes of failure to thrive

Vomiting
- Gastro-oesophageal reflux
- Pyloric stenosis (see Ch. 13)

Malabsorption
- Coeliac disease (see below)
- Cystic fibrosis (see below)

Chronic illness
- Congenital heart disease
- Renal disease
- Tuberculosis

Endocrine disorders
- Growth hormone deficiency

Metabolic disorders
- Galactosaemia
- Phenylketonuria (see p. 208)

Box 12.5 lists other causes of failure to thrive and gives examples in each category.

Coeliac disease

This is a disease that affects the proximal small bowel. It is caused by a sensitivity to the protein, gluten, mainly present in wheat. This damages the villi of the mucosa of the small intestine and results in a reduction of the surface area of the gut for absorption. Nutrients are not properly absorbed and are passed in the stools. Gluten has to be excluded from the diet for life.

Children with coeliac disease present with a wide range of symptoms and the age of onset will depend on the time at which wheat-based cereals were introduced to the diet. 70% have diarrhoea and malabsorption, indicated by pale, bulky, offensive stools. Weight gain is poor and the children are often irritable. There is often abdominal distension due to the fermentation of undigested food in the large bowel. Some children will present with oedema of the lower extremities due to their low level of serum albumin. Diagnosis is confirmed by a jejunal biopsy which should be taken before treatment is started with a gluten-free diet.

The diet controls the symptoms but does not cure the disease. The villi of the small intestinal mucosa return to normal after a few months on a gluten-free diet, but will be damaged again if the diet lapses.

Gluten is found in wheat and rye cereals. Debate has occurred over whether oats and barley need to be excluded from the diet, and they are usually omitted. Cereals and pulses classified as gluten-free include rice, maize, millet, buckwheat, soya and potato. Parents of children with coeliac disease need to be aware that gluten can be 'hidden' and should be advised to read the labels of manufactured foods. They should also be encouraged to join the Coeliac Society.

Cystic fibrosis (see also Chs 3 and 11)

Cystic fibrosis is a genetic disorder with an autosomal recessive pattern of inheritance. 1 in 20 of the population carry the affected gene and 1 in 2000 children are affected. The condition is characterised by chronic pulmonary disease and pancreatic insufficiency. Taylor (1993) identified poor nutrition in cystic fibrosis (CF) as being due to three factors that are interlinked. These are:

- malabsorption
- increased energy demands of the disease
- poor dietary intake.

Over 85% of children with CF produce insufficient pancreatic enzymes to prevent malabsorption of fat (steatorrhoea) and protein. Some children with CF also have insufficient bicarbonate to neutralise gastric acid, which results in the remaining bowel being excessively acid. Consequently enzyme activity is affected, as the enzymes require the correct pH in the bowel to work effectively. However, current research indicates that it is possible to restore normal pH levels in the intestine by the administration of the anti-ulcer drug omeprazole, which blocks the production of gastric acid.

A high-calorie diet with sufficient enzyme replacement to control diarrhoea is advocated (Taylor 1993). This means plenty of foods such as full-fat milk, cheese, butter/margarine, meat, full-fat yoghurt, crisps, chocolate and sweets.

Families who follow 'healthy eating' guidelines will need help to appreciate that their children have needs that are different from those of children without CF. Enzyme replacements contain amylase, which digests carbohydrate, trypsin (protease), which digests protein, and lipase, which digests fat. There are a variety of products available in different forms and strengths to suit the needs of the individual baby and child.

The enzyme replacements should be taken immediately before or with food. As babies are unable to swallow capsules, enzymes can be given in powder form, or the capsules can be opened and the contents mixed with liquid prior to feeding. As most babies will dribble their medicines, the skin around the mouth should be carefully cleaned after administration, as pancreatin can irritate the skin.

From toddler age onwards, capsules can be given. The enzymes are wrapped in an acid-resistant coating, known as enteric coating. The aim is to deliver a higher concentration of enzymes in the duodenum, so the child must be told not to chew the capsules but swallow them whole.

Due to the malabsorption, vitamin supplementation is also required. Usually a multivitamin is given and extra vitamin E: 50 mg in infancy; 100 mg for children aged 1–10 years; 200 mg for those over 10 years.

Children with CF who have severe lung disease often have a poor appetite and find the oral high-calorie supplements unappetising. The nutritional intake of these children can be enhanced by enteral (tube) feeding, which can be via a nasogastric tube or by gastrostomy or jejunostomy.

 For further information, see the Cystic Fibrosis Research Trust publication, *Nutritional Management of Cystic Fibrosis.*

Obesity in children

Obesity is the commonest form of malnutrition in the United Kingdom at present and affects between 2 and 11% of British children. The incidence varies according to the age and the sex of the child. For example, obesity affects:

- at 6 years:
  —1.7 % of boys
  —2.9% of girls
- at 14 years:
  —6.5% of boys
  —9.6% of girls (Stark 1981).

Obesity tends to run in families and both genetic and environmental factors are thought to play a part.

- Children of parents who are not overweight have a less than 10% chance of being obese.
- Children who have one parent who is obese have a 40% chance of being obese.
- Children who have two obese parents have an 80% chance of being obese (Shaw & Lawson 1994).

However, this may not only be due to a genetic factor but may also be affected by family eating habits and lifestyle.

Obesity is caused by energy intake being surplus to energy output. Energy output includes both metabolic rate and energy expenditure through physical activity. The hypothalamus in the brain contains the centres for both hunger and satiety and is also influenced by the appearance, taste and smell of food. Taitz & Wardley describe the 'restrained eater and the unrestrained eater'. The restrained eater will stop eating before he is satiated; this may be due to a voluntary wish not to become fat, or being conditioned to eating a smaller amount of food. The unrestrained eater will continue eating until he is satiated. The amount that children eat will be influenced by the amount and type of food offered by the parents. If the parents are restrained eaters, they will be likely to limit the amount of food offered, so that even if there is a genetic predisposition to obesity, the individual child may remain lean.

Children and adolescents are less active than they used to be and fat children tend to be less active than lean children. It is not clear whether the obesity comes before the reduced activity or the obesity is partly caused by the inactivity. Obese children are often teased at school and will opt out of playground or organised games, at which they do not excel.

Some children may also 'comfort eat'. Being overweight can cause significant distress and many adults will confess to eating more snacks if they are bored or unhappy.

Unless the child and his family are committed to losing weight, it is unlikely that any programme will have a lasting effect. Most programmes will combine a modification of the child's diet with an increase in exercise. Setting target weights can provide an incentive and rewards can be given for achievement. However, it is important not to offer rewards in the form of food. Suitable rewards might be an outing, or for adolescents an article of clothing. If they have been unable to wear fashionable clothing in the past, because of their size, this may be a particularly powerful incentive. Extreme diets are not recommended for children or adolescents, who both require nutrients to grow. Any major change to the diet should be made under the direction of a dietitian.

Deficiency disorders

Iron deficiency anaemia

Iron deficiency is the most common nutritional disorder during early childhood. A survey commissioned by the Department of Health (DoH) and the Ministry of Agriculture, Fisheries and Food (MAFF) examined a sample of children aged 18 months to $4\frac{1}{2}$ years. The children were selected to be nationally representative of the population of Britain. Preliminary results estimate that 12% of children in the age group of 18 months to $2\frac{1}{2}$ years and 6% of the older age group are anaemic (DoH 1994).

The most common cause of this deficiency is dietary, and weaning is a particularly important time. The iron content of the food is important, but the absorption of the iron is equally important. There is an increasing interest in those

---

Box 12.6   Foods which affect iron absorption (Palmer 1993)

Aids to iron absorption
- Vitamin C.
- A small amount of meat or fish will aid the absorption of iron in cereals, vegetables and fruits.
- The iron in breast milk is well absorbed (70%).
- Protein. This is thought to be due to the fact that it will bind with the phytates and reduces their inhibitory effect.

Inhibitors of iron absorption
- Tea, bran, coffee and egg yolk. Tea will reduce the amount of iron absorbed by as much as 60%.
- Both egg and spinach contain a lot of iron, but they also contain substances which inhibit their absorption.
- Only 6% of the iron in a milk formula with 6 mg/l will be absorbed. If the iron is doubled to 12 mg/l, only 4% is absorbed.
- Phytates.

---

foods which aid the absorption of iron and those which inhibit it (Box 12.6).

The symptoms of iron deficiency are listed in Box 12.7. However, many children with iron deficiency anaemia will show no symptoms, so absence of symptoms does not necessarily indicate an adequate intake of iron. It is necessary to ensure that young children are being given sufficient absorbable iron in their diet and, if necessary, iron supplements.

The large number of young children who are suffering from iron deficiency anaemia, often with no symptoms, is leading to discussion of whether there should be a national screening programme and, if so, at what age it would be best to screen. It is likely that more research will be carried out in the near future and a policy formed.

Box 12.7   Symptoms of iron deficiency

- Pallor
- Apathy
- Loss of appetite; this may make it difficult to increase the intake in the diet
- Tachycardia
- Delayed psychomotor development
- Susceptibility to infection

Rickets

Rickets is due to a deficiency of vitamin D, which is stored prior to birth provided that the pregnant woman has sufficient stores herself. Breast milk contains little vitamin D but the full-term infant has sufficient stores to last him until he starts a mixed diet. Vitamin D is synthesised in the skin by exposure to the ultraviolet B radiation in sunlight. Nowadays sunbathing is not advised because of the increased risk of melanoma and parents are advised not to let their children get sunburnt, and to apply creams. However 30 minutes' daily exposure of face, legs and arms during the summer, avoiding the midday sun, is sufficient to replenish vitamin D stores (DoH 1994). Vitamin D is not naturally present in many foods. It is present in oily fish, eggs and some meats. It is also added to infant milks, formulae and many weaning foods.

Rickets is not a common deficiency disease in the United Kingdom, but there are two groups who are at risk and therefore need specific monitoring.

Preterm and low birth weight babies are at risk because of their low stores at birth and their increased growth rate. These infants are usually given vitamin supplements which are continued for at least 1 year.

The other group at risk are the children of Asians living in Britain. There are several reasons for this:

- The diet of some Asians is low in vitamin D, which means that in pregnancy the mother may be unable to pass on sufficient stores to her baby.
- The diet that the infant is given during weaning may also be low in vitamin D.
- The relatively low levels of sunlight in this country, the habit of covering the skin and their skin pigmentation, which appears to inhibit the synthesis of vitamin D in the skin, all contribute to a lack of synthesis in the skin.

With better health education and the advice that Asian women are given, vitamins during pregnancy and supplements to children until the age of 5 years, a reduced incidence of rickets is being recorded.

Food intolerances

Food allergies and intolerances are not well understood and a variety of mechanisms are involved:

- Some are due to an enzyme deficiency, e.g. a deficiency of lactase.
- Some people are affected by the pharmacological properties of certain substances, e.g. the caffeine in tea and coffee, or amines in cheese.
- Some foods, such as strawberries and shellfish, contain histamine-releasing agents and these can cause reactions.
- In some cases there is an abnormal immune response after eating certain foods, and this is probably the most common.

The ways in which food intolerances may be manifest are summarised in Box 12.8.

Cow's milk protein allergy

True cow's milk allergy is not common and the incidence has been decreasing since a peak in the 1960s. The increase in the numbers of babies being given colostrum in the first days of life is thought to be the reason for this decrease (Taitz & Wardley 1989). The condition usually presents between the ages of 6 and 8 weeks with vomiting, diarrhoea and failure to thrive. More acute symptoms are sometimes seen. These

---

Box 12.8   Manifestations of food intolerances

Quick onset
- Anaphylactic shock
- Oedema and urticaria
- Vomiting
- Sneezing
- Colic

Slow onset
- Diarrhoea
- Abdominal pain and distension
- Failure to thrive
- Eczema
- Asthma
- Migraine

infants need to be diagnosed by a paediatrician and referred to a dietitian so that they may be given an appropriate and balanced diet. Some of these infants may also develop an intolerance to soya and may need a formula such as Pregestimil. Often the problems cease when the child is older, so a cow's milk challenge can then be performed. This is carried out in hospital under medical supervision in case anaphylaxis occurs.

Lactose intolerance

This is due to a deficiency of the enzyme lactase. Lactose is the sugar present in milks, including breast milk. Primary intolerance is rare amongst Caucasians. Secondary intolerance occurs when there has been damage to the lining of the gastrointestinal tract. The damage can be done by repeated or prolonged attacks of gastroenteritis, by coeliac disease or where there is a cow's milk protein intolerance. The baby usually presents with frothy, explosive stools when given foods containing lactose. The stools can be tested using Clinitest and will be shown to contain lactose. All foods containing lactose must be excluded from the diet for several weeks until the gut has recovered. This can be quite a restrictive diet and the help of a dietitian is required.

Phenylketonuria

Phenylketonuria is a rare genetic disorder, affecting between 1 in 8000 and 1 in 10 000 births in the United Kingdom. It is an autosomal recessive disorder where there is a deficiency of the liver enzyme phenylalanine hydroxylase. This enzyme is responsible for the metabolism of an essential amino acid, phenylalanine, to tyrosine. Undiagnosed, this leads to a build-up of phenylalanine in the blood and subsequent brain damage. All babies in this country have a Guthrie or a Scriver blood test done between the 6th and 14th day of life, to screen for this disorder. The baby must have had milk feeds prior to the test. There are some children who have atypical phenylketonuria. Their blood levels of

phenylalanine may not be as high as the typical case, so each child must be reviewed carefully.

Phenylalanine is present in all protein foods and, because it is an essential amino acid, it cannot be excluded entirely from the diet; the child needs some phenylalanine for normal growth and repair. The aim is to control the level within safe limits which are:

- 120–360 µmol/l for children up to school age
- 120–480 µmol/l for school-age children
- 120–700 µmol/l for adolescents and adults.

A low-phenylalanine diet is very restrictive and one of the principles is that it must contain a small amount of natural protein, supplemented by a low-phenylalanine substitute such as Minafen or Aminogram. The involvement of the hospital dietitian is essential to ensure that the child gets a balanced diet. Regular monitoring of blood phenylalanine is necessary and should be carried out:

- weekly up to the age of 4
- every 2 weeks between the ages of 4 and 10
- monthly after the age of 10.

The diet is adjusted according to the results.

The age at which the diet can be stopped is as yet unknown. It is now considered a diet for life as neurological changes have been observed in patients who have come off their diet. However, the blood phenylalanine level is allowed to rise to 700 mmol/l in the adolescent and adult in an attempt to make the diet more palatable (MRC 1993).

Girls must be taught from an early age that all pregnancies must be planned and that their blood phenylalanine level must be brought under strict control—60–150 µmol/l—before and during pregnancy to avoid damage to the fetus.

Hyperactivity and food additives

There has been increasing interest in the effects of additives and preservatives in the diet and one theory that has gained significant ground is that additives in the diet can cause hyperactivity in some children. Many, if not most, of the children who are said to be hyperactive are healthy, normal children and there are usually other explanations for their behaviour. If parents are insistent that their child's behaviour is caused by an additive, it is wiser to omit it. The colouring agents E102 (tartrazine) and E110 (sunset yellow) are azo dyes. These and the benzoate preservatives E210–219 have been known to cause asthmatic attacks but less is known about their effect on behaviour (Taitz & Wardley 1989).

CONCLUSION

It is not possible to cover the whole perspective of nutrition, and nutritional and digestive disorders in one short chapter. The children's nurse needs to be well informed and has a responsibility to keep up to date with the latest research concerning nutrition and digestion. A healthy diet is essential in preventing illness and maintaining health. Children who are ill also need to have their nutritional needs met. The references and list of further reading are intended to direct the reader to areas of specific interest.

REFERENCES

Central Statistical Office 1991 Family spending: a report on the 1990 family expenditure survey. HMSO, London
Cystic Fibrosis Research Trust (undated) Nutritional management of cystic fibrosis. Cystic Fibrosis Research Trust, Bromley
Department of Health 1988 Third report of the Sub-committee on Nutritional Surveillance. HMSO, London
Department of Health 1989 The diets of British school children. HMSO, London
Department of Health 1993 Advisory Committee on the Microbiological Safety of Food. Report on salmonella in eggs. HMSO, London
Department of Health 1994 Weaning and the weaning diet. Report on health and social subjects 45. HMSO, London
Department of Health and Social Security 1984 Committee on Medical Aspects of Food Policy. Diet and cardiovascular disease. (The Coma Report) HMSO, London
Duncan B, Ey J, Holberg C J, Wright A L, Martinez F D, Taussig L M 1993 Exclusive breast feeding for at least 4 months protects against otitis media. Pediatrics 91: 867–872
Education Act 1980 Section 22. School meals: England and Wales. HMSO, London
European Economic Community 1991 Directive on formulae. (91/321/EEC)
Garcia J, Garforth S 1985 A national study of policy and practice in midwifery. Available from The National Perinatal Epidemiology Unit, Radcliffe Infirmary, Oxford
Health Education Authority 1989 Diet, nutrition and healthy eating in low income families. HEA, London
Illingworth C, Timmins J 1990 Gripe water: what is it? why is it given? Health Visitor 63: 378
Lucas A, Cole T J 1990 Breast milk and necrotising enterocolitis. Lancet 336(Dec): 1519–1523
Lucas A, Morley R, Cole T J, Lister G, Leeson-Payne C 1992 Breast milk and subsequent intelligence quotient in children born preterm. Lancet 339: 261–264
Martin J, White A 1988 Infant feeding 1985. Office of Population Censuses and Surveys, Social Survey Division. HMSO, London
McClean P, Lynch A B, Dodge A 1990 Comparison of three regimens in the management of acute gastroenteritis in infants. Alimentary Pharmacology and Therapeutics 4(5): 457–464
Medical Research Council 1993 Report of medical research working party on phenylketonuria. Special report. Archives of Disease in Childhood 68: 426–427
Mills A, Magill L, Allen S 1993 Children's dietary habits in hospital. Paediatric Nursing 5(8): 17–19
Ministry of Agriculture, Fisheries and Food 1992 Food and nutrient intakes of British infants aged 6 to 12 months. HMSO, London
National Advisory Committee on Nutrition Education 1983 Proposals for nutritional guidelines for health education in Britain. (The NACNE Report) Health Education Council, London
National Children's Home 1991 Poverty and nutrition survey. NCH, London
Nicholson W 1985 Cracked nipples in breast feeding mothers: a randomised trial of three methods of management. Newsletter of the Nursing Mothers of Australia 21(4): 7–10
Office of Population Censuses and Surveys (OPCS) 1992 Infant feeding 1990. HMSO, London
Oski F A, Landaw S A 1980 Inhibition of iron absorption from human milk by baby food. American Journal of Diseases in Childhood 134: 459–460
Oxby H 1994 When do women decide. Health Visitor 68(5): 161
Palmer G 1993 Any old iron. Health Visitor 66: 248–252
Payne A 1991 Nutrient intake and growth in pre school children. PhD Thesis, Edinburgh
Royal College of Midwives (RCM) 1991 Successful breastfeeding, 2nd edn. Churchill Livingstone, Edinburgh
Savage-King F, Burgess A 1992 Nutrition for developing countries. Oxford University Press, Oxford
Shaw V, Lawson M 1994 Clinical paediatric dietetics. Blackwell Scientific Publications, Oxford
St James-Roberts I 1991 Persistent infant crying. Archives of Disease in Childhood 66: 653–655
Stark O 1981 Longitudinal study of obesity in the national survey of health and development. British Medical Journal 283: 13–17

Stevens F M, Egan-Mitchell B, Cryan E, McCarthy C F, McNichol B 1987 Decreasing incidence of coeliac disease. Archives of Disease in Childhood 62: 465–468

Taitz L S, Wardley B 1989 Handbook of child nutrition. Oxford University Press, Oxford

Taylor C 1993 Nutrition and the child with cystic fibrosis. Paediatric Nursing 5(4): 26–28

Thomas B 1994 Manual of dietetic practice. Blackwell Scientific Publications, Oxford

United Kingdom National Case-Control Study Group 1993 Breast feeding and risk of breast cancer in young women. British Medical Journal 307: 17–20

FURTHER READING

Karmel A 1995 The complete baby and toddler meal planner, 8th impression. Ebury Press, London

Kitzinger S 1987 The experience of breast feeding, 2nd edn. Penguin, Harmondsworth

Pearce J 1991 Food: too faddy, too fat. Thorsons, London

Smale M 1992 Book of breast feeding. The National Childbirth Trust. Vermilion, London

Welford 1994 Feeding your child from birth to three. Health Education Authority, London

USEFUL ADDRESSES

British Diabetic Association
10 Queen Anne Street
London W1M 0BD

Coeliac Society
PO Box 220
High Wycombe
Buckinghamshire

Cystic Fibrosis Research Trust
Alexandra House
5 Blyth Road
Bromley BR1 3RS

National Society for Phenylketonuria (UK) Ltd
7 Southfield Close
Willen
Milton Keynes
Buckinghamshire MK15 9LL

13

The renal system

Marcelle E. de Sousa

This chapter deals with the development and promotion of urinary continence, normal and abnormal fluid balance, the assessment of function of the renal system, the collection of urine samples, the use of catheters and the need for dialysis and transplantation. The reading list at the end of the chapter will guide the reader to texts which detail the many individual diseases of the renal tract which it is not possible to describe separately.

The chapter aims to:
- outline the development of continence in children
- give an overview of fluid balance, with emphasis on the differences between children and adults
- describe the tests that may be required if a child has a disorder of renal function, including the testing of urine
- give an overview of urinary tract infections
- introduce the concept of dialysis.

THE DEVELOPMENT OF CONTINENCE

Voiding the bladder of urine is a complex process which involves the nervous system (brain, spinal cord and peripheral nerves), abdominal pressure and the bladder sphincter. The acquisition of continence requires the learning of both voluntary and involuntary control over the voiding process. Like any developmental stage, continence is acquired at different rates by different individuals. A number of factors will modify the age of acquisition of urinary continence. These include:

- personality and maturational differences between individuals
- genetic factors, which may cause several family members to be late in achieving continence
- illness, both within the renal tract and outside
- differences in parenting styles and cultural norms.

Daytime continence is usually acquired before continence during the night. The normal child of about 18 months to 2 years of age will indicate a wet nappy. This is often a good time to start 'potty training'. Parents will keep a potty handy and may encourage the child not to wear a nappy for periods during the day. The use of the potty after food or drinks, and at other regular intervals, increases the child's awareness of the need to void. Success should be rewarded with praise, but scolding children for 'accidents' is not helpful. The child gradually learns not to pass urine as soon as he or she senses a full bladder, but to hold on to it for a while before voiding. Girls are quicker at learning this skill. Some parents will ambitiously try to toilet train infants of 1 year old or less, but usually this will not be successful.

There is greater variation in the age of acquiring night-time urinary continence than there is in becoming continent during the day. At 5 years old, 15% of children still wet the bed; at 10 years, 7% wet the bed; and at 15 years, only 1% wet the bed (Meadow 1980). Often children will indicate when

Activity 13.1

Talk to some of the parents and ask them how and when they toilet trained their children. Try to find out what made the parents decide on a particular time and strategy. Did they encounter any difficulties?

the night-time nappy is no longer needed. Once again parents should be encouraged to praise success and not to reprimand children for something over which they have not yet learnt control.

Problems of continence

Daytime wetting

Daytime wetting may be due to urge incontinence or urinary tract infection (common) or to a neuropathic bladder or structural abnormality of the lower renal tract (uncommon). The pattern of wetting will often give a clue to the cause. The investigation of urinary tract infection, the neuropathic bladder and structural abnormalities are described later in the chapter. Treatment is directed to the underlying cause. For children with urge incontinence it is helpful for teachers to know that the child may need to be excused in the middle of class to use the toilet. Anticholinergic drugs such as propantheline and oxybutinin reduce hyperreflexia and thereby indirectly increase bladder capacity. Emotional factors may play a part in causing urinary incontinence, and the child with incontinence will often be psychologically affected by the condition. Attention must be given to both the physical and psychological aspects of daytime urinary incontinence.

Nocturnal enuresis

Nocturnal enuresis describes bed-wetting due to lack of bladder control. It may be *primary*, when the child has never learnt bladder control, or *secondary* when control is lost again after a period of night-time dryness. Enuresis may be *continuous*, when it occurs every night, or *intermittent*. This aspect of continence is often a cause of great anxiety to the parent and to the child. The child with primary nocturnal enuresis is more likely to be following a family pattern or to have a maturational delay in the acquisition of bladder control. Psychological factors often play a part in causing secondary nocturnal enuresis. As with daytime wetting, a urinary tract infection, a neuropathic bladder or structural abnormalities may all affect bladder control, although they are a cause of only a small proportion of bedwetting.

Treatment.   Treatment for enuresis begins with trying to establish a cause. Most treatments for children without a physical abnormality are not likely to be successful under about 5 years of age. A continence nurse is an important member of the health care team dealing with children with enuresis. Treatments include reward systems based on star charts, used on their own or in combination with an alarm which wakes the sleeping child at the onset of bladder voiding. A number of different alarms are available, from the 'bell and pad' type to noiseless vibrating alarms (useful if the child shares a room with a sibling) and small pads which fit neatly inside night-clothes. Clear instructions about how to use devices properly, consistency in their use and the back-up of professionals are all necessary to ensure maximum benefit. Drug treatments include tricyclic antidepressants such as imipramine as well as synthetic antidiuretic hormone (DDAVP). Drug treatments are unlikely to produce lasting improvements on their own, and children with enuresis benefit from an approach to treatment which recognises emotional, maturational and physical factors, and emphasises support for the child and family.

FLUID BALANCE

The term 'fluid balance' describes quantitatively the daily intake, distribution and elimination of water by the body. It is a subject of particular importance in children because of the differences in requirements at different ages.

Differences between children and adults

At birth, water accounts for 75% of body weight. The proportion decreases with age as the relative amount of body fat increases, until in the adult, water is about 60% of weight. Water is present both within cells (intracellular fluid or ICF), accounting for 30% of body weight, and between cells (extracellular fluid or ECF), accounting for

between 25 and 40% of body weight at different ages. ECF consists mainly of blood or plasma.

In infants, the amount of extracellular fluid is significantly greater than the intracellular fluid, whereas in adults, the intracellular fluid is greater than the extracellular. The infant also has a relatively small blood volume of 80 millilitres per kilogram of weight. There are other important differences between adults and infants when fluid balance is considered.

The infant has a relatively greater body surface area. It is estimated that the surface area per unit weight of a preterm infant is five times that of an adult, while for a full-term newborn the figure is two to three times that of an adult. This relative increase in body surface area means that there is a greater insensible loss of fluid through the skin. The gastrointestinal tract is also relatively larger, and therefore there is an increased secretion of gastrointestinal fluids. Normally, most of these secretions will be reabsorbed in the colon, but when the child has diarrhoea, there can be a significantly greater loss of fluid.

The infant has a higher metabolic rate than the adult, leading to a greater production of metabolic wastes and also greater heat production. The increased heat production leads to further insensible loss of water through the skin. The infant kidney is also relatively immature and unable to concentrate urine in the way that an adult's kidney can. The infant passes large amounts of dilute urine. When older children or adults become dehydrated, they are able to concentrate urine and pass the same amount of waste products in a smaller quantity of water. The infant's inability to concentrate urine leads to a quicker build-up of toxic wastes if the infant becomes dehydrated.

Activity 13.2

Look at the wet nappies of babies and older toddlers, particularly first thing in the morning. You are likely to discover that the toddler is passing much darker urine than the young baby.

When older children or adults need more fluid, they will feel thirsty and can respond to this. Small babies are only able to communicate by crying and are dependent on adults to meet their need for fluids.

As children grow, their fluid balance becomes more similar to that of an adult and their need for a large fluid intake decreases.

Total daily intake

Water is taken in as drinks and as part of solid foods. In the sick child, intravenous fluids and drugs contribute to the fluid intake. Water is also formed in the body from the metabolism of carbohydrate, fats and protein. Fluid requirements can be calculated on the basis of age, body weight or, most accurately, body surface area (Table 13.1). The total daily intake is arrived at by adding up all the fluids given by whatever route over a period of 24 hours. Unlike adults, small children are not able to tolerate inappropriate fluid intakes because of immaturity of the kidney.

Total daily output

Water is lost mainly in the urine, but also through respiration, perspiration and in faeces. Normal urinary output should be 2 ml per kg per hour. In the sick child there may be exceptional losses, for instance because of haemorrhage, burns and severe diarrhoea and vomiting (Box 13.1). Total

---

Box 13.1   Some important causes of fluid deficit

Inadequate intake
• Bronchiolitis
• Neglect and abuse
• Severe feeding difficulty

Gastrointestinal losses
• Gastroenteritis
• Pyloric stenosis
• Acute bowel obstruction

Losses from renal tract
• Diabetes mellitus
• Diabetes insipidus
• Renal tubular diseases
• Inappropriate use of diuretics

Traumatic losses
• Burns
• Haemorrhage
• Severe systemic infection

---

daily output is calculated by adding up *all* sources of fluid loss over 24 hours (including for example nasogastric aspirate and loss through wound drains).

Daily fluid balance

The daily fluid balance can be calculated by subtracting the daily output from the daily intake. Normally the intake will exceed the output by 300 ml/m^2 of body surface area per day because of insensible losses (through respiration and in faeces). The weighing of sick children is an important aid to managing fluid therapy. Accurate weighing together with charting of fluid intake and losses will identify children receiving excessive or inadequate amounts of fluids.

Dehydration

The term 'dehydration' is used to describe the state in which there is insufficient body water, as a result of either excessive fluid losses or insufficient fluid intake. Dehydration may be described as mild, moderate or severe; the physical signs associated with this are described in Box 13.2.

Table 13.1 Daily fluid requirements in normal children

Age (years)	Oral (ml/kg)*	Intravenous (ml/kg)*
0–1	150	100–120
1–5	80	80
5–10	60	60
10–15	50	50

* These figures worked out from body weight are an approximation of normal total daily requirements. Requirements at all ages are more precisely worked out from body surface area as 1500–2000 ml per m^2 per day.

Box 13.2   **Clinical signs of dehydration in children**

Weight loss less than 5%
• Often no clinical signs

Weight loss between 5 and 10%
• Loss of skin turgor
• Dry mucous membranes
• Sunken fontanelle in babies
• Sunken eyes
• Lethargy
• Oliguria

Weight loss greater than 10%
• Pale clammy skin
• Weak pulse
• Low blood pressure
• Shallow breathing
• Increased core–peripheral temperature gap
• Collapse

Box 13.4   **Fluid replacement in the severely dehydrated child**

Initial fluid replacement
• Intravenous fluid — 20 ml per kg body weight in the first hour
• All or most of this fluid as colloid (plasma or blood)

Subsequent replacement of fluid deficit
• Replace half of fluid deficit in first 12 hours:
   — usually intravenously
   — most as crystalloid
   — choice of fluid depends upon type of fluid and electrolyte loss
• Replace remainder of fluid deficit in following 24 hours
   — intravenously or orally

Continue maintenance fluids
• Intravenously or orally
• At the same time as replacing fluid deficit
• Include any continuing losses (e.g. vomiting)

Fluid replacement

Fluid replacement in the sick child has three parts:

1. to meet daily fluid requirements
2. to correct dehydration by replacing earlier fluid losses
3. to correct for continuing exceptional fluid losses.

The replacement of fluid is accompanied by replacement of electrolytes (especially sodium and potassium), as well as attention to the child's

Box 13.3   **Types of intravenous fluids**

Crystalloid
Dextrose 4% + sodium chloride 0.18%
Sodium chloride 0.9% (normal saline)
Sodium chloride 0.45% (half-normal saline)
Dextrose 10%

Colloid
Human albumin
Fresh frozen plasma
Artificial plasma expanders (e.g. Haemacell)
Blood

Parenteral nutrition
Amino acid solutions (e.g. Vamin)
Fat solutions (e.g. Intralipid)

nutritional needs. As a general principle, if a child is well enough to take and absorb fluids given orally (or through a nasogastric tube), this is the best route to administer fluids. Suitable oral fluids must contain physiological amounts of electrolytes; examples are milk, infant formula feeds and oral rehydration fluids (for instance Dioralyte). Water alone should not be given to replace fluid loss or maintain hydration. Examples of fluids for intravenous fluid replacement are given in Box 13.3.

Intravenous fluids are used in severely ill children and in those not able to tolerate or absorb oral fluids. The replacement of fluids in the severely dehydrated child is done at first rapidly in the first minutes to hours, by the intravenous route, and then continues more gradually over the next 1–2 days, as described in Box 13.4. Abnormal signs such as low blood pressure and an increased core–peripheral temperature gap gradually improve as dehydration is corrected.

Causes of abnormal fluid balance

Pyloric stenosis

Pyloric stenosis is an important cause of abnormal fluid and electrolyte balance in early infancy, with an onset usually between 4 and 6 weeks after birth. The treatment is surgical, but correction of fluid losses and electrolyte imbalance is important before and after surgery. In pyloric stenosis the smooth muscle of the pylorus hypertrophies and obstructs the normal passage of stomach contents into the small bowel. As the stenosis worsens, projectile vomiting develops, leading to loss of fluid and electrolytes. At the time of presentation children may have moderate or severe signs of dehydration, including weight loss, poor urine output, a sunken fontanelle, loss of skin turgor and sunken eyes. The diagnosis is made by palpating the abdomen to find the pyloric 'tumour' (the hypertrophied muscle) especially just after a feed, and it can be confirmed by ultrasound. Most children will have a metabolic alkalosis and hypokalaemia, and will require correction of fluid losses with fluids in excess of ordinary daily requirements as well as intravenous potassium supplements. The improvement postoperatively is usually rapid, and oral fluids (including breast-feeding) can usually be restarted soon after surgery.

Nephrotic syndrome

The nephrotic syndrome comprises oedema, proteinuria and hypoalbuminaemia. It is due to severe loss of protein from blood by the kidneys. The most frequent cause in childhood is minimal change nephropathy. This occurs more frequently in boys than in girls and usually presents between 1 and 5 years of age. Treatment is with immunosuppressants (especially steroids), oral penicillin to prevent pneumococcal infection (to which these children are especially susceptible) and intravenous albumin. Human albumin (20%) is used, given in doses of 5 ml per kg body weight over a period of 3–4 hours. Although these children are often grossly oedematous, their intravascular compartment is depleted of fluid and they are in fact hypovolaemic (as shown by their increased core–peripheral temperature gap). For this reason their fluid intake should not be restricted. In

some special circumstances only, diuretics may be used. A high-protein and low-salt diet is also necessary. When children begin to respond to treatment there may be rapid changes in their fluid balance. Children with nephrotic syndrome need very careful attention to measurement of fluid balance as well as weight, temperature and blood pressure, especially during the early phases of their illness.

ASSESSMENT OF STRUCTURE AND FUNCTION OF THE RENAL SYSTEM

Assessing the renal system in order to determine whether there is any defect or deviation from normal involves some procedures which may be frightening or unpleasant for the child. They should be carried out only by personnel skilled in the procedures, who are also at ease in dealing with children. This service is best offered in a paediatric department. Careful preparation, both physical and psychological, is important for both children and parents, to ensure that the investigations yield the best results. Nurses, doctors and play therapists all have a significant role in this pre-investigative preparation. The use of clear precise explanations, pictures and aids such as dolls is of great value.

The investigations may be either non-invasive or invasive.

Non-invasive investigations

These investigations are painless and usually only the energetic toddler will require sedation.

Height and weight

These must be measured accurately as many children in renal failure do not grow at a normal rate, and may also be underweight for their age.

Blood pressure

Many children with renal diseases will have an abnormal blood pressure (BP). The BP must not be taken in the crying child or in the child who has been running around energetically. Most children dislike the tightening of the cuff and distraction is necessary to keep them calm and relaxed. The appropriately sized cuff is the largest one which covers most of the upper arm, with the length of the bladder being at least two-thirds of the circumference of the arm. Too small a cuff produces an inaccurately high reading. There are several sizes of paediatric BP cuff.

Urine analysis

This is discussed in detail in a separate section (see p. 219).

Radiography

Abdominal radiographs are useful in detecting the presence of renal calculi. Renal outlines can be seen. Spinal defects can also be detected on abdominal or spinal films. The left hand is X-rayed in order to detect signs of renal osteodystrophy and to calculate the bone age in all children with chronic renal disease.

Ultrasound

Renal ultrasound is a painless technique, in which a probe is gently run over the front of the abdomen and then over the back, using ultrasound jelly to ensure good contact. Ultrasound can be used to detect the presence or absence of a kidney and the size of a fluid collection, either within or around a kidney. Cystic disease of the kidney and any pelvic or renal mass can be shown on ultrasound. In children with a history of renal infections, an ultrasound may demonstrate scarring. Obstruction of the renal system can be detected. The volume of urine in the bladder pre- and post-micturition can be estimated. Ultrasound can also be used as guide for renal biopsy.

Invasive investigations

These procedures involve the child being cannulated or catheterised. Children may find these tests frightening or unpleasant.

Blood tests

Important blood indices in children with suspected renal disease include sodium, potassium, urea, bicarbonate, creatinine, calcium, phosphate and haemoglobin. An elevated creatinine is a sensitive indicator of renal failure.

Micturating cysto-urethrogram (MCUG)

The child is catheterised and water-soluble contrast medium is instilled into the bladder. X-ray pictures are taken of the bladder and the ureters. A post-micturition film is also obtained. Catheterisation must be carried out by skilled staff using a lubricated feeding tube. This procedure should not be carried out in a child with a current urine infection or without antibiotic cover. Sedation is not advised as the child has to void the bladder. The MCUG detects vesico-ureteric reflux (see Box 13.8, p. 221) and posterior urethral valves.

Intravenous pyelogram (IVP)

A radio-opaque dye is injected into a vein, and X-ray pictures are obtained of the dye entering and being excreted by the kidneys. Allergic reactions to the dye are a possible complication.

Arteriogram

The anatomy of the renal blood vessels can be demonstrated on X-ray pictures by injecting radio-opaque dye directly into them through a catheter introduced into a femoral artery.

Radionuclide imaging

Radionuclide imaging techniques involve the injection of small amounts of radionuclide-labelled material, which is detected later as it is concentrated by and excreted through the kidney. Detection is by a gamma camera, which is placed close to the abdomen or the back. A DTPA scan (diethylenetriamine pentacetic acid) can assess renal perfusion and obstruction of the renal tract. A DMSA scan (dimercaptosuccinic acid) can assess renal structure and function.

Urodynamics

In this procedure two catheters are inserted into the bladder, and a rectal probe measures pressure. The technique measures the capacity of the bladder and its filling pressure.

Renal biopsy

Percutaneous renal biopsy is used to obtain a tissue specimen for examination under the microscope. This can help to make a definitive diagnosis based upon pathology. It is a procedure which carries some small risk of haemorrhage. The child is fasted and sedated. The child lies on his/her front, local anaesthetic is administered and a trucut needle is inserted through the anaesthetised site into the kidney. The tissue is examined immediately under a microscope. Following this procedure the child is hydrated and is on continuous bedrest for 24 hours, has blood pressure and pulse monitored frequently and urine examined for signs of persistent frank haematuria.

Glomerular filtration rate

The glomerular filtration rate (GFR) is the volume of blood filtered by the kidneys (in millilitres) per minute. There are several methods of measurement, which involve blood and sometimes urine tests.

Collection and testing of urine samples

The testing of urine is the quickest and easiest method of detecting infection and renal disease in children. The problem lies in the collection of urine, particularly in the young child who is not toilet trained.

Initial testing can be carried out in the home, on the ward or in the doctor's surgery. This testing is done using reagent strips which are dipped into the urine and read against a table on the container. Further detailed testing is carried out in the laboratory.

Collection of urine

A 'bag urine' is a urine specimen collected into a sterile bag stuck to the perineum. The nappy is taken off and the genital area cleaned from front to back with sterile saline. The area is dried and the adhesive bag is applied. It is best to leave the nappy off so that the bag can be removed as soon as a specimen is obtained. Drawbacks are leakage from bags, and contamination of specimens with faeces (in about 10% of cases).

A 'clean-catch' urine is a specimen obtained from a toddler who is not toilet trained. It calls for speed. The nappy is taken off, the genital area is cleaned and as soon as micturition starts a sterile receptacle is used to collect the urine.

A 'mid-stream' urine (MSU) is obtained from the older toilet-trained child. The genital area is cleaned as before, although there is a case for not cleaning as only the middle specimen is collected. Younger children may need assistance in putting the container in the right place whilst they are micturating.

Suprapubic aspiration (SPA) is a method of obtaining urine directly from the bladder by needle aspiration. It is a method used only in infants, in whom the bladder is an intra-abdominal organ. This procedure is best done after a feed to increase the likelihood of urine having entered the bladder. The area above the symphysis pubis is cleaned with alcohol, and a needle attached to a syringe is introduced through the skin into the bladder. It is the best method of obtaining uncontaminated urine specimens.

Activity 13.3

Think how you might explain to a 6-year-old child that you need to collect a mid-stream urine sample.

A catheter urine specimen is necessary only in children who already have indwelling catheters or who intermittently catheterise themselves. Other children should not be catheterised to obtain specimens. Catheters can also be inserted into urinary diversions (such as vesicostomies) to obtain a clean specimen of urine.

Testing of urine

Bacteria. Urine is tested most often for the presence of bacteria. This involves both examining the urine under the microscope, and placing some on a bacterial culture medium. The sensitivities to antibiotics can be determined for bacteria which are isolated in this way. This helps to plan treatment for a proven infection (when there is a pure growth of more than 100 000 organisms per millilitre). The presence of white cells in the urine (in excess of 10–50 per microlitre) is another requirement for the diagnosis of infection.

Blood. Blood (haematuria) can be either macroscopic (easily seen by the eye) or microscopic (detected only by testing). Haematuria is caused by:

- renal infections
- renal tumours
- exercise
- congenital abnormalities of the renal tract
- some bleeding disorders.

The urine can either be bright red due to frank haematuria (usually following trauma to the renal system) or darker in colour. Other causes of red urine include dyes present in foods (e.g. beetroot) and some drugs (e.g. rifampicin).

Macroscopic haematuria is often very alarming to parents and the child. However, in more than 50% of children no cause will be found. The parents can be taught to test the urine at home with reagent sticks and record the findings. If the haematuria disappears and the child remains in good health, then nothing need be done. Microscopic haematuria is investigated in the child with other signs of renal disease, or if it persists for more than 1 month.

Protein. The presence of protein in the urine (proteinuria) is normal in small amounts in many healthy people. In large amounts its presence may indicate renal disease. Proteinuria can be assessed by the use of reagent sticks, and a more accurate measure of the amount and type of protein is obtained from a 12- or 24-hour urine collection. The child voids his/her bladder and the collection starts from the next passage of urine. Important causes of proteinuria include infection and the nephrotic syndrome.

Glucose. There are usually very small amounts of glucose in the urine (glycosuria) which are not detected by reagent sticks. Important causes of measurable glycosuria include diabetes mellitus, renal tubular disease such as Fanconi's syndrome, total parenteral nutrition and steroid therapy.

Ketones. Ketonuria (ketones in the urine) is found in children who are fasting, pyrexial or those with metabolic disorders, in particular diabetes mellitus.

pH. The urine should normally have a pH greater than 5.5, and this should be tested for on a fresh sample.

Electrolytes. Electrolytes including sodium and potassium can be measured by the laboratory, and are important in the acutely unwell child with some renal disorders.

Urine tests are summarised in Box 13.5.

Box 13.5 Analysis of urine

Tests using reagent sticks
Glucose
Protein
Blood
Ketones

Tests requiring laboratory analysis
Cell count
Bacterial culture
Quantitative analysis of protein
Electrolytes

CATHETERS

Catheters are flexible tubes, usually introduced through the urethra into the bladder in order to allow the drainage of urine. Catheters may be for either single-use, indwelling or intermittent. They are made from a variety of materials, including silicone-coated latex and newer hydrogel-coated catheters. The latter have been developed to reduce irritation of the bladder mucosa.

Indwelling catheters

Indwelling catheters may be short term or long term. Good attention to hygiene is necessary, both when placing the catheter and in continuing care. Short-term catheters are often used in severely ill children undergoing intensive care or following surgery, including surgery to the renal tract. Children with these catheters require careful supervision of oral and intravenous fluids as well as urine output. Children with long-term catheters, placed for instance to overcome obstruction to outflow from the renal tract, can be ambulant, with the catheter and bag strapped to the leg. Urine must be checked for colour and smell, and a specimen should be sent to the laboratory at least once a week for bacterial culture.

Intermittent catheters

Intermittent catheters are used in children with neuropathic bladders (for instance those with spina bifida) and following reconstructive bladder surgery. Short catheters are used in girls and longer ones in boys. These catheters can be self-lubricating, and may be washed and reused.

Activity 13.4

Consider how you might explain to a 3-year-old child that after he has had his operation, he will have an indwelling urethral catheter for a few days.

The child can be taught by the incontinence nurse to carry out this procedure painlessly and efficiently. It takes patience and a sensitive approach to carry out this training successfully. Cleanliness of the entire system is important. Care must be shown in not being too diligent in cleaning the meatus in boys as this may cause irritation and infection. The positive aspect of this form of management is that children can learn to efficiently empty the bladder, lessening the risks associated with incomplete drainage, and can be dry by day and by night.

URINARY TRACT INFECTION

Infection of the urinary tract (UTI) is amongst the most common bacterial diseases of childhood. Up to 7% of girls and 1% of boys are affected (Berry & Chantler 1986). It is of importance because around one-half of children with UTI have an underlying anomaly of the renal tract. Recurrent UTI, particularly in younger children with reflux, may be a cause of renal scarring.

The symptoms of a urinary tract infection depend upon both the level of infection and the age of the child (Box 13.6). High fever is the commonest and sometimes the only symptom. Abdominal pain is a common symptom and older children who localise pain better may complain of loin pain. Although dysuria (pain on micturition) and urinary frequency occur after infancy as symptoms of UTI, the majority of

---

Box 13.6 Symptoms of urinary tract infection in children

- Pyrexia
- Malaise, irritability and lethargy
- Fits (infants)
- Rigors
- Vomiting
- Poor feeding (infants)
- Anorexia
- Frequency and dysuria (over 2 years of age)
- Abdominal pain
- Loin pain (older children)
- Smelly cloudy urine

children with these symptoms alone will on investigation be found *not* to have a UTI. Because it occurs in all age groups it is important to investigate any young infant with an unexplained febrile illness for possible UTI.

Investigations

Children suspected of having a UTI, or those who have had a previous infection and have a recurrence of symptoms, are investigated by obtaining a urine sample for microscopy and culture as described above. It is important that samples are collected in the correct manner to avoid contamination. In the case of 'bag urine' samples at least two or three are obtained prior to treatment (or a suprapubic aspirate is obtained) in order to be certain of the diagnosis. It is important always to investigate a child suspected of having a UTI and not just to assume that the symptoms are due to infection. Incorrect diagnosis means unnecessary treatment, and could mean the child needing to undergo further invasive investigations.

Treatment

Most children with a UTI can be treated with oral antibiotics, the choice of which will be determined by the sensitivities of the bacteria cultured from the urine. Some children will require intravenous antibiotics, particularly if they are very ill or vomiting frequently.

Recurrent urinary tract infection

Children who have recurrent UTIs require further investigation in order to find any underlying renal tract anomaly and to determine whether the child is at risk of scarring if further infections occur. Different investigations are carried out at different ages (Box 13.7) because the possible risk of scarring changes with age. Children are often maintained on antibiotics until they have completed their investigations (particularly the micturating cysto-urethrogram). Children with vesico-ureteric reflux (Box 13.8) and those with some renal tract anomalies, such

---

Box 13.7 Investigations for the child with a urinary tract infection

Under 1 year
- Plain X-ray
- Renal ultrasound
- Micturating cysto-urethrogram
- DMSA scan

1–7 years
- Plain X-ray
- Renal ultrasound
- DMSA scan

Over 7 years
- Plain X-ray
- Renal ultrasound

Box 13.8 Vesico-ureteric reflux

A micturating cysto-urethrogram is carried out to determine the degree of reflux, i.e. the level to which urine refluxes back up the ureter or into the kidney. There are five grades of reflux:

Grade 1	Contrast enters ureter
Grade 2	Contrast enters ureter, pelvis, calyces—no dilatation
Grade 3	Mild to moderate dilatation of ureter and renal pelvis
Grade 4	Moderate dilatation of ureter, pelvis and calyces
Grade 5	Gross dilatation of ureter, pelvis and calyces

In Grades 1, 2 and 3 reflux, no surgical intervention is necessary; 80% stop refluxing by the age of 2 years. In Grades 4 and 5, 20% stop refluxing by the age of 2 years. The indication for surgical intervention is recurrent breakthrough infections whilst on long-term prophylactic antibiotics.

---

as scars, are placed on continuous prophylactic antibiotics. Suitable antibiotics such as trimethoprim, and nitrofurantoin are given in a small once-daily dose.

DIALYSIS AND TRANSPLANTATION

Children need renal replacement therapy as a result of acute renal failure or when they enter end-stage renal failure. This can be the end result

---

Box 13.9   Causes of renal failure in children

Acute renal failure
- Dehydration
- Haemorrhage
- Septic shock
- Nephritis
- Obstructive uropathy
- Haemolytic uraemic syndrome

Chronic renal failure
- Glomerulonephritis
- Pyelonephritis
- Hereditary nephropathy
- Congenital abnormalities
- Multisystem diseases

---

of a number of renal diseases (Box 13.9). In many paediatric nephrology departments children with chronic renal failure are given renal transplants before dialysis is needed.

Renal dialysis

Dialysis is the movement of solute across a semipermeable membrane. Solutes move from a compartment with a high concentration to one with a low concentration. This can be used to rid the body of solutes such as urea which accumulate in large amounts as waste products.

There are two forms of renal dialysis:

- peritoneal dialysis
- haemodialysis.

With both techniques, there is a need for dietary and fluid restriction and there are often problems with compliance, particularly in adolescents. Psychological counselling and support is an important part of the treatment of these children.

Peritoneal dialysis

In peritoneal dialysis a catheter is inserted into the peritoneal cavity. The peritoneum acts as a semipermeable membrane. Dialysis fluid is infused into the peritoneum, remains there for some hours, and is then removed. The two most common techniques for this are:

- continuous ambulatory peritoneal dialysis (CAPD) which involves four bag exchanges in 24 hours
- automated peritoneal dialysis (APD) with which the child is dialysed overnight.

The main drawbacks of this technique are the risk of infection, especially peritonitis and exit site infections.

Haemodialysis

Haemodialysis is a technique whereby waste products are dialysed out of the blood across an artificial semipermeable membrane in a dialysis machine. This technique requires a method of vascular access (a cannula, fistula or graft). Blood is brought to the dialysis machine through small-volume tubes by a pump and is then returned to the body along similar tubes. Most children undergoing haemodialysis attend a renal unit three times a week.

Renal transplantation

The best treatment for end-stage renal failure is transplantation. Following a successful transplant, children no longer require dietary or fluid restriction, and their quality of life can be significantly improved.

There are two types of renal transplantation:

- a cadaveric transplant, taken from a dead person
- a familial transplant, taken from a living related donor.

Preparation to be a transplant recipient includes tissue typing and blood grouping. Children awaiting a cadaveric transplant will go 'on call'. If a suitably matched donor organ becomes available they will be admitted immediately to hospital for transplantation. Postoperative care of these children is very important. Rejection of the kidney is prevented by the use of immunosuppressant drugs such as prednisolone and cyclosporin. The grafted kidney survives for 5 years in approximately 75% of children.

CONCLUSION

Disorders of the kidney and renal tract are an important cause of illness in childhood. Untreated, they may lead to a deterioration in renal function, impairing the body's ability to regulate its fluid balance and the excretion of waste products. The correct collection of specimens and meticulous attention to the measurement of fluid input and output are of importance in all children, and in particular those with renal disorders. Further information about disorders not covered in this chapter is given in the list of further reading.

REFERENCES

Berry A C, Chantler C 1986 Urogenital malformations and disease. British Medical Bulletin 42(2): 181–186

Meadow R 1980 Help for bed wetting. Churchill Livingstone patient handbook. Churchill Livingstone, Edinburgh, p 1

Postlethwaite R J (ed) 1994 Clinical paediatric nephrology, 2nd edn. Butterworth Heinemann, Oxford

Report of a Working Group of the Royal College of Physicians 1991 Guidelines for the management of acute urinary tract infection in childhood. Journal of the Royal College of Physicians 25: 36–42

Taylor C M, Chapman S 1989 Handbook of renal investigations in children. Wright, Sevenoaks

Whaley L F, Wong D L (eds) 1991 The child with disturbance of fluid and electrolytes. In: Nursing care of infants and children, 4th edn. Mosby Year Book, St Louis, unit X

FURTHER READING

de Sousa M 1989 Renal tract problems. Paediatric Nursing 1(7): 11–12

Gartland C 1993 Partners in care. Nursing Times 89 (28 July): 34–36 (How families are taught to care for their children on peritoneal dialysis)

Hicklin M 1989 Paediatric renal transplants. Paediatric Nursing 1(7): 8 9

Hicklin M, de Sousa M 1995 Nursing support and care. Meeting the needs of the child with altered genito-urinary function. In: Carter B, Dearmun A K (eds) Child health care nursing. Blackwell Science, Oxford

McKenzie J 1989 Haemolytic uraemic syndrome. Paediatric Nursing 1(9): 14–15

Meadow R 1980 Help for bed wetting. Churchill Livingstone patient handbook. Churchill Livingstone, Edinburgh

Postlethwaite R J (ed) 1994 Clinical paediatric nephrology, 2nd edn. Butterworth Heinemann, Oxford

Wright L 1989 Haemodialysis. Paediatric Nursing 1(6): 12–13 (Care of a child requiring haemodialysis)

14

The nervous system

Jim Richardson

In working through the contents of this chapter the student is introduced to the normal functioning of the nervous system in the growing developing child. Major causes of neurological disturbances will be discussed.

The chapter aims to:
- outline the methods the child health nurse might use to assess the health of the nervous system of children
- review briefly the anatomy and physiology of the nervous system in childhood and suggest sources of detailed information on this topic
- describe the process of assessing the level of consciousness of the child and the major causes of disturbances in consciousness
- review the effects of injury of the child's central nervous system and introduce the actions which the nurse might take to help prevent such accidents
- provide a synopsis of the effects of infection of the central nervous system and briefly describe the nursing care needs of the child with such an infection
- discuss the assessment of children in pain and means of providing pain relief
- summarise the common childhood problems of sleep disturbance, crying and toilet training and the role of the child health nurse in helping parents to deal with these issues.

The child health nurse requires particular skills in evaluating the neurological health of a child. The central nervous system develops and grows throughout childhood, and this growth and development is reflected in the different motor and cognitive skills of children of different ages. A knowledge of this pattern of development is a prerequisite to understanding normal central nervous system function. When this is established, departures from the normal pattern can be readily recognised.

REVIEW OF ANATOMY, PHYSIOLOGY AND NORMAL DEVELOPMENT

The nervous system consists of the central nervous system (CNS), the brain and spinal cord, and the peripheral nervous system, the 'circuitry' of the neurological system, which carries messages from the CNS to the organs and extremities of the body and back again. The anatomy and physiology of the nervous system is complex and you will need to devote some time to study of a specialist text such as that by Tortora & Grabowski (1993). A small book by Gwilym Hosking (1982) will also provide you with a thumbnail sketch of the child's nervous system as well as relating this to disorders of this system.

At birth, the baby's brain weighs approximately 25% of its future adult weight, and by the time the child is 2 years old the brain weighs 75% of adult weight (Berger 1988). This indicates the phenomenal growth of the central nervous system during early childhood. To accommodate this growth, the sutures between the skull bones are not yet fused at birth and there are two openings in the skull which can be easily felt. The *anterior fontanelle*, which can be felt in the midline of the skull above the brow, closes gradually in the first 18 months of life, while the smaller *posterior fontanelle*, again in the midline but towards the back of the baby's head, is normally closed by the age of 3 months. The nurse can gain valuable information about a baby's well-being by gently inspecting these fontanelles. The normal fontanelle is flat but may pulsate with the heart beat or bulge when the baby coughs or strains. The fontanelle feels soft and slightly springy from the support of the layer of cerebrospinal fluid which circulates under the arachnoid membrane, cushioning and protecting the delicate brain. If the amount of this fluid is diminished, for example due to dehydration, the fontanelle will be sunken. If, on the other hand, the amount of cerebrospinal fluid is increased or its normal circulation is impeded, the fontanelle may look and feel tense and swollen. This may occur if the baby has hydrocephalus or an infection such as meningitis.

At birth, the baby's central system is immature. The nervous tissue which makes up the circuitry of the central and peripheral nervous system still lacks the myelin sheath of mature nerves. This results in the control of movement being less efficient than in the older child or adult. Also, the control of movement is learnt as the infant interacts with the environment, for example during play, and learns purposeful movement through trial and error. The movements which the new baby makes are often those that are important for the child's survival and are called the primitive reflexes (Box 14.1; see also Ch. 1).

A full description of the infant's reflexes can be found in books dealing with child development such as Sheridan (1975).

The timing and rate at which these reflexes disappear are an important indicator of the health of the infant's nervous system. These signs and the development of purposeful movements and motor skills are used by health care personnel in monitoring the normality of the infant's development.

A full description of child health surveillance is contained in the report, Health for All Children (Hall 1992).

Box 14.1   Some primitive reflexes of the newborn baby

Rooting. When the baby's cheek is stroked the baby will turn her head in that direction and open her mouth. This reflex ensures that the baby can seek the source of food, her mother's breast.

Palmar and plantar grasp. When the baby's palm or sole is stroked her fingers or toes flex to grasp.

Moro reflex. This is a protective reflex which is seen when the baby hears a sudden loud noise or, when well supported, is allowed to fall back a few inches. The baby throws her arms out and extends her fingers.

Activity 14.1

To help to increase your understanding of the surveillance of the infant's motor development you could try to obtain a copy of the personal child health record used by health visitors in your area. These records are now often held by parents in a booklet form.

You may find that a developmental screening tool such as the Denver Developmental Screening Test (Frankenberg et al 1981) is being used by health visitors in your area. Study of the documentation for this test will help you to develop an awareness of the parameters of normal child development.

Although there is a wide range of normal in the development of children, the sequence of development follows certain principles (Lansdown 1984):

• Cephalocaudal (head-to-toe) development is seen in that the infant develops control of the movements of the head and face before those of the trunk or limbs.
• Development is proximodistal, development of the centre of the body preceding that of the extremities. This can be observed in the child gaining gross motor control of the arms before fine motor control of the fingers.
• General before specific development is apparent in that the child masters single, simple movements before complex movements with a series of components.

At all ages in childhood, balance and the ability to control the head, trunk and limbs are important indicators of the neurological health of the child. In the older child, the gait observed when the child walks or runs gives important information about the child's level of development and neurological function. When the child health nurse has a clear understanding of children's development in terms of walking, it is easier to differentiate between normal and abnormal in terms of 'funny walks' and frequent falls.

For further information on the development of walking, see Berk (1991).

In general, child development can be seen to be a continuous process, although the rate can be very variable. The child expends a good deal of energy while developing and most resources are expended on maintaining the most recently achieved developments. For this reason, the most recently acquired skills can be lost if the child's resources are redirected, for example if the child is stressed by illness. This phenomenon, known as regression, can be seen in the child who has recently been toilet trained starting to wet the bed again following admission to hospital.

CONSCIOUSNESS

Assessing the child's level of consciousness

The assessment of the child's level of consciousness is one of the most important parts of the evaluation of a child's neurological health that the child health nurse will undertake—and also one of the most difficult. It is important initially to gain information about the child's normal state and reactions; in this task the assistance of parents, who know the child's normal state best, is invaluable. A general impression can be gained by observing the child carefully, noting the child's level of activity and interest in the environment, and reactions to interaction with other people. When the child has an unstable level of consciousness, continuity of carers becomes even more useful; a small number of nurses can learn the child's baseline state and are then in a position to interpret small changes in the child's consciousness. Again, parents are generally very sensitive to changes in the child's condition.

To assist in the monitoring and recording of a child's consciousness state, the Glasgow Coma Scale (Table 14.1) is widely used and is easy to learn to use. Some sensitivity is required by the nurse to interpret whether a child's failure to respond at any point in this evaluation process may be due to a deterioration in condition or simply due to the child's refusal to cooperate with a strange adult.

You will find further information related to this topic in Chapter 26, which covers the care of the critically ill child.

Assessment of the child's consciousness using the Glasgow Coma Scale is generally combined with observation of the vital signs of blood pressure, pulse and respiratory rate, temperature, and pupil size and reaction to light. Most children's units will have a specially designed chart for use in this form of monitoring.

Activity 14.2

Obtain a copy of the consciousness monitoring chart (Glasgow Coma Scale) from your local children's unit and, working through each part of the chart, clarify *why* each observation is done and what changes in each category of observation might mean. Obtain and read the article entitled *Assessment of Head-injured Children* by Williams (1992), which gives fuller information about the assessment of a child's consciousness level.

Disorders of consciousness

A child's level of consciousness can be affected by very many factors including:

- injury
- infection such as meningitis or encephalitis
- intoxication with drugs, solvents or alcohol
- poisoning with therapeutic drugs, chemical compounds or heavy metals
- metabolic or endocrine disorders such as diabetes mellitus or liver disease
- epilepsy.

Of these factors, perhaps the most important cause of disturbances in consciousness in childhood is injury. Head injuries in children are common, reflecting children's level of activity, tendency to take risks, relative inability to

Table 14.1 The Glasgow Coma Scale

	Adult score (for children over 10 years)		Child score (for children under 10 years)	
Best eye opening	Spontaneously	4	Spontaneously	4
	To speech	3	To speech	3
	To pain	2	To pain	2
	None	1	None	1
Best verbal response	Orientated	5	Orientated	5
	Confused	4	Unconnected words	4
	Inappropriate speech	3	Vocal sounds	3
	Incomprehensible	2	Cries	2
	None	1	None	1
Best motor response	Obeys commands	5	Obeys commands	5
	Localises pain	4	Localises pain	4
	Flexes to pain	3	Flexes to pain	3
	Extends to pain	2	Extends to pain	2
	None	1	None	1

identify dangers and immature motor and balance control.

Head injury

Most head injuries in children are relatively minor though unpleasant. Any child who has had a head injury sufficiently severe to have caused unconsciousness is at some risk of developing dangerous problems as a result. A sudden blow to the head can cause serious problems through two mechanisms:

• The blow may damage the delicate blood vessels within the skull leading to haemorrhage inside the skull. As soon as the sutures between the skull bones have ossified the skull becomes essentially a closed box, any space-occupying lesion such as pooled blood in a haematoma will lead to the pressure within the skull rising with the result that the brain becomes compressed (Williams 1992). This will lead to the child becoming nauseated, disorientated and her consciousness level becomes decreased. The parents of children who suffer even minor head injuries will be instructed to watch carefully for such signs and to seek medical help if any occur. These instructions are often given to parents in the form of a leaflet to reinforce this message. Should a haemorrhage occur, the child could become seriously disabled or even die without prompt treatment (Davies 1993).
• A serious blow to the head can cause the traumatised brain tissue to become swollen and oedematous, resulting in a rise in the pressure within the skull with results similar to those described in the previous paragraph.

Head injuries clearly pose a serious risk to child health (Child Accident Prevention Trust 1989, Avery & Jackson 1993) and the child health nurse, working with families and the community, has a role to play in preventing such accidents (Towner & Barry 1993). One common cause of childhood head injuries is bicycling accidents. A reduction in the severity of these injuries has been achieved by promoting the use of cycle helmets among children. This is a simple health education intervention which can easily be carried out by the child health nurse (Glasper & Skarratts 1990).

Convulsions

A convulsion, whether due to epilepsy (Hart & Shorvon 1990) or the more common febrile convulsion (Hall et al 1990), may cause disruption of a child's consciousness. During a seizure, a child is very vulnerable to injury as she is effectively unconscious and may fall and cause an injury. During the convulsion, the child may have difficulty in maintaining an open airway; also the muscular spasms seen in a seizure may lead to the child injuring herself. In the event of a convulsion occurring, the nurse's most important action is to ensure the child's safety (Platt 1993).

INFECTION

Infections of the central nervous system are relatively rare in childhood but they are very important as they can potentially damage the delicate developing brain and may even prove fatal. The organisms causing such infections may be either bacteria or viruses.

Bacteria—bacterial meningitis

The most common bacterial infection of the central nervous system is meningitis, which is an inflammation of the meninges, the fine membranes that cover and protect the surface of the brain. This infection is usually contracted when the child suffers a respiratory tract or ear infection caused by the bacteria *Neisseria meningitidis* (meningococcus) or *Haemophilus influenzae* (Ross & Peutherer 1987). When this infection occurs in the newborn baby, the offending bacterium is often *Escherichia coli*, which is an organism normally found in the gut. The disease occurs when these organisms are carried to the central nervous system by the bloodstream.

Bacterial meningitis is an infection which typically develops very quickly and, without prompt treatment, can quickly lead to the child's death. For this reason the infection is much feared by the general public, and parents of the child with meningitis will be very afraid at the very mention of this infection; they will need much support and information from the nurse. The child with meningitis will often arrive at hospital having become critically ill within a few hours. The symptoms of this infection include:

- A high fever.
- Irritability.
- Drowsiness and reduced consciousness level.
- A marked sensitivity to light—bright light hurts the eyes.
- Neck stiffness and possibly arching of the back—this occurs because the child seeks, by not moving the neck or back, to avoid stretching the sensitive, inflamed meninges surrounding the spinal cord.
- Children with meningitis caused by meningococcus may have a purpuric rash—this is a very fine purple, pinpoint rash, which appears first on the limbs and does not become pale when gentle pressure is applied to the spot.
- The child may have a very fast pulse and a marked drop in blood pressure—the child may even be in a state of shock.
- The child with central nervous system infection may have a very high-pitched irritable cry. This cry is characteristic to the nurse who has heard it before, but it is often parents who are able to point out that the child's cry has changed. Parents are often very sensitive to their child's different cries and are able to differentiate among cries due to pain, hunger, discomfort, boredom and the cry that simply means that the child wants a cuddle.
- In the young child, the fontanelle may be tense and bulging.

Nursing care of the child with meningitis

All of the steps taken by the child health nurse in caring for the child with meningitis will be directed towards relieving the child's symptoms and assisting the doctor in the investigations required for diagnosis and in treatment.

The nurse will monitor the child's well-being by measuring the vital signs of pulse, blood pressure and respiratory rate frequently. Changes in the values of these signs may indicate a deterioration in the child's condition which warrants rapid further action. The child's neurological state and consciousness level will be assessed frequently using the methods described above; again these observations can give early warning of a worsening in the child's condition. Drugs given to relieve the child's pain will be used with care as many of these can depress the consciousness level, making it difficult to detect dangerous changes in the child's condition. The child's temperature should be frequently measured and steps taken to reduce a high temperature. To achieve this, the child may be given paracetamol, nursed with few clothes in a cool room and, possibly, a fan will be directed over the child's body, avoiding the face. Parents can assist in these strategies to reduce temperature and can derive great satisfaction and reassurance from helping to care for the child. The child with bacterial meningitis will be treated with antibiotic drugs, and these will be given initially directly into a vein; any fluids required by the child may also need to be given by this route. The safe care of the limb in which the intravenous cannula is sited will be an important part of the child's nursing care.

With the introduction of Hib (*Haemophilus influenzae* B) immunisation in the United Kingdom, children are protected against this organism which can cause meningitis (DoH et al 1992).

Lumbar puncture. The nurse may be called upon to assist the doctor in performing a lumbar puncture to help to establish whether the child has meningitis and, if so, the identity of the causative organism. This will allow the doctor to decide upon the most appropriate antibiotic to treat the infection. Performing a lumbar puncture on a sick child is a very demanding task in which the nurse plays a very important role. The test

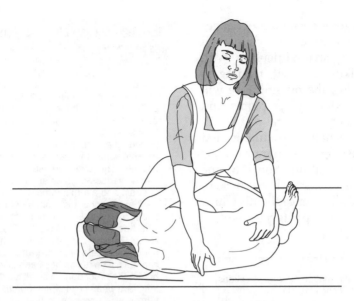

Figure 14.1   Lumbar puncture: position of the patient.

involves the removal of a small amount of cerebrospinal fluid from the spinal column a little below the child's waistline. To facilitate this, the child has to curl into a ball to open up the spaces between the vertebrae (Fig. 14.1). This is obviously very difficult for the small child who finds any back movements painful. A small amount of local anaesthetic will be used to numb the child's skin, but the test remains unpleasant

Activity 14.3

When you have read about the process of performing a lumbar puncture on a child, take some time to consider how the parents of a child undergoing such a procedure can be prepared for the experience. Reserve around 15 minutes for this exercise and sit down with paper and pencil to take notes. Consider what information is necessary to allow the child's parents to form an understanding of what is going to happen. Consider the fears and misconceptions these parents might have and how you can clarify the situation and allay their fears. Take into account the effect that stress and fear might have on the parents' ability to absorb information.

Once you have considered this exercise and taken notes, why not discuss your thoughts with one of your fellow students or your tutor?

for the frightened child. Careful explanation in simple terms of what will happen will help the child to understand this event and perhaps help to secure her cooperation. The nurse will gently help the child into the required position and hold the child securely in this position to avoid any sudden movement. To see their child undergoing a lumbar puncture will be deeply upsetting for distressed parents and some will simply not want to be present. Again, simple explanations of the test, its purpose and how it is performed should prove reassuring for the child's parents.

Viruses—viral encephalitis

Viral infections of the central nervous system are generally less dramatic in their development than infections caused by bacteria. Viruses such as herpes simplex—the cold sore virus—can cause an infection of brain tissue called encephalitis. This is a serious disorder because the infection can damage the brain permanently causing the child to be permanently disabled. The child with this infection will tend to suffer a rather gradual reduction in consciousness level and may appear stunned. The child may also appear to have undergone personality changes and be irritable or aggressive. The child with viral encephalitis may have difficulties with balance and find walking difficult, tending to stagger. In this case also, the nursing care will be directed towards reducing symptoms and ensuring the child's safety. Antiviral drugs will be required and will usually be administered directly into the bloodstream via an intravenous cannula and infusion of fluid. Some of the common childhood infections such as chickenpox and measles can cause an encephalitis which is usually mild and resolves spontaneously.

 For further information on viral infections, see Rudd & Nicholl (1991).

PAIN

Pain is an unpleasant sensation which is a universal human experience (McCaffery & Beebe 1989). The child's perception of pain is a mixture of the physiological sensation of pain and the child's psychological response to pain. The psychological response to pain is learnt and since children may experience pain at any stage in life they begin this learning process early in life. This definition demonstrates that pain is a subjective experience unique to the individual who suffers it.

While the physiological component of pain is common to all children, the psychological component varies widely and is affected by many factors (see Box 14.2).

Pain is, for the most part, an indication of tissue dysfunction or damage. That being so the child health nurse can often anticipate when a child will experience pain, for example following an injury, surgical operation or invasive procedure. The perception of pain will cause the child to display a variety of signs and symptoms.

Signs of pain in a child include:

- increased pulse rate
- raised blood pressure

Box 14.2 Factors affecting a child's psychological response to pain

- Context—the situation in which the child suffers pain and the events leading up to this experience will affect the child deeply. If the pain is unexpected, the sensation can be made to feel worse by the fear and alarm it brings about. If the child is very anxious, this compounds the problem. Also, if the child sees his or her parents upset and distressed, for example following an accident, this can increase anxiety. Increased anxiety then increases distress and a vicious cycle of worsening pain and alarm can be established.
- Past experience and memory of pain will influence the child's response to the perception of pain. The child who has experienced pain will learn to fear its recurrence. Nurses can see this in the child who has to undergo repeated painful procedures such as dressing changes, if no action has been taken to relieve the pain before the procedure. A small child may generalise this fear, and when child health nurses wore traditional uniform it was common to find small children becoming very afraid of anyone wearing a white uniform. The attitude and tolerance of other family members to pain will also influence the child who will tend to reproduce these attitudes.
- Meaning of pain—children, like adults, will tend to be less afraid of pain if they have an accurate understanding of the cause of pain and how and when it will resolve. Depending on the child's stage of cognitive development, it is possible that the child can misunderstand the meaning of pain which will increase the child's suffering. Small children may interpret pain as a punishment, while adolescents may fear that it signals a change in body image or that it indicates a worsening or more dangerous development in their health.
- Culture defines the shared beliefs and attitudes of a group towards phenomena such as pain. The effect of culture on the expression and perception of pain has been classically described by Zborowski (1952). Cultures define what is acceptable behaviour for each gender; in many cultures boys may find that they have to conceal their pain and not give in to expressing their distress.
- Learning ability—the child who has difficulty in understanding the significance of pain will naturally suffer anxiety as a result.
- Personality—children, like adults, vary widely in their reactions to a crisis. Some children will tend to be stoical while others may respond in an exaggerated fashion. These personality types will give very different cues when in pain, increasing the difficulty for the nurse in assessing their pain.

- sweating (after the newborn period)
- pale, clammy skin
- dilated pupils and tear production.

Box 14.3   Behavioural features of the child in pain

The newborn or preverbal child in pain might demonstrate:

- crying
- positioning, facial expressions and movements which suggest distress
- a reluctance to tolerate normal activities such as feeding or play/movement
- a marked dislike of being handled
- an unusual increase or decrease in the time spent sleeping.

When a toddler or pre-school child is suffering pain, the parent or nurse might observe:

- irritability, aggression, low frustration threshold or shortened attention span
- unusual disinterest in normal activities such as play
- unusual quietness or inactivity
- a disturbed sleep pattern—excessive wakefulness or sleepiness
- reluctance to move the affected part, or rubbing or pulling the painful part of the body
- crying or screaming.

Older schoolchildren in pain may display a range of changes in their normal behaviour:

- irritability or aggression
- unusual withdrawal from normal activities, quietness and inactivity
- unexplained upset, fretfulness or distress
- disinterest in normal activities such as play
- low frustration threshold and shortened attention span
- clinginess and tearfulness
- 'guarding' of the affected part and reluctance to move
- changes in the normal sleep pattern.

Features of behavioural change in the adolescent in pain may be subtle and difficult to interpret. These may include:

- unusual postures related to guarding of the painful part
- lethargy and withdrawal
- altered sleep patterns
- visible anxiety and taciturnity.

In addition to these signs, certain features of the child's behaviour can alert the nurse to the possibility that the child is suffering pain. These features are also highly individual and, although classified in Box 14.3 according to chronological age, there is a good deal of variation between children of similar ages. The information should therefore be regarded as rough guidelines only.

Since the newborn baby has a peripheral nervous system which is immature (incompletely covered with its myelin sheath), it was long thought that newborn babies could not experience pain. This, coupled with the view that part of the individual's response to pain is psychological, produced a situation in which it was not seen as necessary to provide small babies with pain relief, even when it could be expected that they would be experiencing pain. This view has been completely discredited by the work of, for example, Anand & Hickey (1987) who showed that even before birth the fetus has the ability to perceive pain during the last 3 months of gestation. These findings highlight the important role of the child health nurse in identifying when the child is suffering pain and taking immediate action to secure relief for the child. Children can be spared much suffering if the nurse can anticipate *when* pain is likely and take steps to relieve pain *before* the child suffers it.

Assessment of pain

Assessing children for the possibility of pain is a complex task due to the subtlety of the signs of pain in many children and the wide variability in the way that children express pain. In this task of assessment, the child health nurse can be greatly helped by the child's parents. Parents have an intimate knowledge of their children's behaviour, reactions and personality and are sensitive to small changes in the child's normal pattern of behaviour which might indicate pain. Great care must be taken, however, to avoid the parents feeling that they are entirely responsible for detecting pain in their child. This is an onerous responsibility and may feel overwhelming, particularly when the parent is stressed and upset about the child's illness or injury. In addition, the parent may have never seen the child suffering severe pain and be at a loss. The verbal child may try to tell the parent or nurse about the experience of being in pain, but if the child is having difficulty in interpreting the pain, what the child says may seem unusual or even potentially misleading. In studying the words children use to describe pain Jerrett & Evans

(1986) met a child who described pain as 'a sausage'!

There are several tools in existence which have been shown by nurses to be helpful in assisting the child to describe the pain experience. These range from the visual analogue scale, which is a measured straight line marked 'no pain' at one end and 'the worst pain imaginable' at the other end. The child can be asked to place a mark on this line to represent graphically the degree of pain. Variations of this principle have been devised for use with small children. The 'Oucher scale' (Beyer & Aradine 1987) shows a series of photographs of children experiencing distress of different levels; the child selects the photograph which corresponds most closely to how the child is feeling. Another simple variant

of this is to show the child a series of drawn pictures of 'smiley faces' progressively ranging from very happy to very sad (Fig. 14.2) and asking the child to select the drawing which shows the way he or she is feeling.

Pain relief

The methods available to the parent and nurse to relieve a child's pain are varied, and their best use will rely on careful assessment of the child's needs and imagination, flair, creativity and persistence on the part of the nurse (Eland 1988). Analgesic drugs are safe to use in helping the child in pain, when the appropriate recommendations for use are observed. Great care will be required, however, in selecting the appropriate means of administering these drugs since children may fear intramuscular injections so much that they will deny suffering pain to avoid a 'needle'. Methods of pain relief that do not involve the use of drugs are summarised in Box 14.4.

Many researchers have noted that children often do not receive adequate pain relief in hospitals (Royal College of Surgeons of England / College of Anaesthetists 1990). The important role of the child health nurse in assessing and treating pain in children is complex and difficult, but success in this challenging task is of utmost importance for the child, the parents and the nurse.

Activity 14.4

When you have looked at a simple pain assessment scale such as the 'smiley faces', take some time to think about what features might make such a scale attractive and interesting for a small child. You might find it an interesting exercise to design your own version of such a scale. You should be careful to preserve clarity and usefulness for the purpose. Do not make it so elaborate that the child using it loses sight of what it is for! When you have done this you could ask the opinion of children you know, such as younger members of your own family.

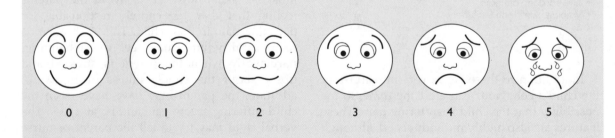

Figure 14.2 A simple pain rating scale for children. It could be explained to the child that, for example, face 0 is very happy because he has no pain (hurt), face 1 hurts a little bit, face 2 hurts a little more and so on. Face 5 hurts as much as you can imagine, though you do not actually have to be crying to feel this bad. The child should be asked to choose the face that best describes how she is feeling. (Adapted from Whaley & Wong 1991.)

Box 14.4 Methods not involving the use of drugs that can be used to help relieve a child's pain and distress

- Information giving—the experience of pain for a child can be made worse by fear of what the pain means and what can be expected in terms of its reduction and disappearance
- Physical comfort:
  —a quiet, calm environment
  —careful handling, support and positioning
  —comfortable clothing and warmth
  —gentle massage
  —cuddles and rocking
- Parental care—'mummy cuddles' and the use of familiar strategies for soothing and relieving distress
- Distraction:
  —listening to music or stories
  —familiar play activities
  —watching videos or television
- Relaxation—older children can be taught relaxation and visualisation techniques

SLEEPING

Sleep can be seen as 'normal unconsciousness' and is an essential activity for all human beings; sleep deprivation has been shown by psychologists to lead very quickly to serious health problems (Oswald 1974). Adults and older children have an established pattern of sleep within a 24-hour period called a diurnal or circadian rhythm—we tend to sleep at night and stay awake by day. This rhythm is established in early childhood as the biological 'clock' is set (Vasta et al 1992). Small babies need around 14 hours of sleep every day and sleep tends to occur in short cycles as babies drowse and wake to feed, play and interact with their parents. As the baby gets older the need for sleep slowly reduces and the child begins to take sleep as nightlong 'blocks'. The sleep requirement slowly decreases throughout childhood until the adult average of 8–10 hours per night is reached in adolescence. The transition in sleep pattern after early infancy can be rather difficult to achieve and many children continue to wake frequently into toddlerhood. Childhood sleep patterns can also be rather fragile and can be disrupted by any

Activity 14.5

After reading further on the strategies used to help the family with a child who has difficulty in sleeping, read Case study 14.1 and make a list of the helpful interventions the child health nurse can make to help this family.

change in the child's routine such as hospital admission, a holiday or even a long journey. Minor childhood illnesses can also naturally disturb the child's sleep pattern, as can nightmares.

For parents, childhood sleep disturbances can be extremely trying (Pfeil 1993). A child who refuses to go to sleep or who wakes frequently in the night and cannot settle can very quickly exhaust the entire family. Health care professionals working in community settings recognise the severity of the problem for the affected family and this has given rise to the establishment of sleep clinics in many localities. With sound, sensible advice, families can help the child with sleep problems to establish a normal sleeping pattern (Bidder & Hewitt 1985).

CRYING

All babies cry; it is their principal means of communicating their needs. Indeed, parents quickly

Case study 14.1 Laura

Laura, aged 3, has never slept well at night. As a small baby she woke every 30–45 minutes to breast-feed. Laura still takes a long afternoon nap and rarely goes to sleep before 23:00. She refuses point blank to go to bed and rarely falls asleep in her own bed; she generally drops off in front of the television. She is still waking five or six times each night and she insists on coming into her parents' bed or on playing with her sleepy mother. Laura's mother is not too concerned about her daughter's sleep pattern as she tends to take a daytime nap with Laura. Her husband, however, is increasingly annoyed and tense about Laura's night-time activities. Laura's sleep pattern is causing serious discord between her parents.

learn to differentiate between, for example, a hunger cry and a boredom cry. The baby who cries often for prolonged periods and who is difficult to soothe can present enormous problems for parents. It is difficult to listen to a baby cry for long periods; parents in this situation will become very anxious and frustrated. Under the age of 3 months, some babies suffer from colic (spasms of abdominal pain), which causes the baby to scream for long periods, typically in the evening (Bax et al 1990). Parents in this situation will need a good deal of support from the child health nurse and other health care personnel. They can be reassured that colic is a self-limiting condition and that it virtually always disappears by the time the baby is 4 months old. In the interim, parents can be advised to use all methods they can think of to make the baby comfortable during attacks of colic; they can check that the baby is warmly and comfortably dressed and that the nappy is clean and dry. Carrying the baby around in various positions, swaddling and gentle massage to back or tummy may soothe the baby. Music may quieten the baby; some families find that the sound of the vacuum cleaner or the washing machine calms the infant! Other babies will settle to sleep in the car. Each baby has her or his own preferences. Antispasmodic drugs have been used in the past but are not recommended for the baby under 6 months. Some parents find that herbal drinks such as fennel, specifically prepared for babies, are helpful. It is rarely beneficial to change the milk used for formula-fed babies. Some babies, especially those who feed very quickly and enthusiastically, suffer from abdominal pain because of excessive amounts of air swallowed while feeding. These babies can be helped by holding them upright and patting or stroking their back until they 'burp'.

Sometimes parents may feel that by continually picking up the crying baby to soothe him or her they run the risk of 'spoiling' the child. The child health nurse can emphasise that small babies cannot be spoiled in this way and that parents should not feel, or be made to feel, guilty when they pick up their distressed baby.

For some families an excessively crying baby can be a severe trial. A self-help group called Cry-Sis has been formed which may provide invaluable help and support for the affected family. The child health nurse can suggest the use of the services of such a group.

CONTINENCE

At birth the infant is incontinent of urine and faeces because the nervous system is not sufficiently mature to allow the conscious control of sphincter muscles. Parents often anxiously wait for the baby to achieve continence, though many do not appreciate that this, in the normal situation, may not be achieved before the child is 3 years old (Berk 1991). There is a wide range of normal timing for the child to be toilet trained and parents can be reassured with information about this fact. The process of learning to be clean and dry is slow and progressive; accidents are common at first and patience is required. In this, as in all questions of development, each child is unique in the rate and timing of achievements. Toilet training is best achieved by taking the process at the child's own pace. A routine can be helpful such as use of the potty after meals or at other times when the parent notices that the child tends to pass urine or stool. It is, however, worthwhile advising against being too rigid in such routines as difficulties can arise when a wilful toddler decides to oppose the parents' intentions (Bidder & Hewitt 1985).

When you have read through this chapter and worked through the activities you should feel that you have achieved the aims stated at the beginning of the chapter. You will by now appreciate the breadth of the topic of neurological health in childhood and the significance of a knowledge of the topic to the child health nurse. By following up the references from this chapter and the texts suggested in the list of further reading you can develop your knowledge in your areas of particular interest.

REFERENCES

Anand K J S, Hickey P R 1987 Pain in the fetus and neonate. New England Journal of Medicine 317: 1321–1329

Avery J G, Jackson R H 1993 Children and their accidents. Edward Arnold, London

Bax M, Hart H, Jenkins S M 1990 Child health and child development. Blackwell Scientific Publications, Oxford

Berger K S 1988 The developing person through the lifespan, 2nd edn. Worth Publishers, New York

Berk L E 1991 Child development, 2nd edn. Allyn & Bacon, London

Beyer J E, Aradine C R 1987 Patterns of pediatric pain intensity: a methodological investigation of a self-report scale. Clinical Journal of Pain 3: 130–141

Bidder R, Hewitt K 1985 If you don't behave ...: practical advice for parents and professionals on the behaviour of young children. The Test Agency, Reading

Child Accident Prevention Trust 1989 Basic principles of accident prevention: a guide to action. CAPT, London

Davies D 1993 Care of the child with neurological needs. In: Carter B (ed) 1993 Manual of paediatric intensive care. Chapman & Hall, London

Department of Health/Welsh Office/Scottish Office Home and Health Department/DHSS (Northern Ireland) 1992 Immunisation against infectious disease, 1992 edn. HMSO, London

Eland J M 1988 Persistence in pediatric pain research: one nurse researcher's efforts. Recent Advances in Nursing 21: 43–62

Frankenberg W K, Sciarillo W, Burgess D 1981 The newly abbreviated and revised Denver Developmental Screening Test. Journal of Pediatrics 99(6): 995–999

Glasper A, Skarratts D 1990 Bicycle helmets—whose responsibility? Paediatric Nursing (Dec): 13–15

Hall D M B (ed) 1992 Health for all children: a programme for child health surveillance, 2nd edn. Oxford Medical Publications, Oxford

Hall D M B, Hill P, Elliman D 1990 The child surveillance handbook. Radcliffe Medical Press, Oxford

Hart Y, Shorvon S D 1990 Epilepsy, 2nd edn. Update Postgraduate Centre Series, Reed Business Publishing Group, Guildford

Hosking G 1982 An introduction to paediatric neurology. Faber & Faber, London

Jerrett M, Evans K 1986 Children's pain vocabulary. Journal of Advanced Nursing 11: 403–408

Lansdown R 1984 Child development made simple. Heinemann, London

McCaffery M, Beebe A 1989 Pain: clinical manual for nursing practice. C V Mosby, St Louis, ch 10

Oswald I 1974 Sleep, 3rd edn. Penguin, Harmondsworth

Pfeil M 1993 Sleep disturbance at home and in hospital. Paediatric Nursing September: 14–16

Platt W D 1993 Nurse-aid: management of neurological emergencies. British Journal of Nursing 2(5): 288–290

Ross P W, Peutherer J F 1987 Clinical microbiology. Churchill Livingstone, Edinburgh, chs 12, 13

Royal College of Surgeons of England/College of Anaesthetists: Commission on the Provision of Surgical Services 1990 Report of the working party on pain after surgery. Royal College of Surgeons of England/College of Anaesthetists, London

Rudd P, Nicoll A 1991 British Paediatric Association manual on infections and immunisations in children, 2nd edn. Oxford Medical Publications, Oxford

Sheridan M D 1975 From birth to five years: children's developmental progress, 3rd edn. Routledge, London

Tortora G J, Grabowski S R 1993 Principles of anatomy and physiology, 7th edn. HarperCollins College Publishers, New York

Towner E, Barry A 1993 Accidental injury in childhood. Paediatric Nursing December: 10–12

Vasta R, Haith M M, Miller S A 1992 Child psychology: the modern science. John Wiley & Sons, New York

Whaley L F, Wong D L 1991 Nursing care of infants and children, 4th edn. C V Mosby, St Louis

Williams J 1992 Assessment of head-injured children. British Journal of Nursing 1(2): 82–84

Zborowski M 1952 Cultural components in responses to pain. Journal of Social Issues 8: 16–30

FURTHER READING

Bax M, Hart H, Jenkins S M 1990 Child health and child development. Blackwell Scientific Publications, Oxford

Berger K S 1988 The developing person through the lifespan, 2nd edn. Worth Publishers, New York

Berk L E 1991 Child development, 2nd edn. Allyn & Bacon, London

Bidder R, Hewitt K 1985 If you don't behave ...: practical advice for parents and professionals on the behaviour of young children. The Test Agency, Reading

Branthwaite A, Rodgers D (eds) 1985 Children growing up. Open University Press, Milton Keynes

Carter B (ed) 1993 Manual of paediatric intensive care. Chapman & Hall, London

Donaldson M 1987 Children's minds. Fontana, London

Glasper E A, Tucker A 1993 Advances in child health nursing. Scutari Press, London

Hall D M B (ed) 1992 Health for all children: a programme for child health surveillance, 2nd edn. Oxford Medical Publications, Oxford

Hall D M B, Hill P, Elliman D 1990 The child surveillance handbook. Radcliffe Medical Press, Oxford

Hosking G 1982 An introduction to paediatric neurology. Faber & Faber, London

Johnston P G B 1994 Vulliamy's The newborn child, 7th edn. Churchill Livingstone, Edinburgh

Mead D, Sibert J 1991 The injured child: an action plan for nurses. Scutari Press, London

Nash W, Thruston M, Baly M E 1985 Health at school: caring for the whole child. Butterworth-Heinemann, London

Rudd P, Nicoll A 1991 British Paediatric Association manual on infections and immunisations in children, 2nd edn. Oxford Medical Publications, Oxford

Sheridan M D 1975 From birth to five years: children's developmental progress, 3rd edn. Routledge, London

Vasta R, Haith M M, Miller S A 1992 Child psychology: the modern science. John Wiley & Sons, New York

Whaley L F, Wong D L 1991 Nursing care of infants and children, 4th edn. C V Mosby, St Louis

While A (ed) 1991 Caring for children: towards partnership with families. Edward Arnold, London

15

The musculoskeletal system

Jonathan Pagdin

This chapter will provide the reader with an understanding of the normal development of the musculoskeletal system of the child. Common causes of immobility will be investigated; these will be separated into acquired and congenital, but because the congenital reasons resulting in immobility are so numerous the reader will be advised on further areas for reading and research. The nursing care of children with immobility problems will be outlined.

The chapter aims to:
- discuss the risks of immobility in children
- outline the commonest acquired cause of immobility in children—fractures
- describe how bones heal
- outline the nursing management of differing types of fracture treatment
- describe a number of common congenital causes of immobility
- discuss advice given to families on discharge
- review the support groups available
- describe the commonly available mobility aids.

The musculoskeletal system has a number of functions in the body; it provides movement, support and protection. It is made up of 206 bones and the ligaments that bind them together, the skeletal muscles and the tendons. It is the musculoskeletal system that gives the body its shape.

SKELETAL TISSUES

Skeletal tissues can be divided into the following groups:

- *Bone tissue.* Bones are made up of two types of tissue (Fig. 15.1):
    - —cancellous bone—this has a 'honeycomb', porous and spongy appearance; it is hard and strong but light in weight; its spaces are filled with red bone marrow
    - —compact bone—this is dense and hard; it forms a shell which gives the bone strength.
- *Fibrous tissue.* A sheet of fibrous tissue, the periosteum, covers all the surfaces of bone except where joints occur. It is a protective covering permeated with nerves and blood vessels servicing the underlying bone.
- *Hyaline (articular) cartilage.* Articular tissue is a smooth connective tissue which is present over the articulating ends of bones where there is a movable joint allowing them to move freely over each other.
- *Adipose tissue.* Bone marrow is a fatty tissue filling the spaces in cancellous tissue.

Bone formation

By the eighth week of the pregnancy, the skeleton of the developing embryo is complete, but is made of cartilage and fibrous membrane rather than bone. This is gradually hardened by the laying down of calcium, which is absorbed from food and transported in the bloodstream to the fetus. Ossification, the conversion of cartilage into bone, begins soon after the eighth week of pregnancy. This process is not completed in all bones until the individual reaches the early 20s when all growth finally stops.

Osteoblasts (bone-building cells) remove calcium and phosphorous from the blood and lay them down as small plates in the cartilage. This process starts in the middle of the shaft of a strip of cartilage—the primary centre of ossification—and calcium and phosphorous are laid down in both directions. Secondary centres appear at each end of the cartilage strip, becoming the extremities of the bone. By birth, there is a strip of cartilage (the epiphysis) remaining between these centres which allows further growth to occur. Cartilage (hyaline) remains as a covering over the upper and lower extremities of the long bones.

Growth of bones

All bones are covered by a fibrous tissue called the 'periosteum'; from this the bone grows in circumference. Growth in length takes place from the epiphyseal cartilage. Bone is a living structure, continually being remodelled by bone cell activity. Old bone is removed by osteoclasts

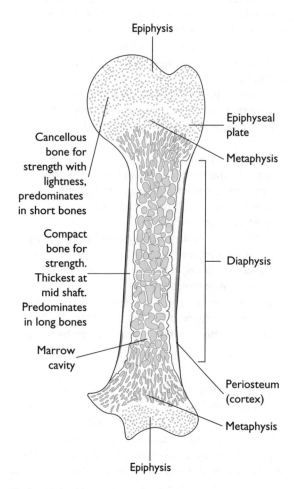

Epiphysis

Epiphyseal plate

Metaphysis

Cancellous bone for strength with lightness, predominates in short bones

Compact bone for strength. Thickest at mid shaft. Predominates in long bones

Diaphysis

Marrow cavity

Periosteum (cortex)

Metaphysis

Epiphysis

Figure 15.1 Normal bone structure.

and new bone is formed by osteoblasts. Bone growth is affected by dietary factors, hormonal factors and physical factors.

Functions of the skeletal system

The skeletal system provides a rigid framework to give shape to the body as well as support and protection for softer structures within it. Individual bones act as levers on which muscles can act to provide movement. Bones serve as storage sites for minerals such as calcium and phosphorous. Lipids are stored in the yellow bone marrow. Bones are also responsible for the production of blood cells, a function that is performed in the red bone marrow (Chandler 1991).

Joints

A joint is an area where two or more bones are in close contact with each other. Joints are held together by bands called 'ligaments'; they are classified according to their structure and mobility.

Fibrous or immovable joints. The bones are held together by fibrous tissue in such a way that no movement is possible, e.g. joints of bones in the skull.

Cartilaginous or slightly movable joints. Here the bones are separated by cartilage; this is compressed allowing slight movement, e.g. the joints between the vertebrae.

Synovial or freely movable joints. These are many and varied but all possess certain characteristics:

- two or more bones from the joint are held together by ligaments
- hyaline cartilage covers the articulating surfaces to prevent friction
- a fibrous capsule encloses the joint and helps to hold the bones in place
- synovial membrane lines the capsule and secretes synovial fluid to lubricate the joint structure.

Synovial joints can also be subdivided as follows:

- ball and socket joints—the rounded head of one bone fits into the cavity of another, e.g. the shoulder or the hip
- hinge joints—the articulating surfaces are shaped to permit only movements backwards and forwards, e.g. the knee or the elbow
- gliding joints—one surface glides against another, e.g. the wrist and the ankle
- pivot joints—one bone rotates on another, e.g. the radius and the ulna
- condylar joints—a condyle (the rounded projection at the end of a bone) of one bone fits into an elliptical cavity of another bone, e.g. the temporomandibular joint.

Function of joints. Joints hold the bones together and allow the rigid skeleton to become flexible and move.

THE MUSCULAR SYSTEM

There are three types of muscle in the body: cardiac, involuntary and voluntary muscle. The term 'muscular system' applies to the voluntary skeletal muscle which forms the flesh of the body. Voluntary muscle is composed of large elongated cells known as muscle fibres; these are bound together by connective tissue into small bundles which in turn are further bound into larger bundles forming the muscle. Each muscle consists of many bundles, or fasciculi, enveloped in a sheet of fibrous tissue (the fascia) which is continuous with the tendon. Tendons are bands of fibrous tissue attaching muscles to the bones; they are extremely strong and flexible. Muscles are attached to each other by sheets of fibrous connective tissue known as aponeuroses. A muscle is usually attached to two or more bones, and either the muscle or its tendon crosses the joint moved by the muscle.

Muscle activity

Muscle tissue is capable of contraction and relaxation but must be stimulated by nerve impulses to contract. Contraction occurs as a result of nervous, chemical, electrical or thermal stimulation of muscle fibres causing them to shorten and pull on the tendons attaching muscles to bones. Relaxation of muscles follows contraction when the muscle fibres resume their former length.

Muscle activity is coordinated; most skeletal muscles work in pairs or groups, where one group antagonises the action of another group to achieve controlled movement. As an example, the elbow works in the following way: in flexion the biceps contract and the triceps must relax to allow the forearm to be pulled up; extension is achieved by the relaxation of the biceps as the triceps contract and pulls the arm down. The erect position of the trunk is maintained as a result of coordination of groups of muscles. Body posture is maintained by good muscle tone and coordinated activity.

COMMON CAUSES OF IMMOBILITY

The causes of immobility in children can be divided into two major categories:

- acquired
- congenital.

ACQUIRED CAUSES OF IMMOBILITY

Fractures

Fractures are a very common reason for acquired immobility in children. They are still the cause of a large proportion of emergency paediatric hospital attendance, despite the increased incidence of asthma. 'Skeletal trauma accounts for 10–15% of all childhood injuries' (Ogden 1984).

A fracture is defined as a break in the continuity of a bone or cartilage, and can occur in any age group ranging from the newborn to the elderly. Usually, fractures are caused by trauma and there is a history of direct or indirect violence (Miller & Miller 1985). However, they can also be caused by repeated stress and strain or be due to pathological reasons.

Box 15.1   Clinical features of fractures (based upon Sacharin 1986 and Duckworth 1984)

Pain
- This is the most common feature.
- It varies with the site and type of the fracture and with the individual.
- The pain may be throbbing or localised.
- It is aggravated by active or passive movement.

Loss of function
- This is due to pain and instability of the fracture.
- The child may be unable to move the limb or can only use it with difficulty.

Swelling
- This is caused by oedema and effusion of blood (haematoma); this varies according to the extent of soft tissue damage.
- Gross swelling implies vascular rupture.
- Swelling takes time to appear and increases over the first 12–24 hours after the injury.

Deformity
- The limb is bent, shortened or has a step in its alignment.
- The deformity is manifested in a number of ways:
  —angular deformity caused by bone displacement
  —shortening of the limb caused by the over-riding of the bone ends at the fracture
  —rotational deformity, usually when the hand or foot has been involved in the injury.

Unnatural mobility
- The fragment distal to the injury can be moved through an unnatural range of movements (usually reproduced when the child is under a general anaesthetic).

Tenderness
- Is always present with a recent fracture.
- Can be elicited at the level of the fracture.

Crepitus
- This is the grating sensation heard and felt when the broken ends of the bone rub together. This feature should *not* be deliberately produced.

The signs and symptoms of fractures

Most fractures are diagnosed from the malalignment of the affected limb and the patient's description of the injury. Many authors describe the clinical features, but they can probably be best remembered under the seven headings given in Box 15.1.

Types of fractures

Fractures can take different forms depending on the force that causes them.

Transverse fractures. These are caused by direct violence.

Spiral or oblique fractures. These are caused by violence transmitted from a distance.

Greenstick fractures. These are found in children where the bone, because it has not completely calcified, is soft and yielding. Therefore, after violence occurs to the bone it bends but does not break completely; the cortex on the concave side of the fracture remains intact. The bone is said to resemble a 'green twig' which is difficult to break cleanly.

Crush fractures. These are caused by strong direct compression of the cancellous bone.

Burst fractures. These are caused by strong direct pressure. They usually occur in short bones, such as a vertebra.

Avulsion fractures. These occur where a tendon or ligament produces traction on a fracture, tearing off a bony fragment.

Dislocated or subluxed fractures. Where the fracture involves a joint, there may be malalignment of the joint surfaces. In children, fractures through the epiphysis (the growth plate) of the bone can occur; these can cause serious problems and may result in interference with, or complete cessation of, bone growth, thus producing a limb deformity.

Open or compound fractures. Fractures may be linked with a wound on the skin surface. Such a fracture is known as an 'open' or 'compound' fracture. Such fractures are potentially open to infection and therefore risk the development of osteomyelitis. To prevent this risk, it is essential to clean and close the wound. In certain cases, 'open' fractures can be linked to internal body surfaces, and the same risk of infection applies. An example of such a fracture is to the pelvis where the bowel may be perforated leading to infection. The nurse must be aware of this risk and observe for it, along with indications of internal bleeding, damage to the bladder and rectum, and less commonly damage to the femoral and sciatic nerves. In children, most pelvic fractures occur in road traffic accidents but the majority will heal in a satisfactory position with simple bed rest. (60% of all fatal pedestrian road traffic accidents occur in children aged between 5 and 14 years (Child Accident Prevention Trust 1992).)

Fractures are further classified as:

• *Stable.* Here the fracture is held in place by the soft tissue attachments, usually the periosteum of the bone itself, and are usually easily maintained in position; greenstick fractures in children can be regarded as stable.
• *Unstable.* The bone ends of a fracture are displaced or have the potential to become displaced. Such fractures need to be realigned (or reduced) allowing the fracture to become stable; however, if a reduced fracture is not held in some way it may re-displace.

Fracture complications

Fractures have the potential to result in many complications which the nurse should be aware of. These complications can be listed as follows;

Infection (see also 'open fractures'). The danger is that the infection will spread beyond the soft tissues, infecting the underlying bone. This can be a particular risk in children, where a large proportion of fractures occur when children are at play or undergoing sporting activities, thus increasing the risk of sustaining other wounds near to the fracture site, or contamination by foreign matter such as dirt, grit or grass. Therefore the nurse must observe for wounds, initiate steps to clean them and ensure that antibiotic therapy is commenced.

Malunion. This occurs when the union (healing) of the fracture takes place in the wrong position. This may be due to poor reduction or inadequate immobilisation or be the result of an unstable fracture. Such a complication, the risk of movement of a reduced fracture, is important in the management of children's fractures and therefore close follow-up is essential.

Delayed union. This happens where the blood supply to the fracture segment is poor and, although the fracture heals, it takes a longer time to do so than expected. Such a complication is usually due to inadequate immobilisation. Delayed union is unusual in children.

Non-union. Here, a fracture fails to unite (heal). This can be due to soft tissues being trapped between the bone ends of a fracture, infection in the fracture, or local bone necrosis.

Avascular necrosis. The blood supply to the bone fragments is disturbed. In some cases, such a condition becomes apparent much later than the fracture itself.

Fat embolism. A plug of fatty matter blocks a blood vessel. The fat deposit may originate from the bone marrow at the fracture site or from the altered state of the fat in the blood. The severity of this complication depends on the size of the embolism and the site where it occurs. If important structures are affected, the patient will show dramatic changes, for example in the brain or lungs.

Damage to structures. In 'complicated' fractures, other structures can be involved causing damage, e.g. to nerves resulting in palsies, or blood vessels resulting in ischaemia.

Compartment syndrome. Such a complication is a specific risk in supracondylar or forearm fracture in children; however, it may occur occasionally in the lower limb. It occurs when bleeding from the fracture takes place in a closed compartment below the deep fascia. Because this is not elastic, the space fills, increasing the pressure, usually on the brachial artery and thereby affecting the circulation to the forearm and the hand.

Circulation can also be disturbed by a displaced bone fragment or a tight plaster cast.

The signs of a compartment syndrome are:

- painful clawing of the fingers
- pain increases on gentle passive extension of the fingers
- the patient feels a burning sensation or paraesthesia
- patchy loss of sensation

- the radial pulse is weak, intermittent or absent
- the fingers are cold and bluish
- the ability to flex the fingers is weak.

Fractures and child abuse

Occasionally fractures in children are the result of physical abuse and the nurse must be aware of this possibility. Children suffering from abuse may present with a number of features:

- The child is generally brought late for treatment and no explanation for the injury is offered, or the explanation is not supported by the presented injury.
- Often injuries are multiple and differ in age; often discovered during a radiographic skeletal survey.
- The site of injury causes suspicion, e.g. not in the usual place of childhood bumps.

Fractures in children caused by abuse are usually as a result of direct blows or twisting of limbs.

Fracture repair/bone healing

The stages of bone healing (Fig. 15.2) are as follows:

- Stages One and Two:
  —The fractured bone bleeds forming a clot.
  —The inflammatory process starts and capillary budding begins.
  —Dead tissue and the clot is removed by phagocytes.
- Stage Three—The migrating cells have osteogenic potential and lay down osteoid, eventually forming bone; cartilage is sometimes laid down as an immediate stage.
- Stage Four—The final aim of the healing process is cortex-to-cortex healing. Such a healing is a slow process requiring the fracture surfaces to be immobilised. Regenerating bone at the fracture site is known as 'callus'.

Healed fractures in children have the ability to 'remodel'. Once a broken bone has healed the

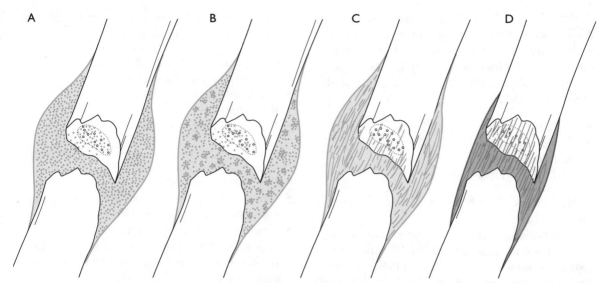

Figure 15.2   Normal bone repair: fracture healing. (A) Stage One: the broken ends of the bone bleed. (B) Stage Two: the blood clots and the broken ends of the bone are joined by the clots. (C) Stage Three: the clots change into 'harder' fibre-like strands. (D) Stage Four: finally the fibres alter into hard new bone or 'callus'.

callus often appears like a bump in the alignment of the bone; however, in time, through osteogenesis and osteolysis/osteoclasis the bump is absorbed. This ability in children means that in certain cases the fracture may not need to be perfectly realigned.

Treatment of fractures

The five Rs summarise the five main aims of fracture treatment (Miller & Miller 1985):

- Resuscitation—of the patient
- Reduction—of the fracture
- Restriction—of movement (immobilisation)
- Restoration—or maintenance of function
- Rehabilitation.

Resuscitation.   Any patient who suffers an injury, no matter what the degree of the injury, is likely to suffer from shock. In the case of fractures, shock is likely to be related to pain and blood loss. The nurse must be aware of the signs and symptoms of shock. The patient may show signs of anxiety and distress, have pallor and cold/clammy skin, a rapid and feeble pulse, shallow breathing and a lowered body temperature.

Usually most fractures in children can be regarded as minor casualties and rarely require resuscitation but the nurse, especially if acting as a first-aider, must be aware of this possibility.

Shock can be relieved in the following ways and these should be considered in the actions of a first-aider:

- careful handling, especially of the affected limb
- temporary immobilisation to relieve pain
- keeping the patient warm.

Reduction.   This describes how the bone ends involved in a fracture are realigned into the correct anatomical alignment. Reduction of a fracture is best achieved if the patient is under a general anaesthetic; this is especially the case with children, hence the large number of children with fractures admitted to hospital, particularly for short stays.

In a number of cases, particularly of children with greenstick fractures, the alignment may be acceptable and the need for reduction is removed.

Restriction. After the fracture has been reduced to a satisfactory position, the limb needs to be held in that position until bony union occurs. The method used to hold the fracture in place varies depending on the site but the methods include:

• traction
• plaster of Paris casts
• internal fixation
• external fixation.

Methods of fracture restriction are addressed below.

Restoration. When fractures are immobilised there is often the risk that the muscles in that limb and associated joints will stiffen; therefore it is important that function is maintained. The patient should be encouraged to exercise all joints, with the exception of those involved in the injury.

Rehabilitation. Once bony union has taken place the method of restriction can be removed. The limb then needs to be exercised to reach its range of movement prior to the injury. With childhood injuries this process usually takes place with little encouragement; however, occasionally the help of a physiotherapist may be required.

Methods of holding fractures

Sacharin (1986) describes two principles in the treatment of fractures:

• prevention of deformity
• allowing growth to proceed normally.

Holding the reduction of a fracture can be done in the following ways:

• stable fractures—some fractures require no means of stabilisation
• splintage:
  —plaster of Paris
  —cast bracing
• traction
• internal fixation
• external fixation.

Splintage—plaster of Paris. Such splintage has the following advantages:

• It is low cost and easily available.
• It is easy to use and apply.
• It is comfortable for the patient.
• It is strong.
• It is permeable to X-rays.

However, it does have some disadvantages:

• It is heavy and warm.
• It may cause pressure problems leading to sores under the plaster of Paris.
• It results in immobilisation of the joints.
• It is difficult to observe; the plaster may hide problems beneath it, e.g. wound breakdown and sepsis.
• There is the risk that toys and small objects may be pushed down the cast, again leading to sores under the plaster of Paris.
• It is not waterproof.

Nursing care when a plaster of Paris is applied. Certain nursing actions and observations must be undertaken when a plaster of Paris is applied. These are as follows:

• The limb should be elevated for a few hours after the application of the plaster of Paris, helping to reduce the amount of swelling that may occur and cause constriction in the cast.
• All plasters should be exposed in the drying period, taking care that pressure is not applied to the wet plaster from the fingers when lifting or turning, and that the cast is not rested on hard surfaces. This is especially important with children who have had 'hip spica' or 'frog' plasters applied.
• The limb should be observed and checked regularly. Miller & Miller (1985) note five important observations when nursing a patient in a plaster cast. These are the five Ps:
  —Pain—throbbing which increases in severity
  —Paraesthesia—burning, tingling or cold sensation
  —Pallor—of extremities and gross swelling of toes or fingers

—Pulse—diminished or absent
—Power loss—inability to use fingers or toes.

Plaster of Paris casts remain in place until the orthopaedic surgeon is satisfied that the fracture has healed. Casts are usually removed in the outpatient clinic, often using a plaster saw. Removal can be a difficult procedure for the child; therefore the procedure must be carefully explained and the child supported throughout removal.

Cast-bracing.   Plaster of Paris or other casting materials are used in combination with hinges or joints to hold the fracture. Femoral and tibial fractures are the most likely to be held in this way; in the case of femoral fracture, bracing may follow an initial period of traction.

Cast braces allow a greater degree of joint mobility and allow the patient to bear weight, which is often encouraged to promote bone healing.

Traction.   Such methods not only hold the position of fractures but may also be used to reduce them.

Traction can be fixed or balanced. In fixed traction, the traction works against the force of the patient's body. The Thomas splint, mainly used in the treatment of fractured femora, is the best example of such of a form of traction (Fig. 15.3).

Balanced traction works by the patient's weight being balanced by an applied load. Simple skin traction and gallows traction (Fig. 15.4) in the treatment of femoral fractures in babies are the best examples of these forms of traction.

Pritchard & David (1990) highlight the following as being the indications for traction:

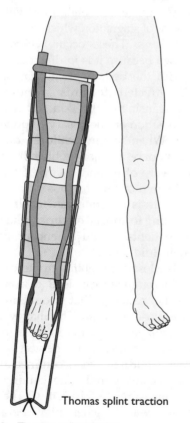

Thomas splint traction

Figure 15.3   Thomas splint traction.

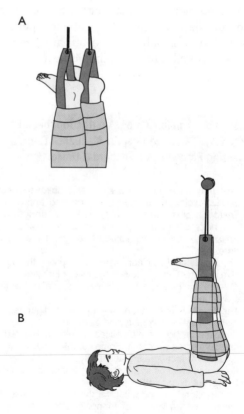

Figure 15.4   Gallows traction.

- relief of pain or muscle spasm
- ensuring that a limb is rested when diseased or broken until healing is done
- maintaining correct alignment
- restoring length where shortening after a fracture has occurred
- reducing dislocation of joints
- maintaining the position of unstable fractures
- as a preoperative measure prior to external fixation
- maintaining position after an operation.

Traction can be applied in one of two ways:

- skin traction—here adhesive strapping is attached along the skin with cords that can be attached to the traction (see Box 15.2); some patients may be sensitive to the adhesive.
- bony traction—the traction is applied through the bone directly by the use of a skeletal pin.

Nursing care of patients on traction. Once traction has been applied, the patient's pain and discomfort is usually relieved but analgesia may still be required. The nurse should be aware of the following problems and take the necessary steps to alleviate them when nursing children on traction:

- *The position of the patient.* Often the position required for successful traction is unnatural and distress is caused to the patient, especially where the patient is required to be 'head down'. Many activities of daily living will be difficult on traction, such as eating, drinking, washing, elimination and learning. Assistance with these needs is essential, as well as maintaining the privacy and independence of the patient.

  The child nursed on traction, once over the initial discomfort and trauma of an injury or operation, is also bound to become frustrated due to the loss of mobility; this can manifest itself as poor or naughty behaviour especially in school-age children. It should be dealt with sensitively but firmly to prevent a general disruption of the ward.
- *Stasis.* Complete immobilisation will lead to several forms of stagnation which are undesirable.
- *Pressure sores.* These occur where the skin breaks down because it is in direct and constant contact with the bed. A great deal of nursing effort is directed towards avoiding sores. Frequent cleansing of the skin and minor alterations in position are necessary to prevent sores occurring. When nursing children on traction, this should not be a major problem but the nurse must be aware of it, particularly if the child is severely injured or unconscious.
- *Kidneys.* Stasis of urine can result in kidney stones, leading to anuria, oliguria or haematuria; therefore patients should be encouraged to increase their fluid intake.
- *Bowel.* The loss of the ability to exercise and the decrease in roughage can lead to constipation; therefore the patient's diet should include increased cellulose and fluid. This may well need to be done in imaginative ways in the care of children. The use of laxatives may be necessary.
- *Boredom.* Children, when confined or immobile, will become bored. The children's nurse must take measures to relieve this. The involvement of the ward teacher, play therapist and nursery nurse is vital (see p. 250).

Box 15.2   Application of skin traction (based on The Royal Marsden Hospital Manual Of Clinical Nursing Procedures (Pritchard & David 1990))

- This may be a painful episode for a child; therefore careful explanations must be made and appropriate analgesia given before the procedure is undertaken, thus helping to gain the patient's cooperation and trust.
- Privacy should be maintained throughout the procedure.
- The limb should be cleaned prior to applying the adhesive skin traction, to prevent the risk of infection.
- The ankle joint is kept free, allowing normal movement of that joint.
- The patella is left free and the leg left in slight flexion, thus preventing deformity and stiffness.
- Pressure on bony prominences should be avoided or pressure sores will result. Some centres may still apply solutions to increase the adhesivity.
- Folds and creases in the strapping should be avoided to prevent discomfort or sores.
- The temperature and colour of the limb is checked to ensure that the tension of strapping is correct.

- *The affected limb.* Constriction of the limb by bandages (see Fig. 15.4) used in the traction may cause disturbance of the following:
    —the circulatory system
    —the muscles
    —the joints
    —the nerve supply.

Internal fixation.   This method of holding a fracture is used for fractures where an accurate reduction is required or when the fracture occurs around joints or when mobilisation of the limb is required. There are many types of internal fixation devices such as screws, plates, intramedullary nails and rods.

Internal fixation has a number of advantages:

- It allows accurate reduction and maintenance of position.
- It allows patient and joint mobility, encouraging rehabilitation and avoiding stiffness.
- It encourages union.
- It reduces time spent in hospital.

However, it also has some disadvantages:

- There is the possibility of introduction of infection.
- It is technically exacting for the surgeon.
- Postoperative complications may occur.
- It requires a general anaesthetic.
- Poor fixation or infection may delay union.
- Surgery is required to remove the device.

Nursing care of a child having internal fixation. The nursing care of a child having internal fixation should include the care of any child having a surgical procedure together with the observations and care required for a patient with a plaster cast.

External fixation.   The use of external devices for the treatment of fractures is becoming increasingly popular with orthopaedic surgeons. There are many different types of external fixation device but they rely on the same basic principles. The fracture is reduced under anaesthetic and imaging control. It is then restricted by the insertion of skeletal pins above and below the fracture; the pins are then attached to the fixation device which lies just above the surface of the affected limb. The fixation device is left in place until the fracture unites and consolidates. It can then be removed, possibly by the child himself, after he has been given analgesia and under supervision. This will depend on the age of the child, and his pain threshold and anxiety level.

External fixation of fractures has a number of advantages; it reduces the amount of time spent in hospital when compared to traction, and it allows earlier and increased mobility. However, it does have some disadvantages, namely the risk of infection via the skeletal pins which could lead to osteomyelitis, and the appearance of the device and the psychological effect this may have on the child and his family. Also, if such a treatment is to be a success, it relies on a great deal of committed self or family care, coupled with a coordinated community support service.

These devices are also used in limb reconstruction and limb-lengthening treatments which are being successfully carried out in many orthopaedic centres throughout the United Kingdom and the world as a whole.

Play in hospital

Many adults see play as a purposeless activity. In fact it is fundamental to a child's social, emotional and physical needs. *Play is work* to a child. Through play, the child learns the skills for living.

Play offers a stimulating environment for physical, intellectual, emotional and social development. Potentially each child's play is the perfect expression of him- or herself as a developing individual. Children use play to cope with distressing situations in life—hospital, death of a relative or pet, starting school, etc. The child who cannot play is severely threatened. The child's need for play is as strong in hospital as at home. Hospitalisation can be very frightening. Visintainer & Wolfer (1975) classify the features of hospital which can worry a child:

1. physical harm or bodily injury in the form of discomfort, pain, mutilation or death
2. separation from parents, especially for pre-school children
3. the strange, the unknown and the possibility of surprise
4. uncertainty about limits and expected 'acceptable' behaviour
5. relative loss of control, autonomy and competence.

Play provides an essential means of helping a child to cope with all these worries. However, encouraging play in hospital is not the same as encouraging play in, for example, a playgroup or in the home. The physiological and psychological stress of illness and hospital can make it very difficult for a child to play in the normal way. Bolig (1984) notes: 'in the absence of familiar persons, objects and routines and with the real or perceived threat of injections, medications and procedures, many children while hospitalised cannot play.'

Therefore it is very important to create a child-oriented environment with appropriate toys and creative materials and the presence of a trusted, permission-giving and responsive adult. This not only includes the nursery nurse and nursing staff; parents too have an important role. Participating in their child's play helps the parents to relax and overcome their own fears and anxieties, thus giving them the confidence to become more involved in the rest of their child's care.

Play and the immobilised child

For children nursed on an orthopaedic ward, who are severely restricted in their range of bodily movements, sometimes for several weeks or months, the practical problems of achieving play have to be overcome. When we place a child in an immobilising device we are taking away the child's independence, freedom of movement and way of discovering his surroundings in order to learn. A child may be in the middle of learning a new skill, for example toilet training. If we immobilise her we could be preventing

her acquiring this skill and in fact cause her to regress; this can be very upsetting and confusing to the child. Many children do adapt quickly to being immobilised, but become frustrated and rebel in various ways. Frustration often manifests through aggressive, disruptive or noisy behaviour and a child can become very demanding. For children on traction or in plaster it is very important that physical and emotional security is provided in what is sometimes a very insecure experience for them; this should be considered when planning play activities.

To keep a child on the orthopaedic ward happy and stimulated can be a problem to the play staff, nursing staff and parents. As immobilised children become more frustrated, their powers of concentration become greatly impaired. Therefore, a greater amount of play activities are needed. These should be interesting and enjoyable as well as encouraging independence, aiding development and continuing the child's learning of life skills. Children need to be provided with as many activities as they might have at home or nursery/school but these need to be adapted to fit the hospital environment and each child's physical constraints.

Examples of play encouraged on an orthopaedic ward

Imaginative/role play. This type of play appears when the child is involved in play with dolls, puppets, soft toys, tea sets, dolls houses, dressing-up clothes, doctor's kits, etc. Through imaginative play, children can assume other roles and learn about other people or situations by 'playing out' these roles, thus reducing fears and anxieties. Children can channel strong/antisocial/aggressive feelings during this play. It can also be used as a way for children to express themselves when language may be limited or they find it difficult to communicate their feelings.

Environmental play/activities. The immobilised child, whose stay on the ward could be for several weeks, may be unable to change his immediate environment; the surroundings in his range of vision remain the same. Therefore, it is important that his environment is changed for him, by moving his bed about the ward or into the playroom, or changing the pictures/posters on the walls around his bed area. It is also important to let the child personalise his bed space, because for some it is 'home' for a time. The child should be encouraged to put up posters of his favourite character or pop group, as well as photographs of family/friends etc. He can make his own mobiles to hang, especially a child who is nursed on his back for most of the time. Environmental play has many values for long-stay patients who cannot leave the ward. It brings the world outside the hospital to them, for example in the form of pictures, posters of the seasons, events, nature, etc. The children can also take part in related activities by making weather charts, pressing flowers, leaf printing, growing seeds (it is good for them to be in charge of something smaller than themselves, and to see that things do re-grow).

Messy play. This includes anything from water, sand, clay, dough, paint, glue, papier mâché, plaster of Paris, even cooking! The greatest value of messy play is that most of the materials used are unstructured and cannot be broken or destroyed. This makes them very versatile and very personal to the child who is playing with them. Children confined to bed or wheelchairs, who may be bored, tense, frustrated or angry, can let off steam by thumping or pummelling the materials without doing any real damage. These materials can also be used in a soothing and comforting way. They can be undemanding. When children are on their way to recovery, but still do not feel like coping with complicated toys, they will play happily in water or sand. Messy play can also be used as a therapeutic tool in preparing children for procedures and to familiarise them with medical equipment. Syringes can be used for water play or syringe painting. The use of plaster of Paris gives the child the opportunity to plaster a doll's leg and later to remove the plaster and see that the leg is still there and is not removed with the plaster. Using clay or dough, bones can be made and broken, then moulded back together to show

Activity 15.1

Devise some play activities for the following children on the ward:

1. an 18-month-old child in a hip spica plaster
2. two 10-year-old boys in traction, who are now well but are to be in hospital for another 3 weeks
3. a 13-year-old girl who has skeletal traction.

how they mend. Through painting, children can communicate their fears and anxieties or show the misconceptions that they may not be able to express through language. This type of play also enables the child to be messy in an otherwise 'clean' environment.

CONGENITAL CAUSES OF IMMOBILITY

There are many conditions which can result in children being immobile or can restrict their mobility. Such conditions are too numerous to describe in this chapter but some, because of the frequency with which they are seen by the paediatric nurse, are worthy of discussion. (The selection of these conditions does not imply that they are of more importance than other congenital causes of immobility.) Unfortunately, it is also necessary to limit each condition to a brief introduction only. However, the paediatric nurse must be aware of how and where to find the necessary information to care for children with disturbed mobility.

The three conditions that will be considered are:

- congenital dislocation of hips (CDH)
- congenital tarus equinus varus
- cerebral palsy.

Congenital dislocation of hips

The normal hip is a major weight-bearing joint of the body. It is a joint of the ball and socket type (the ball is the rounded head of the femur which fits into the socket—the cup-shaped hollow of the

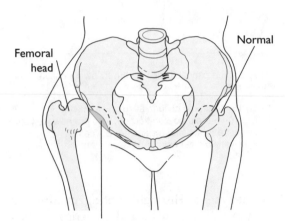

Figure 15.5   Congenital dislocated hip.

pelvis, the acetabulum). In congenital dislocation of the hips this joint is not true (Fig. 15.5).

There are varying degrees of dislocation of the hip:

- *Unstable.* Through manipulation, the head of the femur can be moved in and out of the acetabulum. The shape of the head of the femur and the acetabulum are normal or nearly normal. This condition is often known as 'clicking hips'.
- *Subluxed.* Here the head of the femur is only in partial contact with the acetabulum. There is a lack of development in the shape of the acetabulum.
- *Dislocated.* The head of the femur lies completely out of the joint. The shape and size of the head of the femur and the acetabulum are abnormal and will deteriorate if left out of the joint.

In all of the above there is abnormal laxity of the hip, causing the hip to become subluxed or dislocated usually in utero or immediately after birth.

Causes of congenital dislocation of hips

The incidence of CDH is unclear because many unstable hips can stabilise in the first few days of life, but it is said to be 8–20 per 1000 live births. Incidence is higher in girls than boys.

Hereditary factors may play a part in CDH; possibly there is an inherited characteristic of joint laxity or a shallow acetabulum. Where normal parents have an affected child there is a 1 : 25 chance that a subsequent child will be affected. An affected parent has a 1 : 25 chance of having an affected child, and this is increased to a 1 : 10 chance for further children (STEPS 1992a).

CDH is 10 times more common after breech deliveries, even if the baby has been 'turned' prior to delivery. Overlong pregnancies may also be a factor in the incidence of CDH. Loose ligaments are possibly due to a high level of the hormones released into the mother's bloodstream to prepare her body for labour, helping the ligaments of the pelvis to widen; if the concentration in the fetal blood becomes too high, the baby's hips may dislocate. Some researchers have highlighted a link between the way a young baby is carried and CDH. In North America, in the Indian and Eskimo populations, the incidence is high; here the babies are carried with their legs held in a straight position. In Africa, where babies are carried with their legs in the 'frog' position, the incidence is much lower (STEPS 1992a). CDH is also associated with other congenital conditions such as spina bifida and cerebral palsy.

Prognosis

The prognosis of the condition depends on its severity and when the dislocation is detected. If treatment is started early, when the hip is simply reduced in the first 6 months of life, the prognosis is usually good. Where the condition is more severe and the acetabulum is shallow, treatment is likely to be complex and prolonged, no matter when started. The older the child is when treatment begins the less likely the outcome is to be favourable. A perfect result cannot be guaranteed in any child when treatment starts after the age of 3; however, this does not mean that the child will be disabled or lead a restricted life.

Treatment

Treatments vary widely but can be simplified into two groups: conservative and surgical.

Conservative treatments.   The aim is to hold the thighs abducted so that the femoral head drops into the acetabulum. The constant pressure of the femoral head against the floor of the acetabulum helps it to be moulded and develop properly, therefore stabilising the hip. This can be done in four ways:

Double nappies.   The effect is to keep the legs wide apart.

Splints.   These are usually made from padded malleable aluminium shaped into an 'X' or 'H'. Splints are moulded over the shoulders and under the thighs. Other splints consist of strips and buckles holding the legs in the correct position. Some of the common splints are as follows:

- the Barlow splint
- the Von Rosen splint
- the Craig splint
- the Pavlik harness
- the Denis Browne CDH splint
- the Forester Browne CDH splint.

Splints are usually applied without anaesthetic and are not removed except for examination at hospital visits. Splints are worn for varying lengths of time but it is likely to be months rather than weeks.

Traction.   Traction is used when the severity of the CDH is too much for splints, or the splints have not worked. Traction overcomes the contractures of the soft tissues without undue force. It is used for 2–6 weeks before reduction and is often followed by a period in plaster.

Traction uses adhesive skin traction as in the treatment of some fractures described earlier in this chapter (p. 248). All traction methods use the same principle, gradually reducing the hips by abducting the hips through adjusting the traction. Often this treatment is carried out in hospital, with regular radiological review to monitor progress. Traction can be maintained at home with parental support provided the appropriate circumstances, facilities and support are available to the family.

Types of traction commonly used are:

- the Jones traction frame
- Burns traction
- the Japanese frame
- Alvick traction
- cross traction.

Plaster fixation.   Following a reduction of the hips, usually under a general anaesthetic, a plaster is applied. (This usually follows time spent in splints or traction.) The plaster may require frequent renewal, which is again usually performed with the child under an anaesthetic. This change of plaster also gives the surgeon the chance to examine the stability of the hips. The plaster holds the legs in a 'frog position' and is left in place for around 6 weeks, at which point the stability of the hips is reassessed. If hip stability is satisfactory the plaster is reapplied; if the surgeon has doubts about the hip stability then 'open' surgical treatments will be considered. Plaster treatment usual lasts for 6–9 months, depending on the individual case.

The types of traction used are:

- single hip spica
- double hip spica
- frog plaster.

Surgical treatments.   Surgical treatments are used when other methods of reducing the hip have failed or the diagnosis is made late or the state of the deformity means that conservative methods are unlikely to work. The type of surgery depends on each individual case. Common procedures are as follows.

Tenotomy.   This is lengthening of the tendon surgically. The tendon is located in the groin and its tightness prevents the hip from being reduced.

Limbusectomy.   This procedure refers to the removal of an obstruction in the hip socket.

Open reduction.   This is a surgical operation to place the femoral head opposite to the acetabulum. The leg is placed in a position where the joint is stable and the leg is held by a plaster cast.

Femoral osteotomy (rotational osteotomy). Here the leg is returned to a normal position after an open reduction. The femur is broken and

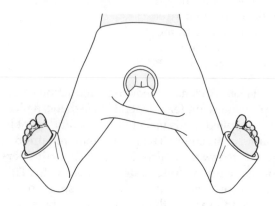

Figure 15.6   The hip spica plaster cast.

rotated into the satisfactory position. The break is held with plates until union takes places and the plates are then removed after about 1 year. The child is usually held in a hip spica plaster (Fig. 15.6) for a number of months.

Acetabulum reconstruction.   These are operations where the acetabulum of the hip is reconstructed.

Nursing and daily care

Plaster casts.   Plaster casts are very cumbersome and uncomfortable for both the child and the parents; for the parents because they have to carry a largely immobile child (immobility is not complete because children soon learn to drag themselves around on the floor) in a heavy plaster of Paris cast. They must be taught how to lift and carry the child before discharge.

Basic care of the plaster follows that already described in this chapter, but the key points are as follows:

• Checks should be made on the circulation, to ensure that it is not being disturbed to the toes.
• Any bleeding immediately after surgery should be noted and marked. Excessive leakage should be reported to the surgeon—this is a sign of postoperative haemorrhage.
• The parents should be made aware of the signs of wound infection under the plaster; this

will be identified by an unpleasant smell from the plaster combined with pyrexia in the child. If this occurs the child must be returned to the hospital as soon as possible.
• The plaster should be protected against being soiled or dampened by excreta. This is done by protecting the plaster in the appropriate areas with waterproof strapping, i.e. 'sleek'. However, this may not stop the plaster becoming soiled slightly.
• The parents should be encouraged to contact the hospital if any cracks occur in the plaster or the plaster softens.

Hygiene care

• Great care must be taken to prevent undue soreness.
• The plaster must be examined for rough edges which may cause skin breakdown.
• A daily sponge down replaces bathing.
• Talcum powder should be used sparingly around the plaster because it can cause excessive irritation to the skin under the cast.
• Hair washing can be a problem and usually becomes a 'two-man' job, one to hold the child over the bath, the other to wash. (Dry shampoo can be used.)
• Nappy area care takes some thought. Terry nappies can be folded or disposable nappies adapted for use; a larger size is often required. Nappies should not be tucked under the cast, so preventing any risk of pressure sores and excessive dampening.

Sleeping.   Younger children are less likely to be affected by the plaster, although 'wind' or colic can be troublesome; therefore 'winding' after feeding is important. Children in casts may only sleep for short periods and often become restless and distressed. Disturbed nights can also result from cramp, itching and the inability to turn over. The actual hospital admission may also disturb the child's sleep pattern. A child in a plaster takes up much more room than one without; therefore the width of the bed will require some thought. Placing the mattress on the floor may be useful and also removes the fear that the child will fall out of bed. Supporting the child in a comfortable position can be done with foam or pillows, but care must be taken to prevent pressure points developing or strain on the cast. The child may require fewer bed clothes since the plaster will act as insulation.

Transport and mobility. This is often a major problem for the family with a child in a hip spica plaster, but the ability to get out of the home is vital for both the parents and the child. Smaller babies will often fit into a push chair with some extra support with pillows. The best form of pushchair is a double one; however, these are expensive. A small baby in a cast may fit into a baby sling, but the parents must be made aware of the strain that this will cause to their backs and shoulders.

Transporting the child in a cast by car is a major problem. Many children can no longer be safely strapped into their car seats; special harnesses are sometimes available, or seat belt exemption can also be obtained.

The child's mobility. Children will learn to pull themselves around on the floor. They may even be able to stand, walk and climb stairs, although all of these activities will cause wear and tear to the plaster. Many families have designed their own aids to help the child be mobile. These usually take the form of some kind of 'tummy trolley'.

Eating and drinking. Some children are able to eat and drink lying on their tummies; others require to be supported in an upright position, either strapped in a normal high chair, or on a bean bag. There are also specially designed hip spica chairs available. A closed cup or a straw is the best method of drinking and prevents too many accidents. Constipation can be a problem for children treated in plaster casts; therefore the appropriate measures should be taken to alleviate this. These have already been discussed (see 'Nursing care of patients on traction', p. 248).

Clothing. This can be a major problem. Usually larger sizes are required; these can be split and then applied using tapes, poppers, Velcro or zips.

Play. Play and activity should be encouraged as much as possible to allow the child to

Activity 15.2

Mary, aged 14 months, is to be discharged home in a frog plaster. Consider the information that her parents need in order to care for her. Mary is not yet potty trained. Her mother has an older child of 4 years and a new baby. She is very concerned that she will not be able to cope with the practicalities of taking the 4-year-old to playgroup, going shopping, etc. What information and advice can you give her?

develop normally and to provide a means of releasing the tension that the child will experience when encased in plaster. Physical and really active play will be almost impossible; the child will have to rely on imaginative or craft types of play. The risk that children in a plaster can become isolated from their friends and peers is a realistic one; therefore normal contact should be encouraged, but games should not be allowed to become too boisterous.

Plasters are normally removed in hospital with the use of a plaster saw. This procedure must be explained to both the child and his or her parents to ease their anxieties and gain their cooperation in the task. After removal, the child will steadily return to normal. Occasionally regimes of physiotherapy may be required.

Congenital tarus equinus varus (CTEV or clubfoot)

Tarus equinus varus is a congenital abnormality of the foot and results in a malformed and irregularly positioned foot or feet. As with other orthopaedic conditions, it varies in its type and severity. There are four types of CTEV:

- talipes equinus—the heel is raised from the ground causing the child to walk on the ball of the foot
- talipes calcaneous—the heel rests on the ground and the front of the foot is raised (the opposite of talipes equinus)
- talipes varus—the sole of the foot is turned

inwards so that the child walks on the outer edge of the foot
- talipes valgus—the foot is turned outwards so that the child walks on the inside of the foot (the opposite of talipes varus).

These different types can be combined into more complex deformities, e.g. talipes equino-varus, where the heel is drawn up and the sole is turned inwards. Other combinations include talipes calcaneovalgus and talipes calcaneo-varus. CTEV is often present in both feet.

Causes and incidence of CTEV

No single cause has been identified, despite CTEV being recorded as long ago as the ancient Greeks; indeed bandaging was used successfully then and is still used as a treatment today. CTEV is often associated with many types of congenital abnormalities and syndromes, i.e. arthrogryposis. It is often inherited; indeed a genetic abnormality is the most likely cause.

In the general population the incidence is 1.2 per 1000 live births, rising to a rate of 2.9 per 1000 amongst the siblings of a child with CTEV (STEPS 1992b).

Diagnosis and prognosis

CTEV is usually identified at birth but with the increased use of prenatal ultrasound screening it is often diagnosed before the baby's birth. (The diagnosis of CTEV in utero may well lead to further screening for more serious congenital abnormalities because it is a component of many syndromes.) The severity of the condition can only be assessed once the child has been born.

Put in its simplest form, the prognosis for CTEV depends very much on the severity of the condition; mild forms are likely to respond well to treatment; more severe forms will probably require more complex treatment and may never result in a foot that looks normal. The aim of any treatment should be that the end result is a functioning foot that is not painful. A treated foot can be said to be at risk of relapsing, and relapse will

tend to occur in periods of rapid growth. Therefore a relapse may take place at any time through childhood, and treatment can go on for many years during the child's life, even into the teenage years.

One of the major difficulties for the parents of a child with CTEV is the problem of getting suitable footwear. This is because the child has a misshapen foot that may need specialist fitting, and where the CTEV occurs unilaterally the difference in shoe size can be as much as three or four sizes.

Treatment

As with many orthopaedic conditions, there are two approaches to treatment: conservative and surgical.

Conservative treatments. The aims of conservative treatments are to educate the malformed foot into an over-corrected position. These treatments are made up of the following:

Physiotherapy. Here the child's parents are taught by a physiotherapist to stretch the ligaments and tendons of the baby's foot. These exercises are then closely monitored by both the physiotherapist and the orthopaedic surgeon. (There are many different stretching regimes.) These exercises are usually carried out regularly by the parents, probably twice daily, and they may result in the child not needing surgery.

Strapping. Adhesive strapping is applied around the foot, up the sides of the leg, and then anchored to the knee so that the foot is in an over-corrected position. Sometimes malleable metal strips are used together with the strapping. The strapping is usually replaced weekly but some parents are shown how to replace it, thus reducing the number of hospital visits. Because the strapping is replaced regularly, meeting the baby's hygiene needs should not be a particular problem, but care must be taken to prevent the strapping becoming wet. The skin should be inspected for sore areas, which should be avoided if possible, or protected if necessary.

When strapping is used as a treatment, it is essential that the parents are instructed to observe for the signs of impaired circulation to the toes, i.e. swelling, discoloration and loss of temperature, and told to return to the hospital if they have any concerns.

Plaster cast fixation. With this method of treatment the baby's foot is manipulated into an over-corrected position by the surgeon or the physiotherapist and then a plaster cast is applied from toes to thigh. The knee must be incorporated in a flexed position to prevent the cast slipping off the leg. The plaster must be renewed regularly to accommodate the baby's rapid growth and to allow accurate monitoring of the position of the foot. Usually the casts are replaced every 4–6 weeks. These casts are applied without anaesthetic in the orthopaedic clinic when casting is used as a conservative 'stretching' treatment.

Parents should be instructed on how to care for their child in a plaster cast, whether it is used as a conservative treatment or after surgery. These instructions should include observing for impaired peripheral circulation (see p. 246–247), postoperative bleeding, infection (often first noted as a foul-smelling cast), and a slipping or damaged cast. If any of these occur, the family should return to the hospital as soon as possible. (The same care should be taken when applying a cast for the treatment of CTEV as for the management of a fracture, i.e. care when the cast is drying, see p. 246). The parents should be consoled with the knowledge that their baby will quickly adapt to having the foot/feet encased in plaster and that normal development should not be impaired in any way. It is important that the parents are instructed to keep the cast dry; a damp cast will be an ineffective cast. Bath times and general hygiene will therefore be difficult, but many strategies have been devised by ingenious parents to overcome these problems, ranging from waterproof coverings to the increased use of lotions rather than water to cleanse the skin.

Splinting. The use of ankle–foot orthoses made from moulded lightweight plastic is now rapidly replacing devices such as Denis Browne splints or Denis Browne boots; however, the function of both is to hold the foot in an over-corrected position.

Surgical treatments. These vary widely in their type and depend on the severity of the condition, but they range from simple soft tissue or tendon releases followed by a period in plaster or orthosis to actual open surgical procedures on the bones of the foot. One recent development in the treatment of CTEV, which is often used when other treatments have failed, is an external fixation device, usually a circular frame called the 'Ilizarov' frame. Such a frame allows the surgeon to slowly alter the position of the foot by stretching the soft tissues or distracting osteotomies (surgical breaks) in the bones of the foot. The new position of the foot is that held by the circular frame until the breaks in the bones have healed naturally.

Cerebral palsy

Cerebral palsy is not a disease; it is a descriptive term for a non-progressive weakness of motor

---

Box 15.3 Cerebral palsy: classification by limbs affected

Spastic hemiplegia
- There is asymmetrical use of the limbs, with one hand being affected.
- There is a lack of reciprocal kicking in lower limbs.
- Walking is not usually delayed because the unaffected side is almost normal.
- Contractures and deformities when they develop affect the wrist, fingers and ankles.
- Epilepsy is more common in this type of cerebral palsy.

Spastic diplegia
- Spastic diplegia mainly affects the lower limbs.
- Spasticity appears in the hips, ankles and muscles of the legs.
- Contracture and deformities affect the hips and ankles.

Spastic quadriplegia
- All four limbs are affected, although the lower limbs are usually more affected than the upper.
- Initially, there is generalised hypotonia followed by rigidity and spasticity by the age of 2–5 years.
- There may be mental retardation and developmental milestones may be delayed.
- Deformities affect the hips and knees more than the ankles.
- Dislocation of the hip may occur.
- Scoliosis may develop.

function occurring in the first few years of life. However, its effects may be progressive as the child develops. It is a congenital condition that affects the child's ability to mobilise. Children with cerebral palsy may also have sensory, emotional or psychological disturbances.

There are three principal types of cerebral palsy:

- spastic (hemiplegic, diplegic or quadriplegic; see Box 15.3)
- dyskinetic
- mixed.

Causes and incidence of cerebral palsy

The incidence of cerebral palsy is 2.5 per 1000 (McClaren & Bell 1990). 50% of these babies have a birth weight of less than 2.5 kg. The main cause has been described as fetal anoxia—lack of oxygen to the newborn baby. Premature infants are prone to diplegia, secondary to periventricular haemorrhage. Birth trauma and postnatal accidents are also regarded as major causes of hemiplegia (McClaren & Bell 1990).

The features of cerebral palsy include delay in motor development, such as in head control (acquired usually at 3 months), sitting without support (usually occurs at around 6 months) and of creeping (usually at around 9 months) combined with the persistence of primitive reflexes. Diagnosis is usually made by a paediatrician.

Hemiplegic spastic patients are usually able to walk independently; 80% of diplegic and quadriplegic patients should be able to walk short distances using aids. There are three musculoskeletal areas where problems may arise: the spine, the upper limb and the lower limb (see Table 15.1).

Treatment

The aim of treatment is to allow the individual to realise his or her full potential. The role of physiotherapy is crucial. Surgery should only be used:

- to correct a developing deformity or one that has not been controlled by physiotherapy
- to correct an established deformity due to contracture
- to correct deformities caused by muscle imbalance, by weakening stronger muscles.

Physiotherapy aims to maintain movement of the joints and prevent abnormal reflex movement. The child should be encouraged by the physiotherapist and medical staff to progress, where possible, through sitting, standing and walking (Sharrard 1984). The child's parents have an essential role in the treatment of cerebral palsy, as physiotherapy regimes are usually maintained by them, once they have been instructed. Splints and braces have limited value. They do not prevent the development of deformities, but they may well improve the child's gait.

Table 15.1 summarises the prognosis and treatment of deformities of the spine and upper and lower limbs in children with cerebral palsy.

ADVICE TO FAMILIES ON THEIR CHILD'S DISCHARGE

The child in a plaster cast

Parents should be given the following advice by nursing staff when their child is discharged:

- Observe for swelling, discoloration, numbness, pain and coldness in the child's fingers or toes. All of these things indicate disturbance of the peripheral circulation.
- The cast should be observed for cracks; if any occur the child needs to return to the hospital for the cast to be repaired and checked to ensure that it is holding the fracture correctly.
- The cast should not be allowed to become wet because this will cause it to be softened and not hold the fracture correctly.
- Children should be discouraged from pushing objects down their casts, especially to try to relieve itches, as these will cause sores under the casts, causing pain or even infection.

Table 15.1 Deformities of the spine and upper and lower limbs in children with cerebral palsy: prognosis and treatment (McClaren & Bell 1990)

	Deformity	Prognosis and treatment
In the spine		
Hemiplegia	Rarely, secondary scoliosis due to leg length inequality	Good
Diplegia	Scoliosis is rare, but may get postural kyphosis	Good, may need a support jacket
Quadriplegia	Scoliosis is common, long C curve, moulded baby syndrome; secondary to pelvic obliquity in presence of hip deformities	In severe cases, sitting and breathing is affected; control from a jacket, moulded seat or final resort to spinal surgery early before the deformity becomes fixed
In the upper limb		
Diplegia	Seldom involved	
Hemiplegia & quadriplegia	Classic flexed elbow, wrist and fingers Internal rotation at the shoulder Forearm pronation and thumb in palm High percentage of sensory impairment	Mildly affected patients have a good prognosis Very little function if severely affected, with poor sensation Conservative treatment with occupational therapy to maximise function Surgery to improve: function, cosmetic appearance, aid hygiene, provide psychological gain
The lower limb in cerebral palsy		
Hip	Adduction, flexion, medial rotation; hamstring tightness, short stride pattern limited straight leg raising in diplegics; weak extensors	Progression leads to dislocation—at risk if abduction > 30° Conservative treatment with intensive physiotherapy Surgery may involve: —adductor release —obturator nerve neurectomy —psoas elongation —psoas transfer —proximal hamstring release —femoral rotation osteotomy
Knee	Flexion deformity due to hamstrings or secondary to hip and ankle deformity	Correct hip and ankle first If overactive hamstrings— lengthen distally If weak quadriceps— transfer hamstrings to patella If weak quadriceps and hip extensor—transfer hamstrings to femur
Ankle and/or foot	Equinus with either varus or valgus ankle; varus/valgus ankle and hindfoot; midfoot break	Dynamic casts or orthoses, physiotherapy If fixed—percutaneous/open elongation of tendon Achilles (ETA) If mobile—orthosis If rigid—fusion

The family should be encouraged to return to the hospital if any of these problems occur or if they have any anxieties; their family GP may also be a useful source of support if problems occur.

Fractures, once reduced and held, must be monitored closely until unification takes place; therefore the child health care nurse must ensure that the family understand the importance of the child attending all outpatient visits.

Support groups

There is a list of the names and addresses of support groups on page 262; most of them supply information, support and advice on care for families of children with specific conditions. They often become valuable support networks for families, ensuring empathetic discussions for parents and children.

Information about mobility aids

Prior to discharge, the child health nurse should liaise with the appropriate physiotherapist and occupational therapist for the family's home district. These may be contacted through the normal health service channels or through the social services department. These professionals will help in provision of aids as well as advising on and administering any necessary adaptations to the child's home.

Mobility aids include the following:

- crutches
- wheelchairs
- pushchairs (especially wide ones when a spica cast is used)
- walking sticks
- cast braces
- monkey poles (to aid movement in bed)
- bath boards
- commodes
- urinals
- slipper bedpans
- ramps
- transfer boards
- stair lifts (if the immobility is permanent).

Box 15.4   Key benefits available to families (STEPS 1993)

- Disability Living Allowance (DLA)—the initial contact address for this is on page 262; Leaflet DS704 provides information.
- Invalid Care Allowance—this allowance is for anyone who spends at least 35 hours a week looking after someone who gets the higher or middle rate of DLA; Leaflet NI 212 provides information.
- Income Support—telephone advice is available on freephone 0800 666555.
- Exemption from Road Tax—to find out if you are eligible for exemption under the disabled passenger's scheme contact the Department of Social Security (DSS) at the address on page 262.
- 'Orange Badge' scheme—you may qualify if you have to transport your child by car because he or she is unable to walk. You may be able to claim a mobility component of the DLA. To apply contact your local social services department.
- Further benefit advice is available from:
  —Local Citizens' Advice Bureaux and other local advice agencies have detailed information about benefits and will give assistance with claims.
  —The Department of Social Security runs a freephone advice line (0800 666555) about benefits.
  —The Disability Income Group offers advice on benefits; they can be contacted on 0181 801 8013.
  —The Disability Alliance can be reached on 0171 247 8776. They also have an advice line (0171 247 8763) at various times of the day.
  —Local charities and other organisations may offer some help, they are best contacted through your health visitor or social worker.
  —The Joseph Rowntree Foundation Family Fund can help families living in the United Kingdom who are caring for a severely handicapped child at home. Information about the fund is available from the address on page 262.
  —Contact a Family is an organisation which supports families who care for children with special needs. They produce a fact sheet about child disability benefits and sources of help and can be contacted at the address on page 262.
  —The Family Welfare Association can help you find funds, though it cannot help with anything already provided by statutory authorities. It administers a variety of trust funds, but applications must be made by social workers on your behalf. They can be contacted at the address on page 262.

In circumstances where the child's immobility may be permanent or long term, the family should be advised that they may qualify for Disability Living Allowance and/or Attendance Allowance (see Box 15.4).

Activity 15.3

John, aged 8 years, has cerebral palsy (spastic quadriplegia). He goes to a special school on a daily basis, but his parents are finding it increasingly difficult to cope with him. Find out what benefits he and his parents may be entitled to and what resources there are to help the family.

Liaison with the child's school is also to be advised. If the immobility is to be long term or permanent then the family should consider their child being statemented by their local education authority as having 'special educational needs'. This can be a lengthy process but, once enacted, it should ensure that the appropriate support and facilities are provided for the child to be educated in mainstream schools.

CONCLUSION

Child health nurses have a varied role to play when caring for children with problems of mobility. Not only will they be ensuring that such children get the appropriate nursing care that their problems dictate, but they will also be involved in providing for other needs. These other needs include help in performing the activities of daily living which will be restricted by the child's immobility. The child may have a problem of immobility for weeks, if not months, and during these periods will need play and stimulation to ensure that development can continue as near normally as is possible and that boredom is minimised. The nurse may also be involved in assisting parents to get the help they need to continue caring for the child at home, even if in traction, a plaster spica cast or splints.

Immobility can be caused by a vast variety of orthopaedic conditions, whether acquired or congenital, and there are many sources of information that the child health nurse can use when caring for, or preparing to care for, such a child. The sources include an enormous number of articles and research papers written by orthopaedic surgeons and nurses, which should be available in most medical libraries.

REFERENCES

Bolig R 1984 Play in hospital settings. In: Yawkey T D, Pellegrini A D (eds) Childs play: developmental and applied. Lawrence Erlbaum, Hillsdale NJ

Chandler J 1991 Tabbner's nursing care: theory and practice, 2nd edn. Churchill Livingstone, Edinburgh

Child Accident Prevention Trust 1992 Fact sheet. Child Accident Prevention Trust, London

Duckworth T 1984 Lecture notes on orthopaedics and fractures. Blackwell Scientific Publications, Oxford

McClaren M I, Bell M J 1990 Neuromuscular diseases in childhood. Surgery 86: 2054–2059

Miller M, Miller J H 1985 Orthopaedics and accidents illustrated. Hodder & Stoughton, London

Ogden J A 1984 The uniqueness of growing bones. In: Rockwood C A Jr, Wilkins K E, King R E (eds) Fractures in children, 3rd edn. J B Lippincott, Philadelphia

Pritchard A P, David J A 1990 The Royal Marsden Hospital manual of clinical nursing procedures, 2nd edn. Harper & Row, London

Sacharin R M 1986 Principles of paediatric nursing, 2nd edn. Churchill Livingstone, Edinburgh

Sharrard W J 1984 Cerebral palsy. Surgery 1(12): 287–290

STEPS 1992a Congenital dislocation of the hips, a booklet for parents. National Association for Children with Congenital Abnormalities of the Lower Limbs, UK

STEPS 1992b Talipes, a booklet for parents. National Association for Children with Congenital Abnormalities of the Lower Limbs, UK

STEPS 1993 Newsletter. National Association for Children with Congenital Abnormalities of the Lower Limbs, UK, Issue 25 (Summer)

Visintainer M A, Wolfer J A 1975 Psychological preparation for surgical patients: the effects on children's and parents' stress responses and adjustment. Pediatrics 56: 187–202

FURTHER READING

Apley G A, Solomon L 1993 Apley's system of orthopaedics and fractures, 7th edn. Butterworth-Heinemann, Oxford

Duckworth T 1984 Lecture notes on orthopaedics and fractures. Blackwell Scientific Publications, Oxford

Roaf R, Hodkinson L J 1980 Textbook of orthopaedic nursing, 3rd edn. Blackwell Scientific Publications, Oxford

USEFUL ADDRESSES

Support groups

ASBAH (Association For Spina Bifida and Hydrocephalus)
42 Park Road
Peterborough
Cambridgeshire PE1 2UQ

Cerebral Palsy Support Group
The Spastics Society
12 Park Crescent
London W1 4EO

Child Growth Foundation
2 Mayfield Avenue
Chiswick
London W4 1PW

Children's Chronic Arthritis Association
c/o Caroline Cox
47 Battenhall Avenue
Worcester WR5 2HN

Contact a Family
170 Tottenham Court Road
London W1P 0HA

Hemiplegia Support Group
c/o Hilary Latham
Hemi-Help
166 Boundaries Road
London SW12 8HG

Osteogenesis Imperfecta Support Group
Brittle Bone Society
112 City Road
Dundee DD2 2PW

Perthes Support Group
Perthes Association
42 Woodlands Road
Guildford
Surrey GU1 1RW

Polio Support Group
British Polio Fellowship
Bell Close
West End Road
Ruislip
Middlesex HA4 6LP

REACH (The Association For Children With Hand
    or Arm Deficiency)
c/o Sue Stokes
12 Wilson Way
Earles Barton
Northamptonshire NN6 0NZ

Restricted Growth Association
103 St Thomas Avenue
West Town, Hayling Island
Hampshire PO11 0EU

Scoliosis Support Group
Scoliosis Association (UK)
2 Ivebury Court
323-327 Latimer Road
London W10 6RA

STEPS (The National Association for Families of
    Children with Lower Limb Deformities)
15 Statham Close
Lymm
Cheshire WA13 9NN

Young Arthritis Care
c/o Kate Nash
18 Stephenson Way
London NW1 2HD

Information on benefits and allowances

Disability Living Allowance (DLA)
Leaflets Unit
PO Box 21
Stanmore
Middlesex HA7 1AY
Telephone advice and help available on
    freephone 0800 666 555

Exemption from Road Tax
Department of Social Security (DSS)
6a Government Buildings
Warbeck Hill Road
Blackpool FY2 0UZ

Family Welfare Association
The Grants Officer
505 Kingsland Road
Dalston
London E8 4AU

Invalid Care Allowance
Leaflets Unit
PO Box 21
Stanmore
Middlesex HA 7 1AY
Telephone advice and help available on 01253 856123

Joseph Rowntree Foundation Family Fund
PO Box 50
York YO1 2ZX

16

The endocrine system

Jean Bayne

From this chapter the student should gain an insight into the normal functioning of the endocrine system. Associated problems most likely to be encountered within the general paediatric setting in the hospital and/or community will also be discussed.

The chapter aims to:
- outline briefly the structure and function of the endocrine system and provide further sources of information
- look at potential problems within the system in relation to the health of the growing child
- discuss physical and psychological problems encountered by the child and family in relation to problems with insulin and growth hormone production.

INTRODUCTION TO THE ENDOCRINE SYSTEM

The endocrine system consists of a series of glands which secrete hormones (Box 16.1) directly into the bloodstream. The function of this system is the maintenance of a constant internal environment, so providing a state of homeostasis in which all cells exist. Endocrine glands are ductless, in contrast to exocrine glands, e.g. salivary and sweat glands, whose secretions pass along a duct.

Control of the endocrine system and release of hormones

The hypothalamus, in the centre of the brain, acts as a link between the endocrine and nervous systems, monitoring and regulating the metabolic state of the body and the autonomic system. It can be considered to be the controller of the endocrine system as it secretes a specific releasing factor to the pituitary, the 'master gland', which then releases the appropriate hormone.

The other means of control over the release of hormones is a negative feedback system. For example the control of blood sugar is achieved by different hormones:

- when blood sugar rises, insulin is produced
- when blood sugar falls, the release of glucagon is stimulated.

The two hormones ensure that normal levels of blood sugar are maintained.

Development of endocrine glands

In order for a child to develop normally, both physically and mentally, and to reach sexual maturity and adulthood, a fully functioning endocrine system is required. The system develops in utero from different areas of the embryo. For example, the anterior pituitary gland develops from a pouch that grows upwards from the mouth. The thyroid and parathyroid glands develop from the membrane which lines the first part of the alimentary canal;

again, pouches grow down towards the area that will eventually become the neck of the fetus. The sex organs develop from the mesoderm of the embryo, close to the cells that give rise to the adrenal cortex. Growth and development of the sex organs is linked to the development of the bladder, urethra and rectum (Lewis 1986). For a summary of hormones produced and their actions, see Table 16.1.

Production of hormones

The production of hormones can be affected by several factors, both internal and external (see Box 16.2). Some of these factors can be controlled, so ensuring that a constant internal environment is maintained. However, excess or deficiency of a hormone can lead to abnormal development and sometimes life-threatening conditions for the child. Hormone production throughout childhood varies according to age and sex and consequent growth and development of the child. Girls grow faster than boys (Tanner 1989) and usually commence puberty earlier.

Links between the development of the endocrine glands, the hormones produced and their action, combined with some of the factors that can affect production, have potential consequences on the health of the developing baby

Table 16.1 Summary of hormones produced and their actions

Gland and hormone produced	Action of hormone
Anterior lobe of pituitary gland	
Human growth hormone	Stimulates growth of bone and muscle
Thyroid stimulating hormone	Controls and stimulates the thyroid gland
Adrenocorticotrophin	Controls cortex of adrenal gland
Gonadotrophin	
Follicle stimulating hormone	Control production of spermatozoa in the testes,
Luteinising hormone	and oestrogen and progesterone in the ovaries
Prolactin	Stimulates lactation and suppresses ovulation
Posterior lobe of pituitary gland	
Antidiuretic hormone	Regulates water absorption from kidney tubules
Oxytocin	Contracts uterus, stimulates onset of labour
Thyroid gland	
Thyroxine (T_4)	Act on all body cells, increase rate food is used up
Tri-iodothyronine (T_3)	and are necessary for growth
Calcitonin	Lowers blood calcium levels
Parathyroid glands	
Parathormone	Regulates level of calcium
Adrenal cortex	
Aldosterone	Facilitates reabsorption of sodium by kidney tubules
Hydrocortisone	Anti-allergenic, anti-inflammatory
Androgens and oestrogen	Necessary for sexual development
Adrenal medulla	
Adrenaline	Prepare the body for action 'fight or flight'
Noradrenaline	
Pancreas	
Insulin	Lowers blood sugar by increasing storage and use by tissues
Glucagon	Increases glucose production
Testes	
Testosterone	Production of sperm, development of male sex characteristics
Ovaries	
Oestrogen and progesterone	Maturation of ovarian follicle, development of female sex characteristics

and child. Further information covering specific conditions can be gathered from suggestions for reading at the end of the chapter. Here, we will go on to investigate and discuss the two conditions most likely to be encountered by the paediatric nurse in the hospital setting or in the community:

- problems with insulin production resulting in diabetes mellitus

- problems with the production of growth hormone.

These are both relevant to the developing child and can have effects throughout his or her life.

For both problems, the chapter will not only look at the effects on the child, but will focus also on the family as a whole and how they all need to cope with potential problems in order to maintain a normal lifestyle.

DIABETES MELLITUS

Facts

1. Diabetes mellitus is the commonest endocrine disorder seen in children. Figures for the United Kingdom for 1988 show a prevalence of more than 20 000 children affected (British Diabetic Association 1988). This is an increase in the under-15 age group to 13.5 per 100 000 per year, nearly double the number for the previous decade (Metcalf & Baum 1991).
2. Both sexes are equally affected in childhood, but in the older age group more women are affected (Day 1986a).
3. Some ethnic groups have a greater tendency to develop diabetes mellitus—Asians and Australian Aborigines have a prevalence of 20 : 100 (all age groups) (Wise 1986).

Types of diabetes mellitus

There are two different types:

- insulin-dependent diabetes mellitus
- non-insulin-dependent diabetes mellitus.

The World Health Organization recognised in 1990 that diabetes in children is different from that in adults. Insulin-dependent diabetes mellitus occurs in younger people (usually less than 40 years) and for this reason we shall concentrate on this topic.

 For further information on non-insulin-dependent diabetes, see Day (1986b).

Causes of insulin-dependent diabetes mellitus

No specific cause has yet been identified. However, it is known that in affected children there is an absence or near absence of insulin. Damage to the insulin-producing cells may occur as a result of a viral illness or infection, or an abnormal reaction by the body against these cells. There is also a tendency for diabetes mellitus to run in families; the actual disease is not inherited, but rather, it seems, the increased chance of developing it.

Normally, insulin is produced in the pancreas (see Table 16.1) when the blood sugar rises, i.e. 30 minutes after the intake of carbohydrate. It lowers the blood sugar by increasing glucose storage and by using it up in the body's tissues. By 2 hours after a meal normal blood sugar levels are restored.

Symptoms and diagnosis

The condition can develop over a period of days or weeks before it is recognised, and at any age. However, often, the younger the child the more rapid the onset and resulting problems. The difficulties in recognising the symptoms in young children or toddlers mean that it may not be until they become ill or lethargic that medical advice is sought (see Box 16.3).

Diagnosis may be made in the family doctor's surgery, an accident and emergency department

---

Box 16.3   Symptoms of diabetes mellitus

After a meal
- Blood sugar increases
- Little or no insulin is produced—therefore blood sugar remains higher than normal
- Blood sugar continues to rise and spills over into the urine
- The child:
  —feels thirsty
  —is tired
  —has glucose in the urine—glycosuria

Over a period of time
- Weight loss
- Frequency of urination
- Nausea—may vomit
- Stomach ache
- Headaches
- Lack of energy and tiredness

If not detected
- Shortness of breath
- Breath smells of pear drops (due to ketosis)
- Dehydration
- Ketones in urine
- Unconsciousness due to ketoacidosis

or the paediatric ward. Depending on the age of the child, how ill he is, his home environment and family background, and the resources available for community care (e.g. paediatric diabetic specialist nurse), he may have been admitted to hospital for stabilisation or cared for totally in the community.

The diagnosis is often a great shock to the family and the child. A great deal of psychological support, supervision and continued education is needed to help the family come to terms with the condition and to care for their child until he is old enough and competent enough to care for himself.

Psychological problems

According to Stillitoe (1988), the incidence of emotional and behavioural problems is higher in children with diabetes mellitus than in other healthy children. This highlights the need for on-going care and supervision for the whole family.

In dealing with the initial diagnosis, it is important to consider the family's religious beliefs and ethnic background, as they will play a role in how the family cope with the disease and the problems they encounter in day-to-day life. It is obviously also important to have clear communication among all those involved in the care of the child and, when necessary, an interpreter must be involved. This will ensure that the family fully understand all explanations and have a chance to discuss specific problems and worries. The importance of good communication between the family and all health professionals involved cannot be overemphasised.

Controlling diabetes mellitus

For children to continue a normal family lifestyle, their diabetes needs to be controlled and homeostasis maintained. The aim of control is to keep a near normal blood sugar and prevent potential complication. This is achieved by:

- administering insulin
- regulation of diet

- regular checks on blood sugar levels.

Control should become part of everyday life and fit into the child's daily routine. As yet there is no cure for diabetes and treatment has to continue throughout life, every day. In view of this, continued care of the child and family is best met by a multidisciplinary team specialising in both paediatrics and diabetes (British Diabetic Association 1991).

Administering insulin

Insulin needs to be given to replace that which the child's body is no longer producing. Insulins are now made synthetically and the doctor will prescribe the type, dosage and frequency of injections best suited to each child. Insulins are available as fast-, intermediate- and slow-acting or as a mix. Insulins and insulin syringes are available on prescription. Insulin has to be given by subcutaneous injection as it is a protein-like substance and would be destroyed if given orally.

The nurse has a major role in ensuring that the child and family learn to draw up the required insulin safely and competently and can then inject it safely. For many parents this is a major skill to accomplish (see Box 16.4).

Rotation of injection sites is important—unsightly lumps will appear if the same site is always used and the insulin will not be absorbed properly. Children should be discouraged from developing a favourite injection site whenever

Box 16.4	Dos and don'ts of insulin injections

- Do ensure that the family know how to store insulin and how to get further supplies.
- Do ensure that there is always spare insulin.
- Do ensure that the child (if able) and at least one adult can safely draw up and give insulin.
- Do not inject in the same site every day; rotate sites—outer arms, buttocks, thighs and stomach.
- Do not ever miss an insulin injection.
- Do always inject before a meal.
- Do ensure safe disposal of needles and syringes at home.

possible. Various pens and devices for administering insulin are now available in place of syringes, and many parents and children find them easier to use, especially those who have a fear of needles.

Regulation of diet

This is the second factor in controlling a child's diabetes. However, it must be emphasised that all aspects of control should become part of normal everyday life and the child and family's eating habits should not be totally disrupted and changed.

Continued education with the involvement of the local dietitian is helpful and important. Dietary restrictions due to the family's religious background, way of life, beliefs and ethnic origins must be recognised and taken into account.

The main emphasis when planning a child's diet is to ensure that it is a balanced mixture of fat, protein and carbohydrate (Day 1986a) and that the child is satisfied and not hungry. A dietary assessment is made and the amount of carbohydrate needed can be calculated, although in many areas advice is based on what the child normally eats and on healthy eating guidelines. The aim is to have *roughly* the same amount of carbohydrate-containing foods each day, over three main meals and three snacks. Snacks between the main meals are important to maintain the blood sugar level, as insulin will still be in the bloodstream. Diabetic foods are expensive and unnecessary.

Problems can arise regarding dietary intake depending on age, likes and dislikes, availability of cooking facilities, family income and where the child spends most of his day. The child's normal routine should be maintained and often snacks can be taken in school break times. Again, good communication among all those involved in the care of the child is essential, as is the education of non-health care professionals with whom the child will spend much of the day. Visits to schools are especially important here.

Depending on local care procedures, regular weight and height checks are made to ensure

Activity 6.1

Food is divided into portions of 10 g of carbohydrates called exchanges/portions/rations/lines. Record all the food you eat in one day, including the amount. Using food value books/diabetic cookbooks and tables, calculate roughly how much carbohydrate you have had.

Increase your own knowledge of carbohydrate values by studying the labels detailing carbohydrate content of packets/tins etc. in the supermarket.

that a normal growth pattern is maintained. Dietary intake and insulin dosage will be altered according to growth and weight gain to ensure that stable blood sugar levels are maintained.

Maintaining regular checks

Blood sugar levels need to be checked regularly to assess the success of treatment. Frequency of tests will be determined by the age of the child, length of time since diagnosis, compliance and past history. The results give an indication of whether enough insulin is being given to balance dietary intake, and whether insulin is being given correctly. Many varieties of blood sugar monitors and finger prick devices are available for use to obtain accurate measurements of blood sugar level. The strips for machines are available on prescription. The child and family should be able to recognise a low or high blood sugar reading and gradually learn to interpret blood sugar level results. Ideally, they should aim for readings between 5 and 10 mmol/l.

If blood sugar levels are high, the urine should be tested for ketones. These are produced when fat is broken down for energy, and spill over into the urine (see 'Complications', p. 269). Again, the test strips are available on prescription. All test results are recorded in a diary which will give an indication of how well the diabetes is being controlled.

Compliance with maintaining regular checks varies from person to person. For parents of young toddlers, it often seems that they are always inflicting pain on their child due to injections and blood tests. For teenagers, blood tests may be another task they have to carry out that makes them different from all their friends. This is an area where all children and families need support and understanding. The nurse should also emphasise the importance of regular checks to avoid problems in the future.

Complications of diabetes mellitus

The aim of caring for children with diabetes mellitus is to keep their blood sugar within normal limits and to prevent hyper- and hypoglycaemia. However, this is never possible all of the time, especially with young children with erratic eating habits and for children in general who, at some time, are going to want to eat at the same time as their friends. Control is especially difficult during the adolescent years.

Hyperglycaemia and ketoacidosis

Hyperglycaemia occurs if insulin is not taken correctly and regularly, or if not enough is given to balance the intake of carbohydrate. Blood sugar also rises naturally when a child is ill. Due to the extra sugar in the blood, glycosuria can also occur. The kidneys usually filter sugar from the blood and then return it, so that none is lost in the urine. However, once blood sugar reaches a certain level, the renal threshold is exceeded, the return mechanism fails, and sugar spills over into the urine. This causes the child to pass large amounts of urine and also become very thirsty. If blood sugar continues to rise, the liver begins to break down fat for energy, resulting in the production of ketones. These are detected in the urine and can be smelt on the breath—the smell is similar to pear drops.

Ketosis (high levels of ketones in body fluids) indicates a virtual absence of insulin and, if left untreated, the child will go on to develop ketoacidosis or a diabetic coma. Hospital treatment is needed to correct dehydration, electrolyte imbalance and to stabilise blood sugar. Hyperglycaemia alone over a prolonged period will result in tiredness, weight loss and lack of

Case study 16.1 Katherine

Katherine, aged 11 years, was diagnosed as having diabetes mellitus at the end of the summer term. This was a great shock to Katherine and her mother, who was a single parent with Katherine's younger brother to care for as well.

Katherine left hospital after 3 days, on twice-daily injections of insulin using a pen device. She was able to give her own injections. Her mother gave some, but found it a traumatic experience. The family coped well during the summer holidays with continued support and education from the community paediatric nurses and medical follow-up at the diabetic clinic.

Katherine started secondary school in the September. Shortly after the beginning of term, she was admitted to the paediatric ward with dehydration and ketoacidosis. She was extremely drowsy and required intravenous fluids and an insulin infusion to gradually correct her blood sugar.

Following discussion when she was better, it appeared that Katherine was fed up with her injections and found it a rush to get ready for school in the morning. She had school lunch with her friends and wanted to eat the same as they did. She admitted to forgetting her insulin injection sometimes. Her mother therefore agreed to give the morning insulin and to supervise blood tests. The school nurse talked to Katherine and her friends about diabetes and diet and explained that a healthy diet was better for everyone. The community nurse devised a revision teaching programme following discussion with Katherine and her mother to go over points they were unsure about. As a result of better communication among all involved, Katherine has been able to stabilise her blood sugar and reduce the possibility of complications.

energy. The child will also be more prone to infections due to the continued presence of sugar in the blood (see Case Study 16.1).

Visual disturbances

Blurred vision can occur as a result of hyperglycaemia, as the high level of sugar in the blood can cause changes to the shape of the eye. Approximately 30% of people with diabetes will experience some kind of visual problem (Hames 1993). It is therefore important for all children with diabetes to have their sight tested and the back of the eye examined, preferably annually. Damage to the retina can occur over several years and, although rare in children, early detection can prevent further complications later.

Damage to feet

Due to long-term diabetes, nerve damage (neuropathy) can lead to decreased sensation in the feet. Ulceration and infection can develop. Foot ulceration is the commonest cause of hospital admission for adults with diabetes (Connor et al 1987).

Therefore, good foot care for children should begin at an early age—feet should be thoroughly dried, toe nails cut straight across and feet measured properly before buying new shoes. Shoes should not rub or be uncomfortable. This is an area for potential conflict between parents and teenagers who want fashionable shoes like those of their friends. Problems such as verrucae or corns should be dealt with by a chiropodist.

Hypoglycaemia

Hypoglycaemia occurs when there is an imbalance between insulin and carbohydrate intake, the latter being too low. Possible reasons are:

* not eating enough at mealtimes
* missing a snack
* unexpected exercise
* giving too much insulin.

It is important for all those involved in the care of the child to be able to recognise the symptoms (see Box 16.5) and take appropriate action. Action must be taken straight away, otherwise

---

Box 16.5 **Signs of hypoglycaemia in children**

* Trembling
* Sweating
* Pallor
* Confusion/aggression/lack of cooperation
* Headaches
* Faintness
* Blurred vision

---

the level of blood sugar will continue to fall, which can lead to unconsciousness and even convulsions in small children. In order to raise the blood sugar, fast-acting carbohydrates should be given immediately (e.g. three dextrose tablets, Lucozade), followed by a small snack of longer-acting carbohydrates (e.g. apple, biscuit, milk). School children should be encouraged to carry their own dextrose tablets and extra biscuits so that they always have something to take.

It is also important for children to have some means of identification, e.g. diabetic card, bracelet or necklace stating that they are diabetic, with details of what to do and who to contact if problems arise. Hypoglycaemia in the very young can happen very rapidly with little warning. If any child does become unconscious no-one should make him try to eat or drink as he will choke.

Glucagon injection is available on prescription and can be administered at home by the parents to increase blood sugar levels. The nurse has a role to play to ensure that the parents know when to give it, how to draw it up and how much to give.

The future

For many families and children affected by diabetes mellitus, isolation from others who are similarly affected and the prospect of lifelong injections plus possible complications are a great strain on their lives. Teenagers in particular worry about future job prospects, forming relationships and having families of their own. For these very reasons, groups such as the British Diabetic Association play an important role in organising local meetings, days out for families and holidays for the children. They also keep families up to date with the latest developments.

Results from the Diabetic Control and Complications Trial carried out in the USA (Barnett 1993) show that maintaining blood sugar levels as near normal as possible over a prolonged period does result in the development of fewer future complications.

Investigation and research into new ways of giving insulin, multidose injections and, it is hoped, a cure continue. Therefore, children and families can be encouraged to hope for fewer complications in later life, due to better care and control commenced at an early age and maintained throughout life.

GROWTH

Babies grow into toddlers, then children and teenagers and eventually fully grown adults—a fact we all take for granted. But what actually makes us grow and what are some of the factors that can cause growth to go wrong?

Facts concerning normal growth

1. The maximum rate of growth actually occurs before birth at about the fourth month of fetal life (Sacharin 1986).
2. Birth weight is doubled by 5 months and tripled by 1 year. By the age of 2 years, children have normally reached half their adult height.
3. From 4 years to puberty, average growth rate for boys and girls is 5–6 cm per year (Tanner et al 1966).
4. Girls grow faster than boys, enter puberty earlier and cease to grow earlier (Tanner 1989). The pubertal growth spurt occurs at around 11 years in girls, 14 years in boys.
5. Growth hormone is required for normal growth from birth throughout childhood.
6. 50–75% of growth hormone is produced at night in deep sleep. The rate of secretion can be affected by exercise and anxiety (Woolston 1991).
7. Taller children secrete more growth hormone than shorter children.

Growth is an indication of a child's well-being and general health (Hindmarsh & Brook 1986). For this reason regular weight and height checks are essential for all babies and children. Weight alone is not a good guide as it is dependent on

Activity 16.2

Ensure that all children have their height measured when you admit them as inpatients.
Find out how to measure young babies accurately when you are in baby clinics.
Learn how to plot height measurements on a growth chart.

nutritional and other factors (Hughes 1989). It is also important to be able to differentiate between weight increase due to healthy formation of bone and muscle and increase due to excess laying down of fat.

Recent trends

During this century there has been a tendency for children to become taller and mature earlier, possibly due to better health care and nutrition, and the eradication of certain diseases. As a result, children reach their final height at a younger age (Hughes 1989). New growth charts for boys and girls for the normal population of the United Kingdom are therefore being prepared to reflect this trend. It is important to take into account a child's ethnic background when comparing heights.

Use of growth charts

Regular height measurements are carried out in GP surgeries, clinics and at school health checks. All children have their height plotted on growth charts (see Apps 1–4). Those that lie outside the 3rd or 97th percentile should be considered for referral for further investigation, having taken the heights of both parents into consideration. Therefore, the importance of accurate height measurements and correct plotting on growth charts cannot be overemphasised.

The endocrine system and growth

As we are concerned with the endocrine system in this chapter, we shall concentrate on problems

---

Box 16.6   Causes of growth problems

- Endocrine disorders
- Chronic systemic disorders
- Problems with absorption of food/nutritional status
- Chromosomal and congenital abnormalities
- Cardiac and renal disorders
- Cartilage and bone disorders
- Psychological disorders
- Irradiation treatment for cancer

---

associated specifically with that system. However, it is worth noting some of the other factors/causes of growth problems (see Box 16.6).

Growth hormone may be over- or under-produced for a variety of reasons; possibly resulting in delayed growth and short stature or in increased growth, the child reaching full adult height sooner than is normal.

Effects of hormones on growth

Hormones work together to ensure that homeostasis is maintained and normal growth and development can occur (see Table 16.1). In normal children, structural growth is under the influence of each child's dietary intake and nutritional stores, together with the body's circulating hormones and their effect on the skeletal system.

The main hormones involved in growth are growth hormone itself and the thyroid hormone, T_4. Growth depends on:

- build-up of protein in the body
- metabolism of carbohydrate
- build-up of energy stores for growth.

These factors are affected by hormones produced by the thyroid gland, insulin, glucocorticoids and androgens, as well as growth hormone.

Release of growth hormone is mainly under the control of two other hormones:

- growth hormone release inhibiting hormone (somatostatin)
- growth hormone releasing hormone (GHRH).

Growth hormone stimulates growth of bone and muscle throughout childhood and adolescence. The growth spurt of puberty and skeletal maturation also depend on growth hormone, T_4 and gonadal steroids.

At the age of 18–24 years the epiphyses of the long bones fuse and it is then impossible for the individual to grow any taller. Problems affecting growth in childhood need to be treated before fusion occurs. If left untreated the individual is affected for life.

Growth hormone deficiency

The causes of growth hormone deficiency may be:

- congenital
- acquired (i.e. following radiotherapy treatment)
- idiopathic (affects 1 : 5000 children in the United Kingdom; Cordell 1993).

Intrauterine growth is not affected, but the rate of growth from birth onwards is slower than normal. Recognition of the problem occurs over a period of time and is the result of accurate measurement of the growing child. Assessment of bone age and failure to produce growth hormone in response to stimulation tests confirm the diagnosis.

Often one of the parents or another member of the close family will have had delayed growth; therefore it is important to have good clear communication with the family throughout assessment and treatment. Boys are more often affected than girls, but as yet no reason has been found (Cordell 1993).

Box 16.7   Features of growth hormone deficiency

- Normal intelligence
- Normal body proportions
- Shorter than peers and classmates
- May have rounder faces and appear facially younger as a result
- May be plumper than classmates

Problems experienced due to growth hormone deficiency

As can be seen from Box 16.7, children with growth hormone deficiency differ from their friends primarily in relation to their height. They may be slightly fatter as growth hormone helps to control fat. However, the physical features can have psychological effects on affected children, due to the way in which adults and peers treat them. Parents can be overprotective and the child can have difficulty in being independent.

Teenagers, especially, can feel different from their friends and left out because they have difficulty in finding fashionable clothes to fit them and being 'one of the crowd'. Teasing and bullying can also be a problem. People who do not know them will treat them as the age that they appear to be (Lindley 1980), which can be very frustrating for the children concerned.

The paediatric nurse involved with the family has a role to play in educating others involved in the child's life and increasing awareness of how the child may feel. Again, good communication among all involved, including health professionals in the hospital and in the community, and other professionals the child comes into contact with, is of great importance.

Treatment

In similarity with the treatment for diabetes mellitus, the treatment for growth hormone deficiency involves replacing the missing hormone. Since October 1985, biosynthetic growth hormone has been available and providing treatment is started at an early age—around 6 years—results are generally good. The dose of growth hormone is calculated according to the child's weight and size and is increased as growth occurs. Depending on local policy, the child will be measured every 3–6 months to assess treatment.

Growth hormone injections. Growth hormone is given daily by subcutaneous injection. The nurse needs to engender confidence in the child and/or family in their own ability to give the injection safely at home. For children with a fear of needles, devices are available which cover the needle so that it cannot be seen when giving the injection.

The nurse can devise a teaching programme in conjunction with the child and family clearly setting out their aims and objectives so they are clear about what they need to achieve and understand. Teaching may take place at the specialist referral centre or in the child's own home.

Presentation of growth hormone. Growth hormone comes in dry powder form with diluent, and has to be mixed shortly before use. As well as ampoules and syringes, many pen devices with cartridges which are easily refillable are now available and are found to be easier to use by many families and children. This especially applies to children with small hands who find the pen device easier to handle, and so they are able to look after themselves and boost their independence. As with other injections required on a daily basis, it is advisable to vary the injection site.

Although growth hormone injections are not required to maintain life, their effect on the child's future size and life must be remembered. Continued contact and support of the family is important to maintain their confidence. Putting them in contact with another family experiencing similar problems is also very helpful.

Everyday life

The importance of the child carrying on a normal everyday life cannot be overstressed. Parents, community nurses and school nurses have a role to play in ensuring that the child does not have problems in school. Starting at secondary school can be an anxious time for parents. Worries should be discussed with the teacher regarding teasing and bullying and also any practical problems, e.g. high benches and stools in science labs, difficulty in doing PE due to the size of equipment. If necessary, other professionals such as the educational psychologist can be involved.

As far as possible, a normal balanced diet should be taken. Research has shown that the greater the deficiency of growth hormone, the greater the likelihood of the child being obese. 30% of children who are deficient in growth hormone are overweight (Cordell 1993).

Puberty

As well as deficiency of growth hormone, many children are also deficient in gonadotrophins which initiate puberty. This is yet another area in which a child/teenager's self-confidence may be threatened, and tact and understanding are needed. If there are no signs of natural puberty, it is normally induced around the age of 14 years (Cordell 1993).

The future

At present, children receiving growth hormone cease treatment on reaching adulthood. Research is taking place into osteoporosis, bone density and muscle mass. At present the only side effects found that result from growth hormone injections are localised skin rashes.

The final height reached by a child is still dependent on when treatment is commenced and the height of the child's parents.

The thyroid gland and associated growth problems

Facts

1. The thyroid gland is situated in the neck, adjacent to the upper part of the trachea, and consists of two lobes joined by the isthmus.
2. It produces T_3 and T_4—hormones that are concerned with normal growth and speed up cell activity.
3. Iodine is essential for the manufacture of these hormones. Iodine is found in food, especially fish, also in the soil in which food crops grow and in water vaporised from the sea to form rain. (Some land-locked countries have a shortage of iodine, and public health measures have to be taken to supplement the diet.)
4. About 2 in every 100 people have an underactive thyroid gland (Hillson 1991), also known as hypothyroidism and myxoedema.
5. Another 2 in every 100 people have an overactive thyroid gland (Hillson 1991), also known as hyperthyroidism or thyrotoxicosis.
6. Goitre is swelling of the thyroid gland and can be due to deficiency of iodine or excess production of thyroid hormones.

Thyroid underactivity in babies and children

Hypothyroidism affecting children can start in utero or shortly after birth.

Congenital hypothyroidism. 1 in 4000 newborn babies are affected (Hillson 1991). Fortunately, routine screening of babies has virtually eradicated the disease, as treatment can be commenced as soon as possible. This is essential because when the disease does start in utero the brain can be affected.

Treatment. Oral thyroxine is given and has to be continued for life. Parents therefore need continued support from diagnosis onwards. In the past, babies who were not treated went on to develop coarse features, large tongues and difficulties in feeding. Mental agility was dependent on the function of the thyroid gland during development of the nervous system and the adequacy of treatment (Sacharin 1986).

Hypothyroidism in childhood. This type of thyroid problem is more likely to have an effect on the growth of a child. In young babies failure to thrive is noted. In older children features commence insidiously and are often due to imperfect development of the gland. The child may stop growing and sexual development and puberty are delayed together with maturation of bone (Bayliss & Tonbridge 1991).

Treatment. Again, oral thyroxine is administered. The catch-up on growth is noticeable but not always complete.

Other endocrine-related growth problems

Other problems that are related to endocrine system dysfunction include premature sexual maturation and precocious puberty, caused by rare diseases of the adrenal glands. The child grows faster and develops puberty at an earlier age than normal.

Cushing's syndrome occurs when over-secretion of adrenal hormones results in obesity and short stature due to arrest of growth. Excess production of androgens results in early pubic hair, acne and excess male hair growth.

These and other causes of abnormal growth and development are complex conditions which require much support and understanding from the child's family. Information can be obtained from the Child Growth Foundation (see Useful Addresses at end of chapter), who also detail support groups for parents and children affected by the various conditions.

CONCLUSION

Conditions and illnesses affecting the endocrine system present problems because of the complex and varied functions of the hormones produced and can affect many parts of the body. However, as a result of advances in medicine and pharmacy many are now treatable, and hormones that the body does not produce naturally can be replaced with synthetic forms.

The day-to-day difficulties faced by the child and family require both physical and psychological care and support from paediatric nurses and other health care professionals in order to achieve compliance with treatment and, above all, maintenance of normal family life.

REFERENCES

Barnett A 1993 Editorial. Diabetes Review 2(4): 1
Bayliss R, Tonbridge W 1991 Thyroid disease—the facts, 2nd edn. Oxford University Press, Oxford
British Diabetic Association (BDA) 1988 Diabetes in the UK. BDA, London

British Diabetic Association (BDA) 1991 What professional supervision should children with diabetes and their families expect? BDA, London
Connor H, Bolton A, Ward J 1987 The foot in diabetes. John Wiley, Chichester
Cordell R 1993 Growth hormone deficiency—a guide. Series no. 2 Child Growth Foundation, London
Day J 1986a Insulin dependent diabetes. Thorsons, Wellingborough
Hames S 1993 Help for the visually impaired. Diabetes Care 2(3): 8–9
Hillson R 1991 Thyroid disorders. Macdonald Optima, London
Hindmarsh P, Brook C 1986 Measuring the growth of children in general practice. Journal of Maternal and Child Health 11(6): 196–199
Hughes I 1989 A practical guide to measurement techniques. Growth Matter 1: 5–7
Keinar C 1989 Growth. Medicine International 21(b): 217–223
Lewis J 1986 The endocrine system. Churchill Livingstone, Edinburgh
Lindley M 1980 Coping with restricted growth. Association for Research into Restricted Growth, UK
Metcalf M, Baum J 1991 Incidence of insulin dependence diabetes in children aged under 15 years in the British Isles during 1988. British Medical Journal 302: 443–447
Sacharin R 1986 Principles of paediatric nursing, 2nd edn. Castlemead Publications, UK
Stillitoe R 1988 Psychology and diabetes. Chapman & Hall, London
Tanner J 1989 Foetus into man, 2nd edn. Castlemead Publications, Welwyn Garden City
Tanner J M et al 1966 Standards from birth to maturity for height, weight, height velocity and weight velocity: British children 1965. Parts 1 & 2. Archives of Disease in Childhood 44: 454–471, 613–635
Wise P 1986 Endocrinology. Churchill Livingstone, Edinburgh
Woolston J 1991 Eating and growth disorders in children. Sage, UK
World Health Organization 1990 Diabetes in Europe. WHO, Copenhagen

FURTHER READING

Day J 1986a Insulin dependent diabetes. Thorsons, Wellingborough
Day J 1986b Non-insulin dependent diabetes handbook. Thorsons, Wellingborough
Ellicot J 1987 If your child is diabetic. Sheldon Press, London
Fletcher R 1992 Lecture notes on endocrinology. Blackwell Scientific Publications, Oxford
Hillson R 1991 Thyroid disorders. Macdonald Optima, London
Hillson R 1992 Diabetes: a beyond basics view. Optima, London
Hillson R 1993 Diabetes: a new guide. Optima, London
Kabi Pharmacia 1993 Growth assessment and management of growth failure in general practice. Kabi Pharmacia, Milton Keynes
Knopfler A 1989 Diabetes and pregnancy. Macdonald Optima, London

Larson G 1988 Managing the school aged child with a chronic health condition. DCI, Minnesota

Laycock J 1983 Essential endocrinology. Oxford University Press, Oxford

Lewis J 1986 The endocrine system. Churchill Livingstone, Edinburgh

North J 1990 Teenage diabetes. Thorsons in association with the BDA, Wellingborough

Pluwridge D Good things come in small packages. University of Oregon Health Sciences Center, Oregon

Shuman N, Sweitzer L 1993 Understanding growth hormone Hippocrene Books, New York

Tanner J 1989 Foetus into man, 2nd edn. Castlemead Publications, Welwyn Garden City

Wise P 1986 Endocrinology. Churchill Livingstone, Edinburgh

USEFUL ADDRESSES

British Diabetic Association
10 Queen Anne Street
London W1M OB8

Child Growth Foundation
2 Mayfield Avenue
Chiswick
London W4 1PW

17

The skin

Jacqueline Denyer   Rosemary Turnbull

This chapter gives an introduction to the importance of the skin in the reflection of the overall physical and emotional health of the child. A brief explanation is given of common skin conditions, and also of the devastating effects of rare genetically inherited skin diseases.

The chapter will:
- list the important functions of the skin in order that recognition may be given to disturbance of such functions in the presence of disease
- outline the appearance of the skin in the newborn and enable the student to identify blemishes that are of medical significance
- offer a brief résumé of basic skin care
- give a short description of common skin conditions, both minor and acute
- provide an introduction to serious genetically inherited skin disorders and the challenge these present to nursing staff.

INTRODUCTION

The skin is the largest organ of the body, but is often not considered to have a large impact on the health of the child; indeed, many dermatological conditions are thought to be 'just a rash'. However, in practice, children with skin disorders may have acute or chronic paediatric problems, with some conditions being a threat to life.

Many skin conditions are painful and many more give severe discomfort as a result of intense irritation. The child with eczema or psoriasis may miss weeks of schooling and integration into a peer group becomes increasingly difficult. Teasing by other children is a major problem for those who look different in any way, and those with skin conditions suffer from the unkind comments of their peers. Many treatments leave the skin greasy and this leads to problems at home and school as clothing and furniture become ruined, and other children and even close relatives avoid physical contact during games and play. This may lead to an altered body image, a problem which can persist throughout life (Price 1990).

Genetically inherited conditions such as epidermolysis bullosa and icthyosis can affect the child's entire well-being with problems affecting mobility, nutrition and psychological welfare.

Children with skin conditions require vast nursing input and careful coordination between hospital and community networks. Often a multidisciplinary approach is essential to ensure that affected children reach their full potential.

There is an increasing need for nurse specialists in the field of dermatology to provide a knowledge base and to teach parents, hospital and community staff the care of each individual sufferer, and to encourage compliance in what may prove to be time-consuming and unpleasant treatments.

Counselling skills, insight into wound healing and currently available products and a knowledge of genetics are also an essential requisite for such a post (Lipman & Deatrick 1994).

THE SKIN

The skin has many functions, the most important being:

- maintenance of body temperature
- transmission of sensation
- waterproofing
- metabolic activity—manufacture of vitamin D
- defence against:

—foreign bodies
—damage
—ultraviolet light (Campbell 1994).

In the absence of disease, skin must be maintained in good condition in order to avoid infections or problems related to dry or broken skin.

The newborn

The full-term infant has many marks on the skin which may cause anxiety for the parent. Time should be taken to explain the nature of such blemishes and the innocence of the majority of them. An information session at prenatal classes is the ideal opportunity to discuss these so that the new mother is not alarmed on examination of her first-born.

At birth, the skin is covered with vernix, a thick greasy substance composed of secretions from the sebaceous glands. This washes away easily, but present thinking is that it should not be washed away because not only does the vernix moisturise the skin it also prevents heat loss from the infant's body—an important consideration in the first hours of life.

Most infants will have milia on the face, most commonly around the nose; these are due to the presence of keratin in the sebaceous and sweat glands (Vullimay & Johnston 1987). They will disappear spontaneously over the first few weeks of life and should never be squeezed, or infection may result.

Birthmarks

Stork marks are very common; they are flat and pale pink. Those on the eyelids or forehead usually fade completely within a few weeks or months. Marks on the back of the head may not always fade completely, but become hidden by hair.

Other birthmarks such as haemangiomata or port wine stains may require medical intervention at a later age.

Mongolian blue spots typically occur in Black

or Asian babies and are flat blue marks over the back and bottom; they may be very extensive. They can be mistaken for bruising and should be documented on the child's record card to avoid any confusion with non-accidental injury (Harper 1990). Mongolian blue spots are present in a very small minority of Caucasian infants.

Cradle cap

A dry flaky scalp can progress to form thick yellow scales which cover the scalp and can have a characteristic cheesy smell. Prevention is better than cure, and shampoo should always be rinsed away thoroughly and the scalp moisturised if it appears dry.

Once cradle cap has developed, initial treatment is by the application of oil. Olive oil is very effective, and application of this must be followed after several hours by gentle encouragement of the loosened scales to separate. Care must be taken not to remove scales adherent to the scalp or permanent hair loss may result. Prescribed or commercial shampoos may become necessary if the condition does not respond.

'Milk spots'

These commonly occur on the face, and sometimes extend to the chest or back at about 4 weeks of age; they are probably nothing to do with milk. They can be inflamed and resemble a miniature version of acne. Again, no action is generally necessary and squeezing may cause further inflammation or even infection.

Nappy rash

Nappy rash will result if nappies are not changed frequently, or if the skin is not cleansed at nappy changes. Modern disposable nappies are designed to hold large volumes of urine without leakage, and the new parent must be encouraged to change nappies regularly and to cleanse the skin as build-up of ammonia can cause ammoniacal dermatitis.

Barrier creams help to prevent nappy rash; commercial Vaseline forms an occlusive layer and is protective and soothing on irritated or broken skin.

Candida nappy rash (thrush) results when the skin has become colonised by *Candida albicans*, a fungal infection. This causes an angry-looking erythematous rash, which may have discrete red spots around the edge of the main rash. If nappy rash does not improve when commercial products are used, then thrush should be suspected. Treatment is by application of an anti-fungal cream or ointment and should be continued for a few days after the rash has disappeared or symptoms may recur.

Oral candidiasis

Oral candidiasis may be associated with candidal nappy rash or occur on its own. It is characterised by small white plaques resembling milk curds which cannot be removed, and bleeding may result if they are scraped off. The plaques are mainly seen on oral mucosal membrane, tongue and gums. Oral thrush can cause pain and discomfort and therefore impair feeding.

Treatment is by use of an oral fungicide such as miconazole gel or nystatin.

Oral candidiasis often results from poor hygiene, for example under-sterilisation of teats and bottles, or may be secondary to antibiotic treatment which reduces the body's normal flora and allows the fungus to invade. Such infections are common in sick or debilitated children or those with impaired immunity.

Suncare

It is gradually becoming more widely accepted that a suntan is not a sign of robust health, can lead to premature ageing and, in some cases, is a causative factor in the development of skin cancer.

Infants should never be placed in the sun. Parents must be encouraged to use a sunshade attachment with the pram or buggy (Foltz 1993). Older children should be encouraged to wear hats and a high factor sunscreen (factor 15 or above) should be applied. Children must never be allowed to use sunbeds.

Basic skin care for dry skin conditions

Daily bathing is generally advised. Bath in warm (not hot) water for approximately 10–15 minutes in the prescribed emollients (see Box 17.1) such as Oilatum or Alpha Keri. Avoid use of commercial soaps or bubble baths, including baby bath preparation, which are often drying, and may be perfumed (Bach 1987). A soap substitute should always be used, such as aqueous cream or Diprobase.

Dry the skin with a soft towel which does not shed. Do not rub the skin vigorously; it should be patted dry, and moisturisers should be applied on top of the slightly moist skin forming an extra barrier to loss of water. Moisturisers should be applied liberally with downward movements to prevent clogging the hair follicles. It must be remembered that the hospital is probably a much warmer environment than the home and therefore moisturisers will need to be applied more frequently.

Box 17.1 Types of preparation commonly used for skin conditions

Emollients. Bathing adds to patient comfort by removing debris and lubricating the skin, reducing dryness and therefore reducing the risk of infection. The effects of bathing in emollients are short-lived; therefore frequent application of moisturiser is required.

Creams. These are water soluble and are easily washed off. They are generally cosmetically acceptable. Some creams contain preservatives to inhibit bacterial or fungal growth, which can act as sensitisers; you should bear this in mind if a rash occurs at the site of application.

Ointments. These are usually greasy and not water soluble and are therefore cosmetically unacceptable to many who wish their treatments to be discrete. Ointments are more occlusive than creams and so encourage hydration (Hunter et al 1989).

Note: It is important to remember when carrying out skin treatments that a cream cannot pass through an ointment, but an ointment can pass through a cream.

Hair should be shampooed separately (i.e. not in the bath) in order to minimise further skin irritation (Thompson 1994), although this may not always be possible with young children.

SKIN CONDITIONS
Infections

The skin is not a sterile field and is covered by a multitude of harmless organisms, or normal flora. Colonisation with pathogenic organisms such as *Staphylococcus aureus* and streptococci can lead to infections such as impetigo.

Impetigo

This is an extremely contagious condition and spreads rapidly in institutions such as nurseries. Treatment is by antibiotic therapy, and spread can be minimised by meticulous washing of hands and by ensuring that everyone has the use of his or her own towel and flannel (Verbov 1988).

Infestations

Parasitic skin infestations are common in childhood. They cause much discomfort and carry social stigma although they are not necessarily associated with poor hygiene. One of the more common infestations is scabies.

Scabies

Infection is transmitted by close physical contact, but the source of infestation may be difficult to identify as the incubation period may be as long as 2 months. Commonly affected areas are between the fingers and toes and in the flexure areas, although the parasites can occur anywhere on the body. When the skin is examined characteristic burrows can be seen as fine grey lines (Fig. 17.1). The itching is intense and secondary infection is a common complication as a result of scratching. Antibiotic treatment will then be necessary.

If the instructions are adhered to, then one course of treatment should be sufficient.

Eczema

Eczema is a dry, painful and irritant condition of the skin, characterised by erythema, small vesicles and papules (see Box 17.2). It is one of the most common skin complaints in childhood.

Classification of types of eczema can be difficult, but the most common types in infancy and childhood are seborrhoeic and atopic.

Seborrhoeic eczema

Seborrhoeic eczema usually develops in the first few weeks of life. It generally starts on the scalp and spreads rapidly to other areas, commonly affecting the face, flexures and nappy area.

It looks painful, but is not generally itchy or sore and causes little distress to the infant. The baby is not unwell (Simpson 1992).

Care of seborrhoeic eczema.   Management is by the general practitioner. The use of soap should be avoided and the infant bathed in emollients, using aqueous cream as a soap substitute. Moisturise the skin regularly, with a bland unscented cream.

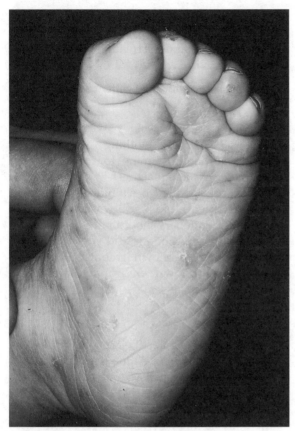

Figure 17.1   Scabies on the sole of the foot.

All members of the family must be treated for scabies, including those showing no signs of the infestation, as the prolonged incubation period makes immediate diagnosis impossible.

Treatment.   Benzyl benzoate is the treatment of choice at the present time, and should be applied as follows:

- The child is bathed and then dried with a towel.
- The prescribed cream or lotion is applied to the entire body, paying attention to the crevices and the areas between fingers and toes.
- The preparation must be left in situ for 24 hours.
- A second application should then be applied without washing off the first application.
- The following day the preparation should washed off.

Box 17.2   Definitions of dermatological terms

Macules.   These are flat circumscribed discoloured lesions of varying shapes and sizes; they are not raised. They can be quite normal, e.g. freckles, or they may result from a disease process, e.g. petechiae.

Papules.   These are raised, firm, circumscribed lesions up to 1 centimetre in diameter.

Nodules.   These are very similar to papules, but are larger and found in deeper layers of the skin.

Vesicles.   These are small blisters usually containing serous fluid. They will disappear and leave no scarring.

Pustules.   These are inflammatory lesions which may be situated superficially in the epidermis or in the deeper layers; they are elevated and contain purulent fluid.

In general, seborrhoeic eczema has resolved by the age of 6 months; however, a percentage of affected infants will go on to develop atopic eczema.

Atopic eczema

This condition can develop at any age, but is not usually seen in infants under 3 months old. Classically it affects the elbow and knee flexures (Fig. 17.2), and the face. The skin is red, inflamed and moist. It is both itchy and painful.

Complications. Constant scratching and rubbing as a result of chronic irritation lead to skin breakdown, which causes lichenification (thickening of the skin). This is a defence mechanism; the body is trying to protect itself from further breakdown.

Scratching can lead to infection, which requires treatment with antibiotics; hospitalisation may be necessary in severe cases. The most commonly seen organisms are streptococci and *Staphylococcus aureus*.

Eczema herpeticum. One the most severe infections is caused by the herpes simplex virus. This resembles an acute exacerbation of atopic eczema, but eczema herpeticum should always be considered when examining a child with worsening eczema, as this infection can be life-threatening.

Early diagnosis is essential since 'complications result from widespread dissemination of virus through the body and multisystem involvement' (Harper 1990). Hospitalisation is always necessary and the treatment is with intravenous acyclovir.

Management of the child with eczema:

- Keep fingernails short.
- Do not overheat.
- Dress in loose cotton clothing.
- Administer antihistamine to reduce itching and so ensure adequate rest.
- Clothes and bed linen should be washed in mild detergent—biological washing powders and fabric softeners should never be used.
- Avoid perfumed lotions and substances, and those containing known irritants.
- Avoid any known environmental trigger factors such as pets.

Treatment:

- Bath the child in prescribed emollients such as Oilatum, Balneum or Alpha Keri, once a day.
- A soap substitute such as aqueous cream must always be used.
- Apply moisturiser frequently to all areas of the body as this will help to alleviate dryness and itching (Spowart 1993).

Icthopaste and Coban bandages. These impregnated bandages are used for children with areas of lichenification. The preparations in the bandages reduce areas of thickened skin by preventing scratching.

Wet wrap bandages. A mild topical steroid may be necessary if the symptoms do not subside with use of emollients. One method of applying steroid cream to children with extensive atopic eczema is via wet wrap bandages.

After application of the preparation to the skin, a layer of wet tubular bandage is applied, followed by a dry layer. Improvement is usually seen within 48 hours, and hospital admission can be avoided. Once the symptoms are controlled, the wet wraps can be used with a moisturiser alone. These must be continued for at least 6 weeks in order for the treatment to be effective, and must be resumed at the first sign of deterioration.

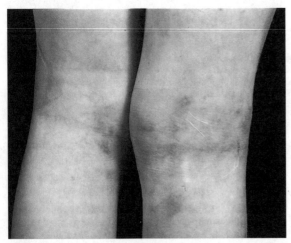

Figure 17.2 Atopic eczema behind the knees.

Activity 17.1

A 3-year-old boy has atopic eczema. What advice on general management would you give to his parents in order to promote a satisfactory quality of life for him?

Psoriasis

This is a chronic relapsing inflammatory disorder, characterised by well-defined red plaques with fine silvery scales. The actual cause of this disorder remains unknown and there is no cure available. Relapses and remissions are spontaneous (Harper 1990).

The normal epidermal transit time is approximately 28 days, but in psoriasis the rate of epidermal cell proliferation is increased and the transit time reduced to 10 days. The pathological findings in psoriasis are summarised in Box 17.3.

There are a variety of different types of psoriasis and therefore treatment is individualised, depending on the type.

Guttate psoriasis

This is mainly seen in children and is often secondary to a staphylococcal tonsillitis or otitis media. There is sudden onset, the skin being erythematous with small papular lesions which will become scaly within a few days or weeks. It is mainly the trunk that is affected and the rash clears within a few months, but plaque psoriasis can later develop (Hunter et al 1989).

Nose and throat swabs should be taken on admission for microscopy, culture and sensitivity testing, and the appropriate antibiotics commenced, usually penicillin V and/or erythromycin.

Pustular psoriasis

This is a rare form of the disorder. It is usually caused by the sudden withdrawal of steroids. For this reason, their use is not recommended in the treatment of psoriasis (Bach 1987). There is initially widespread erythema followed by an outbreak of pustules. The child has the potential to be critically ill with pyrexia, tachycardia and general malaise. The leakage of albumin into extravascular spaces can lead to hypovolaemia (Hunter et al 1989).

Treatment of psoriasis

Coal tar preparations. These are frequently used in the treatment of psoriasis. Although it is not certain why they have a beneficial effect, it is recognised that they inhibit DNA synthesis and therefore must slow the skin cell growth.

Tar-based shampoos. If the scalp is affected, then a tar-based shampoo should be used. However, severe involvement of the scalp will require a preparation that will first soften the plaques. A product such as coconut oil should be applied and left overnight prior to the hair being washed with the tar-based shampoo the following morning.

Dithranol. Dithranol in Lassar's paste slows down skin proliferation and is not absorbed systemically. Treatment with this preparation is messy and time-consuming and is therefore better carried out on an inpatient or day patient basis. The duration of treatment is usually 2–3 weeks. The strength of dithranol used depends on the thickness of the plaques present; strength is therefore reduced as plaques reduce. This preparation burns healthy skin and care must be taken during application. Healthy skin can be protected by applying Vaseline around the plaques before the dithranol is applied.

Retinoids. These are vitamin A derivatives which inhibit cell proliferation. Etretinate, the

---

Box 17.3   Pathophysiology of psoriasis

- Marked thickening of the epidermis
- Absence of granular cell layer
- Retention of nuclei in horny layer
- Accumulation of polymorphs in horny layer
- Dilated capillary loops in the upper dermis

retinoid used in the treatment of psoriasis, is a teratogenic drug and pharmaceutical guidelines must be strictly adhered to. Side effects include fatigue, joint pain and dry lips.

Methotrexate. This inhibits cell replication and is usually taken orally once weekly. Side affects of this drug can include fatigue, mouth ulcers and alopecia. Since liver disorders are a common result of treatment, frequent liver function tests are essential in order to ensure that it is safe to continue drug therapy (Williams et al 1991).

Psoriasis responds well to natural sunlight as the

Activity 17.2

Write your own protocol of care for a 13-year-old girl who requires dithranol paste treatment for psoriasis.

ultraviolet rays produced depress DNA synthesis and therefore slow cell proliferation.

INHERITED SKIN DISORDERS
Epidermolysis bullosa

Epidermolysis bullosa is the name for a group of

Case study 17.1 Jane

Jane is an 11-year-old girl who has suffered from increasing relapses in plaque psoriasis. She was becoming increasingly withdrawn and reluctant to participate in school activities because of the problems with her skin, and was referred to the consultant dermatologist for help with this distressing problem.

Following careful history taking and physical examination it was decided to admit Jane for treatment with dithranol. The proposed treatment was discussed with Jane and her mother and they both agreed that she be admitted for up to 3 weeks, her actual length of stay being dependent on the success of the treatment. Her mother was to remain resident with Jane.

The side effects of dithranol were explained to Jane and her mother, as follows:

- Dithranol stains the skin but the marks will gradually fade on withdrawal of treatment.
- Dithranol will also will stain all contacts (for this reason Jane was advised to bring an old dressing gown).
- Dithranol burns healthy skin. Care must be taken when applying it and she should report any burning sensation to the nurse.
- The actual procedure is messy and lengthy.

Jane had not had this treatment before; therefore a patch test was carried out. A small amount of paste was applied and left in situ for 45 minutes. No complications arose and the procedure was commenced. Dithranol concentrations ranging from 0.05–0.1% were to be used, the strength being increased as her skin tolerated the paste.

Procedure
In a warm room, Jane removed her clothing, keeping on only her pants. Vaseline was carefully applied to all the areas of healthy skin surrounding the plaques in order to protect the

skin. Jane was encouraged to assist in the procedure and she was happy to do so. She was meticulous in her application and keen to explain the rationale to students.

Wearing gloves and a plastic apron to protect ourselves, we applied the dithranol to all psoriatic patches using a spatula and orange stick. The time was noted, as it is imperative to remove the dithranol after the desired time to prevent burning.

Johnson's talc was then used to set the dithranol and to prevent it from smearing. Jane put on a hospital gown and the paste was left in situ for 45 minutes at a strength of 0.5%.

Arachis oil and gauze squares were used to removal the dithranol. A bath was prepared using Baltar and Jane bathed for 15 minutes. Once she was dry she applied Diprobase as a moisturiser. The application of moisturiser was performed twice daily.

Because she has extensive scalp involvement, a coconut oil compound was massaged into the scalp at night and shampooed out in the morning using Polytar. The coconut oil softens the plaques. *Note:* hair washing should be performed separately from the bath to minimise skin irritation.

As her skin continued to tolerate the dithranol, the strength was gradually increased until a 1% concentration was reached. Careful monitoring of the skin was maintained and improvement was noted after 10 days; as the plaques decreased, so the dithranol strength was reduced accordingly.

Jane's face, however, remained a problem as she was unable to tolerate the dithranol even in a very weak strength. She was therefore commenced on a mixture of 2.5% hydrocortisone and 5% tar which proved very effective.

Jane was discharged at the end of 3 weeks and was a much happier and more confident young lady. At the follow-up outpatient appointment she had a much improved body image and was confident to join in school activities without embarrassment.

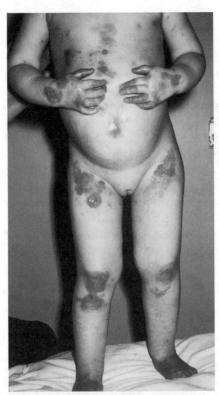

Figure 17.3 Dystrophic epidermolysis bullosa.

rare genetically inherited blistering skin disorders (Fig. 17.3). There are three main types: simplex, junctional and dystrophic.

Epidermolysis bullosa simplex

This is almost exclusively a dominantly inherited condition (one parent has the condition, the other is usually unaffected). There is a one in two chance in every pregnancy that the fetus will also be affected.

The skin blisters in response to everyday trauma but, fortunately, in this type of epidermolysis bullosa, the blisters heal without scarring. The most common type of epidermolysis bullosa simplex is Weber Cockayne, which classically affects the hands and feet. Life expectancy in those with epidermolysis bullosa simplex is in general normal. Walking can be very painful and the choice of occupation is limited in those who are severely affected (Eady 1990).

Junctional epidermolysis bullosa

This is always a very serious condition, comprising several distinct diseases. Inheritance is recessive (both parents are healthy carriers of the defective gene), and there is a one in four chance in every pregnancy that the fetus will be affected.

Many children will die within the first 2 years of life from laryngeal disease and failure to thrive, both resulting from internal blistering. However, a few will survive to adulthood, often with surprisingly little handicap.

Dystrophic epidermolysis bullosa

This condition can be either dominantly or recessively inherited. On the whole, in common with many inherited disorders, the recessive gene causes greater disability.

Children with dystrophic epidermolysis bullosa may become progressively disabled as blistering heals with scarring and contractures develop. In its severest form, there is an acquired syndactyly of the hands (Fig. 17.4), requiring repeated plastic surgery in order to restore and maintain function. Internal blistering and scarring may cause oesophageal strictures and, in

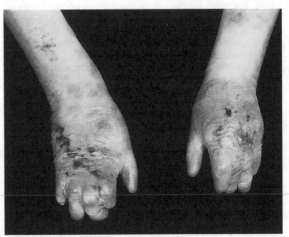

Figure 17.4 Acquired syndactyly of the hands in dystrophic epidermolysis bullosa.

Activity 17.3

What advice and help could you offer to the teenager who has a low self-esteem as a result of a skin condition that causes not only bodily but facial disfigurement?

order to provide sufficient nutrition, gastrostomy feeding is necessary in some cases.

Although in the future it is hoped that some treatment will be available in the form of gene therapy, the present treatment can be only preventive and supportive (Eady 1990).

Management of epidermolysis bullosa

Adequate pain relief must be given as necessary, and each child must be assessed regularly and medication adjusted as required (see Case study 17.2).

Blisters must be burst with a sterile needle or scissors to prevent them from enlarging. Wounds are dressed with non-adherent dressings and padded to reduce pain and prevent further injury. Physiotherapy is vital to minimise disability and maintain mobility (Hough 1990). Adequate nutrition is essential to realise growth potential and aid wound healing. Some children are unable to take sufficient nutrients, as they have very sore mouths, and oesophageal strictures make swal-

Case study 17.2 Sarah

Sarah was admitted to the dermatology ward when she was 4 days old. She had been transferred from the Special Care Baby Unit at her local maternity hospital.

Her mother's pregnancy had been uneventful and the delivery normal but it was noted that Sarah had large areas of skin denuded from both her feet and lower legs at birth. Apgar scores were good and the baby appeared otherwise well. The wounds were dressed with paraffin gauze. Amniotic bands were suspected to be the cause of the lesions.

Over the next few hours Sarah developed blisters from being handled, and blisters and lesions around her upper legs and trunk where her disposable napkin had rubbed. Lesions developed inside her mouth from sucking her bottle.

The initial diagnosis was changed to that of an infection. An intravenous cannula was inserted and antibiotic therapy commenced. Sarah became reluctant to feed, due to pain from the lesions in her mouth, and a nasogastric tube was passed to supplement oral feeding.

Sarah remained afebrile, but there was no improvement in her skin, and blistering continued at sites of friction. It was now suspected that Sarah had epidermolysis bullosa and Sarah and her parents were transferred to the specialised centre.

Following analgesia, the paraffin dressings were soaked off the lesions on her legs; there was a large amount of blood loss as the dressings had adhered to the wounds. The area was then dressed with non-adherent silicone dressings and padded well to avoid further trauma. These dressings were left in place for several days to encourage epithelialisation. Care was taken to ensure that the foot remained in a good position when a dressing was secured.

The adhesive tape securing both the nasogastric tube

and the intravenous cannula was gently removed, using a mixture of liquid paraffin and white soft paraffin. Unavoidably, this resulted in some skin loss.

All the blisters were burst with a sterile needle to prevent them from enlarging and, where necessary, the areas were dressed.

Following application of local anaesthetic gel to her mouth lesions, Sarah fed well from a bottle, taking fortified formula to meet her increased nutritional needs.

Skin biopsy confirmed the diagnosis of epidermolysis bullosa of the dystrophic type, characterised by a tendency for the lesions to heal with scarring, leading to contractures.

Sarah's mother remained resident with her, and gradually overcame her fear of handling Sarah and became proficient at caring for her delicate baby.

Once the lesions were healing, and Sarah's mother able to burst blisters and apply dressings, she was discharged home. Genetic counselling was given prior to discharge and the couple were informed about the prenatal testing that would be available in future pregnancies.

Prior to discharge the clinical nurse specialist visited Sarah's health visitor and district nurse to explain about the rare condition of epidermolysis bullosa and to discuss Sarah's special needs.

Regular visits to the ward over the next few months showed gradual healing of the original lesions on her feet and legs, although, as expected, scarring and contractures were becoming evident and her toes were fusing together. Blistering continued over her body at sites of friction.

Sarah was assessed by the physiotherapist and her parents taught exercises to try to maintain her long-term mobility.

Sarah's weight gain remained good; the dietitian will give continued input and adjust her diet as necessary.

lowing difficult. In this group of children, nutrition is supplemented by gastrostomy feeding (Tesi & Lin 1990). Preventive and restorative dentistry must be practised in order to preserve teeth. It will be impossible for this group of patients to wear dentures, due to the fragility of their gums and subsequent blistering from the prosthesis.

It should be remembered that some children with epidermolysis bullosa have an increased risk during anaesthesia as a result of blistering of the mucous membranes in response to the trauma of intubation.

Prenatal testing in the form of a fetal skin biopsy is available during the 15th week of pregnancy for parents who are carriers of junctional epidermolysis bullosa or the recessive type of dystrophic epidermolysis bullosa. It is hoped that, in the near future, prenatal testing can be carried out earlier in pregnancy by analysis of samples of the chorionic villi.

As it is not at present possible to detect carrier status, parents who are offered testing will already have had a child with epidermolysis bullosa.

Icthyosis

Icthyosis (Fig. 17.5) is a disorder of keratinisation, the skin being extremely dry, scaly and cracked. The disorder is mainly inherited, but can, rarely, be an acquired illness, usually as a feature of a multisystem disorder. Links have been made with metabolic disorders. In its severe form the condition may be incompatible with life. Such infants are described as 'harlequin babies'.

The severe forms are inherited recessively and are usually diagnosed in early childhood (Harper 1990).

Treatment

From the onset of the disorder, the child will require regular intensive skin care. This care is very time-consuming and carers and children, as they mature, must be aware of the necessity for compliance.

The use of moisturising creams is essential as the skin is extremely dry. Keratolytic agents, e.g. salicylic acid and urea preparations, which induce desquamation of the horny layer but do not affect the function of the epidermis, are the main treatments of choice.

Oral retinoids are currently being introduced as a form of treatment. Refer to the earlier description in the treatment of psoriasis for precautions regarding retinoids (p. 284).

As with many disfiguring dermatological conditions it is imperative to seek the advice and involvement of psychologists and other relevant support groups such as the charity, Changing Faces.

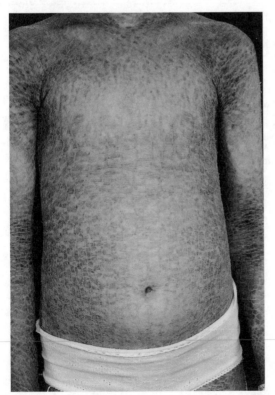

Figure 17.5   Icthyosis.

REFERENCES

Bach J 1987 Eczema and other skin disorders. Grafton Books, London, pp 45, 133
Campbell J 1994 Skin deep. Nursing Times Feb 23: 50

Eady R A J 1990 The classification of epidermolysis bullosa. In: Priestley G C et al (eds) Epidermolysis bullosa: a comprehensive review of classification, management and laboratory studies. DEBRA, Crowthorne

Foltz A J 1993 Parental knowledge and practices of skin cancer prevention: a pilot study. Journal of Paediatric Health Care (Sept/Oct): 220

Harper J 1990 Handbook of paediatric dermatology. Butterworth-Heinemann, London, pp 66, 122

Harper J, Goodyer H 1990 Atopic eczema and infection. Maternal and Child Health (April): 121

Hough F 1990 The classification of epidermolysis bullosa. In: Priestley G C et al (eds) Epidermolysis bullosa: a comprehensive review of classification, management and laboratory studies. DEBRA, Crowthorne

Hunter J A A et al 1989 Clinical dermatology. Blackwell Scientific Publications, Oxford, pp 50–51, 240

Lipman T H, Deatrick J 1994 Enhancing specialist preparation for the next century. Journal of Nursing Education 33(2): 55–58

Marrs R 1990 Living with your eczema. Professional Nurse July: 526–527

Price B 1990 A model for body image care. Journal of Advanced Nursing 15: 585–593

Simpson C 1992 Eczema in children. Paediatric Nursing (June)

Spowart K 1993 Management of childhood eczema. Primary Health Care Journal 3(6)

Tesi D, Lin A 1990 Nutritional management of EB patient. In: Lin A, Carter D M (eds) Epidermolysis bullosa: basic and clinical aspects. Springer-Verlag, New York

Thompson J 1994 Moisturising solutions. Nursing Times (Feb) 23: 52

Verbov J 1988 Essential paediatric dermatology. Clinical Press, London p 48

Vullimay D G, Johnston P G B 1987 The newborn child, 6th edn. Churchill Livingstone, Edinburgh

Williams R et al 1991 Guidelines for management of patients with psoriasis. British Medical Journal 303

FURTHER READING

Bee H 1989 The developing child. Harper & Row, New York

Lin A, Carter D M (eds) 1992 Epidermolysis bullosa: basic and clinical aspects. Springer-Verlag, New York

National Eczema Society Publications. Available from: 4 Tavistock Place, London WC1H 9RA

Priestly G C et al (eds) 1990 Epidermolysis bullosa: a comprehensive review of classification, management and laboratory studies. DEBRA, Crowthorne

Psoriasis Association Publications. Available from: Milton House, 7 Milton Street, Northampton NN2 7JG

Sharvill D 1984 Skin diseases. Gower Medical Publishing, London

Solomons B 1977 Lecture notes on dermatology, 4th edn. Blackwell Scientific Publications, Oxford

Turora G, Anagnostakos N 1987 Principles of anatomy and physiology, 5th edn. Harper & Row, New York

Verbov J (ed) 1979 Paediatric dermatology. William Heinemann Medical Books, London

Weston W L Practical paediatric dermatology. Little Brown, Boston

Whaley D, Wong D 1991 Nursing care of infants and children, 4th edn. CV Mosby, St Louis

Wilkinson J D, Shaw S, Fenton D A 1993 Colour guide: dermatology. Churchill Livingstone, Edinburgh

USEFUL ADDRESSES

Changing Faces
27 Cowper Street
London EC2A 4AP

National Eczema Society
4 Tavistock Place
London WC1H 9RA

Psoriasis Association
Milton House
7 Milton Street
Northampton NN2 7JG

Hearing and vision

Elizabeth J. Mair

In this chapter the normal and abnormal functioning of the ear and the eye in the developing child will be outlined.

The chapter aims to:
- introduce the concepts of screening and surveillance and assessments of hearing and vision to detect normal or abnormal development
- outline the normal and abnormal workings of the ear and the eye with reference to common problems
- alert the nurse to children and families at risk of developing hearing and vision problems
- introduce the reader to services and provisions available for children and families with identified problems
- discuss some conditions that may result in hearing and vision loss and outline nursing care principles
- link in with other topics covered in the book, e.g. care of the child undergoing surgery, language development, communication, impairment, and disability.

INTRODUCTION

Hearing and vision are senses that enrich our lives, and perception is the process by which we read messages that are conveyed by the senses. We learn to use our senses to communicate (see Foong 1992). The growth in perception involves an increase in sensitivity to information in the environment and the ability to register and interpret the information (Bee 1992).

Throughout childhood, health, growth and development are checked to help to enable all children to reach their potential. Hearing and vision are monitored to check for any dysfunction that may impede development in many areas. The checking throughout childhood may be referred to as screening or surveillance.

Screening

Screening has been described as the recognition of disease or defect by the application of tests, examinations or other procedures which can be applied rapidly (Hall 1991), or the determination of incidence or detection of certain specific conditions (Butler 1989). The screening should identify a person who may have a disorder from those who appear not to have the disorder. Such a test is not meant to be diagnostic. There is much debate about the use of, and criteria for, screening tests (Law & Pollard 1994, Holland 1993, Polnay & Hull 1985, McCormick 1983).

Surveillance

There is a grey area between screening and surveillance. Surveillance can be described as the supervision of child health (Illingworth 1991). Hall (1991) describes surveillance as activities initiated by professionals that include:

- oversight of physical, social, emotional health and development
- monitoring of development
- offering intervention when necessary
- prevention of disease, e.g. immunisation
- health education.

The emphasis should be on a partnership between parents and professionals. Surveillance is ongoing and the parent may be seen to be the best person to carry out surveillance of child health. Robertson (1988) describes screening and surveillance as trying to prevent the development of problems by discovering them early.

Hearing and vision problems

Some conditions which affect hearing and vision are life-threatening but many are chronic and call for adjustments in coping from day to day. The terms below are often used in relation to hearing and vision loss; it is important to distinguish between them.

- Impairment means any abnormality of body structure or function.
- Disability means a reduction in ability to carry out a particular task or skill.
- Handicap is the effect of the impairment or disability in preventing the individual from pursuing aspirations, goals and roles in society (Hall 1991).

One of the basic philosophical principles behind concepts of service delivery is that all people, regardless of many factors including level of disability, are entitled to respect, dignity and equality of access to services appropriate to their age (Betts & Meyer 1993).

Hearing and sight are factors that must be assessed by all nurses and every effort must be made to maximise potential and facilitate good use of residual function.

HEARING

The ear is the organ responsible for hearing and can function from before birth. Fetal movement is commonly felt after loud noises, when the fetus responds by means of a startle reaction. Infants may be soothed, alerted or distressed by noise. Babies prefer sounds that are not too intense, and continuous sounds often have a calming effect. Most infants like the rhythm of adult speech (Holt 1991). Children, throughout their early years, have to learn to make sense of

Activity 18.1

Describe the difference between handicap and impairment.

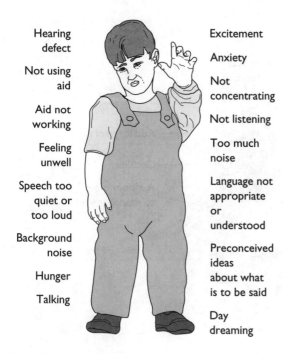

Hearing defect

Not using aid

Aid not working

Feeling unwell

Speech too quiet or too loud

Background noise

Hunger

Talking

Excitement

Anxiety

Not concentrating

Not listening

Too much noise

Language not appropriate or understood

Preconceived ideas about what is to be said

Day dreaming

Figure 18.1 Barriers to hearing.

what they hear and learn to respond with language appropriate to the culture in which they live. Speech development in children is covered in Chapter 1 and, for further information, readers should consult the list of further reading at the end of the chapter. Children also have to learn to listen effectively, although this is a skill that many adults do not acquire! Some of the factors which influence what we hear and how we make sense of what we hear can be seen in Figure 18.1.

For further information on communication and interpersonal skills, see Kenworthy et al (1992).

Hearing is often said to be one of the last remaining senses to be lost when a person is losing consciousness or dying.

Activity 18.2

What would you do if you suspected a colleague was not hearing some of what was said to her and you felt that she was missing important information about the patients?

Workings of the ear

The ear consists of three areas with connecting structures (Fig. 18.2):

• The outer ear in many animals is used to locate sounds and direct them to the auditory meatus or canal.
• The middle ear is a skull bone cavity. The eardrum vibrates and sound energy is transmitted to the fluid in the cochlea via three small bones. The auditory tube ensures that air pressure is the same on both sides of the eardrum.
• The inner ear is embedded in the temporal bone. The cochlea houses the organ of Corti in which vibration produces nervous impulses for transmission to the brain. This part of the ear also houses the organ responsible for balance.

Although not part of the ear, the 8th cranial nerve is important in hearing. This nerve transmits messages to the part of the brain responsible for hearing.

For further information, see Wilson (1990), Tortora (1991), and Tortora & Grabowski (1993).

The pharynx is the muscular back wall of the nose, mouth and throat. The nasopharynx opens into the cavity of the middle ear by the auditory tube. The pharynx is encircled by lymphoid tissue including the adenoids at the back of the nasopharynx and the tonsils between the pillars of the arch of the palate.

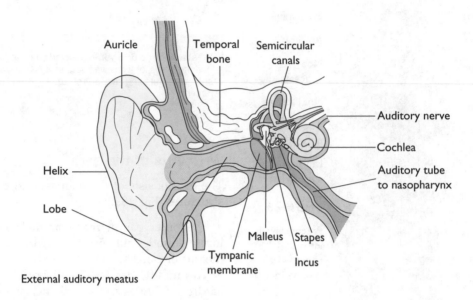

Figure 18.2   Structure of the ear.

Box 18.1   Problems that affect different parts of the ear

Outer ear
- Boils
- Wax
- Foreign bodies
- Inflammation

Middle ear
- Otosclerosis (unwanted bone)
- Infections
- Inflammation, e.g. hay fever

Inner ear
- Injury
- Infection

Nerve
- Anoxia
- Toxic drugs
- Infection
- Injury

Hearing deficits

Hearing depends on a chain of events and can be lost through disorders of any of the structures that contribute to the chain (see Fig. 18.3 and Box 18.1).

The main types of hearing loss are sensorineural and conductive.

Sensorineural hearing loss

Sensorineural hearing loss results from a malfunction in the cochlea, auditory nerve or hearing centre in the brain; the main causes of malfunction are listed in Box 18.2. It may affect one side (unilateral) or both sides (bilateral). The effects of sensorineural loss are more likely to be long term and less treatable than those of conductive hearing problems (Lyall 1989). Children with this type of loss may hear filtered speech; high-frequency sounds are more often lost causing distortion and lack of clarity in what is heard. Without early intervention most children with this type of loss suffer impairment of language acquisition (Hall 1991). Many children with sensorineural hearing loss will be fitted with hearing aids.

Conductive hearing loss

Conductive hearing loss is extremely common. It results in a loss of loudness and not clarity of

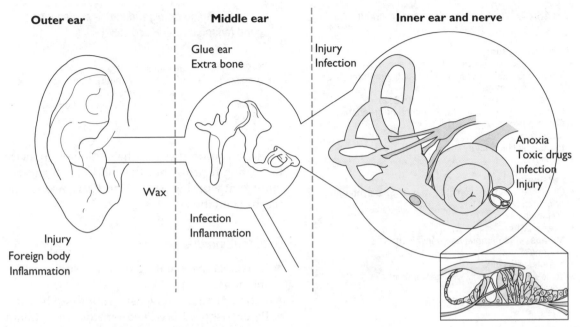

Outer ear

Glue ear
Extra bone — **Middle ear**

Injury
Infection — **Inner ear and nerve**

Wax

Infection
Inflammation

Injury
Foreign body
Inflammation

Anoxia
Toxic drugs
Infection
Injury

Figure 18.3 Factors that may contribute to hearing loss (adapted from Davies 1993).

Box 18.2 Main causes of sensorineural loss (malfunction of cochlea, auditory nerve, or hearing centre)

- Maternal infection, e.g. rubella, cytomegalovirus
- Severe neonatal jaundice
- Dysmorphic syndromes
- Genetic causes
- Asphyxia
- Infection in child, e.g. measles, meningitis (see Swanwick 1989), encephalitis
- Ototoxic drugs, e.g. gentamycin, streptomycin
- Arteriosclerosis
- Accident

Box 18.3 Main causes of conductive hearing loss (impairment of conducting sound waves to cochlea)

- Outer ear abnormality
- Foreign body in canal
- Wax in canal
- Tympanic membrane damage
- Otosclerosis
- Infections
- Chronic otitis media

speech, and is not often long term. Conductive hearing loss may be an air or a bone conduction problem and is an impairment of the mechanisms of conducting sounds to the cochlea; Box 18.3 lists the main causes of conductive hearing loss. In developed countries it is usually due to secretory otitis media (Hall 1991) or some problem with the middle ear— commonly the auditory tube becomes blocked by upper respiratory tract infections or enlarged adenoids. This type of hearing loss is treatable with decongestants, antibiotics or surgery (see later). Often children show a spontaneous improvement as they grow and the parts of the ear get less prone to blocking. The extent of disability caused by having this type of loss is difficult to asses. The referral criteria and management of secretory otitis media are very controversial (Hall 1991; unpublished report).

Another category of children with hearing loss are those who have mixed loss.

Box 18.4   Causes of hearing loss in childhood

Early hearing loss
- Malformation of external or middle ear, e.g. Waardenburg's syndrome, Pendred's syndrome, Alport's syndrome
- Genetic (see Harper 1988, pp. 210–212)
- Maternal rubella—if in first 3 months of pregnancy
- Cytomegalovirus
- Hyperbilirubinaemia
- Intracranial birth injury
- Asphyxia

Later hearing loss
- Otitis media—more common with Down's syndrome or cleft palate
- Meningitis
- Encephalitis.
- Mumps—if 8th cranial nerve involved
- Trauma
- Neoplastic lesions
- Toxic effects of drugs, e.g. gentamycin
- Foreign body

Box 18.5   Guide for parents: infants' response to sound (adapted from Hood 1982)

- 1–2 months   quietens to voice
- 3 months   turns head to sounds on same plane
- 6 months   imitates sounds
- 7 months   turns to sounds made above ear
- 12 months   turns to name

Timing of hearing loss

Hearing loss can happen at any time throughout fetal development, infancy and childhood. Jolly & Levene (1985, p. 314) outline causes of early and later hearing loss in childhood (see Box 18.4).

Testing for hearing loss

The testing of hearing throughout childhood is generally recognised as being useful if done properly. Many different groups may be involved in the surveillance, including health visitors, general practitioners, school and hospital nurses, audiometricians, audiologists and, most importantly, parents and family members. Throughout childhood, any parental concern must be taken seriously and acted upon promptly by testing by the appropriate health professional and referral to a specialist audiological service if necessary.

Activity 18.3

Why can some profoundly deaf people speak?

Health authorities may have different policies for testing hearing, but the child health surveillance joint working party (Hall 1991) made some recommendations.

Birth to 6 months

- Universal neonatal screening using various methods.
- Extra attention for at-risk groups (see below).
- Parents should be asked whether their infant seems to hear. This can be enhanced by use of a check list (Box 18.5; see also Robertson 1988, and Hood 1982, p. 122).

Testing for hearing loss can be done from birth using various methods like brain-stem evoked responses and reflex measurement. From about 6 months, the distraction test, which is a test of detection can be applied. Later on, according to the child's ability, cooperative tests using simple instructions, and performance tests like the toy and picture tests, may be used. From about 3–4 years of age, full audiometric assessment may be possible. Some of the most commonly used tests will be briefly described.

7 months to 1 year

Distraction test. This is usually done by health visitors and trained helpers. It depends on an infant's ability to turn to sounds and requires a certain level of developmental maturity. The people performing the test must be adequately trained and carry out the test to a satisfactory standard in satisfactory conditions. This test should be applied to all infants and is a pass or fail test. A child should not be tested if unwell, especially if there is an upper airway problem. If the child fails on two occasions or the parents express any concerns or the child falls into a high-risk group, the child should be referred for specialist testing.

 For a fuller explanation of the distraction test, see Davies (1993) and Robertson (1988).

18 months to 5 years

Cooperation tests. The McCormick Toy Test is an example of such a test. In it the child is asked to show various small toys which have been matched for sounds, with the tester using a quiet voice. No universal hearing test is recommended between the ages of 18 months and 5 years, but any child whose hearing is in doubt should be referred for diagnostic testing.

 For more detail on cooperation tests, see McCormick (1988) and Robertson (1988).

School-age child

Sweep test. This is a modified pure tone audiogram performed at fixed intensity level. This test may not be performed regularly but should be undertaken if a child experiences learning or behavioural difficulties. (Detailed explanations of specialist tests are beyond the scope of this book.)

Risk factors

There are certain risk factors that must always be taken into account when assessing real or potential hearing problems. Butler (1989) identifies the risk factors as:

- family history of hearing problem
- maternal virus infection in pregnancy
- ototoxic drugs in pregnancy or after birth
- neonatal hyperbilirubinaemia
- preterm delivery
- intensive care when newborn
- mental subnormality
- cerebral palsy
- recurrent otitis media
- pyogenic meningitis
- mumps.

It is important to be aware of the risk factors for loss of hearing when assessing patients. There are also numerous rare syndromes associated with deafness (see Jolly & Levene 1985, Forfar & Arneil 1984). In the older child, exposure to loud noise and, for example, frequent listening to loud noise through headphones may be an explanation for loss of hearing.

Hearing aids and treatment

Once a significant hearing loss has been diagnosed, the approach to care of the child is multidisciplinary, involving audiologists, teachers for the deaf, paediatricians, speech therapists and any relevant professional. The child may benefit from using a hearing aid which can be worn from an early age. Types of hearing aids are listed in Box 18.6.

Hearing aids can improve hearing especially for children with sensorineural loss. They allow children to use what residual hearing they may have by amplifying the sounds. The aids must fit the child, be appropriate for the child and be kept in good working order.

Cochlear transplants are now being performed with varying degrees of success. The implants only treat a symptom and are not a cure (Lyall 1989).

The child and family may be taught sign language (Box 18.7).

Box 18.6 **Types of hearing aids (Sibert 1992)**

- Behind ear
- Body worn
- In ear
- Bone conducting

Box 18.7 **Types of sign language**

- BSL (British sign language)
- Signed English
- Finger spelling
- Makaton (used with children with learning difficulties)

The severity of hearing loss will affect the amount of help a child may need. The type of schooling the child receives may depend on the needs of the child and facilities in the area. The child may be educated in:

- normal school with no extra help
- normal school with extra help and facilities
- special unit attached to a normal school
- special school.

Whaley & Wong (1991) provide a classification of hearing loss, outlining the effect on speech and giving educational recommendations.

The child's needs may be assessed using the special needs statement procedure, which is under review following the Audit Commission report (1992). It is hoped that the parents will be better able to identify whether their child's needs are being met. The aim is for the child to be integrated into the normal system as much as possible, following recommendations made by the 1981 Education Act (Betts & Meyer 1993).

Conditions that may result in hearing loss

Problems with the ears that may result in some deafness are relatively common in childhood. MacFarlane et al (1989) gives the following figures for prevalence:

- mild hearing loss (35–50 decibels) 13/1000
- moderate loss (50–70 decibels) 2/1000
- severe loss (>70 decibels) 1/1000.

Jolly & Levene (1985, p. 315) state that 2% of deaf children have no hearing.

Acute otitis media

This condition occurs when inflammation in the upper airway causes the lining of the auditory tube to swell. If the tube becomes blocked, there may be pain and a reduction in hearing. If the infection spreads up the tube, the pus cannot escape, the increase in pressure in the middle ear may cause pain and fever may result. If, in the presence of other symptoms, the eardrum is visible, and there is little wax present, an ear infection is more likely (Fairey et al 1985). On examination, the eardrum may be tight and dull, the child may present with loss of appetite, vomiting, loose stools, general malaise, pain in the affected ear and fever which if untreated may result in a febrile convulsion (see Ch. 14). If the infection spreads to the back of the ear, then mastoiditis may develop, although this is now very rare. The eardrum may perforate and a purulent discharge from the ear may be seen.

Children are more prone than adults to the development of ear infections as the auditory tube is short, wide and straight. Children also lie down for a large proportion of the time and bacteria and vomit may travel from the nasopharynx into the middle ear. The pharyngeal opening may also be blocked by large adenoids which naturally shrink with age (Jolly & Levene 1985, p. 309). Doctors should routinely check the ears in children who present with any illness or have a history of ear problems. The organisms that cause ear infections most commonly would seem to be:

- *Streptococcus pneumoniae*
- *Haemophilus influenzae.*

It is difficult to collect organisms in the middle ear to culture, but it would seem likely that the organisms are most often those found in the nasopharynx. The treatment of ear infections seems to vary between cultures and remains controversial for reasons like poor response to antibiotics, poor rate of completion of prescribed antibiotics and the risk of ototoxicity (Solomons & Madden 1992, Bain 1989). Bain (1989) cites studies that indicate that antibiotics are not essential in the treatment of all acute ear infections.

Implications for nursing:

- Treatment of any of the above symptoms.
- Administration of analgesics, antipyretic drugs and antibiotics.
- Monitoring for complications, or cross-infection.

Serous otitis media or glue ear

With this condition there is often conductive hearing loss. The most common causes are recurrent infections or allergic conditions. Children more commonly get this condition because of their adenoids which may be large and cause blockage of the auditory tube. Adenoids shrink with age. If the auditory tube becomes blocked, air cannot reach the air-filled middle ear and the cells in the area produce a sterile glue-like substance. This substance restricts movement of the ossicles and hinders the transmission of impulses. As the condition becomes chronic, the decision is then whether to risk perforation of the eardrum or to perform a myringotomy—making a surgical incision in the tympanic membrane and sucking out the exudate. Grommets are small tubes which may be inserted to allow passage of air into the middle ear and drainage. The grommets are intended to stay in position for 6–9 months but often fall out much sooner. The insertion of grommets may not be the best way to treat this condition (Hood 1982, p. 143), but the technique is common and often the child having the procedure is admitted for day surgery (see Ch. 9).

Implications for nursing (see ch. 9)**:**

- Care of the child having surgery.
- Providing information for the child and family about after-care.
- Care of the child having an anaesthetic.
- Post-operative care.

Tonsillitis

Tonsillitis is a condition often associated with hearing problems and ear infection and implies infection of the tonsils. It would seem likely that the organisms which lead to tonsillitis are often the same as those that cause ear infections, namely streptococcal infections. With tonsillitis the child may complain of pain in the throat, have a high fever, appear flushed and have a reduced appetite. It seems that the tonsils provide a first line of defence (Jolly & Levene 1985, p. 308) but often do not function adequately and may harbour the organisms that lead to recurrent infections. Infections can be treated with antibiotics, but if the problems become chronic and result in loss of schooling or prolonged periods of illness, surgical removal of the tonsils may be considered. This procedure is performed much less frequently than in previous decades and is often performed along with adenoidectomy, especially if the child has recurrent otitis media, impaired hearing and mouth breathing.

Implications for nursing:

- Reduction of temperature.
- Administration of pain relief.
- Administration of antibiotics and informing parents of the importance of completing the course.

Care of the child having tonsillectomy and adenoidectomy includes:

- relieving anxiety
- ensuring that the child is prepared for theatre with correct, appropriate information
- protecting the child's safety at all times
- preparing for after the operation—possible soreness, vomiting, bleeding
- after the operation:
  —positioning correctly
  —offering pain relief
  —informing parents to observe for signs of development of problems, e.g. excessive bleeding, infection (see Ch. 9).

Foreign body

A cause of ear problems in children is foreign bodies becoming lodged in the ears. The child may require an X-ray to ascertain the presence of an object in the external ear canal. In extreme circumstances, the unwanted object may have to be surgically removed.

Implications for nursing:

- Being proactive—giving general information regarding potential danger of small objects.
- Care and positioning of a child having an X-ray examination.
- Care of a child having a procedure requiring an anaesthetic.

Referred earache

Often, pain can be felt in the ear if the throat is sore, teeth are erupting or with illnesses like mumps.

Implications for nursing:

- Careful assessment of the patient.
- Being aware of the potential for referred earache.
- Making the child comfortable with appropriate analgesia, in a warm environment or with warm cotton wool.

Looking after the child with impaired hearing

Impaired hearing can be described as the loss of speech frequencies of over 20 decibels (Brunner & Suddarth 1991). The severity of impairment depends on the extent of the defect as well as the age of occurrence, time before diagnosis and adequacy of rehabilitation (Whaley & Wong 1991).

The infant with impaired hearing may:

- have little interest in the environment
- not respond to loud noises
- not turn to vocal sounds at close range
- have minimal vocalisation.

The toddler may:

- have little vocalisation
- show little response to environmental sounds
- have poor speech sounds
- use gestures to express needs.

The pre-school and school child may:

- have tantrums and behaviour problems
- be inattentive and a slow learner.

With a sensorineural loss, the child may talk loudly, whereas the child with a conductive loss may talk in a soft voice. The nurse may meet the child before hearing loss is diagnosed, at diagnosis or after diagnosis. The nurse needs to be able:

- to communicate with the child and family
- to asses normal patterns of language and communication and response to sounds
- to be familiar with types of hearing loss and able to assess whether the child is at high risk
- to report any suspected loss
- to be familiar with community resources
- to facilitate best use of the child's residual hearing and speech, and use aids correctly
- to find out the child's normal routine
- to help support the child and family
- to offer information
- to put the family in touch with other families if appropriate
- to communicate findings to other team members
- to relieve embarrassment if hearing loss is obvious and communication difficult or different
- to be aware that parents may be very protective
- if diagnosis has been recent, to facilitate acceptance and allow grieving to take place (see Ch. 25)
- to be aware of potential altered body image
- to be aware that hearing problem may be secondary
- to be aware that people can mishear, especially if anxious and in a strange environment.

Activity 18.4

What advice would you give to a mother whose 5-year-old child had just had grommets inserted into both ears?

Case study 18.1 Harry

Harry always seemed to be doing well, although his mother thought that something was not quite right. He was a very good baby; he never seemed to cry much and he was always delighted to see his mother or father. He was the first child of Joy, who worked as a teacher, and Philip, who was a business manager. When Harry was 8 months old, he passed his distraction hearing test performed by the health visitor. At the age of 1 year, he was not making many sounds and Joy began to feel anxious. At 18 months, Harry certainly had no words and still did not make much noise, and by now Joy was really beginning to notice that children of a similar age made much more noise. At 3 years of age, Harry had a hearing test after his mother had expressed her concern to the health visitor again. This time, Joy's worst fears were confirmed and Harry proved to be profoundly deaf. The staff at the specialist nursery said that the sooner these children were found the better their communications were likely to be. Joy knew there had been something wrong: she just wished that she had made more of a fuss.

VISION

The eye is the organ concerned with vision. It connects with the part of the brain that makes sense of the visual images via the 10th cranial nerve. In the 1960s Fantz's pioneering work described how infants can organise perceptions enough to show a preference for what they look at (Paradice 1993). Infants were found to have abilities that they had previously been thought not to have. Although the normal infant can see at birth, visual acuity develops in the first year and throughout early childhood (see Holt 1991). An understanding of what can be seen unfolds as thinking areas of the brain cortex mature. We learn to see, and the brain is very vulnerable to the effects of abnormal vision such as a squint or astigmatism up to the age of about 6 or 7 years. This is one reason why early detection of visual defects is vital.

Workings of the eye

The eye is a sphere with a slight bulge in front and a stalk behind (Fig. 18.4). The cornea, or transparent bulge, is covered by the sclera which along with the eyelids serves to protect the eye. Behind the cornea is the pigmented diaphragm supported by muscle, the iris. Behind the iris, again supported by muscle, is the lens. The pupil is the hole in the middle of the iris which allows light to enter the eye and land on the light-sensitive retina. The conjunctiva is the protective membrane that covers the front of the eye and inside the eyelid. It is constantly lubricated with tears which are secreted by the lacrimal gland and drain into the nose via a small opening at the inner corner of the eye.

For detailed anatomy and physiology of the eye, see Tortora & Grabowski (1993), Bowie (1990), Hinchliff & Montague (1988).

The function of the eye is very complex. Impulses from the retina are carried to the brain, which takes several years to learn to interpret the slightly different images from both eyes. Fixation and following of objects should be demonstrable at 6–8 weeks, and following in all directions established by 6 months (Holt 1991). There are several relay stations in the nerve path concerned with reflex activity like adjusting the pupils, as well as functions like maintaining the posture and balance of the body. As an organ of balance, the eye works with the ear and sensation from the muscles and limb joints (see Roberts 1993). Observation of the eye and its response to voice is an important part of the assessment of head-injured children (Williams 1992; see Ch. 14).

For further information about the function of the eye, see Hinchliff & Montague (1988), and Wright (1989).

Disorders of vision

Disorders of vision can be:

- disorders of structure
- disorders of the function of part of the eye

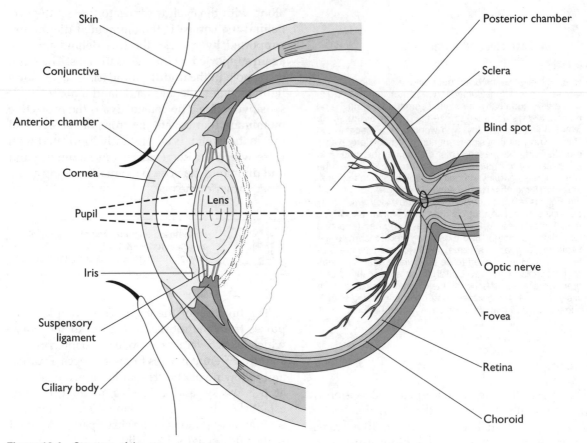

Figure 18.4 Structure of the eye.

* disorder in the passage or interpretation of messages going to the brain.

What we expect to see plays an important role in what we think we see. The relationship between vision and memory and expectation seems to be very strong and complex (Baddeley 1982). Optical illusions are easy to create, and

Activity 18.5

What differences might you find between someone who has just lost their sight and someone who has never been able to see.

Box 18.8 **Defects of vision—when problems can occur**

* Genetically inherited defects, e.g. nystagmus, squint, syndrome (Batten's disease), metabolic disorder (e.g. leucodystrophy), anophthalmia (born with no eyes).
* Antenatal factors, e.g. infection (rubella, toxoplasmosis (Harper 1988, p. 273), toxocariasis (Wright 1990), syphilis), pesticides and the link with anophthalmia (Gilbert 1993).
* Perinatal factors, e.g. prematurity, low birth weight, oxygen therapy, infection.
* Postnatal factors, e.g. injury, accident, retinal haemorrhage from hypertension, infection, inflammatory disorder, poisoning (e.g. lead), disorders such as migraine.

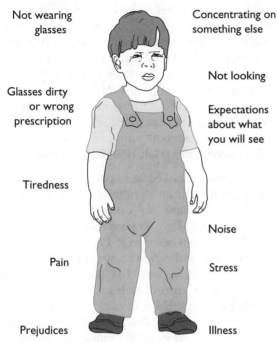

Not wearing glasses

Concentrating on something else

Not looking

Glasses dirty or wrong prescription

Expectations about what you will see

Tiredness

Noise

Pain

Stress

Prejudices

Illness

Figure 18.5 Barriers to seeing.

witnesses at scenes of crimes are notoriously unreliable. The factors that may influence what someone sees are illustrated in Figure 18.5.

The specialised parts of the eye have their own special problems. Problems with the eye and associated structures which result in visual defects can occur at various times during development and growth (Box 18.8). The defects can be caused by congenital factors, disease or trauma. Transient problems such as migraine may also cause visual disturbances.

There are several possible reasons for problems with vision:

- limited or defective visual fields
- impairment of colour vision
- decreased visual acuity
- slight or no vision.

The defects may be:

- ocular, affecting the eye or optic nerve
- cortical, an abnormality in the brain but not the eye

- a refractive error, when the eye does not function as a perfect system.

Risk factors

The nurse must be aware of certain risk factors which may predispose to problems of vision. The risk factors below are adapted from MacFarlane et al (1989):

- family history of squints, ocular disorder before 6 years, wearing glasses before 10 years
- neonatal infections
- perinatal insult
- genetic syndrome and other malformation
- infection
- oxygen therapy as a neonate
- trauma
- child abuse (head shaking or blows).

Disorders of vision are very common (see Table 18.1). Hall (1991) splits visual defects into three groups:

- Serious defects. These cause disabling impairment of vision ranging from partial sight to blindness. The incidence is about 4 per 10 000 (see Harper 1988, pp. 201–209).
- Common and less-disabling deficits. These may be refractive errors which may be correctable with glasses.
- Defects of colour discrimination.

Factors which affect the extent to which a particular defect causes a disability include intelligence, photophobia and field of vision. Partial sight means that there is some residual sight which

Table 18.1 Prevalence of some visual defects (MacFarlane et al 1989)	
Defect	Prevalence (per 1000 live births)
Squint	30–40
Hypermetropia	30
Astigmatism	30
Myopia	10 at 6 years to 200 at 16
Cataract	0.2
Optic atrophy	0.2
Retrolental fibroplasia	0.2
Colour blindness	80 (males) 4 (females)

Box 18.9 Terms used in assessment of vision

Amblyopia. Loss of vision, partial or complete, temporary or permanent, without apparent disorder of the eyes.

Nystagmus. A reflex scanning movement of the eyes. This reflex is partly under control of the organ of balance in the middle ear and if the coordination between this and the eye is damaged nystagmus occurs when the eye should be still.

Visual acuity. How well a person separates visual stimuli.

Refractive error. Refracting structures of the eye do not accurately focus rays of light on the retina.

Myopia or short-sightedness. Difficulty seeing at a distance.

Hypermetropia or long-sightedness. Difficulty seeing close objects. Often causes a child to squint.

Astigmatism. Different degrees of refraction in the horizontal and vertical axes of the eye.

(The last three are examples of refractive errors.)

Activity 18.6

It is worse to loose your sight than your hearing. Discuss.

can be used, and blind means that the person uses methods for education or work that do not require vision (Hall et al 1990). Box 18.9 defines some of the terms that are used in assessment of vision.

Testing vision

The early diagnosis of eye defects in children is thought to be useful for several reasons. Some conditions need early investigation and treatment, for example cataract and retinoblastoma. Problems with the eyes and vision may also indicate disease or ill health in other body systems, for example hypertension. Severe eye problems may lead to behaviour problems, which may be minimised if detected early. The early diagnosis of squint or refractive error is important because, if undetected, there may be a permanent loss of vision.

The question of who should perform the testing is open to debate. Stayte et al (1992) describe a combined system of primary and secondary screening that has been established in response to the need for early treatment of ocular and vision problems. Robertson (1988) states that the more parents are involved with monitoring the vision of babies the greater the chance of early diagnosis of problems. The joint working party on child health surveillance (Hall 1991) recommend:

• Eyes must be looked at as part of the neonatal examination with an ophthalmoscope to check the red reflex, and for cataract and signs of retinoblastoma. This examination may be repeated at the 6-week check. Problems with the eye may be an indication of hypertension.
• Parents must be asked if there is a family history of visual disorders. If so, the child should be seen by an ophthalmologist.
• Parents should be asked at each contact (e.g. by the health visitor) if they have any anxieties about the child's vision. Parents should be asked if their child seems to see, looks, follows moving objects, fixates on small objects.
• Staff should be familiar with the stages of normal visual development and alert parents to signs of visual defect, e.g. abnormal appearance of the eye, poor fixation, wandering eye movements.
• Children with other major defects require a specialist eye examination.
• A test for visual acuity should be performed at school entry and then at 3-year intervals.
• A colour vision test should be carried out between the ages of 9 and 13. Many more males than females are affected by colour blindness (see Table 18.1).

In many areas, health visitors perform tests to screen for visual defects. As well as general observation of the eyes and asking parents about their concerns at each contact, the cover test for squint may be done at 7–9 months and the STYCAR matching test done between the ages of 3 and 4 years. Some professionals feel that orthoptists should be responsible for all pre-school screening, in view of the level of expertise required (Polnay & Hull 1985). In schools, vision may be

---

Box 18.10 **Summary of when to screen**

History—perinatal, 6–8 weeks
Ocular appearance—every contact with a health professional
Parental concern—every contact and invite parent to contact if needed
Active questioning—every contact

---

tested every 2–3 years and the test for colour vision done between the ages of 9 and 13 (Illingworth 1991). These tests may be performed by school nurses, although this practice is of questionable value (Jewell et al 1994). Parents must be encouraged to express any concern at any time. A summary of when screening is done is given in Box 18.10.

The child with vision problems in society

Once a significant loss of vision is diagnosed, special provisions may be made for the child and family. The child and family may need advice and support. Special adaptations may need to be made to the family home to ensure that the environment is safe and to encourage the child to be as independent as possible. The type of schooling the child receives may depend on the needs of the child, and the type of schooling available is the same as for the child with hearing loss. There are special radio programmes for children with visual loss, and talking books and braille books are available to facilitate independence. The child and family may benefit from being in touch with others in similar situations or self-help groups. The problems of labelling people with obvious disabilities must be recognised (see Kenworthy et al 1992).

Activity 18.7

Think of some common sayings that might offend a person with visual problems.

Eye problems

Infections

Tears contain an antibacterial agent, lysozyme, which protects the eye against infection. However, tear production does not begin until approximately 6 weeks after birth, making newborn babies particularly susceptible to eye infections.

In purulent conjunctival exudate or sticky eye there is sometimes swelling of the eyelids but mostly the infection affects the conjunctiva. Often it is caused by amniotic fluid, blood or meconium which gets into the eye during birth. Organisms such as *Neisseria gonorrhoeae* and *Chlamydia trachomatis* must be screened for, although the most common causes are *Staphylococcus aureus*, *Haemophilus influenzae* and *Streptococcus sp.* (Fox 1989). Conjunctivitis is often seen when a child has measles.

Eye infections in this country have few serious complications, unlike the problems caused by parasitic infections in tropical countries and Africa (Kanski 1984). One exception is congenital *Toxoplasma gondii* infection in which vision may be defective or absent (Harper 1988, p.273).

Implications for nursing:

- Correct cleaning of the eye. This should be done with cool boiled water or saline using clean cotton wool. The eyes should be cleaned separately to avoid cross-infection and be cleaned from the inner corner out. Parents and carers should also be taught the correct procedure.
- Correct administration of ointment or drops.

Eye problems in the low birth weight infant

This category of infant (see Ch. 20) demands special consideration as visual problems are common (Schrader 1991). Cataract, squint, myopia and retinal problems must be considered, plus retrolental fibroplasia which is a major cause of blindness (Jolly & Levene 1985, p. 80). The more immature the infant, the greater is the risk of retrolental fibroplasia developing. In this condition, uncontrolled oxygen therapy can lead to prolonged raised arterial oxygen levels, and initial vasoconstriction of arterioles may soon become irreversible. Oedema develops, the retina may detach and an opaque membrane fills the area behind the lens causing blindness. There is some thought that giving vitamin E to all babies under 30 weeks' gestation may protect the eyes from severe disease (Jolly & Levene 1985, p.81).

Implications for nursing:

- Assessing risk, and vigilance in monitoring the infant in this category (see Ch. 20).

Retinoblastoma

This is the most common ocular tumour of childhood. It is bilateral in about one-third of all cases and is sometimes familial. The tumour is congenital and so is seen only in young children, usually about 2 years of age. The growth starts as a nodule on the retina which produces a yellow light reflex visible to the naked eye. A squint is a common feature.

Implications for nursing:

- Careful observation of the eye as part of the initial assessment.
- If the tumour has already been diagnosed, then care of the child with cancer (see Ch. 24).
- Care of the child having surgery.

Ptosis

Ptosis is a condition where there is drooping of the eyelid. This may rectify itself or require surgery, especially if the lid occludes the cornea and sight is obstructed.

Implications for nursing:

- Sensitivity to the child with abnormal-looking eyes.
- Care of the child having surgery.

Congenital glaucoma

In this condition the intra-ocular pressure becomes raised due to poor drainage of fluid in the eye and the eye stretches to accommodate the extra fluid. The condition may be noticed because of an enlarged eye, photophobia, hazy cornea, raised intra-ocular pressure and cupped optic disc. The condition may be treated surgically or with drops.

Implications for nursing:

- Counselling may be needed as the condition is hereditary.
- Care of the child undergoing eye surgery.
- Correct instillation of eye drops.
- Care of the child with impaired vision.

Cataract

The development of a cataract means that there is opacity of the lens causing dimness of vision. The most important cause of cataract development in infants is infection with rubella in the first trimester of pregnancy. The defect is confined to the lens and when this is replaced vision is restored. Corneal transplants can now be performed.

- Giving of pre-conceptual advice regarding rubella immunity.
- Careful observation of the neonate and child for lens opacity.
- Care of the child having corneal transplant surgery.
- Facilitation of organ transplant where appropriate (see Ch. 26).

Squint

A squint or strabismus refers to faulty alignment of the axis of an eye and is due to any disorder that disturbs the ability to use the eyes together. With a congenital squint the muscles and nerves are healthy but the two eyes are wrongly coordinated. The squint may be due to muscle imbalance, for example as a result of trauma where there may have been a bleed into the muscles around the eyes. The most common type of squint in childhood comes on at the age of 2 or 3 and is due to a refractive error, usually long sight. Two different pictures may be produced by the eyes and, in the young child,

Box 18.11   Types of squint (visual axes of eyes differ)

- Pseudosquint—illusion of presence of squint caused by broad epicanthic folds seen in infants
- Manifest squint—constantly present
- Latent squint—only present if tired or unwell
- Alternating squint—child fixates with either eye

Activity 18.8

What care might a child receive following a squint repair in your local hospital?

where the brain is still learning to translate nerve impulses from the eyes into pictures, the picture from one eye may be ignored in order to overcome the problem of double vision. Unless the squint is treated, the brain may continue to ignore the messages rendering that eye useless. There are several different types of squint (see Box 18.11) and any suspicion of a problem should be assessed by a specialist.

The correction of a squint includes correction of focus with glasses, exercises for the eye muscles (orthoptics) which may include patching the dominant eye to encourage use of the weaker eye, and in some cases surgical adjustment of the eye muscles. This type of procedure is especially suited to day surgery (Traynor 1990, Smithson 1993, Strong et al 1992).

Implications for nursing:

- Advising the child and family to use glasses correctly.
- Advising on the importance of assessment by a specialist.
- Advising on the use of patching as directed.
- Care of the child having a general anaesthetic (see Ch. 9).
- Care of the child having eye surgery (see Bowie 1990):
  —avoiding infection
  —correct administration of drops and ointment
  —use of dressings that do not shed fibres
  —careful technique to avoid damage and scarring
  —instructing the child not to rub the eye, if relevant
  —giving analgesia for pain
  —advising parents.

It has been said that many ophthalmic nursing duties are not research based. There are no guidelines for the preoperative preparation of ophthalmic patients and many departments have discontinued routine procedures without assessing the outcomes of changes in practice (Wells 1993).

Looking after the child with severely impaired vision

The nurse may become involved with the child with impaired vision before it is realised that there is a significant problem, at the time of diagnosis or after diagnosis. The infant with impaired vision may:

- show no eye contact
- not follow moving people or objects with his/her eyes
- seem by parents or close relatives to be 'not quite right'.

The older child may:

- squint
- blink excessively
- bump into things and appear clumsy
- rub the eyes and appear to strain to see.

The nurse looking after children with suspected or confirmed vision loss needs to be able:

- to recognise abnormalities in vision and show an awareness of normal development of vision
- to report any suspected abnormalities in appearance of the eye or altered vision using the correct terminology
- to help the family with a child with visual impairment to express concerns and anxieties, and be aware of the grief and feelings of loss which may be experienced

Case study 18.2 Mary

Mary had started to get headaches which were beginning to worry her. One of the teachers told her parents that the quality of her school work was deteriorating and they thought that she was not concentrating as well as she had been in the previous years. Also, some of her friends had commented that she seemed to screw her eyes up to watch television. Mary was 14 and about to start her GCSE courses. The school nurse was approached and permission obtained for Mary to have an eye test. The results of this simple test suggested that Mary was myopic or short-sighted in both eyes. The school nurse advised Mary to go to an optician for a detailed eye test. This test confirmed that Mary was myopic and lenses were prescribed to correct the fault. Once she had chosen the frames, glasses were made up and, when Mary started to wear the glasses, her headaches gradually became much less frequent. The optician explained that headaches frequently accompany the development of eye problems and that myopia often becomes apparent in the early teenage years.

- to provide opportunities for support for the child and family, e.g. introduce them to similar families, be aware of national organisations and local self-help groups
- to be aware of the child's potential and encourage full parental involvement in care of the child
- to help the child to explore her environment, use appropriate toys and meet with other children
- to inform the parents that the child may experience additional feelings of frustration and boredom—give examples of how to cope with these feelings, for example encourage the child to voice frustrations, encourage independence
- to inform the parents that the child may experience some developmental delay in, for example, gross motor skills
- to ensure that any residual vision and all other senses are utilised to the full—provide toys that stimulate hearing, smell and touch, and are appropriate to age and stage of development
- to facilitate relationships with family, ward staff and other patients

- to be familiar with resources in the community, refer families to useful organisations and provide written information and references that may be appropriate
- to liaise with GP, health visitor, school nurse, school teacher where appropriate
- to be aware of the child's normal routine and organise care around this where possible
- to be aware of extra anxieties that may be present due to poor vision and allow for continuity of care given by the same nurse as much as possible.

It is important to treat the child with visual problems as an individual and, like any other patient, assess the type of care that the child wishes to receive.

REFERENCES

Audit Commission 1992 Getting in on the act: provisions for pupils with special educational needs. HMSO, London

Baddeley A 1982 Your memory, a user's guide. Penguin, London

Bain J 1989 Ear, nose and throat disorders. In: Hart C, Bain J (eds) Child care in general practice, 3rd edn. Churchill Livingstone, Edinburgh, pp 170–177

Bee H 1992 The developing child, 6th edn. HarperCollins, New York

Betts C, Meyer G 1993 Children with disabilities. In: Glasper E A, Tucker A (eds) Advances in child health nursing. Scutari Press, London

Bowie I 1990 Wounds to the eye. Nursing 4(15): 24–27

Brunner L S, Suddarth D S 1991 Lippencott manual of paediatric nursing, 3rd edn. HarperCollins Nursing, London

Butler J 1989 Child health surveillance in primary care: a critical review. HMSO, London

Davies P 1993 Diagnosing hearing loss in children. Nursing Standard 7(May 19): 35

Fairey A, Freer C B, Machin D 1985 Ear wax and otitis media in children. British Medical Journal 291: 387

Foong A 1992 Challenging the tower of Babel. Nursing 5(5): 8–9

Forfar J, Arneil G (eds) 1984 Textbook of paediatrics. Churchill Livingstone, Edinburgh, vols 1 & 2

Fox J 1989 Conjunctivitis, keratitis and iritis. Nursing 3(45): 20–23

Gilbert R 1993 Clusters of anophthalmia in Britain. British Medical Journal 6900(307): 340–341

Hall D M B (ed) 1991 Health for all children, 2nd edn. Oxford Medical Publications, Oxford

Hall D M B, Hill P, Elliman D 1990 The child surveillance handbook. Radcliffe Medical Press, Oxford

Harper P S 1988 Practical genetic counselling, 3rd edn. Butterworth, UK

Holland W W 1993 Screening: reasons to be cautious, British Medical Journal 306: 1222–1223

Holt K S 1991 Child development—diagnosis and assessment. Butterworth-Heinemann, London, p 79

Hood J 1982 Problems in paediatrics. M T P Press, London

Illingworth R S 1991 The normal child, 10th edn. Churchill Livingstone, Edinburgh

Jewell G et al 1994 The effectiveness of vision screening by school nurses in secondary school. Archives of Disease in Childhood 70: 14–18

Jolly H, Levene M I 1985 Diseases of childhood, 5th edn. Blackwell Scientific Publications, Oxford

Kanski J J 1984 Clinical ophthalmology. Butterworths, London

Kenworthy N, Snowley G, Gilling C (eds) 1992 Common foundation studies in nursing. Churchill Livingstone, Edinburgh

Law J, Pollard C 1994 Screening: identifying speech and language delay. Health Visitor 67(2): 59–60

Lyall J 1989 Extra sensory aid. Nursing Times 85(50): 66–67

MacFarlane A, Sefi S, Cordeiro M 1989 Child health: the screening tests. Practical guides for general practice 11. Oxford University Press, Oxford

McCormick B 1983 Hearing screening by health visitors: a critical appraisal of distraction tests. Health visitor 56: 449–451

McCormick B 1988 Screening for hearing impairment in young children. Croom Helm, London

Paradice R 1993 How important are early mother/infant relationships. Health Visitor 66(6): 211–213

Polnay L, Hull D 1985 Community paediatrics. Churchill Livingstone, Edinburgh

Roberts A 1993 Systems of life: the eye and vision. Nursing Times and Mirror 39(41): 45–48

Robertson C 1988 Health visiting in practice. Churchill Livingstone, Edinburgh

Schrader B 1991 Visual problems and very low birth weight. Nursing Times 87(4): 55

Sibert J R 1992 A pocket book of social and community paediatrics. Edward Arnold, London

Smithson B 1993 Setting up a day unit in ophthalmology. Nursing Standard 7(51): 25–29

Solomons N, Madden G 1992 Are antibiotic containing ear drops ototoxic when applied to the middle ear? Health Trends 24(2): 64–65

Stayte M, Wortham C, Reeves B 1992 Orthoptists reduce false positive hospital referrals. Health Trends 24(4): 157–161

Strong N, Wigmore W, Rhodes S, Smithson B, Woodruff G, Rosenthal R 1992 Ophthalmic day care surgery: the role of a dedicated day case unit. Health Trends 24(4): 148–150

Swanwick T 1989 Meningitis and the child. Nursing 3(46): 8–9

Traynor T 1990 Day case eye surgery. Nursing Times 86(39): 54–56

Wells H 1993 Preoperative ophthalmic procedures: ritualistic or necessary? British Journal of Nursing 2(15): 755–762

Whaley L, Wong D 1991 Nursing care of infants and children, 4th edn. C V Mosby, St Louis, p 1015

Williams J 1992 Assessment of head injured children. British Journal of Nursing 1(2): 82–84

Wright J 1990 Toxocariasis—the canine threat. Professional Nurse July: 519–521

FURTHER READING

Bowie I 1990 Wounds to the eye. Nursing 4(15): 24–27

Brierley J 1993 Growth in children. Cassell, London

Coleman J 1984 Simon goes to the optician. Adam & Charles Black, London

Daily Telegraph 1993 Hearing aids: screw in skull improves hearing. The Daily Telegraph 25 August: 6

Foong A 1992 Challenging the tower of Babel. Nursing 5(5): 8–9

Forfar J, Arneil G (eds) 1984 Textbook of paediatrics. Churchill Livingstone, Edinburgh, vols 1 & 2

Glasper E A, Tucker A 1993 (eds) Advances in child health nursing. Scutari Press, London

Hall D (ed) Video. Promoting child health. Radcliffe Medical Press, Oxford

Hinchliff S, Montague S 1988 Physiology for nursing practice. Baillière Tindall, London

Holt K S 1991 Child development—design and assessment. Butterworth-Heinemann, London

Kenworthy N, Snowley G, Gilling C (eds) 1992 Common foundation studies in nursing. Churchill Livingstone, Edinburgh

Morris P 1991 Coping with the loss of an eye. Nursing 4(26): 25–27

Neill S J 1990 A Monday to Friday surgery ward. Nursing 4(16): 20–23

Neylon J 1993 Health promotion for school children. Nursing Standard 7(30): 37–40

Pettenuzo B 1988 I am blind. Franklin Watts, London

Roberts A 1993 Systems of life. Macmillan Magazines, London

Roberts A, Gardiner P 1993 Systems of life: the eye and vision. Nursing Times and Mirror 39(41): 45–48

Tortora G J 1991 Principles of human anatomy, 6th edn. HarperCollins, New York

Tortora G J, Grabowski S R 1993 Principles of anatomy and physiology, 7th edn. HarperCollins, New York

Whaley L, Wong D 1991 Nursing care of infants and children, 4th edn. C V Mosby, St Louis

Wilson K 1990 Ross & Wilson: anatomy and physiology in health and illness, 7th edn. Churchill Livingstone, Edinburgh

Wright D 1989 Human biology. Heinemann Educational, London

Speech development in children

Barrett J 1994 Help me speak: parents' guide to speech and language therapy. Souvenir Press, London

Bee H 1992 The developing child, 6th edn. HarperCollins, New York (A classic, readable text which has a very useful section on the development of language in children)

Bruner J 1983 Child's talk: learning to use language. Oxford University Press, Oxford (A small paperback, based on his psychological studies)

Garvey C 1984 Children's talk. (Developing child series) Fontana, London (A clearly written, useful paperback, based on research and written for professionals and parents)

Naremore R C, Hopper R 1990 Children learning language: a practical introduction to communication development, 3rd edn. Harper & Row, New York (An American text, designed mainly for teachers and educationalists)

USEFUL ADDRESSES

Hearing
AFSIC (for children with speech and language impairments)
347 Central Markets
Smithfield
London EC1A 9NH
Tel: 0171 236 3632

Royal National Institute For Deaf People
105 Gower Street
London WC1E 6AH
Tel: 0171 387 8033

Vision
Royal National Institute for the Blind
224 Great Portland Street
London W1N 6AA
Tel: 0171 388 1266

Optical Information Council
Walter House
418–422 Strand
London WC2R 0PB
Tel: 0171 836 2323

General
Advisory Centre for Education
1B Aberdeen Studios
22–24 Highbury Grove
London N5 2EA
Tel: 0171 354 8321

DIAL UK (Disablement information and advice line)
Park Lodge
St Catherine's Hospital
Tickhill Balby
Doncaster DN4 8QN
Tel: 01302 310 123

PHAB (Physically Disabled and Able Bodied)
12–14 London Road
Croydon
Surrey CR0 2TA
Tel: 0181 567 5510

19 Immunity

Amanda Field

Children face a constant battle aginst infection. The body's defence in this battle is the immune system, where invaders are identified and destroyed (Fig. 19.1). There are many children, however, in whom the defence mechanism does not function correctly and these children are known as immune deficient.

This chapter aims to:
- **review the anatomy and physiology of the immune system**
- **describe the problems facing immune deficient children and their families**
- **outline the actions required to overcome the problems faced**
- **introduce the concepts of infection control within the paediatric environment.**

THE IMMUNE SYSTEM

External defences

The skin

The skin is the largest organ in the body; it covers its entire surface and is continuous with mucosa at the body orifices. It is resistant to penetration and has some areas covered with hair, which protects it from damage. The skin is lubricated by sweat and sebum, which contains lactic and fatty acids that helps to provide an acidic environment (pH approximately 5.5). Its surface is colonised by microbes, which can

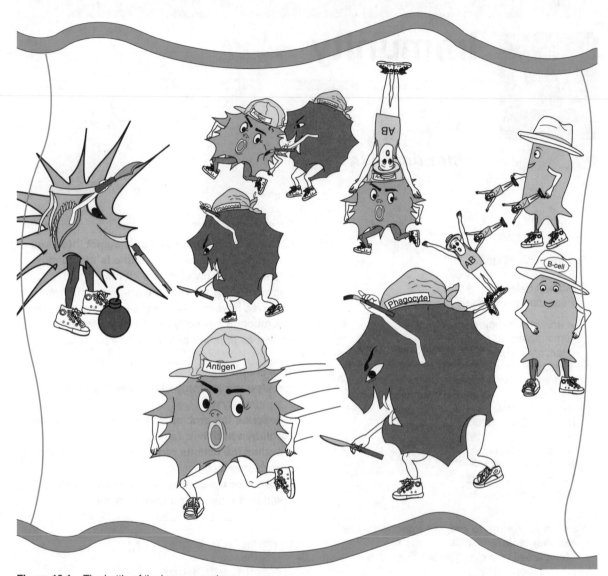

Figure 19.1 The battle of the immune system.

occupy any vacant space and use the available nutrients. Their activities, in conjunction with the acid environment, help to make the skin inhospitable to pathogenic organisms.

The mucosa

This provides the same protection for the internal organs as the skin does for the body's surface. It is not as effective, however, due to its other functions, i.e. the various exchanges—gaseous and digestive—that it has to perform. It aids the defence against infection by constantly renewing its outer layer, and has ciliated cells that sweep away any organisms that may adhere to it.

The respiratory tract

The mucus in the nasal cavity and the turbinates acts as a trap for microorganisms, and the cilia in the nasal passages and bronchial tubes then move the microorganisms to the exterior of the body. If small organisms are inhaled, they are ingested by phagocytic cells that are present in the alveoli, or trapped in the trachea or bronchioles. If trapped, they are moved up the tract by ciliated cells and then either swallowed or exhaled. Sneezing and coughing aid this process.

The mouth

The mouth's defence against infection is twofold.

• The flushing action of saliva, which constantly enters the mouth, and the mechanical action of the tongue remove microorganisms that adhere to the sides of the mouth and teeth.
• The chemical action of the lysozyme in saliva destroys pathogens by digesting their cell walls. The organisms are then swallowed and enter the digestive system.

The digestive tract

The digestive tract has a variety of defences against infection, one being the acidity of the stomach (pH 2.0–3.0), which destroys many pathogens. The small intestine is of an alkaline pH but has many proteolytic enzymes that inhibit microbial growth. The large intestine has a large bacterial content of normal flora, which uses the available food supply and space, while excreting bacteriocins that prevent growth of pathogens. Finally, the peristalsis of the intestine clears bacteria from the system.

The genitourinary tract

The genitourinary system is protected by the acid nature of the tract, which is produced by the normal flora of acid-producing bacteria in the vagina and the acidic pH of urine. The urinary system is also flushed regularly by the action of urinating, and this clears it of any pathogens.

The eyes

The protection of the eye is mainly due to the flushing nature of tears, which clear the conjunctiva and surrounding area. In addition, the tears, like saliva, contain lysozyme (see above).

Internal defences

Lymphatic system

The lymphatic system is similar to the blood circulatory system in that it has capillaries and vessels, and it supplies every tissue that is supplied by a blood vessel, except the brain and the placenta. It has different functions, however, and has unique components—lymphatic ducts, lymph nodes and lymphoid tissue. The fluid it transports is called lymph.

The lymph capillaries pick up excess intestinal fluid, waste products from the cells, microorganisms and debris. The lymphatic vessels then transport the fluid to be filtered and passed back into the circulatory system. Lymph is clear and yellowish and its constituents are similar to those of blood plasma but occur in different concentrations.

Lymph nodes

The lymph nodes are sited in strategic places and they vary in size. They are encapsulated by fibrous tissue and contain reticular and lymphatic tissues which have many lymphocytes. The fluid passes through the nodes and:

• is filtered, removing any particles that are not normally found in serum
• the microorganisms, phagocytes, and damaged or tumour cells are broken down
• activated lymphocytes then collect in the nodes or tissue and multiply, entering the circulatory system to carry out their particular responsibility in fighting infection.

Mucosa-associated lymphoid tissue

In the battle against infection, lymphoid tissue is strategically placed near to the external environment. This tissue, which is mainly filled with lymphocytes, includes Peyer's patches in the ileum, and the nasopharyngeal and palatine tonsils in the mouth.

Thymus gland

This gland lies at the upper part of the mediastinum behind the sternum and extends up to the neck. It is the first organ to produce lymphocytes. It is essential in the immune system because, although it is not exposed directly to the antigens (see Box 19.1) that activate the immune response, it is necessary for the maturation of T cells. The gland grows until puberty, then begins a slow process of atrophy.

Spleen

This organ has functions other than its immunological function. It has blood vessels as well as lymph vessels and, unlike other lymph nodes, lymphocytes enter the spleen via both the blood and lymph vessels. Its functions are:

- phagocytosis of microorganisms and leucocytes
- formation of lymphocytes
- formation of antibodies and antitoxins.

Leucocytes

These are white blood cells and are made in the bone marrow. There are three types of leucocyte:

- granulocytes
- lymphocytes
- monocytes.

Granulocytes.   These cells are phagocytic (see Box 19.1) and have granules in the cytoplasm which contain enzymes that digest organisms, debris and other materials. Three types of granulocyte are distinguished:

• Neutrophils—the first to arrive at the site of an injury and present in increased numbers if there is a bacterial infection. The attraction is due

---

Box 19.1   **Definitions**

Pathogen. A disease-producing agent.

Antigen. A substance that can stimulate the production of antibodies.

Antibody. A substance produced by the blood as a reaction to an antigen.

Phagocytosis. The engulfment by phagocytes of foreign particles or cells harmful to the body.

---

to chemicals released from the infected tissue. They are actively phagocytic for 12–14 hours.
• Eosinophils—2–5% of blood leucocytes. They neutralise histamine, which counteracts the inflammatory action in allergic reactions, and also damage parasites by a protein they release.
• Basophils—<0.5% of leucocytes. They contain inflammatory mediators and are, therefore, important in linking the immune response and the inflammatory reaction.

Lymphocytes.   These are mainly involved in the immune response, and there are two types:

• B lymphocytes (B cells)—found in the lymph system. They develop in the fetal liver and then the bone marrow, carrying a surface immunoglobulin that acts as an antigen receptor. They divide and differentiate in response to an antigen under the influence of cytokines released by T cells (see below). Once activated by an antigen, they enlarge and become plasma cells that produce a specific antibody (see Box 19.1) to that antigen.
• T lymphocytes (T cells, which are further differentiated into:
  —helper T cells, which secrete cytokines that stimulate the activity of other defence cells
  —cytotoxic T cells, which destroy virally infected or allogeneic cells
  —suppresser T cells, which slow or halt the activity of T and B cells.

Monocytes.   These are the precursors of *macrophages*. They are abundant in cytoplasm and have a phagocytic action. They arrive after neutrophils but last longer (active 24–48 hours). They secrete interleukin 1 (a cytokine), which activates the T cell response.

Mediators

Mediators are a group of chemicals, proteins and enzymes that orchestrate the internal defences. They are present at all times in the body but are inactive until the inflammatory or immune system is triggered. Included in this group are interferon, tumour necrosis factor and the interleukins.

Immunoglobulins

Immunoglobulins are protein molecules, known as antibodies, of which there are five different types—IgG, IgM, IgA, IgE and IgD. They have four functions:

- to attack antigens directly, leading to destruction by agglutination, neutralising antigenic substances and lysing the antigen's cell wall
- to activate the complement system
- to activate the inflammatory reaction by histamine release
- to stimulate antibody-mediated hypersensitivity.

Maternal antibodies

These antibodies are passed from mother to child via the placenta and in breast milk. They give protection to newborn infants until their own immune systems are able to develop antibodies on exposure to microorganisms. At birth, the child has the same level of IgG as the mother. The level declines over the following months and the antibodies disappear within 14 months of age. This influences the immunisation programme, i.e. maternal measles antibody remains in the body for several months, providing protection until the time that MMR is given (see Ch. 2 for immunisation schedules).

Response to invasion by microorganisms

The first reaction is the inflammatory response, and it is followed by the immune response.

Inflammatory response

The inflammatory response has three stages.

Cell response. The cell swells and can no longer carry out its normal function, atrophy occurs and it dies. This then stimulates the inflammatory response in surrounding tissues.

Vascular response. Dilatation of blood vessels leads to increased permeability, and fluid

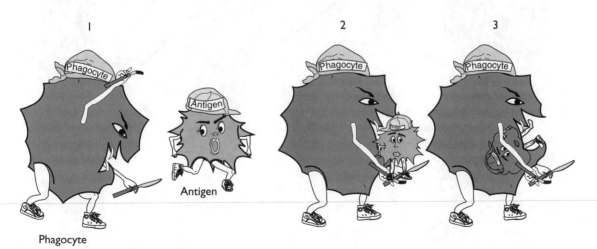

Figure 19.2 Phagocytosis.

leaks into the tissues, causing oedema. This attracts phagocytic cells to the site.

Phagocytosis. Initially, this occurs locally, but if the infection is systemic, it occurs in the lymph and blood systems (Fig. 19.2).

The pattern of inflammation is of heat, swelling and redness caused by vascular injury. Pain occurs, due to pressure on nerve endings by the exudate, which can be clear but may become purulent with dead leucocytes and microorganisms.

The outcome depends on several factors, e.g. age, nutritional status, general health and the virulence of the microorganism. These lead to the next reaction.

Immune response

This is the only response that is specific to the invading organism. It has the following characteristics:

- It differentiates between host and antigen.
- There are specific antibodies for specific antigens.
- It has a memory, thereby allowing a quicker future response.
- It is self-regulating, turning itself off when infection is eradicated.

The immune response has three stages.

Cell-mediated stage. This is directed by all the types of T cells that are activated by the antigenic material released by the action of phagocytes, with the assistance of the mediators.

Humoral response. This response is antibody mediated, and is initiated in two ways (Fig. 19.3):

- The antigen binds to T cells, and the helper T cells will then stimulate B cells.
- Some antigens will directly stimulate B cells into action. The B cells differentiate into plasma cells which produce the specific antibody.

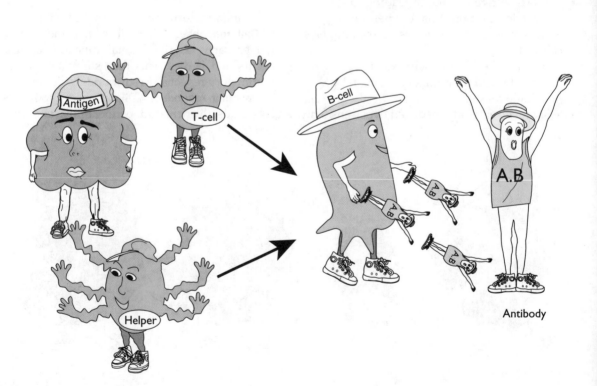

Figure 19.3 Antibody production.

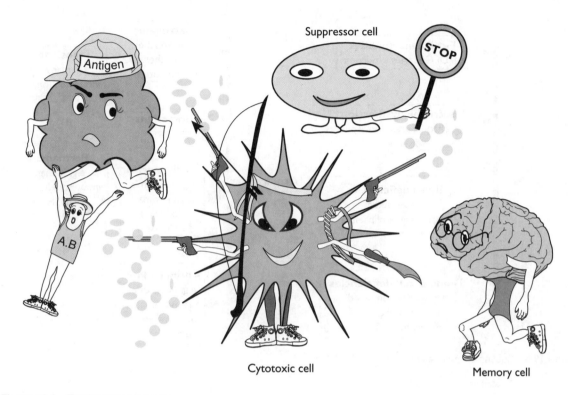

Figure 19.4 The immune response.

The antibody appears on the plasma cell surface and eradicates the antigen by its own action and that of the cytotoxic T cells and phagocytes. The suppresser T cells then halt the immune response when the antigen is destroyed (Fig. 19.4).

Immunological memory. Once the immune system has been exposed to an antigen, the memory B cells retain an immunological memory of the antigen for several years. This enables the antibody response time following future exposure to be considerably reduced. The reaction time (time taken to produce an adequate serum antibody titre) is reduced from 10–14 days on initial exposure to 2–4 days on future exposure.

Immunity

Immunity occurs when specific antibodies are present in the body in sufficient amounts to prevent successful invasion by a specific pathogen. It is gained in four ways:

Natural	Passive	from mother
	Active	from exposure to pathogen
Artificial	Passive	from serum or antibodies
	Active	from vaccine or toxoid.

THE IMMUNE DEFICIENT CHILD

When the immune system does not function correctly, then a child is known as immune deficient. Immune deficiency is caused by a variety of conditions (see Fig. 19.5), and may give rise to many problems for affected children as they become susceptible to disease. Understanding how the immune system works enables us to plan care for an immune deficient child more effectively.

Haematological changes

Normal haematological values for different ages are given in Table 19.1. The immune deficient child has an abnormal blood picture, and can

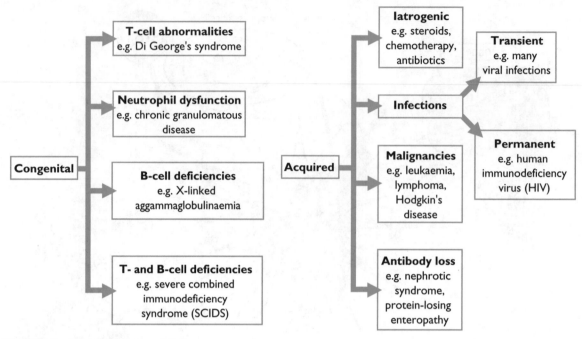

Figure 19.5   Causes of immune deficiency.

become neutropenic, thrombocytopenic or anaemic as a result either of the underlying condition or of its treatment.

- Neutropenia leads to an increased susceptibility to infection and, therefore, strict preventive measures are instituted (see below).
- Thrombocytopenia leads to a derangement of blood coagulation, and so the risk becomes that of haemorrhage, which may be minor or life-threatening.
- Anaemia causes a variety of problems, poor carriage of oxygen around the body leading to tiredness, dyspnoea and paleness. To treat this, blood transfusions are often required. The blood needs to be screened to prevent passive transmission of cytomegalovirus. During the transfusion, the nurse observes for any adverse reaction, by monitoring the child's temperature, pulse, respirations and blood pressure. Procedures for the frequency of these observations vary from hospital to hospital and local policy should be observed.

A deviation from the pre-transfusion baseline observations may denote a transfusion reaction.

Infection

Fighting infection is the function of the immune system. If this defence is altered in any way then infection becomes a key concern. It is the primary cause of mortality in an immune deficient person. The immune deficient child is susceptible to two types of infection:

- common infections—these become more severe in a child that is unable to fight infections effectively
- opportunistic infections—these are infections that are caused by organisms that would not normally produce any disease process or illness (Table 19.2).

There are two main areas of care with regard to infection:

Table 19.1 Biochemical and physiological tables and functional tests 1989: normal haematological values (all values shown are means with the ranges in parentheses) (adapted from Forfar & Arneil 1992)

Age	Haemoglobin (g/100 ml)	White blood cells per litre	Neutrophils %	Lymphocytes %	Platelets per litre	per mm3
Birth	17 (14–20)	18×10^9 (9–30×10^9)	60 (40–80)	32	100×10^9 300×10^9	100 000 300 000
1 week	17 (13–21)	12×10^9 (6–22×10^9)	39 (30–50)	46		
2 weeks	16.5 (13–20)	12×10^9 (5–21×10^9)	40 (30–50)	48		
6 months to 6 years	12 (10.5–14)	10×10^9 (6–15×10^9)	42 (32–52)	51	150×10^9	150 000
Adult F	14 (12–16)	7.5×10^9 (5–10×10^9)	60 (40–75)	30 (20–45)		
M	16 (14–18)					

- prevention of infection, and this is the prime goal (see p. 324)
- treatment of the infection.

Table 19.2 Common opportunistic infections causing severe and disseminated diseases

Organism	Treatment
Aspergillus sp.	Amphotericin B
Candida sp.	Fluconazole Ketaconazole Amphotericin B
Cryptococcus sp.	Amphotericin B Fluconazole
Cryptosporidium sp.	? Paromamycin—no sure treatment identified
Cytomegalovirus	Gancyclovir Foscarnet
Non-TB mycobacteria	Rifabutin Azithromycin Ciprofloxacin Septrin Amikacin
Pneumocystis carinii	Co-trimoxazole Dapsone Pentamidine
Toxoplasma sp.	Sulphadiazine Pyrimethamine

Treatment of infection

As infection can be life-threatening, early detection is essential so that effective treatment can be commenced as soon as possible. Early detection relies on observation for the symptoms associated with an infection by monitoring the child's temperature, looking for fevers, sweats or rigors.

The pulse will usually increase at the time the child has a temperature, as will the respiratory rate. The respiratory pattern may also alter, i.e. there may be cough, grunting, wheeze, or dyspnoea. The child's behaviour will also give a good indication of the start of an infection; she may be withdrawn, showing signs of general malaise and lethargic. There may also be generalised aches and pains, headaches, nausea, loss of appetite, vomiting, diarrhoea, weight loss and at times confusion or delirium. Any of these symptoms should be reported so that the cause can be investigated and appropriate treatment commenced immediately.

The advances in pharmacology have been such that there are a great number of new drugs to treat infections. It is now possible to fight bacteria, viruses, fungi, and protozoa (see Table 19.2), albeit these may have many side effects. These side effects can sometimes make the immune deficiency greater; for example a side effect of co-trimoxazole is neutropenia. In addition, the drugs often require special recipes for their reconstitution using specific fluids to make them stable. It is imperative that nurses are fully trained in the administration of these medications and have literature available at all times, to ensure safe treatment of the child.

 For further reading refer to ABP1 Data Sheet Compendium 1992–1993 with the Code of Practice for Pharmaceutical Industry.

Investigations.   These are varied and include swabs from any possible site of infection, e.g. nose, throat, ear, etc. Secretions are obtained from the lungs as either a sputum specimen or nasopharyngeal aspirate. X-rays may be performed, and urine and stool cultures obtained. Venepuncture occurs to assess the child's blood picture: blood cultures are used to look for infection; a full blood count monitors white cell numbers; the level of c-reactive protein is assessed; and the erythrocyte-sedimentation rate measured. Any elevation in the rate of erythrocyte sedimentation indicates that the body is responding to an infection. All samples taken will be cultured for all types of infecting organism, which will ensure that the correct treatment is administered to the child.

Nutrition

A balanced diet is particularly important for the immune deficient child. An already damaged immune system requires nutrients to build, maintain and allow it to function and the child also requires nutrients to grow and develop normally. To gain a balanced diet is not as easy as it may at first appear, as many factors hinder the intake and absorption of nutrients.

The immune deficient child has specific problems but also goes through stages similar to any other child, such as having food fads. The child may enjoy a food one day and hate it the next, may not like vegetables or only eat sweet things.

This can be a problem in any child but for a child who has increased nutritional requirements the problem is greater.

It is important to help such children to enjoy food by making it fun; this can be done by playing with food, providing foods they like, making food attractive or allowing them to prepare it. These are all good ways of helping children to eat a range of foods that contain various nutrients.

Infections can lead to a decrease in dietary intake. The mouth may be sore, or oesophagitis may develop making it impossible to swallow. Pneumonia leads to tiredness and breathlessness, making eating difficult. A viral or bacterial gastroenteritis may develop, with eating making the diarrhoea worse or causing nausea. Even if the child is eating a nutritious diet, malabsorption, which may occur with diarrhoea (Guarino 1993), is still a problem. The treatment itself may lead to a loss of appetite, with nausea and vomiting often being induced by chemotherapy or by the methods used to treat the underlying conditions. With any of these, the child cannot or will not eat. This is a dilemma for the carers, because this is the time that the child requires more nutrients and calories to enable the body to fight infection and allow healing of damaged tissue.

There are many interventions that can be carried out to overcome these problems. The child can be offered high-calorie foods and drinks, using supplements and snacks. A milk-based diet can be given via a nasogastric or gastrostomy tube. The type of milk depends on the child's requirements and may include protein- and calorie-rich fluids such as lactulose-reduced formula (Leung 1989). Total parenteral nutrition may be required either as a short-term intervention to boost the child's intake or as a long-term method of feeding.

The multidisciplinary team is of major importance in dealing with this area of care. The dietitian, pharmacist, speech therapists and physiotherapists are essential, and all are trained in areas required to assist with the giving of a balanced diet.

This is an area that often upsets parents; it is the one part of the care that they feel responsible for and they see any problem as a failure by themselves. Communication and rapport with the dietitian is essential, as she will coordinate any intervention required by the whole multi-disciplinary team.

Hygiene

To a child who is susceptible to infections, maintaining the body's natural defences is essential, with the effects of the disease process making this maintenance more of a battle. The skin and mucosal areas are the first line of defence, and good hygiene around these areas may help to alleviate the child's suffering.

Skin care

When bathing the child, ensure that a gentle soap is used on what can be fragile skin, and take care to dry the skin thoroughly; good drying prevents abrasions, redness and soreness. Observing the child's skin at regular intervals enables the carer to detect early signs of skin problems.

The rectal mucosal and nappy area is the site that is most often at risk, due to the frequency of the washes required, the wearing of nappies, the many episodes of diarrhoea, and infections that may occur from the gastrointestinal tract. Observation of the area, changing nappies regularly, washing the area thoroughly, and using barrier creams can help to prevent skin breakdown. In the event of breakdown, use a cream to treat the cause, e.g. nystatin for candidiasis, and keep the area dry. Exposing the area to air will assist with drying and healing of the skin.

Having sore, infected or broken areas of skin is a big discomfort for a child, and this is one of the major and often most frequent problems an immune deficient child will have to face. Prevention, early detection and swift treatment can, therefore, prevent many hours of distress.

Mouth care

The oral mucosa is susceptible to breakdown, and good oral hygiene is essential. Regular visits to the dentist to maintain healthy teeth and gums, observation of the mouth for signs of ulceration and development of an opportunistic infection such as candidiasis, are good preventive measures. Regular brushing with a toothbrush to remove debris is essential. Often, these measures are used in conjunction with an antifungal medication as prophylaxis. If the mouth becomes infected, then the cause needs to be treated. The mouth care regime becomes more regimented, with frequent mouth washes, which ensure that the cavity remains moist. The use of foam swabs alone, however, is ineffective for removal of debris (Howarth 1977) and a toothbrush should also be used. The frequency of the regime depends on the carer's assessment of each child (Millinson 1991).

Isolation

The child with a deficient immune system is susceptible to infection at all times. When the neutrophil count is low, protective precautions need to be even more stringent, and the child is placed in protective isolation (see p. 329). This isolation causes specific problems, socially, emotionally and physically.

How much understanding children have of the reasons for their isolation depends on their age. Younger children may perceive it as a punishment and need constant reassurance and support (Whaley & Wong 1985). Their understanding of the need to stay in the isolation room is limited and active toddlers may run out as a game, making constant supervision necessary. Any explanations required need to be geared to a level the child understands and given repeatedly. If children are older, their understanding is greater but they may feel that their developing

Activity 19.1

How would you manage a child admitted to the ward with diarrhoea of undiagnosed cause?

autonomy and independence have been halted and may rebel (Bater 1989). Allowing children to control their care by letting them plan and carry out procedures such as mouth care may help. Adolescents, who may have been administering many medications and intravenous drugs themselves prior to hospitalisation, should be allowed to continue this practice. This will give children or adolescents control over their lives and will assist with cooperation (Shelley 1993).

Preparation for isolation is essential, as at some point it will occur in the child's treatment. Play preparation with masks, gowns and many aspects of care is vital for all children but especially the young child. Stories putting the child's favourite character in the position of requiring isolation increase understanding and acceptance. The older child and adolescents require more in-depth and often technical explanations. Allowing them to ask questions and giving prompt, careful and honest answers will ensure understanding and will help to gain cooperation in the care required.

Visits to the unit and isolation room are also effective in accustoming children and their families to what will become home for a period of time. Allowing children of any age to decorate the isolation room with pictures and bring cards, audio equipment or computer games will make them feel that it is an extension of their home. Calling the isolation room their bedroom makes it less threatening, while rules such as keeping their room tidy need to be enforced, giving them the responsibility to maintain it as they would at home.

Boredom is a prime complaint about being isolated with the minimum of visitors. Developing a routine and timetable for activities is often a good way to fill a child's day, and schooling and play time are essential components. Activities should be stimulating and appropriate to the child's age.

The development of anyone in isolation can be stunted, no matter what their age. Stimulation is essential, be it visual or tactile. Rooms with windows so that the child can observe life on the outside enable the child to develop socially (Fonger et al 1987). Direct touch is often a

Case study 19.1 Jessica

Jessica who is 2½ years old has acute lymphoblastic leukaemia and is undergoing chemotherapy (Fig. 19.6). She has a mother, father and a 5-year-old brother. She has become neutropenic during chemotherapy, which has caused her to:

a. require isolation
b. develop an opportunistic infection with *Candida albicans* in her mouth.

Her problems are that:

• she is isolated in a cubicle and requires stimulation with play and visitors
• she has a sore mouth and is not able to drink or eat; she is therefore losing weight and is requiring an intravenous infusion via a Hickman line to maintain her fluid balance
• her brother has chickenpox and is unable to visit, causing her great distress.

problem, with carers not wanting to increase the risk of cross-infection. If correct procedures are followed (see p. 329), this is not a problem and cuddling and handling is encouraged to prevent sensory deprivation, which often manifests itself in emotional distress and bad behaviour (Fonger et al 1987). The child may regress to gain more parental attention and support during this stressful time.

Drug therapy

Immune depressed children will require long-term drug therapy, taking medication every day of their lives. Drugs may be oral or intravenous and can be toxic; they can actually inhibit the immune system further.

Getting into a routine with medication is important, and maintaining this routine when the child is admitted to hospital is essential. As children develop, their acceptance of the medication may alter and daily battles may ensue to get them to take their medication. Older children may simply refuse to take it and insist on rationalisation of their regime.

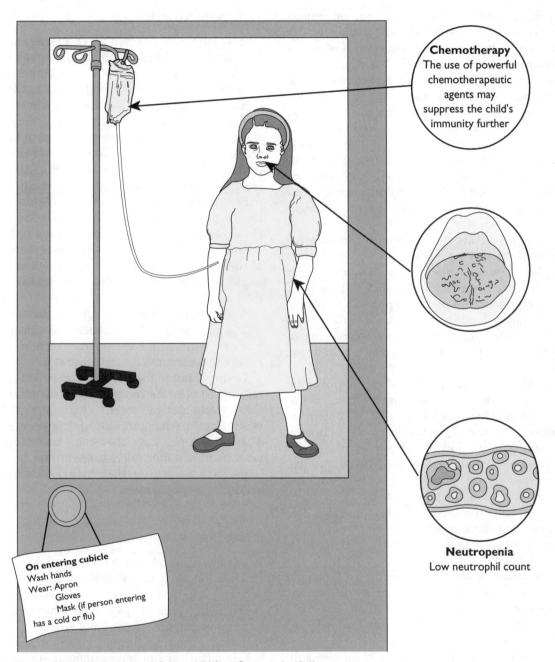

Figure 19.6 Care of the immune deficient child (see Case study 19.1).

If the medication has to be given intravenously, then frequent venepuncture will be needed. Venepuncture is traumatic for any child, but when it has to occur often, it becomes more difficult, and phobias often develop. Therefore the use of central access is preferred for long-term patients, either via a Port-a-Cath or central venous catheter. Using a catheter avoids the use of a needle to puncture the skin and is often the preferred method of access for the younger child (Sepion 1990). The teenager, however, may be less concerned about skin puncture and prefer the Port-a-Cath as there are no tubes to compromise body image. The decision over access is made with the parents and the child. Both types enable blood to be taken easily and medication or feeding to be given over long periods without damaging peripheral veins. Careful management with regard to cleaning of the site is important, as infection is a risk.

The drugs are often immunosuppressive themselves, placing extra strain on an already depleted system, while a medication for another condition, e.g. organ transplantation, may itself be the prime cause of that suppression (Dannie 1993). Often the drugs can be toxic to the child's liver or renal function, so close monitoring of levels is essential to maintain effective and safe treatment.

Giving the parents and the child control of the administration, be it oral or intravenous, is important for the continuation of treatment at home. Education about the drugs, the technique of giving them, and the principles of asepsis, especially if central access is involved, is vital. Supervision and support are critical and the assumption should not be made that the mother or child will want to have this responsibility. The whole procedure involves constant autonomy and safe administration (Charles-Edwards & Casey 1992).

Phobias and non-compliance can be overcome by play therapy and games. Clear explanations and honesty about the medication and how long the child will have to take it will aid understanding.

Administering medication is often the only treatment for many of the conditions that cause immunosuppression. It is essential, therefore, that safe, correct administration occurs in both the hospital and home environment. To achieve this, parental and child support is of paramount importance.

Hospitalisation

Immune deficient children are chronically ill and will require continual care throughout their lives or until the cause is treated. These children will, therefore, need repeated hospital admissions, for minor day care or because they are acutely unwell and when they are undergoing treatment. It is important that they are made to feel at home, are comfortable in the environment and that the environment caters for their interests and needs. Having named nurses and doctors for each patient is important to maintain continuity and the development of interpersonal relationships. However, in reality this is not always possible because of staff movements, but senior members of the team, who are more stable in where they work, become important links for children and their families.

Good communication is vital to convey the child's and family's likes and needs to colleagues. The care required for each particular admission must also be accurately communicated.

Giving children their usual room or bed-space on admission is often comforting as they feel that they belong and can treat it like home. This is reassuring in what can, despite experience, be a stressful time, since they may be unsure of what treatment they will require or may have to undergo a procedure that they are unhappy about, e.g. venepuncture.

Social/peer isolation

Repeated hospital admissions and having a chronic illness lead to disruption of normal social life and development of relationships with peers. Being able to play with other children accustoms the pre-school child to the rules of society, e.g. sharing, forming relationships with non-family members, independence and playing out situations. The risk of cross-infection from peers and protectiveness by families often leads the child to miss out on this area of development. The multidisciplinary team can help to minimise the effects during hospitalisation.

At school, peers become more important and

special friendships develop. With the need to be careful in their activities and the repeated need for hospitalisation, children may feel left out of events. They may worry that their friends may forget them or make other special friends. Visits during periods of hospitalisation are important, as are cards, letters and tapes from school. The teacher or parents can be the liaison for this activity.

For the teenager, the peer group becomes an increasingly important influence on what to do and say, and how to behave. Girlfriends and boyfriends are new concepts and, if the teenager is not present at all times, these normal relationships can fail to develop. Body image and the acceptance of peers are an important part of life. Teenagers may have muscle wasting or alopecia which detract from their body image (Evans 1992) and thus their social standing. Support by peers and the multidisciplinary team is essential to assist them through a difficult period of development.

Education

Missing any time at school can be disruptive and harmful to a child's education. For children who are repeatedly away from school, however, there is an even greater effect on their whole life.

Protection from infections is a vital area in caring for the immune deficient child. The school, where many infections are prevalent, is a dangerous environment. Chickenpox, a common childhood disease, can have a devastating effect on an immune deficient child, who should not attend school if there is any chance of contacting it. This can have serious effects on education, and school work should be sent home to ensure that the child's learning is continual and on a parallel with that of her peers.

During hospital admissions, the maintenance of appropriate schoolwork is essential, as a child may spend many months as an inpatient. Attending the hospital schoolroom to carry out work sent in by her own school should be part of the child's daily routine. Teenagers should continue with work from the same curriculum as their peers, which will prevent isolation and

their falling behind in their course work. It will also enable them to gain qualifications to carry on to adult life (Evans 1992).

Family support

The social, emotional and financial effects on the family are immense. The time that children spend in hospital, or at home when unable to go to school or play group, can be prolonged. These periods often require supervision by a parent, who is therefore prevented from working. Social workers have long been part of the multidisciplinary team and provide expert advice and guidance on what benefits the family may be entitled to claim in order to minimise the financial effects.

Along with the financial problems of not working, there may be feelings of social isolation for the parent whose life revolves totally around the sick child. This in turn puts pressure on the partner and any siblings. Family life can become disrupted with the hospital becoming its centre. Family units such as a Ronald McDonald house (and other similar charitable programmes) are vital to provide a home-like environment and some form of normality. This is especially important if the family live a large distance from the hospital.

Siblings may feel isolated, neglected and forgotten by the other family members. This may lead to regression in behaviour or disruptive episodes occurring to gain attention. The siblings' relationship with their brother or sister may also change; often their attitude is one of anger, but in some cases a sibling may become the carer (Hewitt 1990).

Allowing the extended family, including siblings, to plan, implement and take part in any decisions regarding treatment gives them ownership and control of their child's care. It prevents a feeling of loss and inadequacy when the child is admitted to hospital. Good communication is the essential component in supporting the family and preventing such problems (Fonger et al 1987).

The stress on family life is immeasurable for those caring for a child who has a life-threatening illness, and this often manifests itself in family arguments. Allowing privacy and being aware that arguments can occur, answering questions and listening are all measures that may alleviate some of these stresses. Social isolation for the whole family may result from the fear of society's reaction to their child's diagnosis. They may feel unable to talk to their friends or even to their own extended family. The multidisciplinary team then takes on the role of adviser, listener, source of information and supporter.

Immunisation

The recommendations for an immune deficient child with regard to immunisation are that the child should receive the normal programme with some added precautions. The child should be given inactive vaccines, as the effects of active vaccines cannot be predicted. The immune response requires monitoring as it may not be as effective and full immunity may not be produced.

There are precautions to be taken in respect of siblings, in that active polio vaccine should not be administered to them as this can be transmitted to their immune suppressed sibling.

The use of ZIG or hyperimmune globulin on exposure to chickenpox or measles is advised as prophylaxis. This may not produce an effective immune response, however, and, if the disease develops, treatment should be commenced, e.g. with acyclovir for chickenpox. Acyclovir may also be used as prophylaxis.

Dying

Many of the causes of immune suppression are life-threatening conditions and therefore children have to come to terms with the fact that they may die. Some children are not aware of the consequences of their condition, through either lack of understanding or their parents being unable to tell them that they may or will die.

Supporting the parents at this time is important in coming to terms with this issue. Giving them time to talk, listening, being honest and truthful with answers, all help at this difficult time. Parents often need advice on what to say and how to say it, and just talking them through helps. A non-judgemental attitude is imperative, with sensitive handling of all issues.

Kubler-Ross (1993) identified five stages of dying: denial; anger; bargaining; depression; and acceptance. These will be experienced by all concerned: the children, their families and their siblings. Allowing time for these stages to occur and having some control over the event if and when it is inevitable is important. Issues of where they will die and be buried, and who will have their favourite toys and possessions are all areas that can be addressed and may help in the grieving process. Making a will, writing letters or completing a memory box like the one designed by Barnardo's may help the child. If children are able to do certain things that they have always wished to do, e.g. have a special holiday, this may let them feel in control, while having the knowledge that they will be remembered and that their lives were worthwhile (see Ch. 27).

NURSING MEASURES TO PREVENT INFECTION WHEN NURSING CHILDREN

When caring for a child in either the community or the hospital environment, there are many procedures that can be taken to prevent infection. Children are more susceptible hosts than adults as they may not have completed the immunisation programme or have immunity. There are three principles in the control and prevention of infection:

- eliminating the source of the infection
- halting transmission
- promoting the child's resistance to the infection.

Major areas of prevention and control of infection

Hand washing

One of the most important vehicles in the transmission of infection is the hands, be they of the carer, family members, or hospital staff (Ayliffe et al 1992). Hand washing, if done correctly, proves to be the single most important method of preventing infection.

There are two types of organism that may colonise hands: resident organisms and transient organisms. Resident organisms consitute the normal flora of the hands. Transient organisms are by far the most important type with regard to infection control. They are picked up from other children, equipment or the environment and are passed from child to child.

Many studies (Gidley 1987) prove that technique and frequency of hand washing remain poor despite education. The common areas that are missed during hand washing are the tips of the fingers, the thumbs, the wrist, the palms and the backs of the hands (see Fig. 19.7). It is recognised that a standardised method of hand washing should be adopted by nurses and other health professionals.

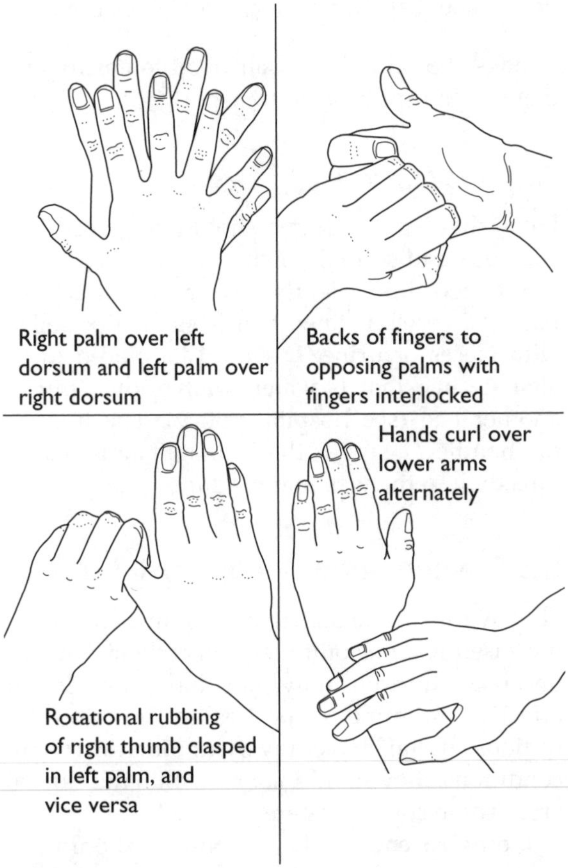

Frequency of hand washing is also a problem. There must be a balance between the appropriate number of washes and an amount that is excessive in that it may cause skin damage, which in itself increases the risk of colonisation by pathogens (see Table 19.2). Appropriate quality of hand washing is, therefore, essential.

What hand washing agent is required is a question that is frequently asked. The answer is that soap and water are effective and appropriate for general purposes. Specialist units such as intensive care areas and infectious disease units require special cleaning solutions (see Table 19.3).

Many reasons are put forward for poor hand washing practices. Training and education are often cited as reasons, as are lack of motivation and availability of appropriate facilities. To promote good practices, an environment that has the correct cleaning solutions available, an appropriate number of sinks with elbow-operated taps, hand towels, hand creams and foot-operated bins is needed. The practitioners should be actively encouraged to carry out effective hand washing practices by managers and peers.

General advice is that hands should be washed:

- at the beginning of a shift
- before and after all patient contact
- before giving medication
- before handling food
- after using the toilet
- after all procedures, e.g. changing nappies, giving bed pans.

Right palm over left dorsum and left palm over right dorsum

Backs of fingers to opposing palms with fingers interlocked

Hands curl over lower arms alternately

Rotational rubbing of right thumb clasped in left palm, and vice versa

Figure 19.7   Hand washing procedures: areas most often missed.

Protective clothing

Gloves.   These should be worn when handling body fluids and blood. They should be changed between patients and should *never* be washed and re-used. On removal of gloves, hands should still be washed, as gloves may be damaged, and the removal technique is not always correct, allowing organisms to contaminate the carer's hands. The practice of wearing gloves combined with effective hand washing has been shown to provide carers and children with greater protection from infection (Linden 1991).

Masks. Masks are used to protect the patient and carer from infections that are transmitted by the respiratory route. However, many research projects have highlighted the fact that they actually offer little protection. Wearing masks will, however, reduce the risk of bacterial spread from the mouth. Filter-type masks should be used in barrier nursing to protect the carer or patient from respiratory infections. They should always be changed if they become moist or the wearer coughs or sneezes (Ayliffe et al 1992).

Gowns. It has often been common practice in protective units to wear gowns when dealing with babies and children who are at-risk, to prevent transmission of infection. However, this is a ritual that various studies have proved to be ineffectual (Larson 1987). The use of plastic aprons, however, is a precaution that can be taken when carrying out practices in which the carer's clothes may become infected, or when carrying out aseptic procedures. They are easy to use, sensible as they are water resistant, and impermeable to organisms. When working with babies, however, remember that plastic aprons are slippery.

It is advised that all protective clothing is discarded when the patient's needs have been attended to; this prevents it from becoming a source of cross-infection (Griffiths-Jones & Ward 1995).

Activity 19.2

For what specific conditions would you wear a face mask?

Disposal procedures

Disposal of waste

The guidelines for disposal of waste are set by the Department of Health (Health and Safety Commission 1982).

- Yellow bags—always incinerated and are for clinical waste, i.e. human tissue and waste that has body secretions on it, for example dressings and nappies. They need to be clearly coded and tied securely.
- Black bags—disposed of in a landfill site. They are for domestic waste, i.e. paper and kitchen waste.
- Sharps bins—for the disposal of sharps and broken glass (see regional policy).
- Cardboard box—aerosol cans, china and bottles can be disposed of in clearly labelled boxes.

Bags should only be half-filled to ensure that there are no spillages in transport.

Disposal of linen

Linen that is not infected should be placed in a clear bag and securely tied.

Infected linen is that from an infectious patient as well as linen that is stained or soiled with faeces or urine. It should be placed in an alginate bag that is water soluble, then put in another bag (see hospital policy). The linen is not handled again as the alginate bag is placed directly into the washing machine.

Staff—when should they work?

Staff within a paediatric environment have an increased responsibility to protect their patients, because children may not have developed effective immune responses to common infections. If staff have any symptoms of certain conditions, they should not be within the clinical area. These conditions are:

Diarrhoea and vomiting. Nurses should not be on duty if they have these symptoms, and should go home if symptoms develop whilst at

Table 19.3 Cleaning solutions: their actions and uses

Cleaning solution	Microbiological action	Use
Detergent		General cleaning
Chlorine-releasing agents, e.g. Milton, Presept	Gram +ve bacteria Gram −ve bacteria Viruses ⎫ Some ⎬ action is related to the concentration spores ⎭ of the solution	Blood spillage Stool spillage Decontamination Feed bottles Hydrotherapy pools NB: can bleach carpet—do not use on urine spills
Clear soluble phenolic compound, Hycolin 1.5%	Gram +ve bacteria Gram −ve bacteria TB Viruses—equivocal	Food spillage Urine spillage Decontamination
Chlorhexidine gluconate 4%, Hibiscrub	Gram +ve bacteria To a lesser extent Gram −ve bacteria	Skin disinfection only
Isopropyl alcohol 60–70%	Gram +ve bacteria Gram −ve bacteria	Rapid disinfection of smooth surfaces

work. If the symptoms continue (see hospital policy), they should consult their GP or occupational health officer to obtain stool specimens and exclude bacterial poisoning.

Sore throat. Severe sore throats with fever may be caused by group A streptococci and require immediate swabbing. Antibiotics should be recommended and staff should not return to work until at least 48 hours after treatment is commenced.

Infectious lesions. Staff with an infected cut or boil need to see their occupational health department. Swabs will be taken and a decision about returning to work will be made. Special care is required if lesions are on the face or hands. If the nurse is allowed to work, cuts need to be covered by waterproof plasters.

Cold sores. A cold sore is caused by herpes simplex virus; staff should not work in any

paediatric environment until the sore has crusted over and dried.

Common childhood diseases (i.e. chickenpox, measles). Immunity can be detected by a blood test. Staff members who are not immune and have been exposed to the illness should not be at work in any area during the infectious period. Different hospitals may require different periods of absence; therefore, consultation of the infection control team is essential.

Head lice. Once treatment has commenced, then staff may work.

Scabies. Staff can work 24 hours after commencement of treatment.

Infection control team

This is a team of staff who are specially trained in microbiology and infection control; it will include doctors and nurses. They provide a variety of services, monitoring infections and outbreaks and giving advice on isolation and nursing care. They are an information source on any infection control matters, and are involved in staff education and the provision of written guidelines and policies.

Activity 19.3

What precautions would you take with your staff if they were caring for a child with chickenpox?

Decontamination

Cleaning. Washing with hot soapy water will remove most organisms from a surface. It will allow for more effective disinfecting and sterilisation as it removes dirt (for cleaning solutions, see Table 19.3).

Disinfection. Treatment with either heat or chemicals will remove vegetative microorganisms and viruses, but not necessarily spores or 'slow' viruses. In a paediatric environment, the commonly used disinfection technique is the use of Milton solution for babies' bottles (for cleaning solutions, see Table 19.3).

Sterilisation. This enables the complete killing of all organisms and spores, and can be carried out by heat, e.g. autoclaving, steam, or by chemicals.

Box 19.2   Notifiable diseases in England and Wales

- Acute encephalitis
- Acute poliomyelitis
- Anthrax
- Cholera
- Diphtheria
- Dysentery
- Food poisoning (or suspected)
- Lassa fever
- Leprosy
- Malaria
- Measles
- Meningococcal septicaemia (without meningitis)
- Meningitis
- Mumps
- Ophthalmis neonatorum
- Paratyphoid fever
- Plague
- Rabies
- Relapsing fever
- Rubella
- Scarlet fever
- Smallpox
- Tetanus
- Tuberculosis
- Typhoid fever
- Typhus
- Viral haemorrhagic fever
- Viral hepatitis
- Whooping cough
- Yellow fever

Aseptic technique

Aseptic technique is a method devised to prevent the contamination of wounds and other sites (e.g. Hickman entry sites), or as protection from infection during a procedure (e.g. catheterisation). Hospitals have their own methods of aseptic technique and these should be consulted. The principle is one of non-touch using forceps or using sterile gloves to clean or carry out the procedures involved.

Notifiable diseases

Some diseases are notifiable by law to the consultant in communicable diseases control (see Box 19.2.). There are slight differences between England and Wales, Scotland and Northern Ireland. This notification allows for monitoring of the frequency and existence of these diseases. The Public Health Department is also informed and will carry out contact tracing and give appropriate advice about prophylaxis. This includes risk areas in schools, play groups and any friends of the child concerned.

Isolation

Isolation has two functions:

- to protect other children and staff from infection
- to protect the child who is susceptible to infection from the environment.

The type of isolation depends on the microorganism involved and how it is spread.

Each hospital has its own isolation protocols (for general precautions, see Box 19.3).

Family education

This is ongoing and is emphasised by all health professionals who are in contact with the family. These include the GP, health visitor, midwife and school nurse. It occurs in a variety of forms with families gaining individual advice from professionals or acquiring information through health promotion campaigns in their health centres. The

Box 19.3   Isolation—general precautions

Protective isolation
Rationale: to protect the susceptible child, i.e. one who is neutropenic

- Isolate patient with door shut, preferably with positive pressure inside the room.
- Gloves and plastic aprons are to be worn when in isolation rooms.
- No persons should enter the isolation room if they have a cold or flu unless it is *absolutely* necessary, i.e. they are parents or key professional staff.
- Filter masks are to be worn on entering by those who have a cold or flu.
- Hands should be washed thoroughly and protective clothing put on before entering room.
- On leaving the room, the protective clothing is removed and hands washed.

Wound/skin precautions
Rationale: the patient has a wound or skin infection

- Gloves and plastic aprons must be worn when changing the wound dressing, in contact with the patient's skin or handling the patient's linen.
- Remove protective clothing when procedure is finished and wash hands with antiseptic hand scrub, e.g. Hibiscrub.
- Dispose of soiled dressing materials into a yellow bag for clinical waste.
- Use an occlusive dressing where possible if a wound is infected.
- Isolation is often recommended.

Respiratory route infection
Rationale: the patient has an infection that is transmitted by the respiratory route

- Isolate the patient with the door shut.
- Gloves and plastic aprons are to be worn when in contact with contaminated items or secretions.
- Masks are to be worn for the infectious period of certain infections, such as pulmonary TB and meningococcal meningitis (see hospital policy).

- Remove protective clothing before leaving the room and wash hands carefully with an antiseptic hand scrub, e.g. Hibiscrub.
- Linen is considered infected and should be placed in an alginate bag inside a linen bag (see hospital policy).
- Sputum and used tissues must be incinerated.
- Restrict staff/visitor entry to room to those who are not susceptible.

Urine precautions
Rationale: the patient has an infection passed by urine

- Disposable latex gloves and an apron must be worn when in contact with the patient's urine, urinary catheter or items contaminated with urine.
- Remove protective clothing when procedure is finished and wash hands with antiseptic hand scrub, e.g. Hibiscrub.
- Any piece of equipment contaminated with urine must be decontaminated before re-use. Jugs, if used, should be heat decontaminated in a bedpan washer, or single-use items.
- For spillage use a phenolic agent, not one that releases chlorine as this reacts with the urine and can produce toxic fumes.

Stool precautions
Rationale: the patient has an infection passed via the stool

- Isolate the patient if diarrhoea is present.
- Disposable latex gloves and plastic aprons are to be worn when in direct contact with the patient or items soiled with faeces.
- Remove protective clothing before leaving the isolation room and wash hands with antiseptic hand scrub, e.g. Hibiscrub.
- The patient must have her own toilet facilities, or bedpans that are disposable are washed in a bedpan washing machine. If these are not available or there is a spillage, use a clear soluble phenolic or chlorine-releasing agent for disinfection.
- Consider linen infected if faecally soiled.
- Heat disinfect crockery/cutlery in a dishwasher.

---

use of school projects or lectures to the children can be helpful. Subject matter includes the need for a balanced diet, sterilisation of babies' feeding bottles, good hygiene, the immunisation schedule and mouth and dental care.

Environmental factors

The child's environment may carry potential hazards with regard to infection and there is

much that can be done to reduce the risk of infection.

Day nurseries/schools

The 1989 Children Act includes criteria that have knock-on effects for the control of infection. The requirement that there are separate rooms for babies and toddlers will reduce the risk of exposure to infection by babies with less-developed immune systems. The need for the staff to have awareness of child development will enable them to understand the risks for the young child. Continuity of staff will reduce the contacts by the children (Ross 1993).

Facilities, such as a separate kitchen where food may be prepared, and good cleaning or sterilisation of equipment and utensils are necessary. Adequate toilet and hand washing facilities that are appropriately sized for the child's ages are essential.

The attendance by children who are sick needs to be controlled. This can be a difficult area as often there are effects on the carer who has to work. However, good communication and understanding can enable a workable arrangement to be made for the child who is unwell.

The hospital

The child who is an inpatient will be a sick child and may well be susceptible to infection. There are many precautions that can be taken to prevent this. Correct isolation procedures need to be active. Young babies require nursing in a cubicle or can be in a communal area with other babies. Each hospital area will have its own protocols, and these should be consulted.

Facilities for hand washing and drying need to be appropriately placed and sufficient supplies of hand wash and towels are necessary. Taps need to be elbow operated and the bins must have a working foot pedal. The required disposal equipment, e.g. rubbish bags, needs to be regularly changed and supplied in appropriate amounts. The correct cleaning solutions are essential and need to be readily available. Domestic staff need to be aware of any requirements to follow during isolation procedures.

Preparation of feeds is often a problem, but with pre-packed bottled feeds the only requirement is for a clean storeroom. Where feeds are to be reconstituted, a milk kitchen is required for the sole use of feed preparation (Ayliffe 1992). Utensils need to be cleaned in hot soapy water and dried.

Staff in paediatric departments should be

Activity 19.4

Devise a nursing care plan for a 3-year-old child who is neutropenic. She has one sibling who is of school age.

screened for their immunity to childhood diseases, e.g. chickenpox and rubella, and immunisation may be indicated.

Toys

The cleaning of toys after use by a child who has an infection is vital to prevent cross-infection. Solid toys should be wiped over by the appropriate cleaning agent. Soft toys should be cleaned using hot, soapy water. Any toy that is heavily contaminated should be destroyed.

REFERENCES

Ayliffe G A J, Lowbury E J L, Geddes A M, Williams J D 1992 Control of hospital infection. A practical handbook, 3rd edn. Chapman & Hall Medical, London

Bater M 1989 Preparing for bone marrow transplantation. Nursing Times 85(7): 46–47

Charles-Edwards I, Casey A 1992 Parental involvement and voluntary consent. Paediatric Nursing 4(1): 16–18

Children Act 1989 HMSO, London

Dannie E 1993 Immunosuppressive agents. Nursing Times 89(4): 34–37

Evans R 1992 Child's play. Nursing Times 88(24): 63–67

Fonger P A, Hort E M, Karn J M, Shiflet J A, 1987 Nursing care of the child with severe combined immune deficiency. Journal of Paediatric Nursing 2(6): 373–380

Forfar J O, Arneil G C (eds) 1992 Textbook of paediatrics, 4th edn. Churchill Livingstone, Edinburgh

Gidley C 1987 Now, wash your hands! Nursing Times 83(29): 40–42

Griffiths-Jones A, Ward K (eds) 1995 Principles of infection control practice. Scutari Press, Harrow

Guarino A 1993 Intestinal malabsorption of HIV infected children: relationship to diarrhoea, failure to thrive, enteric micro-organisms and immune impairment. AIDS 7(11): 1435–1439

Health and Safety Commission 1982 The safe disposal of clinical waste. HMSO, London

Hewitt J 1990 The sibling response to hospitalisation. Paediatric Nursing 2(9): 12–13

Howarth H 1977 Mouthcare procedures for the very ill. Nursing Times (March)

Kubler-Ross 1993 On children and death. Collier Books, Macmillan, New York

Larson E 1987 Rituals in infection control: what works in a newborn nursery? Journal of Gynecological and Neonatal Nursing (Nov/Dec): 411–416

Leung D J 1989 An approach to feeding HIV infected infants and toddlers. Topics in Clinical Nutrition 4(4): 27–37

Linden B 1991 Protection in practice. Nursing Times 87(11): 59–63

Millinson K 1991 Taking care of John's mouth. Nursing Times 87(21): 34–35

Ross S 1993 Creche course in hygiene. Nursing Times 89(29): 59–60, 62, 64

Sepion B 1990 Intravenous care for children. Paediatric Nursing 2(3): 14–16

Shelley H 1993 Adolescent needs in hospital. Paediatric Nursing 5(9): 16–18

Whaley L F, Wong D L 1985 Essentials of paediatric nursing, 2nd edn. C V Mosby, St Louis

FURTHER READING

Ayliffe G A J, Lowbury E J L, Geddes A M, Williams J D 1992 Control of hospital infection. A practical handbook, 3rd edn. Chapman & Hall Medical, London

Brenkley W 1991 Understanding bereavement. Paediatric Nursing 3(1): 18–21

Forfar J O, Arneil G C (eds) 1992 Textbook of paediatrics, 4th edn. Churchill Livingstone, Edinburgh

Gould D 1991 Skin bacteria: what is normal? Nursing Standard 5(52): 26–28

Kendrick R 1993 Teaching children with cystic fibrosis and their families to give IV therapy. Paediatric Nursing 5(1): 22–24

Kreier J P, Mortensen R J 1990 Infection, resistance and immunity. Harper & Row, New York

Kubler-Ross 1993 On children and death. Collier Books, Macmillan, New York

Male D 1991 Immunology. An illustrated outline, 2nd edn. Gower Medical Publishing, London

Pritchard A P, Mallett J (eds) 1992 The Royal Marsden Hospital manual of clinical nursing procedures, 3rd edn. Blackwell Scientific Publications, Oxford

Selekman J 1990 The multiple faces of immune deficiency in children. Paediatric Nursing 16(4): 351–355

Stites D P, Terr A I 1991 Basic and clinical immunology, 7th edn. International Edition. Appleton & Lange, Englewood Cliffs NJ

Whaley L F, Wong D L 1991 Essentials of paediatric nursing, 4th edn. C V Mosby, St Louis

Workman L M, Ellerhurst-Ryan J, Margrave-Koertge V 1993 Nursing care of the immunocompromised patient. W B Saunders, Philadelphia

4

Special client groups

All children need specialised care but, in addition, some children have special needs. This may be because of their age group, for example the premature baby and the adolescent, or it may be because of their specific health problems. This section aims to address the needs of some of these groups.

20

The Special Care Baby Unit

Sue Linnett

CHAPTER CONTENTS

This chapter is designed to give the student an introduction to the care of the sick and preterm neonate.

The chapter aims to:
- introduce the child health nurse to the neonatal intensive or special care unit
- to outline the principles of care of the sick or preterm infant
- provide an overview of common problems of the sick or preterm infant
- discuss the effects on the family of having a child in a special care baby unit (SCBU)
- give an outline of long-term problems.

CARE OF THE BABY IN A HIGH-DEPENDENCY ENVIRONMENT

Appearance of a preterm baby

Even the most immature infants of 23–24 weeks' gestation are formed normally, right down to their tiny fingernails and toenails. A very immature and preterm baby looks very different from a term infant (see Box 20.1 for definitions of 'term' and 'preterm'). The skin is thin and transparent, and can look very red at times. Under 32 weeks' gestation, there is very little subcutaneous fat, making the baby look thin and wasted. The skin may also be covered with a fine coat of hair (lanugo), which will disappear as the baby matures.

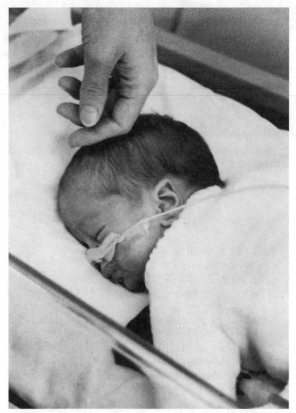

Figure 20.1 Premature baby at 32 weeks' gestation.

These babies will seem to be very floppy as their muscles are weak. It is important for their future development that they are positioned well, preferably with a roll under the hips when prone to keep their legs flexed, and their arms in a position to bring their hands close to the mouth. They should have their position changed regularly.

The umbilical cord will appear large compared to the size of the baby. The bones of the head are very soft and are joined by fibrous tissue. The fontanelles will be much larger than in a term baby. Many units nurse their babies with the baby's head on a water pillow to prevent flattening and elongation of the skull . Although the genitalia are formed early on in pregnancy, in preterm boys the testes may not have descended into the scrotum, and in girls the labia minora are larger than the labia majora.

A method of estimating gestational age has

> **Box 20.1 Definitions**
>
> **NNU.** Neonatal intensive care unit, providing highly skilled medical and nursing care.
>
> **SCBU.** Special care baby unit, providing short-term emergency care and any observation and treatment required in addition to routine care.
>
> **Preterm.** A preterm baby is born before 37 completed weeks of gestation (<259 days) (Fig. 20.1). The length of pregnancy is counted as 40 weeks.
>
> **Term.** A term baby is born between 37 and 42 completed weeks of gestation (259–293 days).
>
> **Post-term.** A post-term baby is born at or after 42 completed weeks of gestation (294 or more days).
>
> **SFD.** Small for dates (or SGA: small for gestational age; or IUGR: intrauterine growth retardation) babies are those whose birth weight falls below the 10th centile for gestational age.
>
> **LFD.** Large for dates (or LGA: large for gestational age) babies are those whose birth weight is above the 90th centile for gestational age.
>
> **LBW.** Low birth weight infants are those weighing less than 2500 g at birth.
>
> **VLBW.** Very low birth weight infants are those weighing less than 1500 g at birth.
>
> **ELBW.** Extremely low birth weight infants are those weighing less than 1000 g at birth.
>
> **Corrected age.** A term used to allow for the effect of prematurity; for instance a baby born at 28 weeks' gestation, when 16 weeks old will be 4 weeks 'corrected age'.

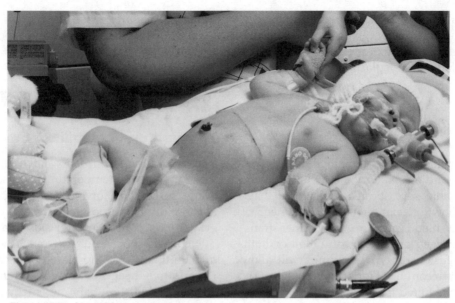

Figure 20.2 Ventilated baby at term.

been devised by Dubowitz et al (1970) and is now widely used in the UK. By the time most preterm infants reach 2 years of age, they are indistinguishable from term babies of a similar age.

Principles of care

The basic aims of a neonatal intensive care unit are to provide a clean, warm, controlled and stable environment, where the sick neonate may be nursed in a friendly atmosphere, including the parents in every aspect of care (see Fig. 20.2).

Infection control

The newborn, and more especially the preterm newborn, has very little defence against infection. The single most effective way of cutting down on infection in the neonatal nursery is that of strict and rigid hand washing and drying procedures (Larson 1987). Parents must be shown the correct method of hand washing, and are usually the most scrupulous of all carers. Staff also need to observe rigid hygiene between handling different babies. All infected or potentially infected babies should be nursed in a closed incubator, or in a cot in a separate room if

an incubator is not needed for warmth. Visitors with or recovering from infectious diseases should be excluded from the nursery.

Temperature control

Newborn infants are only able to maintain their body temperature over a narrow range. Since oxygen is consumed in keeping an infant warm, it is essential to maintain a thermoneutral environment. The temperature of this will vary according to the maturity of the infant and whether the baby is nursed clothed in an incubator or naked under a radiant heater.

The low birth weight infant has difficulty in maintaining body temperature due to a large surface area to body mass ratio and reduced subcutaneous fat. There is also reduced heat production because of inadequate brown fat. A very immature infant may need humidity added to the atmosphere to reduce heat loss through evaporation and help maintain body temperature.

Oxygen therapy

The main aim of oxygen therapy is to maintain normal arterial oxygen tensions. The infant will need careful monitoring while receiving oxygen to ensure that adequate is given but not so much as to cause retinopathy of prematurity (ROP) or bronchopulmonary dysplasia (BPD).

Monitoring

The crux of neonatal nursing is adequate monitoring to ensure a good overall picture of the infant's vital signs with minimal disturbance. Continuous cardiorespiratory monitors should be used. The more sophisticated variety will have modules allowing continuous measurement of temperature, blood pressure, and either trans-cutaneous oxygen or oxygen saturation or both. Neonatal infusion or syringe pumps will allow very accurate recording of input and monitoring of the pressure required to infuse the fluid, enabling early detection of problems. The insertion of an arterial line will allow sampling and/or monitoring of the blood without trauma to the baby.

Nutrition

The fetus gains weight rapidly in the last weeks of pregnancy. When the baby is born prematurely, it is the carers' aim to mimic that weight gain as far as possible. The sucking reflex develops between 32 and 34 weeks of gestation, so, prior to that, nasogastric, orogastric or intra-venous feeding will be necessary.

Handling

The basic principle of handling a sick neonate is don't! These infants need rest and protection from the well-meaning people caring for them. All nursing and medical procedures should be reduced to a minimum, and very careful attention given to vital signs while essential handling is in progress. The environment is also important; loud noises (banging things on the incubator and continuous music blaring) and bright lights are not conducive to rest. The pre-term baby can easily be over-stimulated, causing agitation, distress and possibly periods of hypoxia. It is important that the baby has quiet times, particularly when the mother is present, to allow him the relaxation to focus on his mother's face and voice.

PROBLEMS OF PREMATURITY AND SMALL FOR DATES INFANTS

Temperature instability

Low birth weight infants have difficulty in maintaining body temperature because they have a large surface area for a small body mass and lose heat rapidly. Heat is lost in four ways: conduction, evaporation, convection and radiation.

Neonates should not lose much heat by conduction unless they are placed on a cold surface. Evaporative heat loss may be minimised by ensuring that the baby is adequately dried after delivery and is protected from circulating currents of air. The very immature infant who has highly permeable skin may also need protecting by increasing the environmental humidity. Convective heat loss can be prevented by eliminating cooling air currents around the baby. Heat loss by radiation to nearby objects can be extreme. If the ambient temperature of the nursery is allowed to fall, even if the internal temperature of the incubator is adequate, this will have an effect on the incubator walls, cooling them and thus promoting radiant heat loss. Similarly, in the labour ward or nursery, the baby will lose heat to the environment, unless kept well wrapped.

The neonate will produce heat by metabolising brown fat. Oxygen is consumed during this process. So, if the baby is hypoxic, his ability to maintain his temperature will be compromised. Similarly, a preterm infant has not yet laid down sufficient brown fat to allow adequate heat control. In order to prevent undue heat loss, it may be necessary to use a heat shield in the incubator and put a hat on the baby.

Respiratory difficulties

Respiratory difficulties are the commonest cause of morbidity and mortality in the newborn infant (Wilson & McClure 1992) and may be the

Box 20.2 **Clinical disorders associated with respiratory difficulties in the newborn infant**

- Respiratory distress syndrome
- Congenital heart disease
- Transient tachypnoea of the newborn
- Persistent fetal circulation
- Meconium aspiration
- Acute blood loss
- Pneumothorax
- Hypothermia
- Pneumonia
- Hypoglycaemia
- Diaphragmatic hernia
- Intracranial birth injury
- Upper airway obstruction
- Metabolic acidosis
- Developmental abnormalities
- Muscular weakness

manifestation of a number of clinical disorders (see Box 20.2). Only the most common will be covered in this chapter.

An infant with respiratory distress will be tachypnoeic (60 breaths per minute or more). There may be grunting (forced expiration against a closed glottis), intercostal, subcostal or sternal recession, nasal flaring and central cyanosis (not to be confused with the peripheral cyanosis commonly seen in newborn infants in the first 24 hours of life).

An infant showing signs of respiratory distress should be nursed in a prewarmed incubator and administered oxygen. ECG, respiratory rate, and transcutaneous oxygen saturation levels should be monitored continuously. Further medical investigation is necessary to establish the cause of distress.

Respiratory distress syndrome

Respiratory distress syndrome (RDS) is caused by surfactant deficiency and is the commonest cause of death in the preterm infant. Surfactant is a phospholipid that is produced by type II alveolar cells and, when present in the alveoli, it causes a decrease in surface tension, thereby aiding gaseous exchange, increasing lung compliance and preventing alveolar collapse.

Absence of surfactant causes 'stiff lungs' so the baby is unable to breathe or exchange gases effectively. Production of surfactant begins at about 24 weeks, with a more mature type being produced after 34 weeks of gestation. RDS affects 20% of LBW infants and 65% of VLBW infants (Wilson & McClure 1992).

The incidence of RDS increases if the infant is preterm, male, has suffered from perinatal asphyxia, is the child of a diabetic, or was born by caesarean section. Signs of RDS—respiratory distress with marked expiratory grunting—are seen within 4 hours of birth. These symptoms become worse over the next 24–48 hours. X-ray examination (which should not be done before the baby is 4 hours old) shows a 'ground glass' appearance. The X-ray film can appear very similar to group B streptococcal pneumonia, so the infant should have blood cultures taken and prophylactic antibiotics given until negative results are obtained.

The risk of RDS is reduced where the baby has been under stress in utero, either where the membranes have been ruptured for 24 hours or more before delivery, or there is growth retardation. These effect an early maturation of the lungs, which will also occur where the mother is given steroids antenatally. The exact mechanism by which steroids promote maturation is at present unknown.

In RDS, the main aim of therapy is to maintain oxygenation, prevent a build-up of carbon dioxide and maintain acid–base homeostasis. This may be done by increasing the ambient oxygen or, in the more severe cases, by artificial ventilation, and, above all, minimal handling. The most recent advance in neonatal care is the use of artificial surfactants in the care of infants with RDS.

Complications. Pulmonary air leak, patent ductus arteriosus, intraventricular haemorrhage, lung collapse, chronic lung disease, and retinopathy of prematurity are all potential complications of RDS (many of these will be covered later in this chapter).

Surfactant therapy. Surfactants can be either natural (human or animal) or artificial, and have been shown in numerous trials to be very effective in the treatment of RDS. Results of an international multicentre trial published in December 1992 (OSIRIS Collaborative Group) showed that early administration of surfactant to infants at high risk of RDS prevents both death and chronic lung disease, and reduces the risk of pneumothorax.

Surfactant therapy is the most important recent advance in neonatal medicine. Although first introduced at the beginning of the 1980s, it is now a reality for all preterm babies with or at risk of RDS. Skill is required to administer the drug properly, monitor response and adjust ventilation, so the drug should not be used by inexperienced staff.

Extracorporeal membrane oxygenation (ECMO). ECMO is an invasive procedure, involving the insertion of large cannulae, usually in the neck, to allow blood temporarily to bypass the lungs (and often the heart) in order that the diseased lungs may be given the chance to rest and recover. Although relatively new to the United Kingdom, ECMO has been used elsewhere (particularly in the USA) for some years and survival rates of about 80% have been reported (Krause & Younger 1992).

High-frequency jet ventilation. Conventional ventilation imitates normal neonatal respiration by delivering gas in larger volumes than that of the lung dead space at rates similar to normal respiration. High-frequency jet ventilation injects smaller volumes of gas (sometimes smaller than the volume of dead space) into the lungs at rapid rates (i.e. 300–600 breaths per minute). The exact mechanism by which this method of ventilation works has not been established at present. This is a comparatively new form of ventilation and, at the time of writing, has still to be proven by further clinical trials, but may prove important in the prevention of lung damage following prolonged ventilation (Haney & Allingham 1992).

Patent ductus arteriosus (PDA)

In the fetal circulation, the ductus arteriosus shunts blood from the pulmonary artery to the

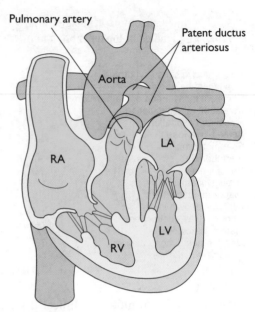

Figure 20.3 Diagram illustrating patent ductus arteriosus: RA = right auricle; LA = left auricle; RV = right ventricle; LV = left ventricle.

aorta, thus bypassing the lungs (see Fig. 20.3). At birth, the ductus arteriosus closes due to a rise in blood oxygen levels and a fall in circulating prostaglandin levels. Failure to close after birth causes oxygenated blood from the aorta, which is under pressure as it leaves the left ventricle, to be pumped back into the pulmonary artery where blood is under low pressure. The ductus arteriosus of a preterm infant tends to close later and less effectively than that of a term baby. In preterm infants recovering from RDS, it may remain open, causing cardiac failure. The first line of treatment is the restriction of fluids followed by drug therapy using indomethacin (a prostaglandin inhibitor) which is effective in about 80% of cases (Archer 1993). Surgical ligation may be necessary in the remaining few.

Apnoeic attacks

Apnoeic attacks are common in preterm infants. If the infant is already unwell, apnoeic attacks may be a sign of deterioration; in a previously well baby they may be the first signs of serious disease. Apnoeic attacks should always be reported and further investigations carried out to exclude underlying disease.

If no problems are identified, the attacks are probably due to apnoea of prematurity. This usually occurs in babies born before 32 weeks of gestation or if the infant weighs less than 1.5 kg. The apnoea is thought to be due to an immaturity of the central nervous system control mechanism, and is treated with oral caffeine citrate or intravenous aminophylline, which are effective respiratory stimulants. The attacks are monitored and usually cease with maturity.

Gastrointestinal and nutritional problems

Feeding is one of the most important aspects of care of the neonate. It is up to the mother to choose whether to breast-feed or bottle-feed. There are several preterm infant formulae on the market now so if the mother is either unable or unwilling to breast-feed there is an adequate alternative.

Feeding

After their stay on a neonatal unit, many preterm babies are able to leave hospital breast-feeding successfully or at least having a mixture of breast and bottle. During the first few days and weeks of the preterm baby's life, the production of breast milk may be the all-important link the mother needs with her baby. It is, however, hard to produce sufficient quantities of expressed breast milk (EBM) to satisfy the baby's needs, especially if it is a long time before the baby is able to suck. The nurse's support is vital at this time, in helping the mother to decide what is best for her and her baby, and then giving the guidance and support necessary.

In the author's experience, most mothers and babies do best on a mixture of breast milk supplemented with a preterm formula. It is best to avoid giving the baby bottles while the mother is establishing breast-feeding, as it can be confusing to the baby to have to master the two different

Case study 20.1 Emma

Baby Emma was born at 2 a.m. at 32 weeks' gestation weighing 1.55 kg. She was making very little effort to breathe and needed intubation and ventilating for a short period. Spontaneous respirations were established by 10 minutes of age and, after a short cuddle with her mother, Emma was transferred to the neonatal unit.

Emma's temperature was only 35.5°C so she was nursed in an incubator, and dressed with a hat on. She required a small amount of oxygen for her first 6 hours but was soon breathing air. Her heart rate, respiratory rate, and oxygen saturation level were being continuously monitored.

Emma's parents were able to visit their daughter 2 hours after delivery; her father brought her mother in a wheel chair. After being shown how to wash their hands thoroughly, they were welcomed into the nursery. They were given a basic explanation of Emma's condition and encouraged to stroke and talk to their daughter.

Emma remained in the neonatal unit until she was 6 weeks old. In that time her parents were gradually encouraged to take over more and more of her care. Her mother was encouraged to express her milk as she intended to breast-feed. All EBM was given to Emma plus some preterm formula until there was enough milk to make this unnecessary. Once Emma was sucking well at the breast, her mother would spend all day on the unit demand feeding. She then came into the mother and baby room for four nights to establish breast-feeding over the 24-hour period.

Emma's parents were overjoyed to be taking their little girl home but somewhat apprehensive as well. The family care sister, who had already met the family, was able to visit for a few weeks while they all found confidence. Once home, Emma never looked back. She is now 5 years old and has just started school.

forms of sucking at the same time. Successful breast-feeding is, of course, dependent on the mother being able to spend most of her day in the nursery while breast-feeding is being established (see Case study 20.1).

Sick newborn babies may well be unable to tolerate enteral feeds because their gut motility will be poor, leading to slow gastric emptying and gut stasis. Parenteral nutrition is appropriate for infants as their sole source of nutrition where there is major gut pathology such as intestinal atresia or necrotising enterocolitis. It is common for a combination of enteral and parenteral nutrition to be used. As the baby recovers and grows, the proportion of enteral feeds increases until the baby is able to tolerate complete enteral feeding.

Necrotising enterocolitis

Necrotising enterocolitis (NEC) is the most commonly acquired gastrointestinal disease amongst sick neonates (Hylton Rushton 1990). Although the causes of the disease are unknown, it is thought that one of the predisposing factors is that of ischaemia of the bowel, making the bowel wall susceptible to penetration by intestinal anaerobic organisms. An infant with this condition, will be generally unwell and, more specifically, will be vomiting bile-stained fluid, have abdominal distension and be passing bloody stools. The infant will be given nothing by mouth and parenteral nutrition will be commenced; antibiotics will be given intravenously. Enteral feeding, preferably with expressed breast milk (EBM), will be started 7–10 days after normal bowel sounds are heard and there is no gastric aspirate, indicating a return to normal bowel function.

Some schools of thought advocate surgical resection of infected areas of gut where medical treatment has been unsuccessful. This can, however, lead to short bowel syndrome where damage has been extensive.

Hepatic immaturity

Jaundice in the newborn is very common and usually requires no treatment. It occurs due to the breakdown of fetal haemoglobin, and the inability of the liver to cope with this in the first few days of life. It may, however, indicate an underlying disease, so should always be adequately investigated. It is commoner in the preterm infant because of hepatic immaturity and increased haemoglobin breakdown. Signs of jaundice in the ill infant, where the onset is within 24 hours of birth, where there is a blood group incompatibility, and where it is prolonged should be carefully investigated.

Phototherapy is indicated according to bilirubin levels, weight or gestation of the baby and age. Phototherapy converts unconjugated bilirubin into a water-soluble form, so that it may be excreted by the kidneys. Where the bilirubin levels are very high, an exchange transfusion may be needed to prevent kernicterus (high levels of bilirubin in the central nervous system may cause brain damage if untreated). Due to the increased awareness of the dangers of high bilirubin levels, it is rare to see a case of kernicterus nowadays.

Phototherapy is a safe procedure, and can be carried out at the bedside. Certain safety measures should, however, be taken. The baby's temperature should be checked regularly, the eyes should be covered and extra fluids given to replace water loss. The stools may become very liquid. Phototherapy is frequently used prophylactically in the very preterm or sick infant. The disadvantage of phototherapy is the separation from the mother. She should be encouraged to take her baby out of the cot or incubator at feed times, even if tube feeding, and to remove eye pads in order to be able to communicate with her baby. Phototherapy blankets may also be used (Savinetti Rose 1990). These make handling and general care of the baby less daunting to the mother.

Renal immaturity

Renal function is limited, even in the term neonate, but even more so in the preterm neonate. The neonate can only regulate fluid and electrolyte balance within narrow limits. There is an inability to excrete large solute loads, and a relatively dilute urine is produced. The sick or preterm baby's intake and output must be very carefully monitored, as fluid and electrolyte balance may be difficult to maintain, and a metabolic acidosis may result.

Immunological disturbances

Defence mechanisms against infection are underdeveloped in the neonate, especially the preterm neonate. The preterm skin is very thin and not robust. The umbilical cord, before it dries up and falls off, is moist and a potential site for infection.

The clinical features of infection in the neonate are non-specific, and any alteration in activity, temperature instability, increase in jaundice levels, disinterest in feeds or vomiting, should be reported immediately. Prophylactic antibiotics may be started after blood tests (culture and full blood count) for infection as babies localise infection poorly, so bacteraemia, septicaemia or meningitis may occur from local sepsis.

Neurological immaturity

Sucking and swallowing reflexes may be immature (these reflexes develop between 32 and 34 weeks of gestation), necessitating nasogastric or jejunal feeding to begin with. Gut motility may be decreased causing fluid intolerances. There may be recurrent apnoea and bradycardia. Preterm infants are also more susceptible to intraventricular haemorrhage (IVH).

IVH is the major cause of death in VLBW infants (Rozmus 1992), both with and without severe RDS, and usually develops within 72 hours of birth. The haemorrhage occurs in the highly vascular area at the floor of the lateral ventricles (the germinal layer) and is usually associated with hypoxia, hypotonia, severe birth asphyxia, pneumothorax or RDS. As the germinal layer involutes early in the third trimester of pregnancy, IVH is rare in infants over 32 weeks' gestation and 1500 g birth weight. IVH may vary from a small insignificant bleed which resolves spontaneously and causes no long-term damage, to a large catastrophic haemorrhage resulting in the death of the baby. Most babies born under 32 weeks' gestation will have cranial ultrasound studies to exclude IVH.

Cerebral hypoxia and/or ischaemia may result in periventricular leucomalacia (PVL), usually found in the watershed areas deep in the white matter where the blood supply from two opposing directions meets. PVL rarely occurs in term infants. Where there is cystic PVL, as seen on ultrasound, there is a high incidence of major handicap.

Activity 20.1

Observe the admission of a baby to the unit. Note down all the procedures carried out in the first few hours and write down the rationale for all the procedures observed. Discuss the admission with the nurse caring for the baby, concentrating on aspects that you did not understand.

PROBLEMS OF A TERM BABY ADMITTED TO THE SCBU

Transient tachypnoea of the newborn

Transient tachypnoea of the newborn (TTN) affects mainly term babies but may affect those born prematurely. It is thought to be caused by a delay in the clearance of fetal lung fluid after birth, but may also be due to a mild abnormality of surfactant. Respiratory distress is seen within an hour or two of delivery. The illness typically lasts for 24–48 hours, and is treated by putting the infant into ambient oxygen to maintain oxygen saturation or transcutaneous oxygen level. Antibiotics are usually given until a more serious, bacterial disease is excluded.

Meconium aspiration

Meconium aspiration is rare other than in the term infant. Meconium staining of the liquor occurs in about 10% of infants delivered at term (Wilson & McClure 1992), and is usually associated with fetal distress. During and immediately after delivery, the infant may inhale the meconium-stained liquor causing trapping of air in the lower airways, and over-distension of the lungs. Meconium is highly irritant and may cause a chemical pneumonitis, as well as there being a high risk of pneumonia.

It is vitally important that a paediatrician is present at all deliveries where meconium staining is seen. The baby's mouth and nose should be sucked out as soon as the head appears on the vulva and, following delivery, the mouth, pharynx, larynx, and the trachea should be sucked out under direct vision. The irritant meconium should be washed out from the stomach to prevent vomiting.

The baby will need to be closely monitored for signs of respiratory distress, and a radiograph will need to be taken. The baby may need to be administered humidified oxygen. In severe cases the baby will need to be ventilated.

Infant of diabetic mother

The infant of a diabetic mother may be large for dates, and has a greater likelihood of complications. Poor antenatal control causes hyperglycaemia in mother and fetus resulting in fetal hyperinsulinaemia and neonatal hypoglycaemia.

Blood glucose levels should be checked as soon as possible after birth, at 30 minutes after birth, and prior to feeds until levels stabilise. Early, frequent feeds will be necessary for the first 48 hours or until the baby stabilises. It is not always necessary to admit these babies to the neonatal unit, as their care consists largely of checking blood glucose levels and feeding.

Drug and alcohol addiction

Drug addiction is common in the larger cities in the British Isles. Due to a lifestyle of self-neglect and poor nutrition, many women who are addicted to narcotics deliver prematurely or deliver babies with congenital infections or intrauterine growth retardation.

In many hospitals, the babies of these women are nursed on the postnatal wards in order to keep mother and baby together. They do, however, need careful observation for a minimum of 2 weeks. Withdrawal symptoms usually appear within 24–48 hours of delivery, but they may not appear for as much as 2 weeks later. An observation chart should be kept, with recordings made every 4 hours of the baby's behaviour. This will give an accurate picture of withdrawal symptoms that need treatment (Merker et al 1985).

Early signs of withdrawal are:

- tremors
- high-pitched cry
- posseting
- irritability

- sneezing
- increased tone
- loose stools
- sweating
- tachypnoea.

Later signs are:

- vomiting
- diarrhoea
- dehydration
- circulatory collapse
- seizures.

Treatment depends on the symptoms. Chlorpromazine is used in most cases and can be gradually reduced, but in the few extreme cases, chloral hydrate and phenobarbitone will be needed to control seizures, which may even sometimes necessitate intubation.

These babies need a lot of love and attention and can be very difficult to nurse on a busy neonatal unit. They seem to be most comfortable when being held, so it may be advisable to have a baby sling available.

Infants born to alcoholic mothers may develop similar withdrawal symptoms and may need sedation. Fetal alcohol syndrome is characterised by:

- growth retardation
- microcephaly
- eye abnormalities
- elongated upper lip
- absent philtrum
- developmental delay
- lowered intelligence
- postnatal growth retardation.

HIV-positive mother

All antibody-positive mothers give birth to babies that are antibody positive. In Europe, approximately 15% of those babies will be HIV positive after their maternal antibodies are lost. This loss occurs at 15–18 months of age.

Fekety (1989) states that it is nearly impossible to rule out HIV infection during the first year of life, so the infant should be managed as though infected, and protected from exposure to infection from others. The baby should be nursed at the mother's bedside where possible and the mother given as much support as is available.

Congenital abnormalities and surgical problems

These can vary from life-threatening malformations such as diaphragmatic hernia, to minor defects such as accessory auricles. The major malformations are important as they account for a large number of neonatal and perinatal deaths and are also a major cause of handicap in childhood and later life. It is very difficult to estimate the true incidence of congenital abnormalities as many are not diagnosed until well after birth.

Congenital malformations needing immediate action at birth are:

- tracheo-oesophageal fistula with or without oesophageal atresia
- diaphragmatic hernia
- choanal atresia
- Pierre Robin syndrome
- omphalocele
- gastroschisis
- myelomeningocele
- encephalocele
- imperforate anus.

Many of these and other malformations will be diagnosed antenatally by ultrasound scan at 16–20 weeks' gestation, and surgery may even be possible in utero.

The majority of neonates requiring surgery should be referred to a regional neonatal surgical unit. When the problem is diagnosed antenatally, it may be possible, and is indeed advisable, to transfer the mother before delivery. This has a two-fold advantage: the baby will have been transferred in the most appropriate incubator, his mother's womb; and the family will be able to meet the staff looking after their baby, and will be on site for visiting postoperatively.

Where it is not possible to transfer antenatally, it is vitally important that adequate explanation is given to the parents before transfer. It will probably not be possible for the mother to accompany her child immediately, although the father should be encouraged to go if possible. The nurse can maintain contact for the mother by phoning the referral hospital, and having the mother transferred as soon as possible.

The baby should be stabilised before transfer and consent for surgery obtained. It is advisable to send cross-matched blood if it is available. The baby must be kept warm. This may be done by wrapping the limbs in warmed gamgee and foil. An intravenous infusion should be set up and careful note made of any fluid loss such as gastric aspirate.

 For further reading on surgical problems in the neonate see Nixon & O'Donnell (1992).

One of the important things to remember when nursing a baby with a congenital abnormality is that the parents will have had an enormous shock, even when the diagnosis is already known to them. Where at all possible, the baby should be nursed on the postnatal ward beside the mother, as the imagined malformation is always far worse than reality. The parents will need repeated explanation and endless patience while they come to terms with their baby's problem.

Birth asphyxia

Birth asphyxia can be caused either by chronic partial asphyxia or acute asphyxia. In the first case, a previously normal baby suffers recurrent episodes of asphyxia during labour either due to incoordinate uterine contractions or episodes of umbilical cord occlusion when wrapped round a fetal part. If such babies are delivered immediately, the respiration will be depressed, but they will probably respond to resuscitation and will be unlikely to have any further problems. If, however, these episodes persist, the fetus will not be able to recover in between, damage will occur to many organs including the brain and, when finally delivered, despite resuscitation the baby will be severely ill and may suffer permanent neurological damage.

Acute asphyxia seen immediately after delivery may be treated by peripheral stimuli. The asphyxia may be due to complications such as previous maternal sedation or prematurity, in which case resuscitation will be necessary.

The appropriate equipment should be available at all deliveries. It is vitally important that it is checked regularly, as with all emergency equipment (BPA 1989).

Large for dates babies

Babies whose weight is greater than the 90th centile for their gestational age at birth may well be entirely normal babies. However, they may also be large due to fetal illness or malformations.

The causes of LFD babies are:

- maternal diabetes
- heavy or large mothers
- postmaturity
- hydrops or ascites
- transposition of the great vessels
- syndromes such as Beckwith–Wiedermann, Sotos, Marshall and Weaver.

Although LFD babies will need careful watching they should be nursed beside their mothers where possible. The important points to note are feeding, weight, jaundice and weaning.

A large baby will need a large quantity of milk right from birth, so it may be difficult for the mother to produce a sufficient quantity of breast milk to fulfil the baby's needs. Supplements may be necessary. Normal babies lose up to 10% of their birth weight. This may be an alarming amount in the LFD baby. These babies are more prone to jaundice in the neonatal period, partly due to possible poor fluid intake especially if breast-fed, but also due to the increased risk of trauma bruising during delivery. The baby may well be ready to be weaned earlier than a smaller baby. This is not a problem as long as weaning does not occur before 3 months and hypoallergenic foods are used for as long as possible.

TRANSITIONAL CARE

This concept was originally pioneered in the United Kingdom by Jean Boxall, Chris Whitby and colleagues (1989). The feeling was that many babies were being separated from their mothers unnecessarily when it would be not only possible but preferable to nurse them at their mothers' bedsides. In some hospitals, a whole ward is given over to transitional care and named the transitional care ward; in others, babies are nursed on the postnatal ward, and are kept under careful observation.

Babies who previously would have been admitted to a neonatal unit on the grounds of weight alone, i.e. weighing 1.8–2.5 kg at birth, and who are otherwise well, may be admitted to transitional care. Basic nursing care is carried out by the mother, who may also be taught such procedures as tube feeding, under supervision. If the baby requires extra warmth for a period of time, there is no reason why an incubator cannot replace a cot at the bedside.

The baby will need more observation than a normal fit term baby, especially immediately after birth, as a careful watch on temperature, respiration and blood glucose will be necessary. However, this is a small price to pay for the increased satisfaction, and confidence of the mother.

It is not always possible for the mother to remain as an inpatient for the period of time necessary to ensure that a small or preterm baby is ready for discharge, so a degree of flexibility is required.

SUPPORT FOR THE FAMILY

For most people, the birth of a baby is a joyous occasion with the whole family being included in this wonderful new beginning. However, when things go wrong this dream is shattered.

The awareness of the need to allow love and affection to develop between mother and infant is not a new concept. Pierre Budin (1900) in his book *Le Nourrison* described a number of mothers who abandoned their infants 'whose needs they have not had to meet and in whom they have lost all interest'. Unfortunately it was not Budin's philosophy that became generally accepted but that of his pupil Martin Couney who believed in the total exclusion of parents from their preterm infants.

It was not until the 1970s that psychologists and paediatricians became increasingly concerned about the effects of separation of the mother and baby (Klaus & Kennell 1982). Early separation can have at least short-term influences on patterns of behaviour in the development of the infant. It may also have long-lasting consequences for the mother and child, and may add to the emotional difficulties of parents who have had abnormal babies.

Antenatal preparation

Most families will have no indication that they are going to have their baby prematurely. The whole experience is a great shock and surprise. The parents may experience a whole variety of emotions: disappointment, guilt, anxiety, anger, horror at the appearance of their baby, rejection, fear, detachment and grief.

It is possible in a few cases to have time to prepare the mother and her partner for what is ahead. If the mother is admitted to the antenatal ward, or for some reason is given warning that the birth will be early, it may be possible to organise a visit to the neonatal unit. This gives her an opportunity to meet the staff and to ask questions. She is unlikely to have been anywhere quite like it before, so a follow-up visit is a good idea to cover all the things she was too overawed to ask. Some units have a photograph album showing the unit, and maybe some 'before and after' pictures, which are particularly useful for mothers who are on bed rest.

Separation at birth

Babies who are very sick at birth will have been swept away before their mothers have had a chance to see them. The resuscitation may well be going on in the same room, so the mother is painfully aware of the tension surrounding her child, and will probably be too afraid to ask what is happening. It is difficult to be aware of the parents when concentrating hard on the baby. It is, however, usually possible to give the mother a quick look at her child before the baby is whisked off to the unit.

It is very hard for the mother left behind, who is often unable to go to her child for a time. The nurse can do much to alleviate her feelings of distress. A photo is always taken on admission for the mother, which the father can deliver if the nurses are too busy to begin with. Parents greatly appreciate someone going to the labour or postnatal ward to give them news of their child. It is important to personalise the message, giving a description of the baby's hair or length of fingers or something else appropriate.

First impressions

It is very frightening for the parents when they walk into the unit for the first time. They are not sure what to expect and can be thoroughly alarmed by the bustle and activity. It will also be difficult for them to see their baby amidst the battery of equipment they are faced with.

At first meeting, a positive, friendly attitude on the part of the welcoming nurse, focusing on the baby's individual characteristics, will do much to reassure. At this stage, only basic information about the baby's condition and the equipment in use should be given, allowing space for questions, and acknowledging the need for future repetitions. A booklet to take away and read will allow parents to have time to take in some of the ward routines and policies.

Parents' feelings

When a baby is born prematurely, the mother and father will not have had the usual time of adaptation and preparation for the changes in lifestyle that becoming parents will involve. They may be faced with a small, sick baby who is a long way from the normal healthy child of their expectations. The sense of loss and grief will be heightened if their baby has to be taken to the neonatal unit. They may feel cheated if the mother did not go into labour, and feel that there never was a real child unless given positive reassurance.

The mother's initial feelings may well be those of guilt as well as grief. She may feel that she has failed both her child and her partner by her apparent inability to produce a normal healthy child. This guilt can be reinforced by the fact that she is not able to look after her child, leading to a withdrawal and reluctance to touch or even visit her child. She may be mourning the loss of her healthy ideal baby, or even a lost twin. This allied with depression may inhibit her ability to form a relationship with her baby. She may even feel that she is actively dangerous to her child, and that the neonatal unit has become a surrogate womb, more successful in protecting the child than herself. All this can conspire to make the mother feel inferior, and much depends on the attitude of the staff; sympathy and understanding will allow the mother to work through these feelings and re-establish her self-esteem.

Drug- or alcohol-addicted mothers will be feeling particularly vulnerable and guilty. It is not the nurse's role to judge but to provide support. These women will need an especially sensitive and understanding approach if they are to achieve their full potential as mothers.

A caring, positive attitude on the part of the staff will do much to make parents feel welcome and included as part of the team looking after their baby. Their relationship with their baby is unique, though they may need help in recognising the special part they play in their baby's life, especially when seemingly lost among the advanced technology of a neonatal unit.

Shared care

Parents will want to be kept up to date on the progress of their child, and they should be reassured that they can visit and phone at any time, day or night. Many little things can help parents see their child as a real person:

- giving the child a first name as soon as possible
- providing a toy to keep in the incubator
- photos of themselves
- in the early stages when cuddles may not be possible, touching, stroking or singing to their baby.

While the baby is sick, having an extra pair of hands for simple tasks such as changing bedding is not only invaluable to the nurse, but a source of real pleasure for the parents. Parents will very quickly, given positive guidance, become proficient in nappy changing, mouth care, and tube feeding.

Parents should be encouraged to talk about their feelings and problems, and to discuss how they feel the baby is progressing. There may be outside influences, such as worry about siblings, financial difficulties or housing, so it may be advisable to bring in other professionals, such as a counsellor or a social worker, who may be able to help.

The family need time together and may feel inhibited by the constant presence of staff. A mother and baby room on the unit will help when the baby is well enough, but initially with a sick baby, the parents must rely on the sensitivity of the staff not to intrude on their time together.

Preparation for discharge

Taking a baby home is a momentous occasion for any parent, but it is even more precious when the baby has been in hospital for some time.

Preparation for discharge begins the moment the baby is admitted to the unit. A sympathetic and tactful welcome when the parents come for their first visit will lay the path for future learning and the gradual handing over of care and responsibility from staff to parents.

The criteria for discharge can vary from unit to unit. However, most commonly, as long as the baby is gaining weight, feeding well, either by breast or bottle, and the mother is confident, the

Activity 20.2

Talk to some of the families on the unit who are about to go home, and make notes about their anxieties. Talk to the more experienced staff about what can be done to reduce the families' worries.

Ask if you can spend a morning in the preterm baby follow-up clinic. Talk to a few mothers and make notes on:

• how they felt about taking their baby home
• what the first few days at home were like
• what they found difficult
• the problems they encountered and what they did to overcome them
• what help they found, e.g. health visitor, general practitioner, family, self-help groups, etc.

Compare the two groups to see if anticipated worries matched the reality, and think of ways to help.

baby is allowed home. Many units have a policy of encouraging mothers to stay a couple of nights in a mother and baby room to get used to their baby over the 24-hour period. This has proved to be of great benefit, even if the baby is not a first child.

It is important in the excitement of going home that everything possible is covered. The baby will probably be prescribed vitamin supplements. The parents will need to be confident in giving these and know where to obtain fresh supplies. There will be a clinic follow-up appointment, and the parents should understand that there will always be someone on the unit who is able to give information or reassurance night and day.

Support at home and long term

The first few days at home can be very frightening and lonely. The parents have become used to the life of the unit, and may well have looked upon the staff as a surrogate family. Now they are all on their own.

The family doctor and the health visitor will have been informed by the hospital, and should visit within a few days of discharge. However, the greatest potential support usually comes from the extended family and friends. The parents can find this quite difficult, as few people will have a very clear idea of what they have just been through, or just how protective they feel towards their child.

Fear of infection and cold may keep a mother indoors for days. A mother who has coped for weeks with the daily trip to the hospital, and running the household round it, may find she is totally disorganised now she has the baby at home. There may be nursing problems with handicapped babies, or the baby may well be unsettled to begin with by the change of environment. In short it can be a very difficult time for the family.

Many units have appointed 'family care sisters' to provide a link between hospital and home. The sister gets to know the baby and family prior to discharge and is then able to provide home support from someone who is familiar to the family for as long as she feels it is necessary.

Voluntary organisations such as Blisslink/Nippers have a very important part to play, providing information written specially for parents, and putting parents in touch with others who have been through similar experiences. Many hospitals have their own local groups providing support in their region (see Fig. 20.4). There are also many groups specialising in specific conditions offering support (see Useful Addresses, p. 355).

When a baby dies

Sadly, not all babies survive. The anguish experienced by all those involved when a realisation is reached that the baby is not going to live is very real to family and carers alike. Nothing can take the pain away, but sensitive loving care can make it more bearable.

When a baby dies so near to birth, there will be very few memories for the parents to treasure. In order to grieve, there must be something to grieve for. Many parents regret not having seen or held their baby, and even more so if the child was malformed, as the imagination is always worse than the reality.

When caring for a terminally ill baby, the

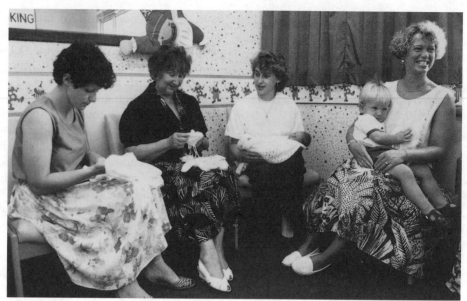

Figure 20.4 Parents' support group meeting.

nurse, as the closest professional involved, is given the opportunity to give the parents a real baby to remember. It will take much care and sensitivity, because part of the grieving process involves denial and withdrawal, and the parents may feel that they cannot bear to allow the child to become a reality because it will hurt far more. The role of the nurse is not to protect them from the hurt—no one can do that—but to help them to work through it.

Parents should be encouraged to spend as much time as they want with the baby, giving him a name if he does not already have one, having photographs taken, touching stroking and talking to him. A christening or blessing ceremony, the baby specially dressed and photos taken to make an occasion of it, can be a precious memory. Parents may also be able to take over much or all of their baby's care. This will help their sense of self-worth, and give them the feeling that they have done something positive for their child. Much of their fear and anger will go as they achieve a greater understanding of their baby's condition and care.

Many mothers speak of a physical unbearable ache in their arms after the death of their child.

By encouraging parents to hold and cuddle their child, this may be to some degree lessened. If babies are terminally ill, it may not be necessary for them to have the usual battery of wires and monitors, thus allowing them the final dignity of normality in their parents' eyes. Many parents, once they have overcome the initial horror of holding their dying baby, look back on the last cuddle in a private room as a very precious time. They may also want to help in laying the child out, dressing him in special clothes.

Respect should always be shown for the religious beliefs of the family. A caring nurse will have found out these practices; for instance Muslims and Hindus do not allow anyone not of their faith to touch the body after death. Parents may receive much comfort from the minister of their religion, so his support should always be offered.

Among the most difficult of situations to cope with, is the death of one twin. The parents have the added problems of grieving for one child, while trying to cope with developing a relationship with the other. Parents need to be given permission to grieve for the dying twin, and may want to spend more time with that one, but feel torn. Where possible, the twins should be in the same nursery as close as possible together to reduce that feeling, and parents should be reassured that they need time and space to grieve for the dying child.

Groups such as the Stillbirth and Neonatal Death Society (SANDS) and the Nippers Bereavement Group will provide a continuing support for parents long after they leave hospital care. They provide booklets for parents to guide them through the initial practicalities involved, but also go into the long-term effects of bereavement, and will continue contact for as long as the family have need of it.

LONG-TERM PROBLEMS
Bronchopulmonary dysplasia

Bronchopulmonary dysplasia (BPD) occurs in infants who have received artificial ventilation, usually for respiratory distress syndrome, and is most common in VLBW infants.

There are many theories as to why this disorder occurs, including lung immaturity, barotrauma from positive airway pressure ventilation, oxygen toxicity, respiratory infections after intubation and increased lung fluid. Dr Southall estimated in 1990 that there may have been up to 730 cases in the UK at that time, and

Case study 20.2 Paul: a mother's account of taking her baby home on oxygen

Our son Paul was born 7 weeks early, weighing 3 lb 14 oz, following an emergency caesarean section for pre-eclampsia. He was taken straight to the Special Care Baby Unit and, by the time my husband arrived, Paul was being ventilated. During the first few weeks of life, Paul went from one crisis to another, the worst of which was a cerebral bleed which resulted in hydrocephalus. It also became apparent that it would be a long time before he would be able to cope without extra oxygen.

He was about 7 weeks old when we were approached about the possibility of taking Paul home on oxygen therapy. I spoke at length to the family care sisters, Pat and Lucy. They were to become my lifeline. To make things easier, Paul now had his oxygen administered via a low-flow meter and nasal cannulae.

I was very nervous at first, but soon gained confidence in setting the low-flow meter to ensure that Paul was getting the correct amount of oxygen (not least because he went a strange colour when he was not). His feeding was an ongoing problem and would continue to be one. I had got used to opening oxygen cylinders and changing his 'prongs' and the time would soon come when we prepared to leave hospital.

I think it was when we first got home that the immensity of our task hit us. We had a little baby (7 lb 1 oz) who was totally dependent on oxygen, and the responsibility for caring for him was all ours (although the unit was on the end of a phone 24 hours a day). The oxygen cylinders weighed 44 lb each and had to be moved from room to room with Paul. I tended to feed him, wash and change him and let him sleep all in the same room in the daytime to make life easier. At night he was in our room with the oxygen cylinder standing nearby and a respiratory monitor attached to his tummy.

During these early weeks Pat and Lucy visited us every day to see how things were progressing and to weigh Paul. Paul's weight was crucial, as failure to gain adequate weight could have been a sign that he was using all his energy breathing and so was not getting sufficient oxygen. Paul made good progress and after a few weeks the visits were reduced to once or twice a week.

I was probably unrealistic in thinking that Paul would only need oxygen for a short time. Our lives seemed to be one long round of feeding and coping with his oxygen requirements. This, coupled with seeing only a handful of people proved to be a great strain. My mother and sister became our saving grace. They soon became as undaunted by the equipment as we were, allowing us to leave Paul in good hands to give us a short break. I sometimes felt that this period in our lives would never end.

Following a short course of steroids, Paul began the slow process of weaning off the oxygen. By the time he was 9 months old, he was well on the way to being off oxygen during the daytime and we became a little more mobile. With all the other worries we had had, it was only when the oxygen dependency was lessening that we started to realise the extent of his other problems, which had resulted from his cerebral bleed. Paul's physical development was very delayed, he had little head control and didn't appear to see very much at all.

The oxygen weaning process took over 4 months and it was not until well after Paul's first birthday that we were able to have all his equipment removed and become a 'normal' family again. At 4, Paul is making good progress (see Fig. 20.5). He is walking, talking and generally making his presence felt. It was an exhausting and lonely time, but seeing Paul now shows how worthwhile it all was.

that after initial hospital discharge, there is a high rate of readmission (60%) and subsequent death (up to 20%) (Southall & Samuels 1990).

The main elements of treatment are to maintain oxygen therapy, preferably using nasal cannulae and low-flow oxygen, and to give as good nutrition as possible to allow for adequate lung growth and repair. There is some debate about the use of vitamin E in the treatment of BPD, and diuretics and fluid restriction may also be indicated. When weaning from ventilation has been difficult, the use of steroids may be appropriate.

Most infants do recover gradually, but continue to have symptoms for the first few years of life, with frequent admissions to hospital. These children also suffer from the disadvantage of prolonged hospital admission and all the developmental problems associated with it. The increased use of home oxygen therapy has allowed earlier discharge and reduced the risks of developmental delay (see Case study 20.2).

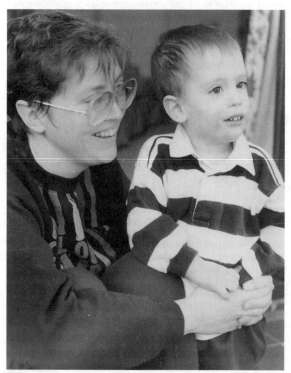

Figure 20.5 Paul at 4 years old with his mother.

Cerebral palsy

In Britain, about 1500 babies are born with or develop cerebral palsy each year (Spastics Society 1992). It is caused by an impairment to the brain which usually happens before, around or soon after birth. The main causes of this are:

- infection during the first trimester of pregnancy
- a difficult or preterm delivery
- cerebral haemorrhage
- congenital abnormality
- genetic disorder.

It is difficult to predict the extent of cerebral palsy, particularly early on. It is important to seek expert help as soon as a diagnosis of cerebral palsy is suspected, as early physiotherapy and support for the family will be of great benefit to the whole family.

Retinopathy of prematurity

Retinopathy of prematurity (ROP) is rare in babies born after 30 weeks of gestation. It is caused by a raised PaO_2 (partial pressure of oxygen in arterial blood) which causes the capillaries of the preterm retina to die, followed by a build-up of new capillaries in the ischaemic area. The damage caused by these capillaries may be minimal, with no discernible difference to the baby's vision, or may be of greater severity, even causing blindness.

Oxygen therapy should be extremely closely monitored especially during times of stress to the baby. As it is possible to prevent further damage occurring with the use of cryotherapy (Dabbs 1993), it is essential that all babies at risk are seen by an ophthalmologist before discharge or transfer back to their referring hospital. The earliest changes are not seen until the baby is 6 weeks old, so all babies should be seen then, even if they are still ventilator dependent.

Sudden infant death syndrome

No adequate explanation for the causes of sudden infant death syndrome (SIDS) has yet been found, although a wealth of research is currently underway. It must be every mother's nightmare, and unfortunately the incidence of SIDS is increased in the VLBW infant and other babies requiring neonatal intensive care (Jackson 1992). The use of home apnoea monitors is advocated by some medical practitioners, but they should not be used indiscriminately. Adequate training and backup must be given to the family before they go home with the monitor, and there must always be someone available to give advice.

Sleep disturbances

Many mothers find that their babies do not settle as well in the quiet and more peaceful atmosphere of the home. This is not very surprising as they have been used to the busy, noisy unit. They will also have to get used to a new routine and new home. Mothers have described all sorts of 'tricks' to get their baby to settle such as turning the vacuum cleaner on or leaving the radio on all the time. Babies are also often discharged just as their voices mature, which will make the mother who has not been warned of this feel that her baby is not happy in her care.

Feeding

All new mothers are worried about whether their babies are getting adequate milk, particularly if they are breast-feeding. The mother of a preterm infant may have been struggling for weeks to establish breast-feeding and will need the maximum of support to continue. As well as support from her health visitor, the help of voluntary agencies may be invaluable at this time. As growth occurs, the baby may go through growth spurts necessitating a marked increase in the amount of feeds. It is important, however, to remember that the baby was born prematurely and an adjustment must be made for this. For instance, a baby born 3 months prematurely will not be ready to start on solids when he is 3 months old; indeed much harm

could result from this as the gut will not be sufficiently matured to cope with anything other than milk. He should not be given solids until 3 months corrected age.

Many preterm infants have difficulty sucking, possibly due to a high palate from prolonged intubation, or more simply because oral feeding was so long delayed. The parents of these babies will need much help and encouragement. Feeding difficulties may continue well into toddlerhood.

Psychological and physical development and schooling

Evidence from long-term follow-up studies indicates that the vast majority of preterm babies surviving today grow up without medical, physical, or intellectual problems. Advances in care have resulted in continuing improvement in outcome for even the smallest and most immature babies. Preterm babies make up only 2% of the number of severely impaired children in the UK (Morley 1988), and even less of the moderately impaired.

Babies who have been in a neonatal intensive care unit should receive close follow-up for a varying length of time depending on the degree of immaturity. This is for a number of reasons:

- to assess growth and development
- to detect complications
- to reassure parents and give continuing advice
- to provide feedback of outcome for future generations
- to detect the emergence of problems generated from new treatments.

Allowances should be made for prematurity for about the first 18–24 months, using corrected age rather than actual age, although developmental assessments are frequently performed at actual age, thus unnecessarily worrying parents.

By school age, most preterm babies will have 'caught up' with their peers. It is, however, thought by some parents that extremely preterm children are still performing to their corrected age by this time and should thus be in the year appropriate to their expected date of delivery.

Family and relationships

Parents

The birth of a preterm or sick infant is an extremely traumatic event. The long-term impact on the family is difficult to assess. The stresses and strains it can place on a couple's relationship are enormous and although most marriages survive intact, some do not. Both parents may find that they are more emotional for some time. They cry more easily, lose their tempers more easily and are generally more irritable. Feelings of anxiety and stress may continue for a long time. Readmission to hospital will bring back all the feelings experienced previously, even if the baby's current problems are relatively minor.

Siblings

The birth of a new baby is threatening to any child and many siblings find it hard to come to terms with their new brother or sister, who takes up so much time and attention. This may well continue long after discharge, as the parents may have been left with a lack of confidence, which manifests itself as overprotectiveness to the extent of the exclusion of other siblings.

Friends and relatives

Close friends and relatives find the birth of a preterm or sick infant very hard to cope with. They are unsure of what to do and frequently withdraw from the situation. Grandparents bear a double load of grief; that of pain for their own child's suffering as well as that of the baby. This can lead to what feels to the parents to be interference, but is in fact an attempt on the part of the grandparents to be supportive. However, the sensitive and positive help from a network of family and friends can prove to be of great help.

REFERENCES

Archer N 1993 Patent ductus arteriosus in the newborn. Archives of Disease in Childhood 69: 529–532

Boxall J F et al 1989 Who is holding the baby? Midwives Chronicle and Nursing Notes (Feb): 34–36

British Association of Perinatal Medicine 1992 Categories of care. Report of working group of the British Association of Perinatal Medicine on categories of babies requiring neonatal care. British Paediatric Association, London

British Paediatric Association (BPA) 1989 Resuscitation of the newborn, Parts I and II. Working party of the BPA, College of Anaesthetists, RCM, RCOG. Royal College of Obstetricians and Gynaecologists, London

Budin P 1900 Le nourrison. Paris. English translation by: Malony W J 1907 The nursling. Caxton Press, London

Dabbs T R 1993 Retinopathy of prematurity. The neonatal nurse's yearbook 1994, CMA Medical Data, Cambridge, pp 3,15–3,17

Dubowitz L M S, Dubowitz V, Goldberg C 1970 Clinical assessment of gestational age in the newborn infant. Journal of Pediatrics 77: 1–10

Fekety S E 1989 Managing the HIV-positive patient and her newborn in a CNM service. Journal of Nurse Midwifery 34(5): 253–258

Halliday H 1988 Care of preterm babies in the first hour. Care of the Critically Ill 4(2): 7–11

Halliday H L, McClure G, Reid M 1989 Handbook of neonatal intensive care, 3rd edn. Baillière Tindall, London

Haney C, Allingham T M 1992 Nursing care of the neonate receiving high-frequency jet ventilation. Journal of Gynecological and Neonatal Nursing 21(3): 187–195

Hylton Rushton C 1990 Necrotising enterocolitis. Part I Pathogenesis and diagnosis. Part II Treatment and nursing care. American Journal of Maternal/Child Nursing 15 (Sept/Oct): 296–313

Jackson S 1992 Sudden infant death syndrome. Midwives Chronicle and Nursing Notes (Aug): 240–278

Klaus M, Kennell J 1982 Parent–infant bonding. C V Mosby, St Louis

Krause K D, Younger V J 1992 Nursing diagnoses as guidelines in the care of the neonatal ECMO patient. Journal of Gynecological and Neonatal Nursing 21(3): 169–176

Larson E 1987 Rituals in infection control: what works in the newborn nursery? Journal of Gynecological and Neonatal Nursing (Nov/Dec): 411–416

Merker L, Higgins P, Kinnard E 1985 Assessing narcotic addiction in neonates. Pediatric Nursing (May/June): 177–181

Morley C 1988 Editorial. Care of the Critically Ill 4: 2

OSIRIS Collaborative Group 1992 Early versus delayed neonatal administration of a synthetic surfactant—the judgment of OSIRIS. Lancet 340: 1363–1369

Rozmus C 1992 Periventricular–intraventricular hemorrhage in the newborn. American Journal of Maternal/Child Nursing 17(March/April): 74–81

Savinetti Rose B 1990 Phototherapy: all wrapped up? Pediatric Nursing 16(1): 57–58

Southall D P, Samuels M P 1990 Bronchopulmonary

dysplasia: a new look at management. Archives of Disease in Childhood 65: 1089–1095

Spastics Society 1992 Your child has cerebral palsy. The Spastics Society, London

Wilson D C, McClure G 1992 Respiratory problems in the newborn. British Journal of Intensive Care September: 287–294

Turner T L, Douglas J, Cockburn F 1988 Craig's care of the newly born. Churchill Livingstone, Edinburgh

FURTHER READING

Avery, Fletcher, MacDonald 1994 Neonatology. Pathophysiology and management of the newborn. Lippincott, Philadelphia

Balfour-Lynn I M, Valman H B 1993 Practical management of the newborn. Blackwell, London

Berry Brazelton T 1984 Neonatal behavioural assessment scale. Blackwell, London

Clinical Standards Advisory Group 1993 Neonatal intensive care. Access to and availability of specialist services. HMSO, London

Cloherty J P, Stark A R 1993 Manual of neonatal care. Little Brown, Boston MA

Dubowitz L, Dubowitz V 1981 The neurological assessment of the preterm and full-term newborn infant. William Heinemann Medical Books, London

Halliday H L, McClure G, Reid M 1989 Handbook of neonatal intensive care, 3rd edn. Baillière Tindall, London

Harvey D, Cooke R W I, Levitt G 1989 The baby under 1000 g. Wright, London

Kelnar C J H, Harvey D 1987 The sick newborn baby. Baillière Tindall, London

Levine M I, Tudehope D 1993 Essentials of neonatal medicine. Blackwell, London

Nixon H, O'Donnell B 1992 Essentials of pediatric surgery. Butterworth Heinemann, London

Redshaw M E, Rivers R P A, Rosenblatt D B 1985 Born too early. Oxford University Press, Oxford

Roberton N R C 1988 A manual of normal neonatal care. Hodder & Stoughton, London

Roberton N R C 1993 A manual of neonatal intensive care. Hodder & Stoughton, London

Stillbirth and Neonatal Death Society 1991 Miscarriage, stillbirth and neonatal death. Guidelines for professionals. SANDS, London

USEFUL ADDRESSES

Blisslink/Nippers (provides support for families of sick and preterm infants)
17–21 Emerald Street
London WC1 3QL
Tel: 0171 831 9393

Contact a Family (links families of children with disabilities or special needs through self-help groups)
170 Tottenham Court Road
London W1P 0HA
Tel: 0171 383 3555

Foundation for the Study of Infant Deaths (cot death research and support)
14 Halkin Street
London SW1X 7DP
Tel: 0171 235 0965
Cot death helpline: 0171 235 1721

National Childbirth Trust
Alexander House
Oldham Terrace
Acton
London W3 6NH
Tel: 0181 992 8637

SCOPE (help and support for families of children with cerebral palsy; cerebral palsy helpline)
12 Park Crescent
London W1N 4EQ
Tel: 0171 636 5020

Stillbirth and Neonatal Death Society
28 Portland Place
London W1N 4DE
Tel: 0171 436 5881

Twins and Multiple Births Association
PO Box 30
Little Sutton
South Wirral L66 1TH
Tel: 0151 348 0020

21 Children with special needs

Mabel G. Doku

This chapter aims to give definitions of special needs, handicap, disability and impairment. It will:

- highlight the different reactions of parents to the disclosure of a handicap
- highlight the nurse's role in supporting the families of children with special needs, and in the training of school nurses and other carers in nurseries and playgroups
- highlight the role of nurses in counselling families, and assessing the needs of parents and the behavioural and psychological changes in siblings
- demonstrate the importance of liaison between the various hospitals involved in the care of the child with special needs
- describe the role of the child development team
- describe the use of medication in children with special needs
- outline the process of notifying education departments and collating reports
- provide preliminary information on the Education Acts to enable further research on current legislation
- encourage the collection of statistics on local trends of disability, the numbers involved and the services available
- provide information on the services available to families of children with special needs
- describe the use of non-conventional therapies
- show the support and services offered by voluntary organisations.

DEFINITION

'Special needs' is a broad, non-labelling term commonly used to describe children with neurodevelopmental delays. These delays/conditions cover a wide range, from developmental delays with undiagnosed cause, through physical disability, hearing and visual impairments, learning difficulties, autism, multiple profound disabilities and degenerative conditions. The Office of Population Censuses and Surveys (1988) estimates that 21 in 1000 children fall under the 'special needs' definition. Previously used terms such as 'handicap', 'impairment' and 'disability' are defined differently by different disciplines and are therefore open to subjective interpretation with its resulting implications for the individual. It is often a major task when definitions of 'handicap' or 'disability' are attempted.

The World Health Organization's (1980) definitions of 'defect/impairment', 'disability' and 'handicap' are given in Box 21.1. Interpretations of these three concepts can be conflicting. The Warnock Report (DES 1978) recommended the use of terminology which actually states the child's specific functional need. Over the years, the term 'children with special needs' has become more favourably used as a vague, non-labelling terminology. For the purpose of this chapter, the 'special needs' of the title includes children with neurodevelopmental delay, visual or hearing impairment, learning difficulties and some with complex medical and chromosomal abnormalities.

Box 21.1 WHO definitions (1980)

Defect or **impairment** is an infection or disorder of the body, intellect or personality.

Disability is defined as a defect which results in some malfunction of individuals' normal life.

Handicap is any form of disability which adversely affects normal growth, development and adjustment to life over a substantial period of time, if not permanently.

The Children Act 1993 broadened the definition of 'children in need' to include children with special needs. Under this Act, social services departments are required to maintain a register of disabled children in their local areas.

Different health authorities adopt different methods of monitoring children who they consider to be 'at risk' of developing a disability. Regular health surveillance through GP or child health clinics will highlight a developmental delay at a very early age. Many areas are compiling lists on computer of children with potential difficulties so that they can be monitored from an early age. Examples of children kept on such lists are:

- those born prematurely—below 28 weeks' gestation
- those whose delivery was traumatic or difficult
- babies with medical complications in the neonatal period
- babies of mothers who have an inherited disorder
- babies showing developmental delay from a very early age (mostly if noticed within the neonatal period).

As a child develops, parents become aware that he or she cannot attain developmental milestones. Most parents will acknowledge a developmental delay by the time a child is 2 years old. In very few instances a parent may alert professionals to a developmental delay or concern about the child, but may then have difficulty convincing health professionals that there is a problem (Audit Commission 1993).

With regular health surveillance programmes, most forms of developmental delay are picked up at the various screening ages. However, there are families who slip through the net and a child may be presented at school with an impairment of speech, hearing or vision, or with a serious physical disability. This mostly occurs in families who move about frequently and find it difficult to attend routine screening programmes. As a result, no one health district gets to know the family long enough before they move on.

The use of parent-held child health records helps the health workers of different agencies to continue surveillance over a period of time and avoid duplication or delay in surveillance programmes. If the book is kept up to date, all developmental screening, immunisation, and health education information is carried by the parents.

There are families who find it so extremely painful to come to terms with a handicap in a child that they continue to believing that the child will 'grow out' of the problem. This presents a major difficulty for primary care teams— GP, health visitors, school nurses and child health clinic doctors. Routine checks and attendance at clinics are encouraged and parents helped to acknowledge the developmental delay.

EFFECTS OF A CHILD WITH SPECIAL NEEDS WITHIN THE FAMILY

Parents' reaction to diagnosis

It is very hard indeed for parents to come to terms with the fact that their baby may have special needs. Parents who are informed early about their baby's diagnosis tend to cope more quickly than those told later. Research has shown that many parents prefer to be informed of a diagnosis as early as in the first week after delivery. There is a danger, however, that knowing about the disability so soon after delivery may 'interfere' with maternal bonding in a positive way. Occasionally, maternal–infant attachment is established very quickly to the point of 'holding on' for the fear of what professionals, family members and friends will be thinking, their expectations and reactions. Occasionally, when bonding is delayed, professionals may attribute the delay to the birth of a baby with special needs. At this point in the postnatal period, it is very difficult to know whether the mother's reaction to a baby is normal or has been affected by her knowledge that her baby has special needs.

In babies where a condition is already diagnosed, e.g. Down's syndrome, services can be geared to offer counselling, practical help and support to the family. These are aimed to reduce stress, anxiety and feelings of guilt which may be projected on the baby. However, few parents have a diagnosis so early and help should be offered regardless of whether the baby's condition has been diagnosed. Some health districts have adopted a system of assessing maternal depression, which is reviewed regularly and at different stages postnatally. The purpose of the assessment is to involve appropriate professionals for support when needed (Brokington & Kumar 1988).

The way that information is given to parents about their child's disability remains vividly in their memories. Unfortunately, some parents find out about the diagnosis by overhearing nurses in conversation or seeing their baby's notes. This should never happen. Strictly speaking, it is not the responsibility of the nurse / midwife to disclose the diagnosis to parents; however, on occasions when a congenital condition is immediately apparent, it may be necessary to do so. In one survey, the diagnosis was told by a sister or midwife in 20% of cases with Down's syndrome (Murdoch 1983). Support workers very much encourage the disclosure of information at an arranged appointment, preferably with both parents (if appropriate) or with the mother and another close family member or a friend. It is also suggested that a professional whose role will be one of follow-up and / or liaison with other agencies should be present with the parents. On a postnatal ward, this could be a midwife, health visitor or social worker, depending on parental preference.

The nurse's role

Ideally, the nurse who is present when information is given will visit and support the parents in the future. The nurse should try to answer questions simply, admit if he or she does not know the answer and endeavour to put the parents in touch with someone who does. The nurse can help the parents to gain confidence in handling their baby by teaching them to do as much as possible for the baby themselves. Nurses should encourage parents to touch and handle their baby when appropriate; in some areas, parents are taught baby massage even when the baby is in an incubator. The birth of a child is a life crisis that certainly involves adjustment in lifestyle. 'Crisis' is defined as a turning point or moment of danger. Realisation that a child is handicapped is an 'added crisis' because so many of the parents' expectations will be completely dashed.

The nurse's role is mainly to listen to parents' concern and to help prepare them with pre-planned questions that they may wish to ask before discharge. Information given should be written clearly in simple non-medical jargon for parents to read over later. Parents should be encouraged to attend a follow-up appointment soon after diagnosis, as they will need time for further explanation of the disability, an opportunity to ask questions relating to treatment and the services available, and counselling.

Sadly, there are some parents who find it impossible to cope with the knowledge that their baby will be disabled. The nurse may find it difficult to accept that parents may reject their baby, but they should be treated with kindness and thoughtfulness. Counselling attempts should be

---

Box 21.2 Handicapping conditions grouped on the basis of time of diagnosis

Group one—the baby's condition is obvious to parents and professionals at birth, e.g. Down's syndrome, spina bifida, skeletal and limb deformities. Bonding with the baby at birth is crucial.

Group two—the condition is not so obvious at birth, e.g. some cases of Down's syndrome, other chromosome abnormalities, some cerebral palsy and microcephaly. Since medical tests may need to be carried out before diagnosis is confirmed, there may be a delay before parents are informed, leading to great anxiety.

Group three—a handicapping condition is observed as the child grows older. This is by far the biggest group and includes developmental delays, most types of cerebral palsy, epilepsy, metabolic disorders, hearing and visual impairment and muscular disorders.

---

left to the expertise of those trained to perform this difficult task and help parents make their final decision. The loss of the 'normal child' that has been expected can lead to the classic searching reaction. Parents' reactions are sometimes different depending on the baby's condition and the time when diagnosis is known (see Box 21.2).

Period of grieving

Parents need space to work through the initial shock of the diagnosis, and information which is given should be allowed to filter through. From the time that diagnosis is confirmed, parents go through stages of grieving, denial, shock, anger and despair (see Box 21.3).

Progress through the various phases depends on the parents' past experience of handicap, their lifestyle, personalities, relationship and, finally, on how they and the baby are treated when diagnosis is given.

Lastly, some progressive neurological conditions present more functional disabilities as the child grows older. This again causes distress to the parents and child, especially if the child is old enough to understand. The dimensions and impact of a progressive neurological condition can be devastating for families. It is essential to offer counselling to parents, child and, where appropriate, siblings in order to allow them to work through their feelings.

Effects on siblings and rest of family

Some siblings of disabled children start to show signs of regression in behaviour as a form of attention seeking. They feel neglected by their parents, who have to spend so much time with the disabled child both at home and attending hospital appointments. The time and effort that is spent on the disabled child renders siblings more vulnerable, resulting in sibling rivalry and behaviour problems. There is a feeling of being left out, embarrassment, fear of chronic sickness or even death of their sibling and fear of giving birth to a handicapped child themselves.

Nurses should be able to assess the needs of a

Box 21.3   Model of psychic crisis at disclosure of handicap (adapted from Cunningham 1979)

Parent is told
↓

Psychic crisis	Manifestations		Needs
1. Shock phase	Emotional disorganisation, confusion, paralysis of actions, disbelief, irrationality	Can last from 2 minutes to several days	Sympathy and emotional support
2. Reaction phase	Expression of: sorrow, grief, disappointment, anxiety, aggression, denial, guilt, failure, defence mechanisms	A process of reintegration through discussion	Listen to parent, catharsis through talking out. Sympathy but honesty. Facts on cause
3. Adaptation phase	Realistic appraisal; parents ask; 'What can be done?' This is a signal of readiness to proceed with; 'How can we help?'		Reliable and accurate information on medical and educational treatment and future
4. Orientation phase	Parents begin to organise, seek help and information, plan for future		Provide regular help and guidance in treatment

Crisis over

sibling both developmentally and psychologically. Regular liaison with other agencies where siblings attend, such as playgroup or school, may help the children to be more open about their fears and feelings. There are psychotherapy units where families will be offered therapy and advice on how to prevent and manage behaviour problems arising in siblings. In some areas, there are groups being formed for siblings of children with special needs to meet and share experiences, and also to enable them to do enjoyable activities together.

Commonly reported ways in which a child's disability affects the family include:

- outdoor activities are restricted
- social life is absent
- there is a feeling of being 'tied to the house'
- there are baby-sitting problems
- life is disrupted
- there are marital problems

- other children:
  - —get less attention
  - —have their activities restricted
  - —are resentful
  - —are under pressure
  - —become 'little carers' and miss out on being children themselves
- all family members are subject to:
  - —stress/nerves/worry
  - —frustration/temper
  - —psychosomatic illness.

There are, however, families who say that their disabled child enhances their lives and the lives of the people who know the child; 'their child brings out the best in people'.

Genetic counselling

The parents of a child who presents with complex medical problems and developmental

Case study 21.1 Baby A

Baby A was born to a healthy 27-year-old mother. An initial diagnosis of Down's syndrome was made and the parents were informed within 1 hour of birth by the paediatrician on duty. The mother reported that she knew immediately at delivery that there was something wrong with her baby. On the postnatal ward, she was given a side room where her husband and the rest of the family members had unrestricted visiting times. The local child development team was informed and contact was made with the paediatrician, social worker and health visitor.

Initially, the parents wanted the baby to be adopted, and so all social services procedures for adoption were commenced. The parents, however, changed their decision at the last minute. Baby A was placed with temporary foster parents for the first 6 weeks and regular contact with the parents was encouraged. The couple were offered intense counselling and a helper was provided in the family home for a few hours each day.

The baby's mother became extremely ill for the first 3 months after delivery, with unexplained severe headaches.

She had extensive neurological investigations, which failed to find any abnormality. Baby A had gradually been reintroduced into the family. The father refused to discuss the idea of handicap in his baby; his comment was, 'My son will be fine'. There were two other children who were healthy, although lately the middle child had developed psychosomatic illness (frequent soiling and abdominal complaints) and regression in behaviour.

Mother and the two siblings are now coping extremely well with baby A, who is 2½ years old, walking unaided, eating well and gaining weight steadily. He has no recognisable speech and so has been taught to communicate with Makaton signing, which the rest of the family are also learning. He has started to attend a local day nursery and his mother is very pleased with his developmental progress. Regular surveillance by the local child development team will continue and a full educational statement will be prepared. Involvement of a speech therapist, occupational therapist, physiotherapist and the health visitor/nurse will continue until he starts full-time education.

delay should have access to genetic counselling (0.5% of all disabilities are caused by chromosomal abnormality). This is available to all parents of children with disability where there is the risk of an inherited disorder being passed on to future children. It helps to identify people who are apparently healthy but who risk transmitting inherited disorders to their children. Families should be offered information about the investigations available and have access to up-to-date advice about future risks. This is a stressful period for families, and it is recommended that one professional, usually a nurse, who is viewed by the family as a person of trust should be present at such appointments. In some regional units, the genetic counselling service has a specialist health visitor or nurse who visits the family and remains in contact until all investigations are completed. In areas where this service is not available, the professionals involved can decide who would be the key person to liaise with the family's local district hospital.

The professionals involved need to take into account the family's religious beliefs and whether a termination would be considered. The use of amniocentesis to detect Down's syndrome is available to women aged 35 years or older. In some districts this age limit is lower, or the test can be done at the request of a mother with a previously affected child. Recently, there are more advanced screening methods available including specialised radiology and ultrasound to detect fetal abnormalities.

It is a great dilemma for families if the fetus is found to be affected by a chromosomal abnormality and parents then have to decide whether they wish the pregnancy to be terminated. Nurses can counsel the family and guide them through the decision they make without being judgemental in their approach. Whatever the parents decide, the final outcome is very painful indeed. Some mothers have been known to change their minds at the last minute about termination. Nurses need to be very supportive at such times.

CHILD DEVELOPMENT TEAMS

In the early 1950s, paediatricians had recognised the need for centres to assess children with disabilities, although different health authorities adopted different methods to monitor such children. Some of these centres monitored children with specific disorders and did not assess all children with disabilities. The Sheldon Report (DHSS 1967) recommended health authorities to review their arrangements for the assessments of children with disabilities. The Court Report (DHSS 1976) went further and recommended that it should be the responsibility of each district to organise formally a multidisciplinary team for assessing and monitoring all 'handicapped' children. These were the beginnings of the district handicap teams as they were then named. The Warnock Report (DES 1978) favoured the use of 'child development centre' instead of 'district handicap team' as a title. It was felt that the latter suggested specialising in disability rather than development, regardless of whether that disability was minor or severe. The initial recommendation of the Court Report was that teams should comprise a consultant community paediatrician, a health visitor for handicapped children, a specialist social worker, a principal psychologist and a teacher with experience of handicapped children of nursery and infant school age. In areas where a teacher is not part of the team there are close liaison and coordinated review meetings with education departments or personnel. The report made no mention of therapists, namely physiotherapist, occupational therapist and speech therapist, nor suggested that they form core group members of the team.

Assessment and treatment

The rationale for setting up child development teams is to provide integrated multidisciplinary assessment, treatment and monitoring of all children with disabilities. Team members assess children jointly or individually depending on district resources and practice. Regular meetings are held to discuss clinical information and update of a child's progress. In order for team members and doctors to offer a comprehensive treatment, children may be referred to specialised units for investigations which are not available from the local district hospital—these may include genetic tests, special muscle tests, investigation by urodynamics clinics, cardiac and liver specialists, bone marrow units and many more. All of these separate appointments in addition to attending follow-up appointments at local clinics and district hospitals put further strain on family life.

Key worker

The Warnock Report (DES 1978) recommended that there should be a key worker or named person who parents can contact for various queries and use as their advocate. The professional chosen as a key worker varies from child to child depending on the child's disability. In most teams, the person who has the most frequent contact with the family is selected as the key worker. This may be a therapist, a social worker or specialist health visitor. The role is to bring concerns and queries from parents to the attention of the team, and liaise between various agencies. He or she can direct the parents to sources of information and help them to find appropriate counselling if needed. Occasionally, the key worker can act as a direct link with the local education authority. It should be borne in mind that, although the team might choose a member to be the parents' advocate, whoever is chosen should also be someone the family trusts and feels comfortable with. Criteria for choosing a key worker should therefore be flexible so that parents' wishes are taken into account.

Case discussion/planning meetings

In order to facilitate effective communication among all disciplines involved with the family, regular meetings are convened to share information and highlight any gaps in services. They also give parents the opportunity to meet all of the professionals involved. The nurse may need to advise parents of the format of the meetings. The usual times for these meetings to be held are soon after diagnosis is confirmed, following team members' assessment or at any stage when parents request a meeting. All of the professionals involved are encouraged to work in partnership with the parents in order to achieve a co-ordinated service for the child.

Lastly, child development teams also act as a district resource and information centre for disabled children and their families. The team members contribute to the in-service training of all professionals in the district who play a part in the care of disabled children.

Table 21.1 summarises the services and specific support available at the time of diagnosis and to meet the future needs of the child and family.

CHILDREN WITH PHYSICAL DISABILITY

Causes

Occasionally, a child's physical disability may not become apparent until much later in the child's life, when delayed physical development may be manifest. The disability may be due to intrauterine, perinatal or postnatal causes. Generally, the causes of physical disabilities can be divided into four main groups:

- physical disability due to cerebral palsy—may be mild, moderate or severe.
- disability caused by specific chromosome abnormalities which affect physical development, such as 3M dwarfism syndrome
- disabilities caused by spinal abnormalities such as spina bifida
- disability caused by neurodegenerative conditions.

Management

Medical treatment and physiotherapy

Routine follow-up of physically disabled children continues for many years to avoid and prevent complications. Medical follow-up in orthopaedics, paediatrics and wheelchair clinics will be continued, with regular assessment and review. For the majority of children with physical disabilities, follow-up by a physiotherapist will continue to prevent further physical complications.

Adaptations at home or school

The family with a physically disabled child may need to be rehoused in a property that is more suitable for the care of the child. There may need to be major adaptations to the home, such as building ramps, fitting a chair lift, making doors wider to accommodate a wheelchair, and providing various bathing aids. The occupational therapist will assess the child's needs and suggest suitable adaptations and equipment. Various aids may be needed to help the child with physical disability, such as electric communication equipment, special switches and typewriters to aid communication.

Day care provision will be encouraged in order to aid peer group integration. Special

Table 21.1 Guide to early support services (adapted from Cameron & Sturge-Moore 1990)

Need	Implementation
Early support	Telling parent of a diagnosis, hospital policy, assessment, child development centre (counselling, parent-to-parent schemes, early intervention (Portage), immediate referral to community support)
Communication and information	Information booklets, special interest group
Community support	GP, health visitor, social worker, peripatetic specialist team, assessment centres, special needs registers, specialist health visitors, key worker, referral to voluntary group
Social interaction	Play facilities (including integrated opportunity playgroups and holiday schemes), day care, pre-school nurseries, respite care, ethnic minority support, transport services available
Education	Assessments, schooling, advisory services, parents' support groups, information packs

chairs and standing frames will be provided both at day nursery and in the child's home in order to continue treatment. Once a child is older and can manage to propel a wheelchair, advice will be given jointly by the phsiotherapist and occupational therapist as to a suitable wheelchair. Many children with physical disability are integrated into mainstream schools where ramps are already built for wheelchair access. If the child has had a full educational statement (see 'Education' p. 366), there may be a helper provided to aid with toileting, feeding and moving 'swiftly' within the building. Depending on the severity of the disability, a child may be educated in a school specially designed for physically disabled children (see 'Education' p. 366).

Leisure and sports

Local sports and recreational activities sometimes lack access for wheelchairs and this further ostracises the child with physical disability. Often parents may need to travel further in order to find suitable sporting activity. The British Sports Association for the Disabled recommends either medical or technical classification to be based on functional ability as opposed to type of disability. Swimming, horse riding and gymnastics are some of the sports that children with physical and learning difficulties enjoy.

CHILDREN WITH PHYSICAL DISABILITIES AND LEARNING DIFFICULTIES

Causes

- Chromosome abnormalities that are apparent at birth, e.g. Down's syndrome.
- Neurodegenerative conditions such as Hurler's syndrome where the child becomes both physically and intellectually more disabled as the condition progresses.
- Other chromosomal and metabolic abnormalities which present with severe developmental delay much later in life. Examples are fragile-X syndrome and tuberous sclerosis.

Case study 21.2 Baby B

Baby B was born at 40 weeks' gestation. Pregnancy had been uncomplicated. Both parents are healthy and have a son. When baby B was delivered, there were immediate and obvious signs of limb deformity. The baby was referred for an orthopaedic consultation. Initially there was concern that the baby might have a dislocated hip joint and she was therefore put in a plaster of Paris cast from the waist down to above the thigh (frog plaster). Close contact, handling, cuddling and nappy changing were extremely difficult because of the position of the plaster.

Before discharge home, there was involvement of a local paediatrician, occupational therapist, physiotherapist and a speech therapist. The nurse working with special needs children remained in close contact and visited the family initially until they settled at home. The nurse also liaised with the family's health visitor and two other specialised hospitals involved with baby B's medical management. At this stage, genetic investigation had confirmed a rare combined chromosome 18 and 21 abnormality which would result in the child being severely physically disabled. Because of the number of specialised doctors involved, from three different hospitals and other local professionals, it was felt necessary to have a case discussion with the family when the baby was aged 10 months. This meeting gave all the professionals involved in the care a chance to share information with the parents, decide on a key worker and discuss plans for future medical/surgical intervention.

At the age of 2 years, baby B started at a specialised day nursery part-time, which was her mother's choice. The education authority had been informed of her special needs and a full educational statementing of her needs was in progress. Cognitively, she is a bright girl, smiles responsively and has lots of single words; a developmental check at 15 months was satisfactory apart from her physical delay. She bottom-shuffles adequately and occasionally in her baby walker manages to move about the house well. Various equipment for seating, feeding and bathing is provided in the home. The family house needed further adaptation for safety and to allow baby B to move about freely. It is not clear at this stage whether she will be able to attend a mainstream school with a helper or attend a school for physically handicapped children.

Management

Some of these children present with complex medical, social, psychological and developmental delays. Handicapped children and their families require the resources of a multidisciplinary team approach. The care of such children with complex needs sometimes appears complicated due to the number of professionals and hospitals involved.

Many parents of children with severe learning difficulties will seek to know the diagnosis of a child's condition no matter how severe. Parents prefer to have information that they can explain to relations and friends about their disabled child, although many have to accept that there is no known diagnosis for their child. This does not mean that the child cannot be helped.

Public reaction to a handicapped child can have adverse effect on both the child and family members. If the handicap is not obvious, the public have expectations that the child behaves in a certain manner. Failure to achieve such norms leads to parents having to explain the child's behaviour patterns. On the other hand, if the handicap is obvious, the child and family will be exposed to a wide range of reactions from guilt, annoyance, or sympathy to helplessness. Even today, public reaction can be expressed as overt sympathy when in contact with a handicapped person. Parents experience difficulty in dealing with negative attitudes of family members and the public to the handicapped child. The known handicapping condition can camouflage many other underlying medical problems in the child. Research on the incidence of depression in teenagers and adults with severe learning difficulty has highlighted many undiagnosed depressions.

Some children with severe learning difficulty, especially if the condition is due to a progressive cause, may present with seizures very early on in age or later in life. Non-compliance with medication can be a problem, although this mostly occurs in older children. Nurses have a role in educating parents about seizures, outlining the signs to look for, recording them and stressing the importance of regular use of the anticonvulsants.

The Warnock Report (DES 1978) recommended that children be grouped on the basis of functional abilities such as mild/moderate or severe learning difficulties. Children with severe physical and learning difficulties will have full educational assessment (see below). The Education Act 1993 promotes integration into mainstream schools with full-time support. However, a child may need to attend a special school (see below) if he or she needs constant attention.

EDUCATION

Notification and statementing process

The Warnock Report estimated that 20% of children will have special educational needs at some time during their school life. Children have such needs:

- if they have significantly greater difficulty in learning than the majority of children of their age, or
- if they have disabilities which either prevent or hinder them from making use of educational facilities of a kind generally provided in schools within their area of residence.

It is the duty of the local authority to ensure that suitable educational provision is made for children who have special needs. Each health authority has a responsibility to inform the education authority of a child's educational needs. This notification can be made once the special needs have been identified (Education Act 1993). Parents will need to be prepared for the time that the process of full educational assessment involves, the impact this will have and the reports to be collated from the professionals involved. Parents are encouraged to be partners in the planning, assessment and placement of their children into schools.

During the multiprofessional assessment there will be an educational report as well as medical, psychological, therapists', social and nursing assessments of the child's needs. A decision about the type of school that will meet

Case study 21.3 Baby C

Baby C was born at 37 weeks' gestation. During the pregnancy, there had been concern about the baby's slow growth and at 34 weeks an ultrasound scan confirmed microcephaly.

At birth there were obvious signs of microcephaly with a head circumference of 32 centimetres. There were extreme feeding difficulties in the neonatal period which necessitated nasogastric tube feeding. The baby developed seizures in the first week of life and was transferred to the Special Care Baby Unit. With the use of anticonvulsants, seizures were well controlled. Before the baby was discharged home, his mother was taught how to tube feed and administer medication. Initially, she needed lots of support until she felt comfortable and confident to pass and test the nasogastric tube. The family was visited by a paediatric community nurse who guided them during the settling-in period. When the baby was 10 months old, after repeated hospital admissions with chest infections, vomiting and uncontrolled seizures, a diagnosis of diabetes insipidus was made following extensive investigations. He was discharged home on desmopressin, 0.05 millilitres twice a day by nasal

spray. The parents were reintroduced to the team of paediatric nurses, who taught and supervised them in the use of the nasal spray. They were informed of the signs to look for, especially if baby C suddenly became dehydrated. He adopts an opisthotonos position which makes feeding, caring and positioning extremely difficult. The occupational therapist made special wedges to support his back in order to get him into an upright position.

At the age of 21 months a diagnosis of spastic quadriplegia was confirmed. He is interested in his surroundings but will not attempt to reach toys. He has no speech and remains extremely difficult to feed. His weight has always remained low and therefore extra milk feeds are given by nasogastric tube at night. The dietitian has advised that dietary supplements and extra calories should be added to his feeds. It is being considered whether a gastrotomy operation may be of benefit because of the frequent chest infections that result from gastric reflux. The nurse will remain in contact with the family and other carers at nursery and later in school in order to train them in feeding, administering both nasal and oral medication, suctioning and correct positioning.

the child's educational needs is made when all of these reports have been collated. The child then becomes the subject of a statement, which specifies the requirements (from the local authority) as to how the educational needs are to be met. It explains the right of parents to appeal and the annual reviews to be carried out by the school.

Types of school

Provided identified resources are met, children who have had full educational statementing can be integrated and educated in local mainstream schools. The majority of children with moderate/mild learning difficulties or physical disability can be integrated into mainstream schools with support. Occasionally, parents of children with physical disability choose to have their children educated under the conductive education system developed in Hungary by András Petö.

There are, however, some children whose needs are extreme and for whom special educational provision has to be made. Parents must be approached with great sensitivity when there is

a need to discuss the subject of special schooling. There are parents, however, who have to be persuaded that their child can be accommodated in a mainstream school, because they prefer the protective, caring environment of the special school.

Special schools

Special schools provide education for children whose physical diabilities and/or learning difficulties are such that they cannot profit fully from education in a mainstream school. The type of special school is selected according to the child's needs.

• Schools for the physically disabled are housed in single-storey buildings with easily accessible entrances, have specially adapted classrooms and are supplied with communication aids and computers.

• Schools for children with learning difficulties differ depending upon whether they cater for children whose condition is moderate or for those whose condition is severe. The type of school a child attends is determined by the child's intellectual ability and the care that is needed during the day.

• Singular specific disorder schools include language units, units for the hearing impaired and the visually impaired, and schools for autistic children.

Parents as partners

The Education Act 1993 recommends professionals to work in partnership with parents. All processes throughout the full educational assessment should be explained in detail to parents. Usually, there is one key worker who acts as the parents' advocate, to guide and explain different stages of the educational assessment. This key worker may be a therapist, a social worker, a health visitor or an educational psychologist. Once a school has been decided upon, parents will need to be prepared for the separation and settling-in period. The key worker/nurse can arrange to visit the school with the parents and child and to meet the school nurse. This helps to explain procedures in the school and allows parents to ask questions of concern, especially where nursing care such as suction, feeding and medication is involved. Children who attend special schools have transport arranged between school and home. Parents may choose to take and collect their child if they have transport of their own. Children with severe visual impairment or hearing difficulties may attend specialised units which are some distance away from their place of residence. Often, as these children grow older, they have feelings of isolation because they have no school friends living locally. These may be reduced if they are encouraged to attend local clubs, go swimming, or take part in after-school activities which encourage socialising with children of the same age group.

SERVICES FOR CHILDREN WITH SPECIAL NEEDS

There are services available to help families to cope and organise their lives so that they are as near to 'normal' as possible. During visits or contacts with families, the nurse or other professional can assess a family's needs and advise on the available local resources. The frustration for parents having to battle through various systems where resources are limited are a far too common experience. The nurse should enquire whether the service is available in their local district and be able to answer the following questions:

• Who is entitled to use the facility?
• How often are the sessions?
• How much does it cost?
• Are there opportunities for socialising that would benefit both child and family?
• Is there ongoing family support?

A visit may be arranged with parents to some of the facilities/centres.

Transport

During the initial stages of investigations and treatment, families sometimes feel that they spend most of their days in hospital outpatient departments. Very few specialised areas do clinics jointly; however, wherever possible, joint appointments should be arranged. Financial assistance with transport to and from hospital is available to ease financial worries. Information should be given if this service is available within the health district or local borough. Most families on income support can claim transport fares to attend hospital appointments.

Orange/yellow badge. Special parking permits are available through local boroughs for people with permanent disability and their carers. Application is made through social services.

Taxi card. This allows disabled children and their carers to obtain reduced fares in taxis—a fixed lower fare is paid for a specific mileage travelled.

Other transport services are available depending on local resources, e.g. Dial a ride and Tripscope.

Day care

Specialised day centres offer assessments of children and continue therapy over a period of time. Day nurseries run by social services departments offer day placements for children and help with their progress to further school placements. There are local playgroups, and mother and toddler groups, which enable a gradual process of integrating children with special needs with their peer groups. They also offer enormous support to parents who meet and discuss issues on disability and normal development with other parents.

Home learning

In some districts, toy libraries are run by voluntary organisations, and a home teaching scheme known as 'Portage' may be available. The scheme may be run by educational psychologists, although in some districts it is carried out by a trained health visitor or Portage worker. The input and goals in this scheme are set at the child's developmental level. The great benefit is that a small task is taught and mastered before a more complex task is introduced, thereby allowing the child to gain new experiences each time. This helps the family to see improvements, even if they are very slight. Another advantage is that the Portage worker visits the child's home regularly and provides regular support for the parents.

One drawback to this scheme is that workers occasionally abide by a very rigid check list system derived from the original document (Portage Early Education Programme 1985). This is a colour-coded booklet with six sections under headings of 'Infant stimulation', 'Socialisation', 'Language', 'Self-help', Cognitive skills', and 'Motor skills', which are developmentally sequenced from 0–6 years. The list offers a rough guide to the future curriculum and acts as a method of ongoing recording/assessment. The potential for such a check list to cause distress should be borne in mind and each child's input altered accordingly.

Financial benefits

There are financial benefits available to help families with a disabled child. A weekly disability allowance is paid to the carers looking after the child. This is divided into care and mobility components. Whilst the care component is paid from any age when special needs are identified, the mobility component is not paid until a child is aged 5 years or over. A single payment may be available from charities such as Family Fund for purchase of equipment, for example a washing machine or cooker. Families should be encouraged to discuss with a social worker which benefits they are entitled to. Some child development centres have their own social worker.

Respite care

Historically, the notion of children having respite care in other family homes was not looked upon favourably. This explains the lack of statistical information about children under 15 years and respite care provision. Although the prevalence of this belief has reduced considerably over the

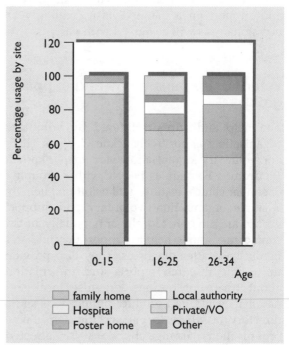

Figure 21.1 Sites used for respite care provision (adapted from Frazer et al 1991).

past 20–30 years, it highlights society's preference for institutionalising handicapped people. In 1991, in a report by Frazer et al, it was stated that 90% of children under 15 are cared for at home. Figure 21.1 gives an indication of the types of respite provision used in the past in that a large number of individuals in the older age groups are cared for outside their family homes.

Respite care provision is now accepted by families as a way of relieving carers at home. Parents, initially, may not be keen on their child going into another family's home. There is a feeling of inadequacy and guilt, and it should be explained to them that respite care is a positive resource available to relieve them occasionally of the total care of their child. Although the child may go to a respite carer, the aim is to achieve integration into the family and their local community. Respite care is available in different formats. In some areas it is arranged on a daytime basis; in others the child stays overnight or for a weekend. The length of time children spend in respite care varies from area to area. The Crossroads Care Attendants Scheme offers help and support on a planned basis, regularly or occasionally as will be agreed with parents.

Voluntary organisations and support groups

The help and support offered by voluntary organisations is positively acknowledged. There are voluntary organisations for many known syndromes. Sometimes people with a grouping of similar clinical features will be offered help by a single organisation. Voluntary and support groups are run either locally or nationally. Initial contact may aim to help to support the child and family soon after diagnosis. They also provide up-to-date research reports and information about treatment options, organise local and national events, and produce publications and a directory of where to get specific help. Some organisations arrange holidays for affected children and operate befriending schemes. Examples include:

• Contact a Family—links families who have children with very rare disabilities or special needs, through self-help groups. Examples are the Down's Syndrome Association, the Williams Syndrome Association (Williams syndrome is also known as infantile hypercalcaemia), the Autistic Society, and many more. Contact a Family now have a directory that lists all the support groups in the country.
• National Children's Bureau—brings together representatives of voluntary organisations and statutory authorities in the medical, educational and social work fields who are concerned with the care of children.
• In-Touch—offers information and contacts for parents of all children with special needs.

As well as national organisations, there are some local groups aimed at meeting the needs of their population.

A check list of services to be considered when visiting or meeting families is given in Box 21.4.

Box 21.4   Check list of services available to families of children with special needs

- Early support schemes
- Parent-linking schemes, parent befriender schemes
- Counselling
- Specialist health visitor or nurse for children with special needs
- Special needs service
- Information packs and guides to local services
- Specialist services—speech, physiotherapy, occupational therapy, psychologist
- Early intervention schemes
- Care attendant schemes
- Baby sitting
- Respite care schemes
- Toy libraries
- Integrated opportunity groups
- Parents and toddler groups, playgroups, adventure playgroups
- Parent support group
- Holiday play schemes
- Parents in partnership scheme—parents' involvement in education
- Swimming, trampolining, horse riding
- Transport facilities

NON-CONVENTIONAL THERAPY OR ALTERNATIVE MEDICINE

As more and more alternative forms of treatment are known of, families of children with special needs, either diagnosed or not, are seeking help and advice from alternative medicine. The following list is not exhaustive but all treatments are known to be tried on children with severe physical disabilities and learning difficulties:

- ostéopathy
- homeopathy
- craniopathy
- Kerlands Foundation treatment
- Petö Institute conductive education system
- faith healing
- shiatsu.

There are no scientific research findings to prove how these non-conventional therapies work; however, parents are keen to try them and unbiased information should be given by the nurse if parents enquire. If there are reasons to believe that any of these methods may be harmful to an individual child, then the parents should be told and encouraged to discuss its use with the child's paediatric consultant.

REFERENCES

Audit Commission 1993 Extract from report on research among parents with disabled children. ICM Research, London

British Sports Association for the Disabled 1990 National year book. BSAD Information Service, London

Brokington I F, Kumar R 1988 Motherhood and mental illness. Wright, London

Cameron J, Sturge-Moore L 1990 Ordinary everyday families: action for families and their young children with special needs, disabilities and learning difficulties. Mencap, London

Children Act 1993 HMSO, London

Cunningham C C 1979 Parents counselling. In: Craft M (ed) Tredgold's Mental retardation, 12th edn. Baillière Tindall, London

Department of Education and Science (DES) 1978 Report of the Committee of Enquiry into the education of handicapped children and young people. Special education needs: the Warnock Report. HMSO, London

Department of Health and Social Security (DHSS) 1967 Report of the Committee of Inquiry into Child Welfare Service. (Sheldon Report) HMSO, London

Department of Health and Social Security (DHSS) 1976 Fit for the future: report of the Committee on Child Health Services. (Court Report) HMSO, London

Education Act 1993 HMSO, London

Frazer R, Sacks B, Rhodes J 1991 People with mental handicap in the North West Thames Region. Extracts from: Dimensions of mental handicap—Research Report. Department of Public Health and Epidemiology, London

Klaus M H, Kennell J H 1976 Maternal–infant bonding. C V Mosby, St Louis

Murdoch J C 1983 Communication of the diagnosis of Down's syndrome and spina bifida in Scotland—1971–81. Ment Defic Res

Office of Population Censuses and Surveys (OPCS) 1988 Disability studies. HMSO, London

Portage Early Education Programme—Checklist 1985 NFER–Nelson, Windsor

World Health Organization 1980 International classification of impairment, disability and handicap. WHO, Geneva

FURTHER READING

Bone M, Meltzer H 1989 The prevalence of disability among children. Report 3. In: OPCS Surveys of disability in Great Britain. HMSO, London

Buckman R, Sabbagh K 1993 Magic or medicine. Pan Macmillan, London

Department of Health and Social Security (DHSS) 1979 Report of the Committee of Enquiry into Mental Handicapped Nursing and Care. (Jay Report) HMSO, London

Department of Health and Social Security (DHSS) 1983 The classification and measurement of disablement. HMSO, London

Office of Population Censuses and Surveys (OPCS) Disabled children—services, transport and education report 6. HMSO, London

Saks M 1992 Alternative medicine in Britain. Clarendon Press, Oxford

World Health Organization Working Group 1980 Early detection of handicap in children. WHO, London

22

Adolescents

Sharon Goodchild

CHAPTER CONTENTS

The period of change from being a child, dependent on adults for food, clothing, security and guidance, to fully independent adulthood, is a difficult stage in most people's lives.

Adolescence is a time of great change and is fraught with problems—emotional, psychological, physical and social. Adolescents are often considered to be the healthiest group in our society; however, they have very special needs which are often overlooked by the medical and nursing professions.

The chapter aims to:
- discuss the meaning of the term 'adolescence'
- outline the physical, psychological and social changes that occur, and look closely at the impact of this important stage of development on both the child and the family
- discuss how illness and an admission to hospital can magnify these problems
- discuss how to meet the needs of adolescents in hospital, where they should be nursed and whether there is a need for specialist adolescent units in this country
- review two important issues in adolescence—teenage pregnancies and attempted suicide.

WHAT IS ADOLESCENCE?

Adolescence is often described as a 'passing phase' by weary parents, teachers and health professionals. We often hear people talking about teenagers and saying: 'He'll grow out of it—it's just a phase he's going through'. The word 'adolescent' itself is often used in a negative way to denote a type of behaviour, and teenagers themselves see it as an insult to be called 'an adolescent'.

Adolescence is seen as a transition between two important periods of life—childhood and adulthood. This very belief, however, implies that adolescence has no value of its own, and indeed this seems to be reflected in our treatment of adolescents in hospital (Müller et al 1986).

Adolescence is, however, a period which lasts up to about 10 years—a long time to be called 'a passing phase'!

The term 'adolescence' is difficult to define and, indeed, in the literature available, the range of definitions and theories is vast. There is also little consensus among psychologists, doctors and writers regarding a definition.

One view is that adolescence refers to that period between childhood and adulthood when the child not only changes physically, but develops the attitudes and interests that will eventually make him an adult (Gordon 1981). It has also been suggested that it is a period of 'storm and stress', a time of conflict between biological and cultural forces (Weisfield & Berger 1983), beginning with puberty and ending when full adult status has been achieved. The question of when 'full adult status' is achieved is a difficult one, however, and one which will be discussed later.

It is generally accepted today that adolescence is a process rather than a period. It is no longer seen as a stage of development that is fixed, either in time or in its manifestations (Swanwick & Oliver 1985); rather it is a transitional process through which individuals pass from childhood to maturity over a period of time which varies from person to person. This process is characterised by many personal changes—physical, social, psychological and cognitive, occurring between about 10 and 20 years of age.

Many pass through this process with very few problems, but many young people experience the transition from childhood to adulthood, and from dependence to independence, as a time of confusion. According to Mackenzie (1988): 'Adolescence is a time of great change, a time for decisions, for adapting and assuming responsibility'.

An admission to hospital can exacerbate these normal life stresses, making adolescents one of the most testing groups to care for in hospital. We will next discuss in more detail the physical, psychological and social changes that occur in this stage of development, and highlight the problems faced when an adolescent is admitted to hospital with an acute problem or an illness or handicap that is long-standing.

Physical changes

Physiologically, adolescence begins around puberty, with the onset of menstruation in females and the production of live sperm in males. The exact physiological explanation for the onset of puberty is unknown, but it is believed to originate in the hypothalamus, with the resultant stimulation of the pituitary gonadotrophic hormones—luteinising hormone (LH) and follicle stimulating hormone (FSH). These hormones stimulate the ovaries to secrete oestrogen and the Leydig cells of the testes to secrete testosterone. The action of these hormones brings about the development of the secondary sexual characteristics. These body changes occur relatively quickly: it takes approximately 2–3 years to change physically from child to adult, and there is great individual variation both in terms of the age at which the growth spurt occurs and the rate of change. So the adolescent not only has to cope with problems of maturity such as responsibilities and academic pressures, but also has to cope with them within a 'new' body image.

Physical development in the adolescent is of great importance, not only in itself, but for its emotional and social overtones. Writers, including Coleman (1984), suggest that the adolescent has two main body images:

• 'own body image'—the way he or she thinks he or she looks

- 'ideal body image'—the way he or she would like to look.

The body changes in adolescence may cause feelings of inferiority and embarrassment, which adolescents may try to overcome by attempting to make their bodies appear better. They may exercise a lot, or spend more money and time on clothing and appearance. An admission to hospital can threaten to change the body image and make the gap between their own body and ideal body image even greater. Any illness or injury which affects appearance or sexuality can be devastating for the adolescent; a single facial spot can be a cause of great concern and even an appendicectomy scar can lead to emotional turmoil.

Adolescents with a physical handicap also become increasingly aware of their looks and body image as they grow up; they become more aware of their disabilities and the effect these may have on their lives. During the period of adolescence they may have feelings of resentment, frustration, anger and inferiority as they realise that they are 'different' from their peers. One example of this is of a girl with Crohn's disease who had an ileostomy formed at a very young age. She coped very well until she reached adolescence, when she had problems coming to terms with her altered body image and her sexuality. Consider also adolescents who have been paralysed in road traffic accidents, and the problems they will face in coming to terms with their handicap. At a time when they are becoming acutely aware of their changing body and are forming relationships with the opposite sex, they no longer have control over what happens to their body, or so it seems, and become dependant on others for its care. And what happens to their relationship with their family and peers, their new-found independence and their hopes, plans and dreams for the future?

Psychological and social changes

For psychologists, adolescence is not so much an age range in which physiological change takes place, but rather a developmental process. During this period or process, psychological changes take place so that adult behaviours take over from the more childish ones. A variety of adjustments are made during this time which may take months or years in each individual, and the transition from child to adult is not always smooth.

Perhaps the most influential approach to understanding adolescence is Erikson's (1965) work on psychological development. He identified the central problem of adolescence as establishing a sense of identity: 'Who am I?' In the literature, the theme emerges that adults are people who have to some degree gained a sense of their own identity, while adolescents are still in the process of doing so. Marcia (1982) describes identity as: 'An internal, self-constructed, dynamic organisation of drives, abilities, beliefs and individual history'.

The search for identity

Acquiring an identity is a dynamic process which begins when the infant first recognises its separateness from the primary care giver, and progresses by means of a series of developmental phases. Adolescence seems to be a crucial phase in which changes occur in relation to identity (Müller et al 1986). Adolescents form their own identity in many areas, namely values, morals and thought processes, politics, friendships, sexuality and relationships. Obviously these identity changes may continue into old age, but according to Marcia (1982), the importance of identity in adolescence is that this is the first time that physical development, cognitive skills and social expectations coincide to enable young people to understand their past and begin to decide upon their approach to the future. Often, the process of developing identity is not conscious, and decisions are rarely taken irrevocably. As a result, there is often conflict with parents as adolescents break away from the home environment and establish their own values.

It has been said that adolescents, unlike children and adults, have a set of specific developmental paths that they must follow before they can shed the remnants of adolescence (Kuykendall et al 1985). This is all part of establishing a sense of identity. The way in which an adolescent copes with finding his or her sense of identity is dependent on many factors, not least personality, exposure to temptations, support and guidance from parents and specific life events such as hospitalisation.

The role of the peer group

In their bid for independence—emancipation from their parents—adolescents turn to one another for security, help and support. Consequently, the role of the peer group becomes increasingly more important, serving an essential function, wherein its members use each other to explore and evaluate values, attitudes and behaviour. The 'group' may be socially or antisocially formed, but it determines the behaviour of its members. To feel secure, adolescents must feel accepted by their group, and therefore they will tend to conform to the demands and practices of the group, whatever these may be (Roberts 1987). Pressure to conform to the group norms can be immense, as to go against these means running the risk of disapproval. Thus it becomes very important to affiliate by doing the 'in' things, e.g. dressing the same and having the same ideas and beliefs. Depending on the group norms, young people may find themselves feeling pressurised to participate in the exploration of alcohol, drugs, solvent abuse and smoking.

Relationships with parents

As the peer group becomes more important, parents and other adults become less so, and conflict develops—a tug of war between dependence and independence. Outwardly, adolescents may appear not to need their parents; however, inwardly they still value their approval (Mackenzie 1988). Adolescents may complain that their parents do not understand them and that they treat them like children, while the

Activity 22.1

Can you remember how you felt as a teenager? Write down these feelings and any problems you may have encountered with your parents, siblings, etc. Then, working in a small group, share and discuss your feelings, and how you overcame or dealt with any problems.

parents complain that their children do not listen. Thus, for parents, the period of adolescence can be a particularly trying time and one which creates a dilemma—while they continue to feel responsible for their children, and care deeply what happens to them, they find they have decreasing influence and authority. 'They may be puzzled and upset that previously amenable, polite children may become quarrelsome, impertinent, no longer interested in family activities and generally make everyone else's life a misery' (Roberts 1987).

Achieving independence from parents is seen as a developmental task for adolescents (McKinney et al 1977). When making this transition from dependence upon parents to emotional independence, adolescents face a dilemma because they need to feel that their thoughts and feelings are their own, and not necessarily in accordance with those of their parents. The adolescent's tug of war between independence and dependence is aggravated greatly when he or she is admitted to hospital. A vicious circle can develop with the parents anxiously wanting to protect their child while the adolescent is torn between needing their support and his or her independence. For example, it may make some adolescents feel more dependent if it is necessary for their parents to start or continue physical care. On the other hand, an enforced separation may actually help some teenagers to gain independence.

The handicapped child. For the handicapped child, physical independence may never be possible, but emotional independence and maturity must be encouraged (Duberley 1981). Some research by Anderson & Clarke (1982), comparing adolescents with spina bifida or cerebral palsy with unaffected adolescents, discovered that parents found it very difficult to enable their disabled children to be independent, especially if mobility or continence was a problem. Parents can become overprotective towards their children and may feel very hurt if their help is rejected. The adolescent may feel that he has total control over his life, but resent the fact that, under the age of 16, he cannot sign a consent form for surgery or procedures. So there is an ongoing struggle.

Intellectual development

Not only does the adolescent develop physically and emotionally but also intellectually. Piaget & Inhelder (1958) describe the adolescent years as 'formal operational'. A younger child needs concrete or real situations in which to solve problems, whereas adolescents become capable of thinking in abstract or hypothetical terms, and can now imagine 'as if' situations relating to illness and injury, which are not actually part of their experience of life so far.

The adolescent becomes capable of all the forms of logical thought that an adult commands. This development of reasoning brings with it the questioning of religious and political views, and often the challenging of parental attitudes and behaviour. To parents and carers, adolescents can seem rebellious and argumentative; according to psychologists, however, it is important that they pass through this stage in order to find their own identity. Hence, adolescence is also a time for experimenting and testing family or community norms and values. Children with a chronic condition such as diabetes may suddenly resent the restrictions the disease puts upon them and rebel against treatment and care.

Choosing employment and developing academic and vocational skills are important features of adolescence. It can be acutely distressing if hospitalisation disrupts plans and examinations. Adolescents may, as a result, find themselves behind with work at school or may be unable to obtain employment due to repeated stays in hospital. They may feel that they have 'let their parents down' or 'failed them' in some way. Today, due to the socioeconomic climate, there is a feeling of insecurity as it is difficult to know whether there will be jobs available when young people leave school, either with or without educational qualifications. This insecurity places a great burden on young people. In some areas of the country, youngsters may well wonder whether effort at school is really worthwhile if they are to be faced with the prospect of very little, or no, work to go to afterwards. When adolescents are admitted to hospital, therefore, it is important that all carers—doctors, nurses and others—are aware of these life stresses facing them.

ADOLESCENTS IN HOSPITAL

In our earlier consideration of the nature of adolescence, the image emerged of adolescents as confused, peer oriented, self-conscious, questioning individuals. They need privacy, space, individual attention and much love to help them, under the best circumstances, through the transition from childhood to adulthood. How much support then, do the same adolescents need when they are also sick, in pain or frightened by strange procedures? This part of the chapter discusses how we can try to provide this support and meet the needs of the adolescent in hospital.

When adolescents are admitted to hospital, they often find that they must give up the independence that they are trying to attain. They have been removed from their family and friends, and now face a new environment in which they perceive themselves as having little control. Loss of body control, frequent examinations and embarrassing physical procedures tend to undermine their sense of pride and identity. They must also experience a great deal of anxiety related to a fear of the unknown. They may have a poor understanding of their illness or be concerned about the possible effects of the illness or surgery upon their physical appearance. 'Young people are often far more concerned about social losses and change in the "images" which result from their hospitalisation and treatment than about the illness itself' (Jackson 1973).

So, considering all the information so far, how can we as health care professionals minimise the negative impact of hospitalisation and illness and help maintain the normal process of adolescence? Box 22.1 helps to answer this question. It looks at four nursing interventions and areas of care:

- establishing a trusting nurse–adolescent relationship
- promoting social interaction, involvement in groups and contact with significant others
- helping adolescents identify their own personal qualities
- helping adolescents make a successful transition

from the hospital environment back into the home, school and community.

The suggestions for the care of the adolescent given under these headings are by no means the only solution, but it is hoped that they will encourage all staff to question their own beliefs and lead them to have a greater awareness of adolescents' special needs and their response to them.

Where should adolescents be nursed?

The question of where adolescents should be nursed and whether there is a need for specialist adolescent units has caused much controversy over the years. Provision for adolescents in

---

Box 22.1 Nursing interventions

Establishing a trusting nurse–adolescent relationship
- Provide a safe environment with well-defined and consistently enforced limits.
- Find ways of assisting adolescents to develop their own set of rules and attitudes without compromising others; for example, establishing rules for lights out and morning waking.
- Provide consistency of care givers.
- Involve adolescents in the planning of their care. Allow choices when feasible.
- Encourage self-administration of medication.
- Encourage adolescents to ask questions about their health status and treatment plan.
- Stress confidentiality of the information received.
- Respect privacy and fear of embarrassment.
- Give adolescents understandable and reliable explanations of procedures, treatment, etc. Reinforce information that has already been presented.
- Clarify any misconceptions concerning care/treatment.
- Avoid negative criticism.
- Provide positive feedback.
- Serve as a positive adult role model for the adolescent.

Promoting social interaction, involvement in groups and contact with significant others
- Encourage visits from parents, siblings, peers and other significant persons when appropriate.
- Provide telephone for maintenance of family/peer contacts.
- Encourage letter writing.
- Encourage involvement in hospital/unit activities—school, occupational therapy, physiotherapy, etc.
- Provide somewhere for peer interaction with games for groups (e.g. a pool table), magazines, television, etc.
- Assist the adolescent and family to accept help from others when needed.

- Encourage persons of the same age with similar problems, to share experiences. Initiate a discussion group.
- Avoid overprotecting the adolescent and encourage the family to do the same.

Helping adolescents to identify their own personal qualities
- Provide positive feedback.
- Explore strengths and activities with the adolescent.
- Emphasise abilities and disabilities.
- Provide adolescents with check lists, calendars, charts, etc. to monitor personal progress.
- Teach adolescents about their health problems and how to manage them successfully.
- Encourage self-care as much as possible.
- Provide information relevant to the priorities of adolescence, e.g. fact sheets concerning aspects of health care and sexual development/education.
- Encourage adolescents to dress in their normal clothes if appropriate. Provide mirrors and encourage use of cosmetics, shaving equipment, etc.

Helping adolescents to make a successful transition from the hospital environment back into the home, school and community
- Assist adolescents in thinking through how they might respond to inquiries about their illness, hospitalisation, appearance, etc.
- Liaise with the community group, e.g. school, workplace, youth group, and provide information/education about the adolescent's illness, treatment, changes in appearance, etc.
- Assist in identifying support sources—self-help group, support group, family, friends, church and other available community resources.

hospital in this country is often inadequate and neither the children's ward nor the adult ward is the appropriate environment for meeting their special needs.

Some 40 years ago, children of all ages admitted to hospital were sometimes cared for on an adult ward. It was realised at the time that the hospital care of children was quite different from that of adults and that the environment of the adult ward was detrimental to a child's physical and emotional well-being. The report of the Committee on the Welfare of Children in Hospital (the Platt Report; MoH 1959) stated that children required separate accommodation and facilities. Now, most children are cared for on children's wards, except in special circumstances (e.g. when intensive care is needed) and health professionals are very aware that children have special needs in hospital.

Many people now feel that we are facing a situation similar to that of 40 years ago, in that adolescents have special needs and should be cared for in their own ward or unit, with people of their own age (Burr 1993, Wheeler 1981). The special needs of adolescents were addressed in the Platt Report, which states: 'Separate accommodation is required for those who have left childhood but have not yet entered adulthood ...'. However, despite the special problems faced by adolescents in hospital, which were again referred to in the more recent Court Report (DHSS 1976), 'it is estimated that between 50% and 70% of adolescents are placed inappropriately in adult wards' (NAWCH 1990). According to the literature, it would seem that the allocation of a patient to a particular area of the hospital, whether to a children's ward or to an adult ward, may well depend on bed availability or to policies which state, for example, that someone over 16 years old is an adult and under 16 years old a child. But, since the term 'adolescence' is difficult to define in chronological terms, it is difficult to judge when a child becomes an adult. There is no clear-cut ending to adolescence (Müller et al 1986).

In 1965 and 1977, the World Health Organization Expert Committee recommended that the age limits of adolescence should be 10–20 years, with a subdivision of early adolescence from 10–14 years, and later adolescence from 15–19 years. The law, on the other hand, reflects society's perceptions of adult status; we may marry at 16 years of age, hold a driving licence at 17 years and vote at 18 years. However, we know that people mature and develop physically and psychologically at different rates. Some 16-year-olds may indeed consider themselves to be adults, but so also do many who are 13, 14 or 15 years old! Others may not mature until much later. Therefore, it is impossible to generalise—we should not label youngsters according to their age; rather, each adolescent needs to be considered, and treated as an individual.

The Court Report (DHSS 1976) recognised that adolescents should be considered as a distinct group for health care provision, and yet in the 1990s there are very few adolescent units in this country (Box 22.2).

Some hospitals do set aside beds or a 'bay' on general paediatric wards for adolescents, but often adolescents who are admitted to hospital today may still find themselves next to a young baby or toddler or on an adult ward where the average age is often over 60.

The children's ward

The children's ward may be inappropriate for adolescents for many reasons. Firstly, the peer group is very important to adolescents—they need and prefer to be in the company of individuals of their own age. Also, the Charter of the National Association for the Welfare of Children in Hospital (now Action for Sick Children) clearly states:

Box 22.2 Existing adolescent units in 1992

1. Wexham Park Hospital, Slough
2. The Chelsea and Westminster Hospital, London
3. St Mary's Hospital, Manchester
4. Northern General Hospital, Sheffield
5. Royal Preston Hospital, Preston
6. Bristol Royal Hospital for Sick Children, Bristol
7. Royal National Orthopaedic Hospital, Stanmore
8. Nuffield Orthopaedic Centre, Oxford

'Children shall be cared for with other children of the same age group' (NAWCH 1984).

Secondly, the atmosphere on the children's ward may not be congenial to adolescents. They may not like the crying babies and the generally noisy surroundings. They admit, however, that they make plenty of noise themselves but say this is of a totally different kind!

Often there is nowhere on the children's ward for adolescents to go to study, listen to music and be with their friends. The 'playroom' is generally full of children's toys and books, and there are very few books and games suitable for the teenager. Also, the posters and paintings of 'Donald Duck' and the 'Care Bears' may have lost their appeal at this age!

Adolescents value their independence and freedom and may resent the restrictions imposed upon them on the children's ward. It is important also to remember that some youngsters leave school at the age of 16 and are working in the 'adult world'—so is it really appropriate for them to be looked after on a children's ward?

Adolescents need privacy and space, which is often lacking on the paediatric ward, but which is important at a stage when the young person is aware of, and can be easily embarrassed by, changes in body image. There are normally curtains which can be drawn around the bed area, but they provide very little privacy in practice. Locks are needed on bathroom doors, and separate bathrooms need to be provided for boys and girls; but, in reality, are such facilities available on all adult wards?

Even young patients with prolonged conditions such as diabetes, cystic fibrosis, asthma or hydrocephalus, on reaching adolescence, may no longer wish to come to the children's ward they have known for years, and where they know the medical and nursing staff. Their needs as adolescents are different from those of a child, and will alter and develop as they pass through adolescence.

The adult ward

The adult ward, on the other hand, is not equipped to care for the adolescent effectively and is not the best alternative to the children's ward. Firstly, the age difference is a major problem. The majority of patients on a general adult medical or surgical ward are over 65 years old, and their needs are vastly different from those of the adolescent. The noise produced by the youngsters creates an unsuitable environment for the elderly. Similarly, the environment which is suitable for the over-65s is not a suitable nursing environment for the adolescent (Burman 1985). The Platt Report (MoH 1959) stated: 'in our view it is even more important that adolescents should not be in a position to overhear some of the conversation of an adult ward.' Adolescents are at an impressionable age and may be upset and frightened by the illnesses witnessed on an adult ward, and may not understand some of the things they see and hear.

The British Paediatric Association working party in 1985 concluded: 'For the older patient the activities of the adolescent may be unacceptable, whereas for the adolescent the sights and sounds of a ward containing much advanced or degenerative disease are unsuitable' (BPA 1985, p. 3: 2.3).

An opposing view, however, is that it may be rather narrow-minded to think that adolescents function exclusively within their own peer group; community services programmes are now being carried out in schools, and a changing culture is giving adolescents more opportunity to meet and relate to people of all ages.

The adolescent unit

If adolescents are not nursed on paediatric wards or adult wards, is it feasible to have specialist adolescent units?

Activity 22.2

What facilities are needed on an adolescent ward?
If an adolescent ward/unit is to be opened in your hospital, consider what facilities would be required for the teenagers, e.g. area for study. Draw up some guidelines or 'ground rules' for their stay in hospital.

It is generally desirable that adolescents should have their own accommodation so that the common problems, and interests of the group may be taken into account …

(MoH 1959)

In 1959, when these words were written, the country was experiencing a bulge in the adolescent population due to the post-war baby boom (Blunden 1989). As Rosemary Blunden asks in her article, given the current falling numbers of adolescents, the increased sophistication of young people, and the developments in nursing, how relevant is the statement today?

Other work has shown, however, that there are still sufficient adolescents to merit a special unit. In 1986, Pollach & Fry estimated that 8.3% of the population was aged between 10 and 15 years. Adolescents are the healthiest age group in the population and yet there are a surprising number of them in hospital at any one time, though scattered among the specialities (Gordon 1981). The report of the working party on the needs and care of adolescents (BPA 1985) estimated that in the age group 11–15 years the approximate requirement for hospital beds is 7.5 per 100 000 total population, and therefore suggested that a district serving 200 000 people should have enough adolescents to fill a 15-bedded ward.

Many reasons have been put forward for the poor provision of adolescent units in this country. The most commonly stated reason is lack of finance. There are just not sufficient funds available to build, or develop adolescent units, and money is channelled into other specialities. However, more children are being nursed at home and, where children's wards are underused, it has been suggested that space could be made available in some districts to develop an adolescent ward (BPA 1985).

The question is also raised of whether it is feasible to nurse young people requiring a variety of specialities on the same ward, e.g. adolescents with neurological and cardiac conditions, psychiatric disorders and gynaecological problems. Here, it is argued that the medical and

Activity 22.3

Is there a need for an adolescent unit in your area? Conduct a survey, on your own or working in a group, looking at the numbers of teenagers in your local area and how many were admitted to hospital each year. Find out how many were nursed on the children's ward and how many on the adult ward.

nursing needs are so specialised that they require the expertise of a specialist unit (Burman 1985). However, as Dr Burman explains, there is no need for the patients to be deprived of the benefits of an adolescent ward during the day or when they are no longer requiring the intensive care of the specialists. According to a British Paediatric Association working party (BPA 1985): 'Adolescents requiring hospital in-patient care should be in wards specifically for them and this consideration is usually of greater importance than the needs of system specialists'. However, the working party recognised that it may be difficult to integrate adolescents with psychiatric problems on an adolescent unit, and it may be wise to nurse an adolescent admitted for termination of pregnancy on an adult ward due to the emotional effect this may have on the other teenagers.

Providing separate adolescent units may be the solution to meeting the adolescent's special needs in hospital, and this is the sentiment shared by many writers and health professionals. However, this is not always possible and the ward may not be suitable for all adolescents. Adolescents are not children and yet they have not quite reached adulthood. They are a distinct group with separate health care needs. Considering the vast physical and emotional changes they are facing, adolescents need to be assessed and treated as individuals. It is vital, therefore, that nurses, in all areas of the hospital, provide sensitive care for adolescent patients so that their admission to hospital, their stay, and their re-integration into society on discharge may be less traumatic.

NAWCH, as part of their Quality Review Series, published *Setting Standards for Adolescents in Hospital* in 1990 and this contains check lists as well as examples of good practice. This document is useful reading for all concerned in the provision and purchasing of adolescent care.

THE ADOLESCENT AND CONSENT

The issue of consent is extremely important in nursing and health care generally today, and there has been much debate concerning adolescents giving consent for their treatment and care (see Ch. 7).

Adolescents and their parents usually agree on whether to consent to the medical treatment that is suggested to them. However, problems can arise when the views of adolescents and their parents are in conflict. Consider the case of a 14-year-old boy who has leukaemia. He has endured aggressive chemotherapy and radiotherapy in the past, and now he has relapsed and faces further unpleasant treatment. He refuses to have more treatment, however, although realising that this decision means he might die. His parents, on the other hand, do want their son to be treated and expect the medical and nursing staff to comply with their wishes. Who has the right to decide whether the adolescent should be treated, and has he the right to refuse?

The general law governing the age of consent is inconsistent: legally, adolescents under 18 years of age are considered to be 'minors'. Only when they become 18 can they vote, make and sue upon contracts and decide about life choices, including where to live and work. It is, however, possible to marry legally at 16 years of age and have sexual intercourse.

Since the Family Law Reform Act 1969, minors between the ages of 16 and 18 years may be treated as if they had attained their majority in that they have a statutory right to give consent to treatment (including medical, surgical and dental care, anaesthesia and diagnostic procedures). However, the Act is silent on minors aged under 16 and their right to consent to their treatment. In the Gillick case of 1985 (see Ch. 7), the judge said that 'the court should ascertain the wishes and feelings of the child concerned (considered in the light of his age and understanding)'. It was held that contraceptive advice could be available legally to under-16s, without parental consent. Although this case was particularly concerned with contraceptive advice, it has been taken to set a much wider legal precedent over the issue of consent for the under-16s. According to the Department of Health guidance on the welfare of children and young people in hospital (1991), 'the consent of the child and the parent or guardians should be obtained to treat children under the age of 16, save in an emergency ... Even where younger children do not have the required understanding, they should be provided with as much information as possible and their wishes ascertained and taken into account'. The report continues: 'if, in the opinion of a doctor, a child below this age has achieved sufficient understanding of what is proposed, the child *may* consent (or refuse to consent) without the parent's knowledge or support'. This raises the question of the age children have to be before they can weigh up choices and be trusted to make sensible decisions for themselves. Also, what is 'sufficient understanding' and how can anyone tell when a child has it?

The law states that the age of consent is 16 years, but age is a crude way of defining competence. At the age of 15 years, 11 months and 29 days a minor would not be able to consent to treatment, but on his 16th birthday he would.

Lord Scarman said, during the 1985 hearing of the case of *Gillick* v. *West Norfolk and Wisbech Area Health Authority*: 'If the law should impose on the process of growing up fixed limits, where nature knows only a continuous process, the price would be artificiality and a lack of realism in an area where the law must be sensitive to human development and social change'.

Also, it is not to be assumed that a person is competent if he or she makes the 'right' decision. After all, who decides what the 'right' decision is? The parents? The medical staff? This idea violates the patients' autonomy, as it ignores the private, individual reasons they have for their decisions (Charles-Edwards 1991). A minor or child is considered competent to give consent, if he has an understanding of the nature, purpose and consequences of treatment. A report entitled *Making Health Care Decisions*, which was published in the USA in 1983 (cited in Kennedy & Grubb 1989), suggested that the ability to make decisions should be described as:

- possession of a set of values and goals
- the ability to communicate and understand information
- the ability to deliberate and reason about one's choices.

The level of understanding required here can be achieved by most adults and indeed most 14-year-olds. Weithorn & Campbell (1982) demonstrated that most 14-year-olds have the same level of competence to make decisions, such as consent to treatment, as most adults. Piaget & Inhelder (1958) also stated that children reaching the developmental age of 12 enter into the stage of 'formal operations'. They become able to reason about hypothetical abstract situations, review possibilities, think about their thoughts and see problems from perspectives other than their own.

So, if adolescents under the age of 16 are able to make their own decisions about their medical treatment, what moral and legal rights do their parents have? They have a duty of care to their children and, while children are young, parentalistic behaviour is justified. But as children mature and develop autonomy, the rights that their parents have over them decrease (Fig. 22.1). Although parents may wish to continue to exercise their parental right to make decisions for their children, it needs to be decided whether the adolescents themselves are competent to make their own treatment choices.

The Gillick case was so notorious and highly publicised because the dispute concerned giving contraceptive advice to girls under the age when sexual intercourse becomes legal. Contraception is a form of medical treatment and, therefore, if it is legal for doctors to give contraceptive advice to girls under 16, it means that girls or boys under 16 may meet the criteria for competence to give or refuse consent to medical treatment of any kind. The Lords decided in this case that understanding is the key element of competence. The adolescent must be capable of understanding the nature, purpose and material risks of the proposed treatment before giving or withholding his consent.

Anyone involved in caring for adolescents should review the extent to which they involve them in decisions regarding their treatment. 'To ignore their views, either implicitly or explicitly could be to lack respect for a child's autonomy and to ignore their competence to make legally valid decisions' (Charles-Edwards 1991).

TEENAGE PREGNANCIES AND SEX EDUCATION

Children today are far more sexually aware, through the media and peer pressure, than they were 20 years ago. One study in America showed that 50% of all teenage women have had sexual intercourse by the time they are 17 years old (Kantrowitz 1987). In Britain, a 1990 health education survey of 10 000 16- to 19-year-olds found that 31% of 16-year-olds had had full sexual intercourse, rising to 70% by the age of 19

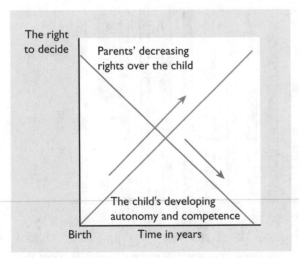

Figure 22.1 The increasing autonomy of the child over time.

years (RCOG 1991). This has led to increased concern among health professionals and parents over the increased number of pregnancies and sexually transmitted diseases in the adolescent age group. The number of teenage pregnancies accounts for a large proportion of all pregnancies. For example, in 1988, 8.5% of the total number of maternity cases in the United Kingdom were in the under-20-year-old age group (Alcock 1992). The rate currently stands at nearly 10 per 1000 girls in the 13- to 15-year-old age group. Figure 22.2 shows conceptions in young women aged under 20 and under 15 years between 1970 and 1987.

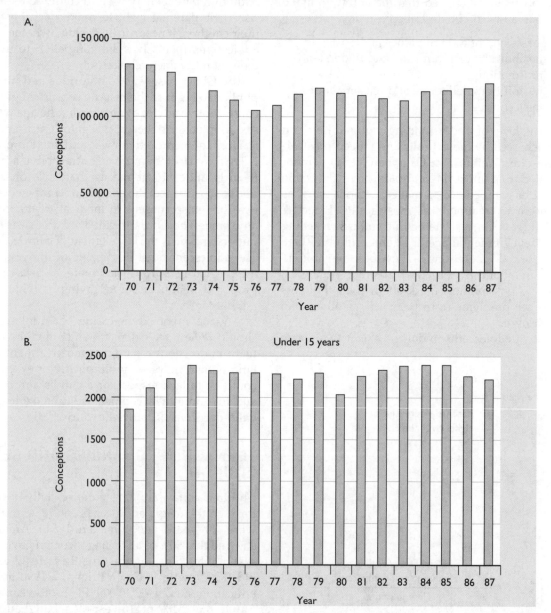

Figure 22.2   Number of conceptions annually from 1970 to 1987 in young women aged: (A) under 20 years; (B) under 15 years. (Source: OPCS 1991.)

The graph in Figure 22.3 may give a clearer picture; it shows changes in conception rates from 1970 to 1987 in 14- to 17-year-olds. This shows that the conception rate is increasing in all age groups. The most worrying are the 14-year-olds; although this group is small, the risks are higher.

Teenage sex is seen to be a normal stage of development (Strasburger & Brown 1985). Experimentation is a typical and expected behaviour of adolescence. Interest in the opposite sex, both as friends and as 'dates' increases during the teenage years. Teenage pregnancy, in particular in girls under 16 years of age, can be a traumatic experience medically, socially and emotionally. Physically and psychologically, the young girl is not prepared for it. Pregnancy in such a young girl carries the risk of many medical complications; for example there is an increased risk of miscarriage and intrauterine growth retardation. What may be more important, however, is the emotional impact pregnancy has on a teenage mother and her family. Pregnancy can lead to isolation, family breakdown and loss of education and a secure future. The period of adolescence is difficult enough by

itself. Add to this the developmental pressures imposed by pregnancy and impending parenthood, and the problems are compounded. The Government White Paper, *The Health of the Nation* (DoH 1992), identified teenage pregnancy as an aspect of health that needs to be tackled on an urgent basis. The target is to halve the present rate of conception amongst the under-16s by the year 2000. In order to reduce this rate, there needs to be increased awareness of the problem, provision of sex education in schools and comprehensive family planning services. Sex education needs to be included in the curriculum for students as young as 12 years old. Also, contraceptive usage must be encouraged and contraceptives should be easily accessible to those who wish to use them.

Despite the rulings of the Gillick case (1985) many general practitioners are reluctant to advise and prescribe contraceptives for girls under the age of 16, without parental consent. However, the impact on pregnancy at such a tender age far outweighs any ethical, moral or legal consideration and, in the interest of the child's health, suitable advice and contraception should be provided (Ranjan 1993).

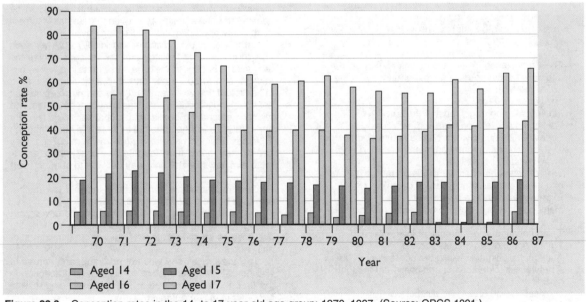

Figure 22.3   Conception rates in the 14- to 17-year-old age group: 1970–1987. (Source: OPCS 1991.)

Comprehensive sex education not only comprises teaching about the biological aspects of sex. It should also impart to teenagers responsibility for their own sexuality, respect for self and others, and include discussions on relationships, commitment, emotions and love. While informed sex education may neither increase nor decrease the incidence of sexual activity, it is at least likely to enhance understanding and respect between the sexes.

ATTEMPTED SUICIDE

Teenage years are not easy. All adolescents have to try to live with conflicting feelings and emotions, new ideas and many physiological changes. Many teenagers simply cannot cope with these changes and have eating disorders, become depressed, and may even contemplate suicide.

Teenage suicide is on the increase. Since 1970, the suicide rate for adolescents between 15 and 19 years has risen by 44%, compared with a 2–6% increase for the general population. In general, girls are more likely than boys to attempt suicide, but boys are more likely to succeed. The main reason for this is that

boys tend to choose more lethal methods of suicide, e.g. hanging, jumping and carbon monoxide poisoning. Girls, on the other hand, tend to choose drug overdose as their method of suicide.

For some adolescents, suicide is seen as the only solution to their problems (Teicher 1970). It may be that they are unable to cope with the physical changes that occur in puberty, possibly because they are unable to face growing up and becoming adults. Other writers, including Gilead & Mulaik (1983) have suggested that adolescent suicide may be a response to a developmental crisis and the adolescent's diminished capacity to cope with a new developmental phase. Various studies have shown that suicidal adolescents have more difficulty with solving problems than adolescents who are

---

Case study 22.1 Jane

Jane, aged 16 years, was admitted to the adolescent bay at 21.00 hours on a Thursday evening, after taking 16 paracetamol tablets. She was drowsy on admission but could easily be roused. Fortunately, the paracetamol levels were within normal limits but Jane needed to be admitted for close observation overnight and assessment by the duty psychologist the following day.

Jane was quiet and withdrawn initially but was soon able to discuss her feelings and the reasons behind the overdose. It transpired that she had exams in a few weeks and felt pressured by her parents, particularly her strict father, into doing well. Jane had also started sleeping with her boyfriend aged 21 years, and was concerned that she might be pregnant. She did not feel that she could talk with her parents, and when she did try to talk to her mother on Thursday afternoon after coming home from college, they had an argument. Jane felt that she could not take any more and saw that the only way out was to take an overdose.

Jane regretted this immediately and told her mother who took her to the casualty department.

On Friday morning, Jane and her parents saw a psychologist who felt that Jane was not suicidal, but took the overdose as an immediate way out without thinking rationally about it.

To Jane's relief, she was not pregnant, and agreed to visit her GP with her mother to discuss contraception in the future. Jane continued to see the psychologist, with her parents, as an outpatient.

Box 22.3 Suicidal signals/problems

- Feeling depressed, indicated by changes in eating and daily habits, poor school performance, apathy and withdrawal
- Loss of self-esteem
- Feeling sad and angry most of the time
- Feeling hopeless, worthless and helpless
- Behaviour changes, which can be subtle or dramatic, e.g. sudden crying for no apparent reason, giving away favourite possessions
- Loss of someone or something important, e.g. death of a loved one (or anniversary of death)
- Extreme isolation and no support
- Major change, e.g. move to new area, new school, break-up of family through separation/divorce
- Talking about suicide, directly or indirectly
- Writing about death and suicide
- Auditory hallucination telling the adolescent to die
- A previous suicide attempt and continued thoughts of suicide
- Intoxication with drugs and alcohol

not suicidal. They seem unable to think logically and clearly about the problem and see suicide as the only way out. It is estimated that more than 80% of all those who die from suicide give out signals of how they are feeling before they commit suicide. Suicide may also coincide with a bereavement or important event. Writers, including Holinger (1978), Patten & Valente (1977), and Schneidman & Faberow (1961), have all listed high-risk symptoms indicative of suicide.

Some of their ideas are summarised in Box 22.3. It is important to point out that any of these symptoms can occur in isolation in the non-suicidal adolescent and be part of the normal process of growing up. However, when they occur together at any given time, the teenager may be unable to handle his or her feelings and emotions, and contemplate suicide.

Nursing care

It is very important for the suicidal adolescent to be cared for in an appropriate environment. The general paediatric ward can present problems as such wards tend to be very busy and there may not be enough time to spend with an adolescent. Ideally, an adolescent who has attempted suicide should be nursed on an adolescent unit or in an area of the ward allocated for teenagers.

The first few days after an attempted suicide can be crucial. When the adolescent is first admitted it is important to ensure that he is physically stable. Following an overdose, for example, a stomach washout may be required, which can be extremely traumatic. Once stable, he may remain an inpatient for a few days, whilst an accurate assessment of the background to the suicide attempt and his mental state is carried out by the child psychologist and other members of the medical team. The adolescent needs to be looked after by nurses who are aware of an adolescent's special needs. In a study by Martin Hicks (1988), it was felt that the nurses caring for these patients needed three main attributes: consistency; listening skills; and

self-awareness. Also important are a sense of humour, empathy and flexibility. It is important to be able to develop rapport and thereby good communication lines with the suicidal adolescent. If possible, he should be looked after by one or just a few nurses, so that a trusting relationship can develop. Only then will the teenager feel safe and free to talk about his problems.

ACKNOWLEDGEMENTS

The author would like to thank Claire Evans, St Peter's Hospital, Surrey, for her assistance with this chapter.

REFERENCES

Alcock K M 1992 Teenage pregnancy and sex education. The British Journal of Family Planning 18: 18–92
Anderson E M, Clarke L 1982 Disability in adolescence. Methuen, London
Becker-Fritz T, Barbee M A 1993 What are the warning signs for suicidal adolescents? Answers Professionally Speaking 13(2): 37–40
Blunden R 1989 An artificial state. Paediatric Nursing 1: 12–13
British Paediatric Association (BPA) 1985 Report of the working party on the needs and care of adolescents. BPA, London
Brykczynska G 1989 Consent. Paediatric Nursing 1: 6–8
Burman D 1985 The paediatrician and the adolescent. In: Too young or too old—how and where should adolescents be nursed? NAWCH, London
Burr S 1993 Adolescents and the ward environment. Paediatric Nursing 5(1): 10–13
Charles-Edwards I 1991 Who decides? Paediatric Nursing 310: 6–8
Coleman J C 1984 The nature of adolescence. Methuen, London
Department of Health (DoH) 1991 Welfare of children and young people in hospital. HMSO, London
Department of Health (DoH) 1992 The health of the nation: a strategy for health in England. Cm 1986. HMSO, London
Department of Health and Social Security (DHSS) 1976 Fit for the future: report of the Committee on Child Health Services. (Court Report) HMSO, London
Duberley J D 1981 Adolescence (Introduction). Nursing, the Add-on Journal of Clinical Nursing 24: 1027
Edgar E D 1988 You are not alone! Journal of Pediatric Nursing 3(4): 276–279
Erikson E 1965 Childhood and society. Penguin, London
Family Law Reform Act 1969 HMSO, London
Gilead M, Mulaik J 1983 Adolescent suicide. A response to developmental crisis. Perspectives in Psychiatric Care

21(3): 94–101

Gillick v. West Norfolk and Wisbech Area Health Authority [1985] 3 All ER

Gillies M 1992 Teenage traumas. Nursing Times 88(27): 26–29

Gordon R R 1981 The adolescent in hospital. Nursing, the Add-on Journal of Clinical Nursing 24: 1045–1050

Hicks M 1988 Not child's play. Nursing Times 84(38): 42–44

Holinger P C 1978 Adolescent suicide. An epidemiological study of recent trends. American Journal of Psychiatry 135: 754–756

Jackson D W 1973 The adolescent and the hospital. Pediatric Clinics of North America 20: 903

Kantrowitz B 1987 Kids and contraception. Newsweek 109 (16 Feb): 54–65

Kennedy I, Grubb A 1989 Medical law: text and materials. Butterworths, Sevenoaks

Kuykendall J et al 1985 Adolescents in hospital. In: Too young or too old, how and where should adolescents be nursed? NAWCH, London

Mackenzie H 1988 Teenagers in hospital. Nursing Times 84(32): 58–61

McKinney J P, Fitzgerald H E, Strommen E A 1977 The adolescent and young adult. The Dorsey Press, Illinois

Marcia J E 1982 Identity in adolescence. John Wiley, Chichester

Miller S A 1987 Self-esteem in the hospitalized adolescent. Issues in Comprehensive Pediatric Nursing 10: 187–194

Ministry of Health (MoH) 1959 The welfare of children in hospital. Report of the Committee on Child Health Services. (Platt Report) HMSO, London

Müller D J et al 1986 Nursing children: psychology, research, and practice. Harper & Row, London

National Association for the Welfare of Children in Hospital (NAWCH) 1984 Charter for children in hospital. NAWCH, London

National Association for the Welfare of Children in Hospital (NAWCH) 1985 Too young or too old—how and where should adolescents be nursed? NAWCH, London

National Association for the Welfare of Children in Hospital (NAWCH) 1990 Setting standards for adolescents in hospital. NAWCH, London

Office of Population Censuses and Surveys 1991 Birth statistics. Series FM1 No 20. HMSO, London

Patten C L, Valente S M 1977 A suicide assessment and intervention. Appleton-Century-Croft, New York

Piaget J, Inhelder B 1958 The growth of logical thinking from childhood to adolescence. Routledge & Kegan Paul, London

Pollach M, Fry J 1986 Common sense paediatrics. McGraw Hill, New York

Ranjan V 1993 Pregnancy in the under-16s: waking up to the realities. Professional Care of the Mother and Child 3(2): 34–35

Roberts D A 1987 Adolescence. Nursing, the Add-on Journal of Clinical Nursing 24: 914–919

Royal College Of Obstetricians and Gynaecologists (RCOG) 1991 Report of the RCOG Working Party on Unplanned Pregnancy. RCOG, London

Schneidman E S, Faberow N L 1961 The cry for help. McGraw-Hill, New York

Strasburger V C 1985 Normal adolescent sexuality. A Physician's Perspective 1: 101

Strasburger V C, Brown R T 1985 Adolescent medicine. A practical guide. Little Brown, Boston

Swanwick M, Oliver R W 1985 Psychological adjustment in adolescence. Nursing 40: 1179–1181

Teicher T 1970 Children and adolescents who attempt suicide. Paediatric Clinics of North America 17: 687–696

Weisfield E, Berger J M 1983 Some features of human adolescence viewed in evolutionary perspective. Human Development 26: 121–133

Weithorn L, Campbell S 1982 The competency of children and adolescents to make informed treatment decisions. Child Development 53: 1589–1598

Wheeler M J 1981 Adolescents and health care. Nursing 24: 1028–1030

World Health Organization (WHO) 1977 Health needs of adolescents. WHO Expert Committee Technical Report Series 609. WHO, Geneva

World Health Organization Expert Committee 1965 Health problems of adolescence. WHO Chronicle Vol. 19. WHO, Geneva

FURTHER READING

British Paediatric Association (BPA) 1985 Report of the working party on the needs and care of adolescents. BPA, London

Edgar E D 1988 You are not alone! Journal of Pediatric Nursing 3(4): 276–279

Eiser C 1993 How teenagers cope with chronic illness and compliance. Maternal and Child Health 18(5): 148–150

Gillies M 1992 Teenage traumas. Nursing Times 88(27): 26–29

Kuykendall J et al 1985 Adolescents in hospital. In: Too young or too old, how and where should adolescents be nursed? NAWCH, London

Mackenzie H 1988 Teenagers in hospital. Nursing Times 84(32): 58–61

National Association for the Welfare of Children in Hospital (NAWCH) 1990 Setting standards for adolescents in hospital. NAWCH, London

Roberts D A 1987 Adolescence. Nursing, the Add-on Journal of Clinical Nursing 24: 914–919

23

Children with mental health problems

Andrew Dickson   Douglas Fraser

This chapter concerns itself with the mental health problems of children and their families, and will endeavour to increase the reader's awareness of the complex nature of children's emotional and psychological problems.

The chapter aims to:
- introduce the student to the concept of mental health development
- discuss the ways in which children's mental health problems are categorised
- discuss the needs for intervention in families of children with mental health difficulties
- summarise the recognised treatment methods available in child psychiatry
- give an overview of the multidisciplinary approach to care
- discuss the extended role of the nurse within child psychiatry.

INTRODUCTION

The provision of health care facilities for children with mental health problems has only been established in this country over the past 30 years. Professionals working in this field require specialised training and a high degree of expertise. Post-registration training in child and adolescent psychiatry is a prerequisite for such work. Many will also be educated in various skills based on treatment programmes, such as family therapy and behaviour therapy.

The incidence of child psychiatric disorders has been described in various research documents and texts. For the purpose of this chapter the authors will consider referrals to the Department of Child and Family Psychiatry at Yorkhill Hospital in Glasgow during the year 1994–1995.

The number of referrals is indicative of the number of children suffering from mental health problems in all areas of the country. Glasgow has a population of 900 000 people of whom 190 000 are under 18 years old. During the past year, 850 new referrals were made to the community outpatient departments, there were 1200 attendances of children at the various programmes, and 30 children were treated as inpatients. The recent health advisory document, *Together We Stand* (HAS 1995), indicates that it is generally accepted that, in a total population of 250 000 of which 20–25% are aged 0–18, one might expect between 5000 and 12 000 children to have a mental health or psychiatric disorder at any one time. The overall level tends to be higher in the older age groups because some disorders persist and others arise in older children.

This chapter sets out to briefly describe the diagnostic categories used in children's mental health and its multifactorial nature. It includes intervention and treatment models which are currently being used and highlights the importance of good case management. It also looks at the various organisational aspects of the service, covering multidisciplinary team work, liaison work and the role of the nurse in child mental health services.

This is a brief introduction to child and family psychiatry and it is recommended by the authors that additional texts should be studied for a more in-depth knowledge of the material covered in this chapter.

For further reading, see Hoare (1993).

EMOTIONAL HEALTH DEVELOPMENT

Emotional development occurs in tandem with all other areas of normal development. Many areas of child development are easily recognised and identifiable. It is therefore quite easy to measure emotional development against expected normal rates of development to determine whether there is any abnormality requiring intervention. Cognitive development can be measured against academic achievement or psychometric testing, and so can be compared readily to generalised norms. Emotional development is more difficult to quantify, making it difficult to establish norms and so diagnose when deviations from these norms are occurring. Chess & Hassibi (1978) state that periods of child development strive to find the lawful relationships among various aspects of development and the mechanisms through which changes emerge. There are still differing opinions concerning the 'lawful relationships' which occur in early stages of childhood development, particularly within infant emotional development. As these children cannot talk and describe the level of their emotional health, emotional development has mainly been based on observation and interpretation of infant and early childhood activity.

It is reasonable to assume that emotional development will follow certain patterns and processes which correspond with physical development. Emotional and mental health development do not occur down a pathway exclusive to themselves, but take place in combination with all the other major areas of development. Difficulties in one area of development may therefore have knock-on effects in other areas. For example, difficulties in emotional development may affect motor development, perception, language acquisition and concept formation.

This may go some way to explain the multifactorial nature of the difficulties expressed in later life by children within this category. One of the more obvious links which can illustrate why emotional development can affect other areas of normal child development, is the relationship between emotional state and ability to socialise or socialisation. Children who through a variety of factors have become socially withdrawn, or excessively shy, will have difficulty in their capacity to seek contact with other children of their own age. Development of social skills and establishing a sense of identity in relation to others is hindered, or indeed does not begin to develop. As these children get older and go to nursery or junior school, the difficulties may become magnified, resulting in their having problems in establishing any normal social interactions. This can then affect or create new areas of emotional/psychological distress/trauma within them.

It is important to indicate, at this stage, the critical nature of the immediate environment on child development. In the early years, children are exclusively reliant on those around them to meet their needs. Initially, the interventions of carers are as basic as making sure that the children are adequately fed, cleaned and nurtured. As children develop, the carers' input is widened to include teaching and educating them in developing life-skills. It is reasonable to assume that dysfunctions within the group of carers will reflect on their ability to provide care, nurture and education for their children. This can result in both abnormal physical development and abnormal mental/emotional development. Children may begin to express inappropriate emotions such as anxiety, aggressiveness, and overactivity. This might influence the carer(s) to continue to respond in inappropriate ways, which can further cement the mental/emotional distress.

Theories of emotional development

There are various theories concerning child development, and various opinions about the level of importance of different theories. The degree of combination between them varies with the background and beliefs of the individuals who practice or follow them. Chess & Hassibi (1978) have provided an excellent introduction to the major theories and split them into three areas:

1. psychoanalytic theory
2. development theory, mainly through Piaget's theories
3. learning theory.

Psychoanalytic theory. Two major exponents of psychoanalytic theory were Sigmund Freud, initially, and later Melanie Klein, who took up the ideas of Freud and expanded and developed them. Their theories were based on observation of infants and young children. From these observations certain psychoanalytic principles were developed as a means of measuring normality/abnormality and explaining or interpreting the emotional/psychological content behind the observations. Further information can be gleaned from the many available works by Freud and Klein, or indeed from interpretations of their works, particularly *Therapeutic Working With Children And Young People* by Copely & Forryan (1987).

Piaget's theory of developmental psychology. Although questioned by many theorists, this attempted to give another explanation of emotional development and was particularly revered by educationalists. Piaget's principles remain relevant reading for those wishing to gain an understanding of the theories behind child development. Piaget attempted to describe the mechanism by which man, therefore child, comes to develop an accurate image of the physical world and his place within it. The major difference between Piaget's theory and the psychoanalytical theory is that Piaget does not view the infant as a passive receptive organism which understands its environment through the contacts it receives. Piaget discusses the fact that intelligence and emotional development is the outcome of active adaptation to the external world, i.e. children have a proactive as well as a reactive component to their development.

Learning theories. These can be crudely grouped as the more behavioural forms of theories which explain development. Those interested in learning theory state that child development can be viewed as a gradual modification of the behaviour of the newborn infant into the more socialised adult form. Both the emotional and psychological development of children are very much influenced by the nature of the society of which they are part. There will be components of the psychoanalytical and Piaget theories that are common to all aspects of children regardless of the society in which they exist, but the central key to development will be society itself.

This introduction to very complex topics serves as a means of introducing the material that comes after it. It should always be taken into account that particularly within psychiatry/ psychology and psychotherapy there is a great deal of continuing debate about even fundamental principles which determine normal and abnormal child development. This chapter can only provide more material for debate, rather than give exclusive answers to many of the questions which it will raise for individuals reading it.

DIAGNOSTIC CATEGORIES OF CHILDREN'S MENTAL HEALTH PROBLEMS (MULTIAXIAL CLASSIFICATION)

Single factors are rarely responsible for psychiatric disturbance in childhood (Hoare 1993). More often there are a multiplicity of circumstances interacting with each other, resulting in the disturbance.

The three main elements that can be identified are:

- constitutional, i.e. genetic, temperamental, disease at birth or trauma during birth
- environmental factors, i.e. family, school, local environment
- physical health, i.e. chronic illness, terminal illness, neurological diseases/mental illness.

As psychiatric disturbance in children is normally multifactorial, it is important when formulating and diagnosing a child's difficulties to have a model which reflects these factors. This is described in the World Health Organization classification of diseases (WHO 1978, 1992), where a clinical descriptive approach is used to diagnosis, and disorders are categorised along five separate dimensions (Rutter et al, WHO 1978):

- axis 1—clinical psychiatric syndromes
- axis 2—specific delays in development
- axis 3—intellectual level
- axis 4—medical conditions
- axis 5—abnormal psychosocial situations.

In axis 1, the classification covers all psychiatric disturbances for a variety of age ranges, including adults. However, it also includes specific descriptions of psychiatric disturbances found in childhood.

Some examples of psychiatric disturbance found in children are given below.

Axis 1—Clinical psychiatric syndromes

Conduct disorder. There are two main types within this classification: socialised and unsocialised conduct disorder. Both of these can be defined as persistent antisocial behaviour, either in the company of the peer group or by the individual. The common symptoms include temper tantrums, oppositional and defiant behaviour, hyperactivity, aggression, stealing, lying, and truanting. It is different from delinquency in that the latter is legal terminology for a young person who has committed a criminal offence.

Enuresis. This condition refers to the involuntary passage of urine where there is no physical abnormality; it may be either nocturnal or diurnal. The term *primary enuresis* is used to describe a child who has never gained full bladder control and has been bed-wetting continuously. *Secondary enuresis* is the term used when there has been at least a 6-month period of dry beds and there has been a recurrence of bed-wetting later in the child's life. Nocturnal enuresis is more common than diurnal.

Encopresis. Encopresis is the inappropriate passage of faeces, again in the absence of any physical cause. The condition can range from a slight soiling of underclothes to the smearing of faeces on furniture and walls.

Emotional disorders. These can best be understood as abnormalities and disturbances of mood and affect and can be recognised in children presenting with anxiety and fearfulness, misery and unhappiness, sensitivity and shyness and social withdrawal, or relationship problems. The term 'emotional disorders' includes a number of states, such as acute anxiety states, phobia states, school refusal, depression or obsessive compulsive disorder.

Hyperkinetic disorder. This disorder presents with the features of poor attention span and distractibility. Children are usually disinhibited and poorly organised. They are also impulsive and have marked mood fluctuations, and can often present with aggressive behaviour. There are also delays in development of specific skills, and peer relationships are often poor.

Childhood autism. Kanner's original (1943) description of 11 children with 'an extreme autistic aloneness' has not been improved upon. He observed that these children have an inability to relate in an ordinary fashion to either people or situation, and also described 'an anxiously obsessive desire for the maintenance of saneness'. The three main features, which are essential for diagnosis, are:

- failure to develop social relationships
- language retardation
- restricted repertoire of activities.

These difficulties are normally evident before 30 months (Hoare 1993).

Asperger's syndrome. This condition was originally described by Asperger in 1944 and shows some similarities to childhood autism. However, the conditions differ in two main aspects. There is no general intellectual retardation in children with Asperger's syndrome and their language development is normal. These children are described as distant, aloof and lacking in empathy; other features include aggressive outbursts and sensitivity to criticism (Kendall & Zealley 1993).

Axis 2—Specific delays in development

This category describes specific delays in the child's biological development and the main elements which have to be considered. These are:

- reading retardation
- arithmetical retardation
- other specific learning difficulties.

These elements of the child's difficulties are not due to intellectual impairment or poor schooling. Some examples are given below.

Developmental speech and language disorder. Commonly there is a delay in the development of normal word sound production, resulting in defects of articulation. The child can also use substitution for consonants and there may be a delay in the use of the spoken language, e.g. developmental articulation disorder, dyslexia.

Specific motor retardation. The main feature of this condition is a serious impairment of motor coordination.

Mixed developmental disorder. This is a mixture of developmental and specific motor retardation. It is usual for the motor clumsiness to be associated with some degree of impaired performance of visual spatial cognitive tasks, e.g. clumsy child syndrome, developmental coordination disorder, developmental dyspraxia.

Axis 3—Intellectual level

This criterion is used in order to understand the child's intellectual capacity and capabilities. A child's intellect can often be assessed by means of psychometric testing or using other clinical evidence which is available. It ranges from within the normal range of variation to profound mental retardation.

Axis 4—Medical conditions

This refers to physical illness and disability in relation to the psychological well-being of children. Illness or disability can often affect a child's development. Many illnesses or disabilities inevitably limit or restrict a child's ability and opportunity to acquire everyday skills and to develop interests or hobbies. Children with chronic illness or disability and their families are more at risk of developing psychological or emotional disturbance.

Examples may include:

• Asthmatic children are less able to participate in exercise, and this could have an effect on their development in relation to peer group functioning.
• Children suffering from diabetes have dietary restrictions, and this can often cause complications in the management of these children by their parents, who have to restrict what food their children can eat. As many diabetic children have to inject insulin, they are sometimes shunned or ridiculed by their peer group.
• Children with epilepsy can also have their activities restricted, and this can have implications for their everyday life; for example flashing lights can bring on seizures. This condition also carries a great deal of stigma and can result in isolation as peer relations may be poor.

Axis 5—Abnormal psychosocial situations

This category concerns itself with associated abnormal psychosocial situations which are abnormal in both the developmental and social circumstance. It includes 16 aspects which directly or indirectly may affect the child's emotional and psychological well-being. Some of the main aspects are:

• mental disturbance in other family members
• discordant family relationships
• over-involvement by one or both parents
• inadequate parental control

Activity 23.1

Think of children with a chronic illness whom you have cared for. Make a list of the restrictions that their illness imposes on their lifestyle and consider whether this is likely to have an impact on their self-image or self-esteem.

• lack of affection
• distorted communications
• anomalous family situations.

It also refers to inadequate living conditions and psychosocial disturbances which the child may experience outwith the family environment. They include:

• stresses at school
• social transplantation or migration
• discrimination and persecution.

It is frequently the case that children who are referred to psychiatric services, although often the identified patient, may well be a product of a dysfunctional family process, e.g. over-involvement, discordant family relationships.

Having considered the multifactorial aspects of a child's presenting difficulties, the reader will begin to understand that none of the WHO categories can be understood in isolation. In other words, the child may well be presenting with symptoms that are the result of a traumatic major life event which the family has experienced, i.e. death of a close family member, separation or divorce of parents, or unemployment resulting in loss of financial security.

Another quick check list to aid understanding of the severity of the child's presenting problems is to consider the three main aspects of a child's environment:

• family
• school
• community.

Should the child be presenting difficulties in all three areas, then the nature of the problem is more severe than if difficulties are confined to only one area.

The mental health problems of children can be best summarised by reference to Dr P. Hoare's book, *Essential Child Psychiatry*, as abnormalities of 'emotions, behaviour or relationships which are sufficiently severe and persistent to handicap the child and their social or personal functioning

Activity 23.2

Describe the components of the diagnostic evaluation and the multi-axial diagnostic classification used in child psychiatry.

and/or to cause distress to the child, the parents and to the people in the community'.

INTERVENTION MODEL

The treatment of children's mental health problems has, like all other areas of psychiatry, evolved over the last 20 years. However, the approaches have evolved more rapidly over the last 10 years. There is now a greater understanding of the factors that can result in children's mental health problems. Particular emphasis is placed on the multifactorial nature of the causative factors. This has resulted in changes in the professional approach to assessing and treating these difficulties. It has also resulted in a broadening of the strategies used to assess and treat these conditions.

We will now look at a simple model which attempts to explain the multifactorial nature of children's mental health problems (Fig. 23.1). This model will then be used to illustrate the different treatment strategies which are used.

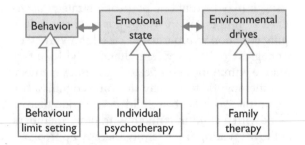

Figure 23.1   Intervention model of mental health problems in children.

Behaviour

It is usually a child's behaviour that initially brings him or her to the attention of the services. Inappropriate behaviours can be noticed at home, within the neighbourhood, in schools or nurseries, and in the general practitioner's surgery. Inappropriate behaviour very quickly alerts the outside world to something being amiss. If behaviour is viewed as a child's means of communication, then the situation makes even more sense. For example, when a child is misbehaving in a classroom situation, it is reasonable to assume that there is an internal reason for this. At the other end of the scale, an extremely withdrawn child is communicating his internal world in a different way. It is not surprising to know that one of the major approaches within child psychiatry was to attempt to modify or change behaviours. A wide variety of behavioural approaches have been, and still are, practised throughout the country. Behavioural practices can range from the basic strategy of attempting to extinguish inappropriate behaviour and encourage appropriate behaviour through a reward system, to more sophisticated behavioural approaches which involve cognitive behavioural therapies. Imagine a child who has frequently been admitted to hospital with non-specific headaches or stomach pains where the physical factors have been ruled out. It is important to understand that the pains may be related to feelings and then the child can be provided with strategies for dealing with these feelings when they arise, instead of complaining of headaches or stomach pains. It should also be remembered that in a hospital setting there will be a natural degree of limit-setting, regardless of the level of disturbance of the child. There will be an environment within the hospital, within which the child must function. (See 'Organisation and systems', pp. 403–408.)

Emotional state

As we see in our model, there is a relationship between behaviour and emotional state. Behaviour is a means of communication; therefore, disturbed behaviour is a means of communicating a disturbance. It would therefore be reasonable to assume that the behavioural disturbance reflects a mental health disturbance. To clarify this, we can call it a disturbance of emotional state. Here, we are clearly outlining a relationship between the behaviour and the emotional state. It is the feelings, or emotions, that are the important factor in the inappropriate behaviour. To understand the behaviour, we must understand the emotional functioning of the child. If this can be achieved, there will be a greater understanding, and a more effective strategy can be devised to manage the behaviour. One of the main strategies of intervention at this stage would be for the nurse therapist to have a clear understanding of the child's perception or understanding of his/her past, present and future. The strategies to understand and communicate with a child are fully covered in basic psychotherapy textbooks.

 For further reading, see Hoare (1993).

The intervention a nurse therapist may make would very much depend on the skill level of that nurse and includes simple observation of a child over a given period of time. A large amount of information and understanding can be gained by observing how children interact with their peers and adults, in particular their parents and relatives, and how they spend the time when they are on their own. It should be emphasised that observation is a skill and thought should be given to how these observations are recorded, and what use is made of them. As nurses become more skilled they can become involved in more therapeutic interventions. These may involve individual sessions with a child of an hour's duration where particular emphasis is placed on the inter-

actions between the child and the nurse therapist. (See 'Treatment and interventions', pp. 397–403.)

Environmental drives

If we return to the intervention model (Fig 23.1), we see that there is a relationship between the emotional state and the wider systems (environmental). Behaviour does not occur at random, just as disturbance in the emotional state does not occur at random. The model shows that there is a relationship between the disturbed emotional state and some factor within the child's world. The child may be experiencing feelings which he cannot understand, but there may be clear reasons for this within the outside world. In general, the major environmental drives which affect emotional state are the child's immediate family and close relatives. The other major environmental drives are the neighbourhood and school. If changes were made in these environmental drives, they may alter the emotional state which may in turn result in an improvement in behaviour. The most common treatment strategy of environmental drives is a family therapy approach. There are a variety of family therapy approaches and many are long-standing. (See 'Treatment and interventions', pp. 397–403.)

The nurse also has a role liaising with the community services, such as social work, health visitors, GPs, schools and other agencies. It is important that all these agencies are functioning in a coordinated fashion to ensure successful intervention.

Due to the complex multifactorial nature of the cases, it may be that one particular strategy or intervention in isolation would not be enough. It is quite common in a particular case for a variety of strategies to be used simultaneously to effect change within the complicated system. A member of a therapeutic team may do some cognitive behavioural work with a child or psychodynamic work with a child in tandem with other members of the team adopting a family therapy approach.

The nature of the model can also be highlighted by use of case studies (see Case studies 23.1 and 23.2).

Case study 23.1 Susanne

Susanne, aged 8, has frequently presented at casualty departments with stomach pains which have had no physical basis. Recently she has been complaining of low mood and feeling that she wants to die. Her mother and father have a fragile relationship, although at present there have been no separations. The child has been admitted to hospital to determine whether there are any psychological reasons for her stomach pains, and also because of her recent thoughts of self-harm. A short assessment period occurred where therapists got to know the child and the family in more detail and were able to devise a formulation and treatment plan. The formulation stated that there were serious problems within the marital relationship between the parents. It was increasingly likely that they would separate. Susanne was very concerned about what was happening and the matter was not being explained to her. She was coping with her confusion by presenting with somatic complaints, such as stomach pains etc.

There were three points of intervention:

- Some cognitive behavioural work was done with Susanne at the beginning of the therapeutic work. This made the connection between the physical symptoms she was experiencing and her emotional state.
- Individual play therapy was practised to understand her perception of what was going on in her world. During these sessions she was able to state that she was extremely concerned that her mother did not love her father and they were going to leave her. She felt that if she was ill, then they would concentrate on her and not their own difficulties.
- Intervention was done at the stage of family therapy to:
  a. assess the state of the marriage, and
  b. allow the adults to make decisions and then be able to explain them to Susanne in a way that she would understand.

This case study serves to illustrate the multifactorial nature of the work and, therefore, the need for multifactorial approaches. The simplicity of the model and the simplicity of the examples stated do not accurately reflect the complexity of the work, but give an initial understanding of the complex area.

Case study 23.2 John

John, aged 7, presented with severe conduct disorder in school and at home; exclusions from school were compounded by numerous hospital admissions and frequent family moves due to his father's type of employment. John's diagnosis was accurately determined as severe emotional disorder due to a combination of specific learning difficulties (making him unable rather than unwilling to learn without special help), coupled with lack of emotional warmth from both parents in tandem with major life event changes (hospital admission, moving home). This lack of warmth resulted in John being given an inadequate explanation for either his hospital admission or the sudden moves, resulting in a fearful and anxious child.

Interventions
- Behavioural. Limit-setting to contain any excessive conduct disorder, helping to improve self-esteem and feeling of safety in John.
- Individual psychotherapy. To establish John's perception of the situation, i.e. his understanding of further frequent hospital admissions and frequent moves of home.
- Wider system—environmental drives. To establish with his family that John's 'real' difficulties are emotional rather than behavioural and to 're-focus' them to deal with this. To also seek an educational establishment more suited to John's educational needs.

teachers, will often find themselves working with children and their families. This work is extremely important and offers counselling, support and advice to families. However, family therapy is a focused skill which one has to be trained in, and involves the therapist being familiar with family assessment and treatment techniques which are intricate and complex.

Family therapy was first introduced into this country in the late 1950s and remains closely identified with child and adolescent psychiatry. It is often the case that children who present with emotional difficulties are seen as the presenting problem of a dysfunctional family system, i.e. children who have been traumatised due to divorce, separation, bereavement or abuse. In other cases, the family dysfunctions can be poor parenting or problem-solving, or inadequate communication systems. Family therapists will often work with the structures and hierarchy of the family, which may have broken down. Such breakdown can create situations which make it

TREATMENT AND INTERVENTIONS

Family therapy

Working with families in child psychiatry is inevitable and therefore family assessment and therapy skills are extremely useful. Family therapy, however, should not be confused with working with families. Professionals, i.e. nurses, doctors and difficult for children and young people to grow and develop, e.g. poor behaviour controls, lack of warmth and confusion of roles. The child may adopt the role of a departed or absent parent, thus creating a parental child who feels she has the authority and control of an adult.

It is important before engaging in therapy with a family to assess the difficulties. Then an opinion can be formed which will identify the areas of family dysfunction that need to change. Family therapy has various schools of thoughts including problem-centred family therapy, structural family therapy, analytical family therapy, and integrated models of family therapy.

For further reading on family therapy, see Barker (1992).

Problem-centred family therapy

This work was pioneered by the McMaster Group in Canada who developed an explicit model of problem-centred therapy. This was developed from a study of normal families and the emphasis is on assessment. It concentrates on six dimensions of family functioning which are:

- problem-solving
- communication
- roles
- effective responses
- effective involvement
- behavioural controls (Will & Wrate 1986).

Structural family therapy

This looks at the family's organisational structure and the various relationships within it, taking into consideration the developmental and environmental factors. The theories which it supports are structural techniques such as family sub-systems and boundaries and the regulation of emotional intensity. It also makes good use of diagrammatic information in models to describe

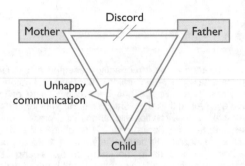

Figure 23.2   Diagram describing discord between parents in which the mother communicates unhappiness via the child.

the family system. An example of this is triangulation of children where there is discord between both parents (Fig. 23.2).

For further reading on structural family therapy, see Minuchin (1974).

Analytical (psychodynamic) model

This was pioneered by Robin Skynner from the Tavistock Clinic in London and looks at the psychodynamic approaches to family work. The main aspects of this model provide valuable concepts for understanding difficulties in family relationships and it permits a depth of meaning to interpretative work with families where this may well be appropriate. This, therefore, can

Activity 23.3

Select a child who is well known to you and has presented with an emotional or behavioural problem. Does the child have difficulties within the family, within the school or within the community?

Draw a family tree, looking at the hierarchy and the relationships within the family.

enable the therapist to have a greater under-standing and tolerance of family anxiety/dynamics within the session. A brief and simple example can be to explore the parents' own childhood and adolescence in order to under-stand their present function.

For further reading on analytical family therapy, see Skynner & Cleese (1993).

Integrated model

The integrated model is a combination of the three preceding models, where the therapist will use his or her skills to assess the family from a problem-centred, structural and psychodynamic model and will also use the same extensive skills in order to change and modify the family's dynamics and functioning.

Behaviour therapies

Behaviour therapies are used in child and adolescent psychiatry as an individual technique to resolve or improve the child's presenting difficulties. There are a number of behavioural therapy techniques; however, they can be best understood as belonging to one of three main categories:

- exposure techniques including desensitisation and modelling
- operant techniques including reinforcement, extinction and punishment
- cognitive behavioural techniques.

A common exposure technique used for chil-dren suffering from anxiety or phobic states is the use of a desensitisation programme. The pro-gramme involves a graded and gradual expo-sure to fearful situations or objects. This is used in conjunction with relaxation and anxiety management techniques.

Case study 23.3 Jamie

Jamie, aged 6, was referred by his GP with behavioural disturbance and mood swings. Assessment of the family revealed that they were a recently reconstituted family of just over 2 years. Jamie's biological mother had died of cancer just prior to his fourth birthday. His father met his present partner shortly afterwards and they had married 6 months later. His stepmother was diagnosed as having Crohn's disease, which was exacerbated by stress, and suffered from frequent ill health due to this. During the initial family assessment, it was discovered that Jamie's parental grandparents had acted as surrogate parents after his mother's death, during his father's grief, and at the present time still enforced some of their own behav-iour controls on Jamie.

Some of the dynamics and difficulties which arose from the assessment of this family was that the step-mother was not recognised as Jamie's legitimate parent by his paternal grandparents. This had an adverse effect on the parents, who had little opportunity to establish their own relationship and were therefore not able to deal with the issues surrounding their status as a reconstituted family. These issues included, good parenting, communi-cation, effective involvement and the establishment of roles. The paternal grandparents constantly imposed their own controls and authority on the family and treated their son (Jamie's father) as if he were a child. It was revealed later that he had not been able to establish his indepen-dence from his parents. This friction and acrimony led to a deterioration in his wife's condition and therefore compro-mised her new position as a wife and stepmother.

Work with the family was carried out to establish firm limits and boundaries between them and the paternal grandparents in order to establish them as an indepen-dent family unit. This enabled them to establish their role as a parental couple. Some marital work was also carried out to enable the couple to spend some time together to reinforce their own relationship, which in turn supported their independence as a family unit.

Positive reinforcement

This is one of the commonest models used with children. The method, which involves the use of star charts, contracts and diaries, promotes the development of desirable behaviour through a reward system for particular behaviour. The most common condition treated with this tech-niques is bed-wetting/enuresis. The therapist would in the first instance ask the child or parents (if required) to keep a diary of the bed-wetting. A star chart is then introduced to measure and monitor the child's progress. The

Case study 23.4 Linda

Linda, aged 13, was referred to the service by her GP after having been treated by several agencies for a chronic school refusal problem, which had been ongoing for approximately 1 year. When Linda was first seen by her therapist during the summer months, it was discovered that her father had died of a heart attack 1 month earlier. Linda found herself being confined to the family home and was losing contact with her friends and peers. The mother, who was obviously grief stricken, was now focusing more attention on her daughter and was becoming over-involved and more protective. This resulted in Linda regressing in her behaviour. She was now sleeping in her mother's bed and became anxious and upset if she was not constantly in her mother's presence (separation anxiety).

Assessment at the school indicated that prior to the summer holidays, and her father's demise, Linda had attended school on a sporadic basis and, when she did attend school, she was allowed to use a storeroom where work was brought to her, rather than attend classes. This storeroom overlooked the car park where her mother and father sat in the family car until school finished. This allowed Linda the opportunity to observe her parents throughout the school day.

After initial assessment, a contract of work was set up with Linda, her family and the school. This encompassed a desensitisation programme with Linda, which was set up with Linda, taking into account her wishes and realistic aims and objectives. Initially, this included driving to the school, sitting in the car and discussing her anxieties. Gradually Linda moved on to walking round the school and increasing the time spent there by short periods. The reinforcement for Linda was in the form of conquering and managing her fears. During the process, anxiety management techniques and relaxation exercises were used to allow her to cope. A cognitive behavioural approach was also used to help Linda address her difficulties in relation to her fears of school, i.e. her acute anxiety. Symptoms of palpitations, flushes and sweating were seen by her as symptoms of a heart attack, similar to that which had killed her father. This obviously was a negative element which required to be constantly addressed, challenged logically, and supported by the positive element of her return to school. Linda was also afraid that whilst she was away from the family home, something dreadful would happen to her mother, leaving her and her elder brother parentless. Again, these fears were born out of the tragic death of her father and reinforced earlier fears that she had had in relation to her parents, which had no logical basis.

After a period of 12 weeks of treatment and support of the school and family, Linda was successfully reintegrated into school and completed her Standard and Higher Grade examinations.

child is rewarded when sufficient stars have been gained. Rewards can be material, social or privileges. Goals and objectives should be realistic and achievable.

Cognitive behaviour therapy

The principal theory behind this technique involves the individual's cognition and thoughts concerning himself, his environment and the effects that will have on his future (Shaffer et al 1985). These thoughts are of a negative nature and continually reinforce the individual's low opinion of himself. For example: 'I am not liked by my teacher; therefore, that means no-one likes me at school.' The objectives and treatment are:

- to train the child to record and monitor the maladaptive thoughts and the resulting behaviour
- to offer alternative explanations for the situation
- to encourage a more appropriate behaviour
- to evaluate the outcome of the treatment.

Psychotherapeutic methods

Play can certainly be described as a mirror into the world of the child. Play is an expression of:

- the child's understanding of the outside world
- the child's internal world.

Psychotherapists put great emphasis on understanding play. To understand this topic in great detail, it is certainly advisable to be familiar with the early principles of Sigmund Freud and, more importantly, the later work of Melanie Klein and Anna Freud. There is no doubt that whatever the individual's opinion of psychotherapy there is some merit in seeing play as a means of communication and therefore available for interpretation. Nurses who are not trained in analysis, or are sceptical of analysis, can still work extremely well with children on psychotherapeutic principles. This is best summarised by explaining the difference between directive and non-directive play therapy as a means of taking initial, but significant, steps down the long road of understanding psychotherapy.

The relationship between the individual and the child, and the environment in which that relationship occurs is very important for the success of directive or non-directive play therapy. If at all possible, the following conditions are required:

1. Individual sessions should take place in the same room.

2. This room should ideally be bare with only reasonable, planned furniture; it should not be cluttered with toys and play equipment that have been used with other children. Everything used in the session should, ideally, be taken into the room and taken out again at the end of the session.

The play equipment used should be carefully considered, rather than gathered together at random. It would be advisable to get some understanding of what the child's interests and likes are prior to any sessional work commencing. However, it is important that there is a wide range of play equipment that stimulates all five senses available to the child for the session. It should range from things which are pleasant to things which are more unpleasant. For example, it would be suitable to have a number of cuddly, warm animal puppet figures, such as a polar bear or hedgehog, and also to have other figures which are less pleasant to the eye or to the touch. It is usual for therapists to build up their own collections of play equipment over time. They may gather equipment which they particularly favour or has worked well in the past. However, in general, therapists tend to behave like magpies and collect a great deal of equipment which they find suitable and which they can disregard should the child be uninterested. There should also be a range of equipment which allows free expression, such as pens, pencils, paint and paper. Some of the more recent innovations which have been extremely useful are the mobile play figures which can be utilised in a number of different settings.

3. The time of the session is also quite important. If at all possible (this is one of the hardest things to organise) the session should happen roughly at the same time and place. If this is not possible, then certainly the length of the session should remain consistent. In general, it seems that sessions tend to last between 45 minutes and 1 hour. It is important to get over to the child that this is the child's time and, regardless of how the child tends to use this time, the time will remain consistent. Therefore, if a child appears bored it is very important not to stop the session in response to a request to do something else. Conversely, it is also important to finish the session on time, again so the child sees the time spent with the therapist as significant and important.

Leaving the room is something which should not be encouraged. It is common for children to ask to go to the toilet when they are bored or want to find a way of relieving themselves, not just physically but also emotionally, from a difficult situation. A child may want to leave or run out of the room, particularly if he is expressing emotions which he has difficulty coping with. This illustrates again the significance of interesting play equipment.

On leaving the session, it is useful to show the child where the play equipment and work that has been done is stored as a way of reassuring him of the importance of the session and also of its confidentiality. It would be a lie to tell a child that anything that is said in the session will be kept confidential, as this is clearly not the case. It is useful to say to him that anything that he says or does in the session will be between the therapist and himself. An exception to this would be if the therapist considered that because of what the child has communicated, some harm may result to the child or a member of his immediate family. Although this is not entirely satisfactory, it does help some children.

More creative touches such as the child's own appointment card or calendar to illustrate when the next session will occur are always useful. The more creative the individual the greater the likelihood there is of sessional work being interesting and successful.

Non-directive therapies

Non-directive therapies are particularly useful during an assessment stage of working with a child. In non-directive therapies the therapist plays as small a role as possible within the sessions and concentrates as much as possible on observation. Obviously, if the child wishes the therapist to participate in some of the play, the therapist should do so. It also may at times be important for the therapist to ask for clarification about a name or age or sex of a particular character within the play.

The benefit of this form of therapy is in the observation. It is important that the therapist is aware that the child may be functioning at a very subtle or subconscious level. Seemingly minor or unimportant events may in fact be very significant. The therapist should write down the content of the session, in as much detail as possible, as soon as the session has been completed. This enables two things; firstly the therapist, at leisure, can think in more detail about what occurred during the session and, secondly, if she or he has access to experienced supervision, there is more information to present from these sessions. The therapist should then be able to see whether recurrent themes exist within the sessions and gain some understanding of what may be the significance of these. In doing this, the age and cognitive ability of the child have to be taken into consideration. The great debate which exists surrounding non-directive therapy is how far should interpretations be taken. There is at present no definitive answer to the question of interpretation within non-directive sessions. However, it would be reasonable to assume that recurrent themes are significant to the child and those which reflect situations which may be known about from other sources such as family meetings and case notes are doubly so. It would be practical to assume that the best way to approach the issue would be that once certain themes have been developed then hypotheses can be provided to explain these themes. These hypotheses can then be tested out in a more directive approach, using directive therapies.

Directive therapies

As the name implies, these therapies are led by the therapist, although there is still a great deal of scope for flexibility within them. For example, it may be that during non-directive work the theme of violence in the home has reappeared time and time again. It would be reasonable to design a more directive therapy to explore this area further. For example, some directive work could be done on anger, i.e. Who gets angry in the house? What happens when people get angry? What makes people scared? What makes a child angry or frightened? If the theme is non-productive, it is very easy to switch to another area. If the theme is productive, then issues can be pursued more vigorously, as there is more certainty that the information being provided is significant.

There are a number of excellent books which act as work books. These can be extremely useful in directive therapies. Examples of these are *This is Me* by Merrill Hamil, *My Secret File* by John Asthrop and *The Anti-Colouring Book* by Susan Striker & Edward Kimmel. These books provide general directive information and they are extremely useful, particularly with older children. More specialised directive material is available: for example, *I Know the World's Worst Secret* (a child's book about living with an alcoholic parent) by Doris Sandford with pictures by Gracie Evans; *The Very Worst Monster* by Pat Hutchins, which looks at a new child coming into the family and sibling rivalry; and *What's Under My Bed?* by James Stevenson, which is a way of explaining night fears.

Thus, we get an understanding of the steady progression between directive and non-directive therapies. The scope for both types of work is huge and very much depends on the skill and adequate supervision of the individual. Without suitable supervision and skill training, nurses should not undertake these forms of work.

Group work with children and their families

Like all other therapies, there are a wide variety of approaches to and strategies for group work with children and their families. Groups can range from specialised activity groups right through to very specific groups aimed at treating a particular symptom or condition. There are a number of areas to consider before deciding on which form of group to pursue.

Initially, it is very important to decide whether the group should be open or closed. If the group contains the same members throughout the period of the group, this is known as a closed group. In an open group, decisions have to be taken as to whether the group should fluctuate in numbers and members. This may be due to the actual nature of the establishment wanting to run the group. For example, in an inpatient unit there may fluctuating numbers in the population, making it difficult to run a closed group. Fluctuating groups or open groups tend therefore, to be more practical.

The second most important consideration is the age range of the children within the group. Age range must take into account cognitive ability as well as chronological age. It is desirable that some assessment of the possible group participants should take place prior to the group being organised, to ensure that the group composition is based on knowledgeable decisions. Examples of the variety of groups include:

1. *Specialised activity group.* Over the past 3 years in Glasgow, the inpatient unit has been running a series of puppetry workshops on a weekly basis. This involves the making of puppets, the writing of stories, and production of the material which has been made. Whilst many of the activities are based on enjoyment, it is clear that there is great scope for puppetry to be used within individual and group work. When skills have been developed by both staff and children, puppetry is used in individual sessions, to assist assessment and treatment.

2. *Cognitive behavioural anxiety management group.* A directed group was devised to work with children who had been admitted to hospital with non-specific stomach aches and headaches or other physical symptoms which, after thorough investigations, were shown to have no physical basis. It was concluded that these children were having difficulty in coping with levels of anxiety, and this was being expressed in physical symptoms. A group was devised around a number of similar children with the goals of:

   a. gaining understanding of the connection between feelings and physical symptoms

   b. giving the children strategic management strategies to cope, should these feeling arise again.

3. *Group activities with children and their families.* In this instance there are two groups, one for the mothers and one for the children. The children's group consists of pre-school hyperactive children and it is facilitated by a number of therapists who model appropriate responses to hyperactive children. The mothers' group is run with similar work strategies being put to them. The advantages are that mothers can see strategies working successfully and learn from the model strategies practised by the professional facilitators. This allows the adults to discuss more complex issues.

ORGANISATION AND SYSTEMS

The multidisciplinary team

> A satisfactory child and adolescent mental health service requires a wide range of assessment and treatment provisions and is only possible when contributions are available from the full range of relevant professionals.
>
> (HAS 1995)

Although the structure, role and function of multidisciplinary teams has been changing over the years, the basic principles underlying practice remain the same. Effective child psychiatric services rely on the professional skills of different disciplines being brought together to carry out both complex assessments and effective treatment interventions. This is managed by recruiting a number of professionals from different backgrounds, most commonly child psychiatrists, psychologists, psychotherapists, nurses, social workers and occupational therapists. All of these professionals offer different contributions to the multidisciplinary team and these will be briefly described.

Child psychiatrist. Psychiatrists have, in addition to their general psychiatric training, spent a number of years specialising in child and adolescent psychiatry. They not only offer their medical knowledge, but also provide a valuable diagnostic service to this specific group. In addition, they offer treatment programmes and consultation services.

Clinical psychologist. Psychologists are graduates who will do a further 4 years' generic training, working with people who have emotional and psychological difficulties (HAS 1995). If they wish to specialise in child psychiatry, they will often have had additional training/experience in working with children. They offer a variety of treatment programmes from both a behavioural and psychodynamic model. They also provide psychometric testing to assist in the assessment process.

Child psychotherapist. Psychotherapists receive a 4-year postgraduate training in communication with children and adolescents. This enables them to understand the feelings and thoughts of young people, and thereby more effectively understand the roots of emotional and behavioural problems. Their work is informed by psychoanalytical theory and knowledge of child development. Their work is normally on an individual basis with children.

Occupational therapists. The degree course in occupational therapy enables occupational therapists to analyse a child and family's function or dysfunction in areas of daily living. They are trained to devise a therapeutic activity for children and their families in relation to identified problem areas.

Child psychiatric nurses. Child psychiatric nurses working in the sub-speciality of child psychiatry should, if possible, be trained in either professional studies, three modules (Scotland), or ENB603 (England). Nurses will provide valuable input to teams in both inpatient and outpatient settings. In the inpatient department they offer not only therapeutic roles for the children and families with whom they work, but also provide a therapeutic setting which encompasses structuring the environment, providing an appropriate social backdrop. They are also able to continuously monitor the progress made by children in the inpatient departments.

Nurses in outpatient teams are often trained in therapeutic techniques such as family therapy, group therapy and individual psychotherapy. They also liaise closely with other services and agencies who contribute to the child's well-being, i.e. social work department, school, and voluntary agencies.

    For further reading, see Wilkinson (1983).

Social workers. Social workers normally have a degree in social science and follow this with a postgraduate training in social work. Social workers working in the field of child psychiatry normally have specialist therapeutic skills in both counselling and family therapy and offer expert advice in legal and statutory aspects of child care.

Although all the disciplines have their own training and special training in child and family psychiatry, their goals and functions can sometimes overlap. However, a good multidisciplinary team should offer a comprehensive assessment package and a wide range of treatment models, including individual and group psychotherapy, marital and family therapy, an activity-based approach, psychopharmacological treatment, and liaison and consultation services.

Nursing and social work

It is important to examine nursing relationships with other members of the multidisciplinary team. Nurses may be involved in child care proceedings and therefore require a knowledge of how the system works. This section describes the important work carried out by nurses in relation to their social work colleagues in a variety of settings, including area social work teams, hospital social work and residential workers.

Social workers have important statutory responsibilities including child protection work, preparing court reports and providing supervision for children and statutory care and control orders, and also the maintenance of standards of care for children in residential settings. Social work departments provide a number of services which include social work area teams, children's homes, and residential assessment centres. They also provide social work services within hospitals, particularly in paediatric hospitals where their role is extremely important in relation to children and their families.

An important piece of legislation is the Children Act 1989 which was implemented in England and Wales in 1991. This Act revised the law in relation to children's rights. The main aspects of this law are to protect children while recognising their rights and looking after their interests, i.e. 'children are separate parties with their own right of representation in legal proceedings'.

In Scotland the Children Act was introduced in 1995. Prior to this, the Social Work Scotland Act of 1968 was in place and this legislation already placed the emphasis on the 'best interest of the child'. The Social Work Scotland Act includes the children's hearing system (in England the equivalent is the juvenile court) which is administered by a Reporter who normally has a background in either law or social work, or both. The Children's Panel consists of lay people who are trained and supported by the Reporter and his/her department. Referral to the Reporter and the Children's Panel can be made by anyone, including professionals, parents and the police.

The parents of the referred child have the right to challenge and question the referral and may be referred to the Sheriff Court for a 'proof hearing'.

The children's hearings are empowered to carry out one of three options:

- dismiss the case
- make a supervision order (voluntary or compulsory)
- make a residential supervision order (place of residence).

Legislation also requires that reviews are carried out once a supervision or residential order has been implemented.

Child psychiatric nurses working within community settings will often participate in this system in two ways:

- by furnishing the Panel with reports and an opinion followed up by recommendations of what is in the child's and family's best interest
- by seeking advice and support from the Reporter about a child whom the nurse may wish to refer to the hearing system.

Social work area teams.   It is part of the remit of nurses working in child psychiatry to liaise and be involved in joint working with social workers from area teams. This is often necessary as the local authority social worker carries the responsibility for the implementation of legislation regarding children. Nurses are also required to attend and contribute to case conferences in various social work department child care provisions, including children's homes, residential schools and assessment centres. They will often represent the views of their colleagues within the psychiatric team.

Relationship between nursing and education

Local authorities have a statutory responsibility to provide education for children and young people up to the age of 16 years. Nurses within both inpatient and outpatient services work alongside education in different ways.

In the inpatient department, the child will

attend a school provided by hospital education. This is a valuable resource in two ways:

- It fulfils the child's educational needs whilst away from school and will assist in his return to the normal school setting on discharge.
- Teachers can assist in assessment of the child's difficulties, especially in identifying specific learning difficulties which may be contributing to the child's condition.

It is important that the nursing and teaching staff make every effort to work together in providing a suitable and therapeutic environment during the child's stay in hospital.

Nurses working in outpatient clinics work with a defined outpatient case load. They will be much more involved with schools and nurseries within their 'patch'. Schools are a valuable source of information during the assessment period, providing information on the child's peer group relationships, relationships with adults and academic achievements and abilities. Nurses working in community settings may also be involved in the treatment of children and young people within schools, i.e. school refusers/phobics. They also provide advice and support to educational staff on children and young people with serious emotional and psychological difficulties. This usually involves the nurse working with the educational psychologist attached to the school.

Community care

In the past, child psychiatric services have been mainly provided from a hospital setting; however, in recent years in line with community adult psychiatry services, child psychiatry has moved into community models, establishing a role for community psychiatric nurses and nurse therapists. As well as a qualification in child and family psychiatry, many of these nurses have additional therapeutic training, i.e. family therapy, counselling, group work. The clinical model should ideally offer a service to a defined area. This allows the service to be more accessible to

children and their families and to promote a user-friendly image, which should enable de-stigmatisation of the service. Another benefit to service delivery is the ability to liaise and establish working links with other services and agencies who have an involvement with children and families, e.g. health visitors working with children under 5 years and their involvement with mothers who may suffer from postnatal depression.

As these clinics are established within specific areas, the nurses are able to gain a greater knowledge of the community where they are working and therefore identify areas of specific need which may have an effect on children's emotional and psychological health and well-being, i.e. economically deprived areas, areas of high unemployment and areas of poor service provision. In addition, nurses are able to familiarise themselves with the provision of services within their area. These would include child care provision, special education facilities, intermediate treatment groups, truancy projects, etc. During the course of this outreach work, the nurse is able to educate established and potential referrers to the service in how to make best use of child psychiatric provisions.

Integrated model

Many agencies offer a variety of expertise and fulfil many roles in providing physical and mental health care to allow children and their families an opportunity to develop and grow in a healthy manner. It has been recognised in recent years, that when purchasing child and adolescent psychiatric services, there should be a joint commissioning body in order to make best use of resources and expertise. It has been suggested that joint commissioning interests could be set up between health care, social care and education. Joint commissioning of services would allow for an assessment to be made of current service provision and how to make more effective use of current resources. This would allow joint assessment of population needs, individual needs and the need for research and

Activity 23.4

Draw up a list of all the agencies which may be involved in the various aspects of children's mental health. How many agencies interact with each other to the benefit of the children and their families?

development. It could also identify the training requirements of staff working in various services and agree a joint strategy. This would lead to joint service planning, which in turn would allow for joint care planning/care management and care programming.

Inpatient and day services within a hospital

The provision of inpatient and day services has been approached in a variety of ways throughout the country over the past 10 years. There has been no set national standard or method of working for inpatient and day services and indeed the services have tended to function according to the local opinions, philosophies and resources available within local areas. However, a general description can be provided of the nature of the main organisational systems which occur in inpatient and day services within child psychiatry.

Setting

The setting of the inpatient/day service can vary. In the main, the positioning of the services within health authorities was very much dictated by the availability of space, rather than discreet premises being identified or discreet premises being purposefully built for child psychiatry. Some inpatient/day service departments are based within a main hospital complex, such as a paediatric hospital, as seen in Birmingham and Glasgow, or within a major psychiatric hospital, as seen in Strathaven Hospital in Cupar.

Other services may find themselves located outside hospital premises and be situated either on their own or in combination with child health centres. These departments take on the appearance of discreet clinics rather than ward areas within a hospital.

Staffing

The skill mix and professional qualifications of staff working in child psychiatry have varied from area to area. It has been traditional for some hospitals who have child psychiatric departments within a paediatric setting, to have employed mainly paediatric trained nurses to cover the ward. In other areas, for example psychiatric hospitals, the central qualification has been RMN rather than RSCN. It is clear that the most suitable nursing staff are those who have a variety of basic qualifications. This is particularly true for child psychiatric units within paediatric settings where a larger than average number of children with psychiatric/psychological problems coupled with physical illness occur.

Training

It is interesting to note that in respect of working with children, child psychiatry has for a long time been the only child speciality where it is not required to have additional training to the first level qualification. It is recommended that nurses working in a general paediatric hospital should have a basic nursing qualification plus the RSCN qualification, or have done the Child Branch of Project 2000. At present the only available, nationally recognised course is the English National Board Course, ENB603, which is a 1-year full-time course (or it can be done on a part-time basis) in child and adolescent psychiatric nursing. However, since the peak of the mid- to late-1980s, the number of centres offering this course has been reduced steadily and the number of centres offering the course full time has also declined.

Range of services

Inpatient and day services themselves can vary. The most common facility is inpatient units which require 5- or 7-day cover. Units that operate over 5 days tend to work on the principle that the parents need to be involved in the care of the child, in particular in evaluating whether any progress is being made. The hospital environment is recognised as being unnatural compared with the child's own natural environment. However, a 5-day unit cannot cater for severe cases where a child or family require 7-day care. There may be additional problems arising from the distances that some families have to travel to attend the service. Both 7- and 5-day units can offer a combination of inpatient and day services, and the day services can range from attendance for 1 day a week for a particular specialised programme, such as for hyperactivity or communication disorder, to 5-day attendance for assessment or more generalised treatment.

Multidisciplinary team working

The multidisciplinary team concept is very important in child psychiatry. Inpatient and day services may have their own discreet multidisciplinary teams or may share members with other multidisciplinary teams, such as outpatient departments or specialised services.

Philosophy

It is therefore clear that the philosophy of how the inpatient/day service runs is very much influenced by the location of the unit, the training of the staff and the make-up of the multidisciplinary team.

THE EXTENDED ROLE OF THE NURSE

As with all areas of nursing over the last 10 years, there have been traumatic changes in the role of the nurse within child psychiatry. Particular emphasis is being placed on value and auditing the exact nature of what each professional does. With this in mind, it is very important for nurses within child psychiatry to establish very clearly what they do and develop skills to increase their ability to function within multidisciplinary teams. If this were to happen, nurses would become a very valuable resource and a very cost-effective asset, as nursing is the least-paid of all professions working within child psychiatry. It is obvious from discussing areas within the multidisciplinary team concept and nurses' relationships with other professionals that there is a great deal of overlap in child psychiatry. One good illustration of this is in the field of family therapy. It is clear that what is required to be a family therapist is training in family therapy skills and then practising the skills developed. It really should not matter from which professional base the individual comes. The defining factor is who is the family therapist, and this should be more influenced by the amount of family therapy training and experience the individual has. Medical personnel will remain the most usual professionals in diagnosing and providing treatment; however, the field beyond this is much more open. For example, would it be preferable to have a psychologist with no family therapy training practising family therapy or a nurse who had extensive family therapy training?

Psychiatric nursing, like all other specialities, has developed a greater community component. Nurses are, therefore, more often being expected to work within multidisciplinary teams where they have a much higher degree of independence. The nurse practitioner role in child psychiatry is well on the way to complete development. Nurses today are acting as case managers, where they have greater responsibility for the management of the particular case they are working on. This responsibility for management is from referral to closure, including formulation and discharge. It is interesting to note that, perhaps, the independent practitioner has already arrived, although this is not fully recognised because of the way the present system operates.

To achieve further development in the role, the main priority must be to improve the level and consistency of training that nurses working in this speciality receive. Things are done very much on a piecemeal basis and there is a definitive need for:

1. A major, or at least much larger, child psychiatry component within the present Project 2000 training schedule. This could both occur within the Child and Mental Health Branches.

2. A nationally recognised further training package that is available to any nurses who are working within the special field of child psychiatry. This would ensure that a basic standard of competency was being achieved, and a recognised qualification would put nurses in a stronger position to participate more fully within multidisciplinary teams.

Finally, as well as being educated themselves, it is vital that child psychiatric nurses become educators, not just about issues concerning their role within the teams they work in but their role within hospital or community settings. It is evident that even in areas which contain child psychiatric units or departments there remains a great deal of ignorance and lack of understanding about what child psychiatric nurses actually do. They are commonly described as 'glorified baby-sitters': 'You just play with the children.' The second major aim is in educating the general hospital population about the child psychiatric nurse's role. This will help develop further understanding of the importance of the psychiatric/psychological or emotional health of the child and the way in which this influences the recovery of a child from physical illness. It may also result in earlier identification of children who suffer from mainly psychological rather than physical problems. For example, a child who may be expressing emotional pain through somatic complaint, such as tummy aches or headaches, may be referred more quickly to the service which is best equipped to help a child with that particular problem.

To conclude, we are looking for the ideal child psychiatric nurse having a clearer identifiable job description. This nurse will have basic qualifications and skills supplemented by a nationally recognised training. She or he will be a manager, clinician and educator of child psychiatry.

REFERENCES

Chess S M D, Hassibi M M D 1978 Principles and practice of child psychiatry. Plenum Press, London

Children Act 1989 HMSO, London

Copely B, Forryan B 1987 Therapeutic working with children and young people. Robert Royce, London

Health Advisory Service (HAS) 1995 Child and mental health services. Together we stand. HMSO, London

Hinshelwood R D 1989. A dictionary of Kleinian thought. Free Association Books, London

Hoare P 1993 Essential child psychiatry. Churchill Livingstone Medical Division, Longman, UK

Kendall R E, Zealley A 1993 Companion to psychiatric studies, 5th edn. Churchill Livingstone, Edinburgh

Rutter M et al (undated) A guide to a multi-axial classification scheme for psychiatric disorders in childhood and adolescence. Institute of Psychiatry, De Crespigny Park, London

Shaffer D et al 1985 The clinical guide to child psychiatry. The Free Press, Collier and Macmillan, London

Social Work Scotland Act 1968 HMSO, London

Will D, Wrate R 1986 Integrated family therapy. Tavistock Publications, London

World Health Organization (WHO) 1978 ICD-9. WHO, Geneva

World Health Organization (WHO) 1992 ICD-10. WHO, Geneva

FURTHER READING

Asthrop J 1982 My secret file. Penguin, London

Barker P 1992 Basic family therapy. Blackwell Scientific Publications, Oxford

Barker P 1995 Basic child psychiatry. Blackwell Scientific Publications, Oxford

Cattanach A 1994 Play therapy—where the sky meets the underworld. Jessica Kingsley, London

Fitzpatrick P, Clarke K, Higgins P 1994 Self esteem. (The Chalkface Project) available from: The Chalkface Project, PO Box 907, Milton Keynes, MK5 6JB

Gajewski N, Mayo P 1989 Social skills strategies book A. Thinking Publications, Auclaire, USA

Gajewski N, Mayo P 1989 Social skills strategies book B. Thinking Publications, Auclaire, USA

Hamil M 1978 This is me. DLM, USA

Hoare P 1993 Essential child psychiatry. Churchill Livingstone Medical Division, Longman, UK

Hutchings S, Comins J, Officer J 1991 The social skills handbook (practical activities for social communication). Winslow Press, Bicester

Hutchins P 1985 The very worst monster. Bodley Head, Middlesex

Jampolsey G G, Taylor P 1978 There is a rainbow behind every dark cloud. Celestial Arts, Berkeley, USA

Martin F M, Murray K (eds) 1982 The Scottish juvenile justice system. Academic Press, Edinburgh

Minuchin S 1974 Families and family therapy. Harvard University Press, Cambridge, Mass

Sandford D 1887 I know the world's worst secret.
  Multnomah Press, Portland, Oregon
Sgrol M S 1982 Handbook of clinical intervention in child
  sexual abuse. Lexington Books, Boston, Mass
Skynner R, Cleese J 1993 Families and how to survive them,
  2nd edn. Methuen, London

Stevenson J 1983 What's under my bed? Springbourne
  Press, Essex
Striker S, Kimmel E 1979 The anti-colouring book.
  Scholastic Publications, New York
Wilkinson T 1983 Child and adolescent psychiatric nursing.
  Blackwell Scientific Publications, Oxford

24

Children having oncology treatment

Ginny Colliss

In working through the contents of this chapter the student is introduced to the care of the child having oncology treatment. The main areas relating to the nursing care of the child will be discussed.

The chapter aims to:
- **outline the management of childhood cancer nationally; this will include trials, informed consent, and randomised treatment**
- **indicate the effects of diagnosis on the family, and the support available, both in hospital and the community**
- **provide a synopsis of treatment options, outline the effects of the treatment and describe the nursing care needs of the child**
- **outline the educational needs of the family when caring for the child in hospital and at home**
- **indicate the side effects of treatment both in the short and long term**
- **suggest essential reading to support the knowledge gained from this chapter to assist the nurse in caring for children with cancer and their families.**

INTRODUCTION

Childhood cancer is rare; only 35 per million of the population aged between 0 and 16 years are affected. Of all cancers, only 1 in 200 are in children and it is quoted that a general

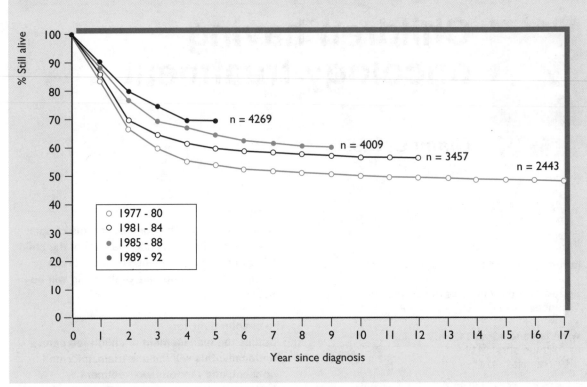

Figure 24.1   Survival of UKCCSG patients 1977–1992 (adapted from Stiller 1993).

practitioner will meet only two children with cancer in his working career. However, by the year 2000, 1 in 1000 young adults will have survived childhood cancer (Meadows et al 1986). The overall survival rate is now 70% (Fig. 24.1), with a wide variation depending on the type of cancer.

A major 5-year study (1992–1997) is being undertaken by the United Kingdom Children's Cancer Study Group (UKCCSG) in an attempt to identify facts that might lead to further knowledge about the incidence of the disease. The group plans to investigate possible links between childhood cancer and environmental factors—radiation, X-rays, magnetic fields, power stations, chemicals—and to study the effects of these factors on both parental germ cells (ova/sperm) and the child during development in the womb and after birth. It will also consider the possibility that some childhood cancers may arise as a rare and abnormal response to infection.

There is evidence to show that children treated at regional centres have a better prognosis than those treated in local hospitals (Audit Commission 1993). This means that the child and family may have to travel some distance for initial diagnosis and the start of treatment, but by sharing care with the local hospital the amount of travelling can be reduced. It is also an advantage and of benefit to the children if the regional team visit the local hospital to share their expertise. Many units now have specialist oncology nurses, as part of the team but working in the community. They may be funded by the hospital or by charitable organisations (e.g. Cancer and Leukaemia in Childhood Trust (CLIC), Cancer Relief). All are trained paediatric nurses; many hold the ENB 240 paediatric oncology certificate and the district nurse qualification. They establish links with shared care

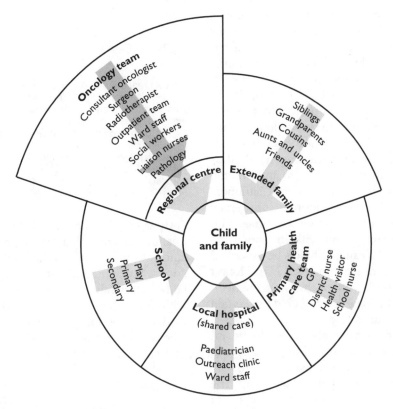

Figure 24.2   The team approach to childhood cancer.

hospitals and the primary health care team—general practitioners, school nurses, paediatric community nurses, health visitors, district nurses and, in some areas, paediatric Macmillan nurses. They extend the hospital into the community by giving care at home—taking blood, giving chemotherapy and supporting the family, especially if palliative/terminal care is needed.

It is essential that resources in the community are used wisely. The family needs only a limited number of people to be involved, but those who are involved should have liaised effectively with the appropriate specialists.

There are 22 centres in the United Kingdom that are part of the United Kingdom Children's Cancer Study Group (UKCCSG). Regional centres vary—some having purpose-built oncology units with or without bone marrow transplant facilities while others still share space with general medical and surgical patients. Although a purpose-built unit is ideal, children with cancer are not put at risk when cared for in a mixed ward. It is important to make sure that appropriate measures are taken to reduce the risk of infection, and the staff are appropriately trained.

The team is quite extensive (Fig. 24.2), but this is essential to ensure that the child at the centre receives effective treatment. Ideally, a large proportion of the nursing staff will hold the paediatric oncology certificate ENB 240 (Ch. 5).

SUPPORTING THE FAMILY OF THE CHILD WITH CANCER

There is probably no occasion more firmly imprinted on the memory of the family than the time that parents are told that their child has cancer. This may be by their general practitioner, the local paediatrician, or the oncologist at the regional centre. The impact of the word 'cancer' often blunts their ability to retain information at the initial interview, and the nurse may frequently be asked questions later that she feels unable to answer. For this reason it is important that a nurse is present at this interview, to repeat details when asked. A number of centres now use taped interviews when breaking disturbing news, thus enabling parents to listen again to information that was lost in the distress of the situation. Children also need an explanation in appropriate language, for they have to contend at times with parents who are upset, and with investigations and treatment which cannot always be described as pleasant (Eiser & Havermans 1992). Honest factual information is vital at this stage, remembering that not all will be remembered but certain things will stand out clearly.

The rest of the family also need to be informed, and in particular the siblings. They will understand, and take the truth well, if words are used that are appropriate to their age group. The use of the play specialist to help here could prove ideal and she will provide a link for the future months of treatment. The grandparents and the older relations frequently find the diagnosis harder to accept, as they feel that the child is in the wrong age group to be affected. Many units have support groups for both parents and siblings (Stone 1993, Hewitt 1990).

WHAT IS CANCER?

Cancer is the growth of abnormal cells. Growth may be in one place causing a lump, a solid tumour, e.g. brain tumour, or abnormal cells may be found in the circulation, e.g. leukaemia.

Solid tumours

The solid tumour in a child is usually a sarcoma, whereas in adults it is generally a carcinoma. A sarcoma can be found anywhere in the body, for example in bone, muscle or brain, and can be formed at any age from the baby to the teenager.

Case study 24.1 Nicola

Nicola, aged 5 years, had increasing pallor over several weeks. 4 days before admission she was knocked over and suffered a cut lip with excessive bleeding. She developed bruising on her face and back.

A blood count was performed and leukaemia was confirmed:

Haemoglobin	6 g/dl	
White blood cells	187×10^9/l	90% blasts
Platelets	52×10^9/l	

Fortunately, chemotherapy is far more effective in treating sarcomas than carcinomas; therefore the cure rate in children is far higher than it is in adults. Solid tumours start in one place in the body, but as they grow, pieces too small to be seen with the naked eye may break away and be carried by the blood to other parts of the body where they 'seed' and grow (metastasis). Common sites for metastases are the liver and lungs.

Leukaemia

Leukaemia is the most common form of cancer in childhood. It is the growth of abnormal white

Case study 24.2 Gareth

Gareth, who is 3 years old, has been ill on and off for the last 6 weeks with pains in his abdomen and neck. He was admitted to his local hospital with suspected appendicitis. His full blood count was normal at this time and he was sent home with symptoms resolved. 2 weeks later he was seen by his GP with pains in his chest and a stiff neck and left jaw, but was playing happily. Nothing was found. He was followed up by his GP and everything was satisfactory. At the weekend, a fortnight later, his symptoms recurred and a provisional diagnosis of juvenile arthritis was considered. The following Monday he was seen by his GP for tests.

A blood count was performed and leukaemia was confirmed.

Haemoglobin	8.3 g/dl
White blood cells	3.6×10^9/l
	(blasts seen in peripheral blood)
Platelets	153×10^9/l

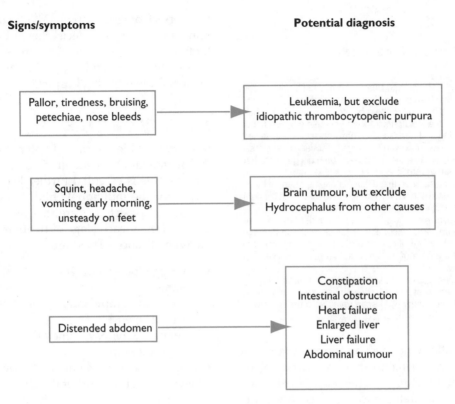

Figure 24.3   Signs and symptoms leading to a diagnosis of childhood malignancy.

cells—lymphocytes in acute lymphatic leuk-aemia (ALL) and myelocytes in acute myeloid leukaemia (AML). Myeloid leukaemia is more common in adults than in children.

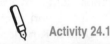

Activity 24.1

John, aged 2½ years, has been unwell for several weeks—he has been tired and lethargic and looks pale. He has several bruises to his legs, but so did his sister at his age. He has been taken to his doctor as a follow-up to a recent ear infection. The decision is made to under-take a blood test.

The result is:

Haemoglobin	4.6 g/dl
White blood cells	$64 \times 10^9/l$
Platelets	$60 \times 10^9/l$

In what way has the potential diagnosis of leukaemia affected his count, and what will his nursing needs be for the next 24 hours?

White cells are produced in the bone marrow and originate from stem cells. All cells in the bone marrow are immature and are called blasts, e.g. megakaryoblasts, lymphoblasts. They mature within the marrow, and then enter the circulation. In ALL some of the lymphoblasts are abnormal and unable to mature into lympho-cytes; indeed they are unable to serve any pur-pose to the body at all, and all they do is multiply. Eventually they become so numerous, that they fill the marrow cavity and crowd out the normal cells. As the abnormal cells increase still further, they diffuse from the marrow into the circulation. At this point, the effect of their circulating in the system is likely to produce symptoms that will cause a blood test to be performed, and the abnormal cells will be found in the peripheral blood. As normal circulating blood should contain only mature cells, the child will need further investigations.

Case study 24.3 Robert

Robert, aged 5 years, had been a normal child until 1 year ago. His mother then became concerned that his walking and balance had changed. He held his head to the left. He had been seen by the local paediatrician because of episodes of pallor, vomiting and headaches. These episodes only lasted 24 hours and were followed by a rapid recovery. A diagnosis of abdominal migraine was made—as both his grandmother and aunt suffer from migraine. He was also seen by an ear, nose and throat surgeon at a different hospital when he failed his hearing test at school. He was found to be deaf in his right ear and this was thought to be congenital.

A couple of months ago he banged his head in the playground and was unconscious for several minutes. He was admitted overnight to the surgical ward of a third hospital, under the care of the neurosurgeon, but discharged the next day.

Most recently, over the last 2 weeks, he has had early morning headaches, slight drowsiness and vomited. A computed tomography (CT) scan revealed a brain tumour.

For the child who has developed signs and symptoms requiring further investigation, the route to the doctor (general practitioner, paediatrician, or paediatric oncologist) is very varied and not always straightforward. Childhood cancer is rare, and it is often a combination of circumstances, signs and symptoms that lead to

---

Box 24.1 Investigations and initial management of a child referred with a possible diagnosis of acute lymphoblastic leukaemia

- Intravenous line + fluids to protocol
- Full blood count—to confirm blast cells in peripheral blood
- Samples taken for:
  —chromosome study (abnormalities can relate to prognosis)
  —childhood cancer study
  —viral titres (chickenpox and measles, and others)
- Blood transfusion to correct anaemia (after blood tests taken)
- Planned procedure under local, short-acting or general anaesthetic:
  —bone marrow aspirate (to confirm leukaemia and identify type)
  —lumbar puncture (to exclude leukaemic cells in cerebrospinal fluid)

---

the correct diagnosis (Fig. 24.3). This must be remembered, as it affects the attitude of the family when the opportunity comes to share the care of the child with the primary health care team and the referring hospital.

ASPECTS OF CARE

It is impossible in this chapter to cover the different treatments required for all childhood cancers; this is essential further learning whilst caring for the individual child. However, there are certain aspects of care that are relevant for the children at each stage of treatment whatever the type of cancer. These are:

- investigation and diagnosis
- treatment
  —chemotherapy and its side effects: neutropenia
  —surgery: biopsy/removal of tumour
  —radiotherapy
- long-term management and follow-up
- psychosocial support of the child/parents/siblings.

Investigation and diagnosis

It is important that all investigations are completed at a regional centre once the possibility of a malignancy has been raised. This ensures that the tests are consistent with those laid down in the protocols planned by the experts and managed under the aegis of the United Kingdom Children's Cancer Group or the Medical Research Council.

The investigations and initial management of a child who may have acute lymphoblastic leukaemia are given in Box 24.1. This is a basic list of investigations; other more specific tests may also be carried out.

Box 24.2 lists the investigations and initial management of a child with a possible diagnosis of neuroblastoma. The results will confirm the diagnosis and show the extent of disease and therefore the treatment required. The 'stage' of the disease will also give an indication of the

---

Box 24.2 Investigations and initial management of a child referred with a possible diagnosis of neuroblastoma

- Intravenous line
- Urine collection for vanillyl mandelic acid (accuracy is vital as this hormone is excreted almost exclusively by neuroblastomata) (Bell 1991)
- Planned procedure under short-acting or general anaesthetic:
    —bone marrow aspirate
    —trephine bone biopsy
- Bone scan (to determine extent of disease)
- CT scan (to show anatomical extent of tumour)
- Biopsy of tumour
- Glomerular filtration rate (baseline test to assess renal function prior to treatment)
- Pain management

---

ultimate prognosis, e.g. Stage 4 neuroblastoma has a 30–40% survival rate whereas Stage 1 has a 60% survival rate. Pain, caused by marrow and multiple site involvement, is a significant feature of neuroblastoma.

Treatment

Planning

Once all the investigations have been performed, and the diagnosis confirmed, a plan of action will be explained to the family, which will involve chemotherapy, surgery or radiotherapy, or a combination of the three. Childhood cancer, unlike adult cancers, is especially sensitive to chemotherapy. Research has shown that for the child under 3 years, there are long-term side effects from using radiotherapy to the brain and spinal column (Jannoun 1983). It is known to affect normal growth and endocrine function, but has also been shown to affect intellectual development. However, there may be occasions when there are no other alternatives for this age group.

Treatment can last from approximately 6 months to 2 years depending on the diagnosis. Certain cancers necessitate almost continual hospitalisation, e.g. AML or Stage 4 disease rhabdomyosarcoma/some B-cell lymphomas. This is due to the chemotherapy being administered over several days, the effect of the treatment on the child and the supportive care required during this period, and the fact that as soon as the child has recovered, the next course of chemotherapy is due.

Helping the family to plan. The family needs to be able to plan for this time; this means making arrangements for the siblings to be cared for and, where necessary, continue their schooling. Parents need to sort out their work—both parents may have jobs and may have to choose who is to have time off. Babies in the family will need either to stay with a parent or be cared for by a reliable friend or relative. If the baby is kept in hospital, there is an added responsibility for the parent who will need help from the staff. For those who have either short stays or day visits, the planning can be just as great because the disruption is intermittent.

The role of the social worker is important here. For children under 21 this service is centrally funded (by the Malcolm Sargent Cancer Fund For Children) and most units will have at least one MS social worker. They aim to give support to the family, which may be by helping in planning how to cope during treatment, and assisting with financial problems and travel expenses. They are also seen by the family as being members of the team, who are working with those giving the treatment. As a result, parents voice their concerns more openly, and problems can be aired.

Trials

Trials of methods of treatment are essential in order to compare and contrast results. In the United Kingdom the trials are coordinated by the United Kingdom Children's Cancer Study Group (UKCCSG) or the Medical Research Council (MRC). There are also links with Europe through the Society of International Oncology Paediatricians (SIOP). These groups plan protocols for different cancer treatments and evaluate the results. Changes to the protocols are made to benefit future children. For example, in the late 1980s UKALL10 was the protocol used for children with ALL. All children were given 2 years' treatment with a variation only in the timing and frequency of an intensification block of chemotherapy. The trials randomised the children to one of four options. However, girls aged between 2 and 10 years with a low presenting white cell count were thought at that time to have a better than average prognosis and did not receive the intensification block. The results from that treatment were evaluated and at least two factors emerged:

• girls, who had been considered to have a better outlook and had therefore received less intensive treatment, had not done as well as expected
• out of the four options, the children receiving more intensive treatment had done better overall than the others.

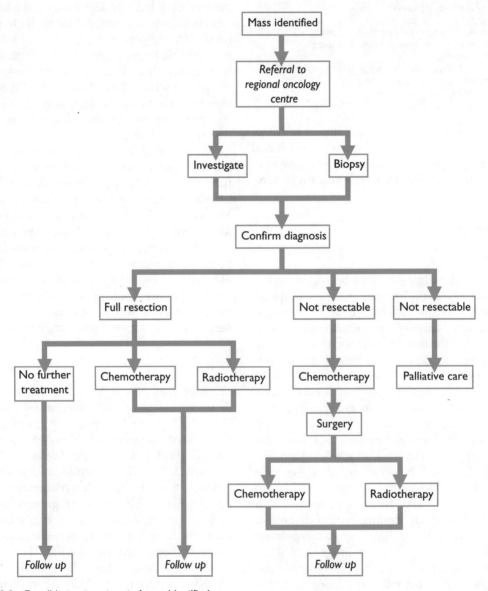

Figure 24.4 Possible treatment route for an identified mass.

The present protocol, UKALL11, has been adapted from those results, and has already been updated.

Informed consent.   It is the responsibility of the consultant to ensure that the parents have the planned treatment explained to them, and the different aspects of treatment if a randomised trial is taking place.

In order to take part in randomised trials it is essential that the parents understand what is involved. It is not easy at this stage in the illness for them to take in the details proposed. An information sheet is available to give added back-up information before they have to decide. Some parents find it impossible to take the 'risk', whereas most feel that it is the appropriate way forward (Ruccione et al 1991).

Randomised trials.   Randomised trials take place in an attempt to identify better outcomes for the patient when there is more than one option of treatment. They ensure the collection of data for a set protocol and, by using several centres, have a greater number of patients taking part. Once the parents agree, the trials coordinator is contacted, and the randomised course of treatment is confirmed.

Note: There may be a need for exclusion from the trials for clinical reasons. The consultant in charge is then able to decide the most appropriate treatment for the individual child, and the decision is often made as the result of considerable discussions with other experts in the field.

Types of treatment

Once the diagnosis is confirmed, the treatment can begin. For solid tumours, surgery and radiotherapy will be used in conjunction with chemotherapy, depending on the site of the cancer (Fig. 24.4).

Bone marrow transplant is used as a rescue when high-dose chemotherapy, with or without total body irradiation, is given as the treatment of choice, or as the final part of a course of treatment (Williss 1993, Thompson 1990). The transplant may be:

- autologous—using the patient's own marrow

- allogeneic—using marrow from a matched sibling
- mismatched—using marrow from an unrelated donor.

This treatment is used for certain types of leukaemia and some solid tumours.

A recent development is to harvest peripheral stem cells instead of bone marrow, and transplant the stem cells This procedure is in its infancy, but may become part of several protocols in the future.

Administration of chemotherapy

Only by nursing children who are receiving chemotherapy for different types of cancer, can the individual begin to understand the numerous drugs, protocols, methods of administration, and particular observations needed while treatment is in progress. This section aims to give broad guidelines, which will be consolidated during clinical placement. There will also be variable local policies applicable.

It is essential that the child's weight and height are measured accurately, as doses of the majority of the drugs used in chemotherapy are calculated on the basis of the surface area of the body rather than on the weight alone.

Intravenous access

This may be gained via:

- peripheral veins
- central lines, e.g. Hickman, Broviac, Port-a-Cath
- long lines.

The essential factor is to ensure the safe administration of the drug or fluid required. Poor venous access, age, needle phobia, or the need for high volumes of fluid are all reasons for the use of a central line (Fig. 24.5), which is surgically inserted (Sepion 1990). It may also be local policy to use central lines. However, there are disadvantages, and the options should be fully considered.

Using a 'long line', a method in frequent use in treatment of the neonate, a tiny catheter can be

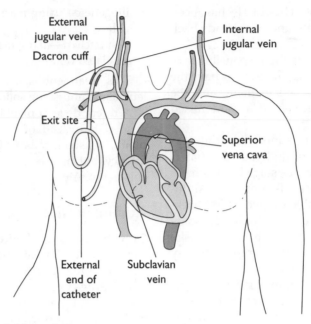

Figure 24.5 Position of central line catheter.

threaded up a vein, as a temporary measure for several days, and removed once the treatment is completed. The most important observation for the nurse is to ensure that the fluid is safely infusing into the vein.

Central line management. There may be variations in central line management between different units but the principles are the same (Box 24.3). The majority of parents become experts too

---

and can manage the line both in hospital and at home (Fig. 24.6). For those children whose parents do not feel able to manage, but for whom it is felt to be the appropriate treatment, the management of the central line at home will be arranged through liaison with the local hospital, the primary health care team, in particular the paediatric community nurse, and the oncology team.

Extravasation policy. Chemotherapy agents may be vesicants (substances that cause blistering) and can cause severe damage if they leak from the blood vessel into the surrounding tissues (extravasation). It is essential that the site of insertion of the intravenous cannula is checked frequently, and that all staff know the local

---

Box 24.3 Central line management

Points to remember:

- asepsis at all times
- management of the site dressing
- management of blockage
- check prior to administration of chemotherapy
- education of family:
    —dressing
    —flushing line
    —taking bloods
    —bath
- signs of infection.

Activity 24.2

Box 24.3 provides a list of important points to remember when using a central line. Using your local policy, identify the ways in which these are taught.

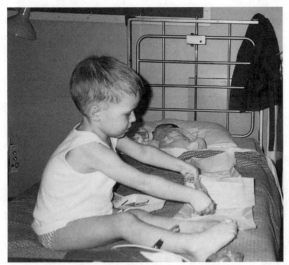

Figure 24.6   Child assisting with central line care.

policy if a leak occurs (RCN 1995). It is also a reason why central lines are used, but these too can become displaced, though rarely.

Drug dose and preparation

In the majority of units now, the preparation of cytotoxic drugs takes place in a central area (usually the pharmacy). If this is not the case, then a suitable area should be available to ensure the protection of those preparing such drugs. The drug and dose will have been decided and calculated in accordance with the protocol. Information regarding side effects can be obtained from either the protocols available on the unit, or drug formularies. The drugs may be administered as a bolus injection, a short intermittent infusion, or a continuous infusion.

Timing.   It is important that the drug regime is completed to time as the protocol has been planned in detail. For this reason infusion pumps that control the rate are frequently used. It is ideal to have a pump that has pressure regulation so that it will alarm if the infusion site is at risk. It is dangerous to increase the rate of infusion above the prescribed rate, as this may lead to toxic levels of the drug in the circulation.

Handling of chemotherapy and body fluids. Local policy will apply. There is no evidence of absorption of chemotherapeutic agents through the skin, but it is prudent policy to take sensible precautions.

Effects of treatment with chemotherapy

Vomiting

Vomiting a few hours after administration of the cytoxic drug is the least pleasant side effect of treatment.

Anti-emetic management.   There are effective anti-emetic drugs now available, which should be used. Local policy will apply. Alternative approaches to symptomatic management are the use of:

- acupressive bands
- play therapy
- diversional therapy
- massage/aromatherapy.

Tumour lysis syndrome

If there is widespread disease at presentation, i.e. 'bulky' lymphoma or high-count ALL, the child is in danger from the effects of treatment (Oakhill 1988). As the tumour breaks down, cells are destroyed and, in particular, potassium is released. Intracellular waste is excreted in the urine and this can lead to renal failure (Ch. 13). The child will require close monitoring of electrolyte and fluid balance, and cardiac monitoring, and transfer to the intensive care unit may be considered (Ch. 26).

Effects on normal cell development

The aim of chemotherapy is to destroy the cancer cells. As a side effect it affects normal cell development and may give rise to a number of disorders (Fig. 24.7). There are three specific areas that are likely to cause concern:

- hair loss
- mucosal damage
- bone marrow suppression.

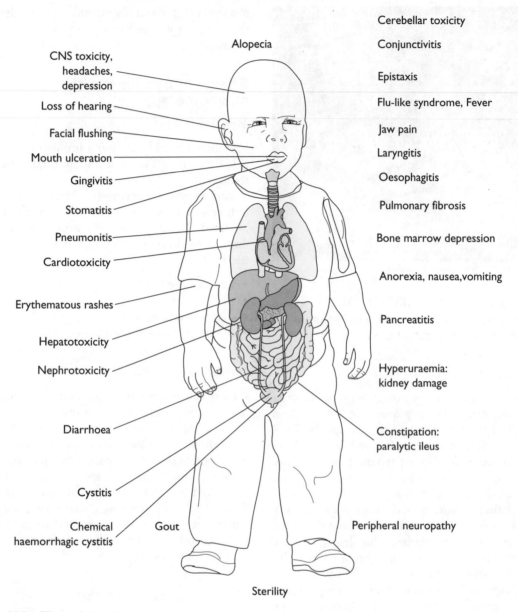

Figure 24.7   Effects of chemotherapy.

The hair loss depends on the drugs used and where in the cell cycle the drug has its effect. Mucosal damage and bone marrow suppression occur at around 7–10 days after administration of the chemotherapy, or earlier if the treatment is intense.

Mouth ulcers/mucositis

The extent of ulceration is related to the intensity of the chemotherapy, and may lead to mouth ulcers only or to extensive mucositis of the gastrointestinal tract.

Mouth care both regular and effective is essential, and can be simple teeth cleaning to the use of antiseptic mouth washes and antifungal agents (Campbell et al 1995). Good fluid intake, ideally by mouth, also helps. For the child with extensive mucositis, the symptoms can be severe—there is difficulty in swallowing, abdominal pain and severe diarrhoea. Pain control is essential, and a morphine infusion is ideal. Total parenteral nutrition will be required in extreme cases to rest the gut.

The blood count

Bone marrow suppression results in a reduction in the numbers of circulating red cells, white cells and platelets (Table 24.1).

Red cells. Anaemia will occur as a result of treatment and transfusions will be required. Unusual tiredness is usually related to anaemia, but both pyrexia and infection (see below) are also tiring.

White cells. As the white cell count falls and the neutrophil count becomes virtually non-existent (neutropenia), the child is at risk of infection. Sepsis has in the past been one of the causes of death during treatment, but with present-day management this is rare. In some units prophylactic antibiotics are given when neutropenia is expected.

Platelets. As the platelet count falls, the child is at risk of bruising and bleeding. Each centre has a platelet count level at which platelet transfusion will be given. This is when the count is below $20 \times 10^9/l$ and the child has significant bruising or bleeding or is pyrexial. It is important to examine the child carefully for new bruises more than once a day.

Reduced immunity to infection

Sites of infection. Whereas the person with a normal neutrophil count will form pus if there is infection, the neutropenic child will, at most, have a reddened area. It is important that the nurse and the parents understand this and report such findings, observing especially old sites of intravenous access, injection sites and sores. If the child has diarrhoea, then the anus should be checked regularly as any crack can become infected. An old-fashioned but effective method of reducing this risk is to dry the area with a hair dryer after a bath, to ensure that it is not left damp. There will be a local policy for infection screening for the neutropenic child.

Environmental risk factors:

Food. This is an area of considerable discussion, and local policies apply. These are led by the bacteriology department, but relate in particular to uncooked food—for example salads and fruit.

Flowers. Again local policies apply, but the risk is especially in the water, which may not get changed. However, more recently the organisms that are on the plants are making flowers suspect.

Table 24.1	Blood values		
	'Healthy' child	Newly diagnosed ALL	Neutropenic
Haemoglobin	11.6 g/dl	6.0 g/dl	12 g/dl
WBCs	$5.6 \times 10^9/l$	$187 \times 10^9/l$	$1.7 \times 10^9/l$
Neutrophils	$3.1 \times 10^9/l$	$3.74 \times 10^9/l$	$0.17 \times 10^9/l$
Lymphocytes	$2.5 \times 10^9/l$	$12.2 \times 10^9/l$	$1.5 \times 10^9/l$
Blasts	Nil	$169 \times 10^9/l$	Nil
Platelets	$335 \times 10^9/l$	$52 \times 10^9/l$	$19 \times 10^9/l$

Activity 24.4

Jane has just completed her 3-day course of chemotherapy for a bone tumour. Her parents are told that the maximum effect of treatment will be felt 10 days later when she becomes neutropenic. What advice should the family be given so that they know what to watch for during this time?

Mixing with others. As has been said earlier, many units are mixed, so the children are already mixing with another group. The family will be told if their child should not mix, for example at school or going to the supermarket. It is important that they understand why their child might be 'at risk'.

Infectious diseases. Chickenpox and measles are major hazards to the immunosuppressed child. In the past they were a major cause of death. Fortunately the measles, mumps and rubella (MMR) immunisation uptake has been excellent, reducing the number of potential contacts for a vulnerable child. The drug, acyclovir, has revolutionised the management of chickenpox—both the illness and contact with it. It is important that the degree of contact with the infection is identified, so that appropriate prophylactic treatment can be given (Ch. 19). The immunocompromised child is also vulnerable to opportunistic infections such as *Candida*, cytomegalovirus and organisms causing pneumonitis.

When is a hospital admission necessary?

Again local policies apply but the general rule is that hospital admission is needed when the child is unwell or needs treatment. This means that the child may need blood or platelet transfusions, and is at risk of bleeding or of overwhelming infection. Ease of access, transport and distance may decide at what point admission is necessary. The parents are told that pyrexia is the specific indicator, accompanied by a relevant low neutrophil count, and that intravenous antibiotic therapy is then commenced.

Pyrexia. The standard set for intervention with appropriate antibiotic cover for the neutropenic child is a temperature recording of 38°C twice within 4 hours or 39°C once when the neutrophil count is below $0.5 \times 10^9/\mathrm{dl}$. Antibiotic treatment is decided locally in conjunction with the bacteriology department and may include prophylactic cover once the child is expected to become neutropenic. A full infection screen is carried out, remembering especially to culture samples from any reddened areas which may prove significant. It may be that no organism is cultured, but as long as the child is at risk, twice-weekly screening takes place.

What to do if the count does not recover. Sometimes the neutrophil count takes a long time to recover. If the delay is greater than can be considered acceptable, a bone marrow aspirate will be performed, to assess the function of the marrow and exclude relapse. Some protocols are now including the drug G-CSF (granulocyte colony stimulating factor) to minimise prolonged or profound neutropenia. The aim is to encourage the bone marrow to make granulocytes, which include neutrophils (see Ch. 19), so G-CSF is not given simultaneously with cytotoxic drugs.

Information

It is vital that the child and family are given as much information as possible regarding the treatment. They will need to know:

- the specific side effects of drugs, i.e. constipation, mood changes, peripheral neuropathy, discoloured urine
- whether nausea and vomiting will persist, and what to do if it does
- the care of the Hickman line/Port-a-Cath at home, i.e. flushing, dressings
- the timing of further treatments
- the need for blood counts between or before courses of treatment
- the effects of treatment on the bone marrow and therefore on the blood count
- the significance of each blood cell and the

signs and symptoms to look for, i.e. bruising, bleeding, anaemia

- the use of blood products
- what 'neutropenia' means, when it will occur, what they should do and who to contact
- the importance of mouth care and monitoring of temperature when the child is neutropenic, and when antipyretics and antibiotics would be used
- when the child can return to school and the significance of contact with chickenpox/measles
- when hair loss will occur and whether a wig can be obtained in time
- about nutrition and weight loss
- what effects there may be on the child's body image (see Price 1993)
- how to maintain discipline and the psychological management of the child and siblings
- who they can rely on for support.

Written information is imperative when the parents take the child home from hospital. They must have literature that they can refer to when the immediate support of the hospital is no longer available.

Surgery

In the adult, surgery is often the first choice of treatment for solid tumours. Chemotherapy is, however, an excellent agent in childhood cancer and, unless complete removal of the tumour is the option of choice, it is likely that a biopsy will be performed to confirm diagnosis and treatment begun, using chemotherapy in the first instance. The size of the 'lump' can be used as an indicator of the success of chemotherapy, and surgery will remove the tumour at some stage during the planned management.

There will be concerns for the family in addition to those expected for the child undergoing surgery (Ch. 9), as this is a momentous event. For the child having surgery for a Stage 4 neuroblastoma, the operation can take up to 8 hours. The outcome, depending on how successful the

surgery was, may have implications for further treatment options or the prognosis. Sometimes the surgery can be disfiguring, for example facial tumours, although fortunately amputation has become less used as the treatment for bone cancers. It is also possible that, at this stage, the surgery takes place on a different ward or even in a different hospital. It is important that contact is maintained by the oncology team to provide continuity of care and emotional support.

Radiotherapy

The radiotherapy department is commonly used by adults, which means that it is essential that the needs of the children are communicated and firm links are established.

Radiotherapy involves a dose of radiation being 'beamed' at the site for a very short period of time—a few minutes. The dose is large when compared with that needed to make an X-ray, and aims to destroy the ability of the cell to grow and divide. It also damages normal cells. It is essential that the child remains still during the treatment and, for the young child, a general anaesthetic may be necessary, although it is possible with patience and adequate explanation to get children as young as 2 years to have treatment without anaesthetic.

Preparation

It is important that the child and family understand about radiotherapy. They need to understand about the machinery and how the rays 'travel'. The treatment is planned over a period of time—from 10 days to 6 weeks as the protocol demands. The radiotherapy consultant will explain the plan and give an explanation of what to expect, both during treatment and after. It is an opportunity for the family to ask all the questions that come to mind. Many units have a video about the treatment which shows what to expect. As the treatment is for such a short time each day, families living some distance away may prefer to live at home and travel in each day. Some units have houses that are ideal for this, where the family can lead a near normal life but not have to travel long distances (e.g. CLIC House in Bristol; Sick Children's Trust, Hospital at Home in London).

Planning

The treatment area is carefully identified and usually marked with an indelible pen. For children having treatment to the head, a mask is made to enable the child to be kept in perfect position during the few vital minutes. The planning takes time but it ensures safe treatment.

Management of the treatment area

The most important point to remember is that the marks must not be washed off. The family will be given instructions as to what they can do, but the main points are:

- wash the treated area with unscented soap
- do not use lotions, perfumes or deodorants
- use a high-factor suntan lotion if the area is exposed.

Side effects

Many of the side effects relate to the area being treated; for example, if the head is treated, hair loss is inevitable in the treated area. Nausea and vomiting may occur but anti-emetic medication can be prescribed.

Management at home

The child may find the treatment very tiring; some of this can be related to the travelling if the child is attending the hospital daily. For this reason it may be beneficial to stay at or near the hospital. Children having radiotherapy to the head appear to have a 'sleepy' period about 6 weeks after completion of treatment. This sleepiness can cause great anxiety, as it may have been a symptom prior to the initial diagnosis.

There should be good liaison with the oncology team, who will also see the child regu-larly in their clinic throughout the course of radiotherapy. Once the treatment is completed, follow-up is usually returned to them.

Day-to-day care

From a very early stage, the child and family rapidly become experts in their diagnosis and treatment, and this can be quite threatening to the inexperienced nurse or doctor. There are certain aspects of care that need to be addressed:

Nutrition

It is important that the child is weighed regularly so that any significant alteration is noted. Children will gain weight as a side effect of treatment with steroids, but of greater concern is weight loss. This is usually due to poor eating, caused by loss of appetite (chemotherapy can affect the tastebuds, making food no longer appetising), mucositis, and nausea. The longer the period of poor nutrition, the more likely it is that intervention is required. This can be addressed in steps:

- appealing meals
- nutritional supplements
- enteral feeding or total parenteral nutrition.

The earlier this potential problem is raised with the family, the less distressing it is when intervention is required (Ch. 12).

House rules

It is hard for a family to maintain discipline, when faced with a child with a potentially life-threatening illness, and at times they may need help. The presents pile up at the end of the bed, and the child can make demands that would normally be refused. Children do benefit from boundaries and feel safe if treated as normally as possible. It needs confidence to send children back to school and let them play with friends as they did so recently before admission. The hospital team must support the family, and visits both to the home and school are part of the work of the team.

Management of the family

The disruption to normal family life cannot be underestimated. Attending a regional centre far from home, other children left with friends or relatives, husband and wife taking it in turns to stay with the sick child, trying to hold down a job; all add to the problems. The nurse needs to be aware of the parents' need for time alone together, and for the siblings to be included and made to feel special too. Sibling groups can be a way of helping them to understand what is happening. This major change in the life of the family will affect its members in different ways, which may at times seem inappropriate, but are their ways of coping. Parents at different stages of treatment act as an informal group to an official support system in many units.

The adolescent

The impact on older children and teenagers is considerable. They are seen as on the threshold of life, and are able to consider the options personally. They are also able to refuse treatment and have the right to give their consent to treatment (Children Act 1989, Fowler 1988, Palmer 1994, Peck 1992). The right to privacy is especially important to them and it is ideal if special facilities are available to them (Ch. 22; Burr 1993, Evans 1993).

How to cope with the long-term outlook

Once the family return home, for short or long periods between treatments, the significance of the cancer hits home. Support is needed, and is provided by both the primary health care team and the local hospital. Communication between the teams is vital and the use of a 'shared care book' is one way of keeping all informed (Hully & Hynes 1993). The liaison nurse and the Malcolm Sargent social worker provide essential links.

LONG-TERM OUTLOOK

Prognosis

The family will have been given a prognosis at an early discussion, as there are certain diagnostic indicators. There are other factors that will also affect the prognosis—especially bacterial and viral infections.

Length of treatment

The protocol will indicate the length of treatment required, or the number of courses needed. Delays can occur as a result of neutropenic episodes. Alterations are made if the response to treatment is not as expected. Once treatment has been completed, follow-up is maintained on a long-term basis at extended time intervals as time passes.

Table 24.2 Long-term side effects of treatment

Side effect	Cause
Growth	Radiotherapy to head
Endocrine function	
Sterility	Chemotherapy—certain drugs only
Thyroid dysfunction	Radiotherapy to neck
Intelligence	Radiotherapy to head (deep X-ray treatment to brain in child aged under 3 years)
Renal tubular damage	Chemotherapy—certain drugs only
Cardiotoxity	Chemotherapy—certain drugs only
Further malignancy	Certain chemotherapeutic agents Radiotherapy

Long-term side effects of treatment

It is vital that children are followed for many years and into young adult life. Some of the long-term effects of treatment are only now becoming evident (Table 24.2).

The need for long-term follow-up has been well demonstrated by the experience of a few pregnant girls who developed severe problems in labour many years after treatment with potentially cardiotoxic drugs. As a direct result, the method of administration of these drugs has been changed, and regular cardiological monitoring now takes place.

'Cure'

Although 'cure' is the aim, it is more correct to consider the child who no longer has symptoms as being 'disease free'. The longer the time from diagnosis, the less likely it is that recurrence will occur. However, there are some cancers that do relapse years after completion of treatment.

- Relapse in leukaemia does respond to further treatment, and protocols give intensive treatment. The prognosis is fair.
- Recurrence and secondaries also occur in solid tumours. The effectiveness of treatment will depend on the histology of the recurrence and the amount of treatment given previously.

There will always be a proportion of children who will not get a response to treatment. At this point, time needs to be spent with the family to ascertain their wishes as the caring moves into the terminal phase (Ch. 27). Effective control of symptoms is the aim and close liaison ensures this.

One must accept that successful treatment is not always possible and that the quality of life is also important. At all times the family must feel able to discuss this, among themselves and with the oncology team, so that appropriate decisions are made together.

Caring for the child with cancer is demanding but rewarding. The nurse can establish a relationship with the family through a critical period in their lives. There are happy and sad times, and the children are, without doubt, exceptional.

REFERENCES

Audit Commission 1993 Children first—access to tertiary centres. HMSO, London, p 22

Bell S 1991 Neuroblastoma screening in babies. Paediatric Nursing 3(1): 16–17

Burr S 1993 Adolescents and the ward environment. Paediatric Nursing 5(1): 10–13

Campbell S T, Evans M A, MacTavish F 1995 The Royal College of Nursing paediatric oncology nurses' forum: guidelines for mouth care. RCN, London

Children Act 1989 HMSO, London

Eiser C, Havermans T 1992 Children's understanding of cancer. Psycho-oncology 1: 169–181

Evans M 1993 Teenagers and cancer. Paediatric Nursing 5(1): 10–13

Fowler M 1988 Pediatric informed consent. Heart and Lung 17(5): 584–585

Hewitt J 1990 The sibling response to hospitalisation. Paediatric Nursing 2(9): 12–13

Hully M, Hynes J 1993 Using parent-held records in an oncology unit. Paediatric Nursing 5(8): 14–16

Jannoun L 1983 Are cognitive and educational development affected by age at which prophylactic therapy is given in acute lymphoblastic leukaemia? Archives of Disease in Childhood 58(12): 953–958

Leukaemia Research Fund (LRF) 1993 Dictionary of leukaemia and related diseases. LRF, London

Meadows A et al 1986 Medical consequences of cure. Cancer 58: 524

Oakhill A 1988 The supportive care of the child with cancer. Wright, Sevenoaks, ch 5: 76–89

Palmer S 1994 Providing information to adolescent oncology patients. Paediatric Nursing 6(5): 18–22

Peck H 1992 Please don't tell him the truth. Paediatric Nursing 4(2): 12–14

Price B 1993 Diseases and altered body image in children. Paediatric Nursing 5(6): 18–21

Royal College of Nursing (RCN) 1989 Safe practice with cytotoxics. Scutari Projects for RCN, London

Royal College of Nursing (RCN) 1995 Guidelines for paediatric oncology training in the giving of intravenous drugs, including cytotoxics, 2nd edn. RCN, London

Ruccione K, Kramer R, Moore I, Perin G 1991 Informed consent for treatment of childhood cancer: factors affecting parents' decision making. Journal of Pediatric Oncology 8(3): 112–121

Sepion B 1990 Intravenous care for children. Paediatric Nursing 2(3): 14–16

Stiller C A 1994 Malignancies. In: Pless I B (ed) The epidemiology of childhood disorders. Oxford University Press, Oxford

Stone M 1993 Lending an ear to the unheard: the role of support groups for siblings of children with cancer. Child Health Journal 1(2): 54–58

Thompson J 1990 The child and bone marrow transplant. In:

Thompson J (ed) The child with cancer: nursing care. Scutari, London, pp 109–125

Williss J 1993 Bone marrow transplant. Continuing Education Article 702. Paediatric Nursing 5(2): 28–33

FURTHER READING

Audit Commission 1993 Children first. HMSO, London

Braithwaite A 1989 I have cancer. Dinosaur Publications, London

Brazier L, Trapp A, Yates N (undated) Simon has cancer. Victoria Publications, Newcastle upon Tyne

Brunner L, Suddarth D 1991 The Lippincott manual of paediatric nursing. HarperCollins, London

Cancer Research Campaign (undated) Welcome Back! CRC, Manchester

Cowlishaw S (undated) Jenny has a tumour. Premier Print Services, Nottingham. Available from Malcolm Sargent Cancer Fund for Children

D'Angio G, Sinniah D, Meadows A, Evans A, Pritchard J 1992 Practical pediatric oncology. Edward Arnold, London

Ekert H 1989 Childhood cancer: understanding and coping. Gordon & Breach, Reading

English National Board for Nursing, Midwifery and Health Visiting 1993 The nursing of children. ENB Publications, Sheffield

Focchtman D, Foley G 1982 Nursing care of the child with cancer. Little Brown, Boston

Glasper A, Tucker A 1993 Child health nursing. Scutari Press, London

Hague A 1985 Leukaemia. Price Stern Sloan Publishers, Lederle Laboratories, Hants

Hockenberry M, Coody D 1986 Paediatric oncology and haematology. Mosby, St Louis

Jackson A (ed) (undated) Hodgkin's disease. BACUP, London

Jackson A (ed) (undated) Non-Hodgkin's lymphomas. BACUP, London

Kenworthy N, Snowley G, Gilling C 1992 Common foundation studies in nursing. Churchill Livingstone, Edinburgh

Leukaemia Research Fund (LRF) 1991 Acute lymphoblastic leukaemia. LRF, London

Leukaemia Research Fund (LRF) 1991 Acute myeloid leukaemia. LRF, London

Leukaemia Research Fund (LRF) 1991 Bone marrow transplant. LRF, London

Leukaemia Research Fund (LRF) 1991 Leukaemia in children. LRF, London

Leukaemia Research Fund (LRF) 1991 The lymphomas. LRF, London

Leukaemia Research Fund (LRF) 1993 Dictionary of leukaemia and related diseases. LRF, London

Lewer H, Robertson L 1983 Care of the child. Macmillan, London

Lilly (undated) Cytotoxic chemotherapy. Lilly, Basingstoke

Neuroblastoma Society 1990 Neuroblastoma—a booklet for parents, 3rd edn. Neuroblastoma Society. Available from: Neuroblastoma Society, Woodlands, Ordsall Park Road, Retford, Nottinghamshire DN22 7PJ

Pinkerton C, Cushing P, Sepion B 1994 Childhood cancer management—a practical handbook. Chapman Hall Medical, London

Richardson A 1992 Manual of core care plans for cancer nursing. Scutari, London

Silkstone J, Hague A 1985 When your brother or sister has leukaemia. Price Stern Sloan Publishers, Gosport

Stevin M (ed) 1990 Coping with hair loss. BACUP, London

Stevin M (ed) 1990 Understanding chemotherapy. BACUP, London

Stevin M (ed) 1991 Acute lymphoblastic leukaemia. BACUP, London

Stiller C A 1994 Malignancies. In: Pless I B (ed) The epidemiology of childhood disorders. Oxford University Press, Oxford

Thompson J (ed) 1990 The child with cancer: nursing care. Scutari, London

Trapp A (undated) Into and out of the forest. Victoria Publications, Newcastle upon Tyne

Trapp A (undated) Our cancer. Victoria Publications, Newcastle upon Tyne

United Kingdom Children's Cancer Study Group (UKCCSG) 1987 A parent's guide to children's cancer. UKCCSG, London (Only available from UKCCSG, Bennett Building, University Road, Leicester LE1 7RH)

Whaley L F, Wong D L 1982 Essentials of paediatric nursing. C V Mosby, St Louis

USEFUL ADDRESSES

Cancer and Leukaemia in Childhood Trust
CLIC House
11/12 Freemantle Square
Coltham
Bristol BS6 5TL

Cancer Relief
15–19 Britten Street
London SW3 3TZ

Malcolm Sargent Cancer Fund for Children
14 Abingdon Road
London W8 6AF

Sick Children's Trust
Hospital at Home
Guildford Street
London WC2

Children with chronic illness

Lucy Godman

This chapter introduces the student to the care and support of children with chronic illness and their families.

The chapter aims to:
- identify the factors that affect the adjustment of the child and the family to the illness
- describe ways in which the child and family can be helped to live with the illness
- consider the needs of the adolescent with chronic illness and the transition from paediatric to adult care.

ADJUSTMENT TO ILLNESS

According to Knafl & Deatrick (1986), adjustment to illness is dependent on:

- the diagnosis
- age of onset of illness
- the nature of the condition
- external support.

In addition, the cognitive ability of the child and his/her family affects the child's adjustment to the illness.

There are many complex reasons why some children adapt 'well' and others 'less well' to illness; some findings and ideas will be discussed here.

Parental adaptation

The adaptation of parents affects the adaptation of the child as well as of the family. Knafl & Deatrick's (1986) research into normalisation suggests that children take the cues from their parents on how to react to illness. This suggests that parents who minimise illness will have the effect of influencing their child to do the same. Similarly, the parent who reacts anxiously will influence the child to react in a similar manner.

Cultural aspects

In his study of aspects of health and illness, Helman (1990) identifies cultural responses to stressors as well as ritual ones within the context of the illness, for example responses to pain which vary with culture. Whilst it would be unhelpful to suggest that all people from a certain culture behave in a particular manner, it is to be noted that different cultures have differing concepts of health and illness. This not only affects the response to illness in the form of attitude towards it, but also the behaviours surrounding the illness. Thus culture, in its widest sense, is an important area to consider when assessing the effects of illness on the child and family. This is most simply done by asking what the particular illness means to the family and their friends.

Normalisation

The analysis by Knafl & Deatrick (1986) of the work of other researchers points to a fairly well agreed idea of normalisation by families of children with chronic illness. That is, the ability for families to be accepted as normal within their communities, which is a vital element of coping with chronic illness. Normalisation is seen as:

- engaging in usual parenting activities
- limiting contacts with similarly situated others
- making the child appear normal
- avoiding embarrassing situations
- controlling information.

Theory of adaptive tasks

Canam (1993) puts forward an alternative approach to adaptation by parents. He postulates a series of adaptive tasks that must be completed by the parents in order for adaptation to occur (see Box 25.1).

The child's ability to understand illness

Having noted the importance of the parents' role in a child's adaptation to illness, though not separating the two, it is important to consider the child's ability to understand illness. Bibace & Walsh (1980), Eiser (1985) and Rundahl Hauck (1991) have written extensively on the cognitive ability of children with regard to health and illness. Each points to the cognitive ability of children affecting their understanding. Therefore a

Activity 25.2

Return to the list you made earlier when carrying out Activity 25.1. How many of the factors that you identified then relate to the cultural aspects mentioned, the normalisation process described, and the theory of adaptive tasks? Also consider the cognitive ability of the child; was he or she more advanced in some areas than you would have expected?

knowledge of cognitive development is a vital tool in comprehending the child's understanding. However, a child who is exposed to illness may have an advanced understanding compared to his/her peer group (Rundahl Hauck 1991).

HELPING THE CHILD AND FAMILY TO LIVE WITH ILLNESS

Many of the problems that are experienced by sick children and their families are illustrated in the case history that introduces Activity 25.3.

Professionals exercise a strong influence on the way a child's illness is perceived and, according to Knafl & Deatrick (1986), their ability to inform the family of all aspects of the illness is a vital part of this. If normalisation does not occur, there is a risk of disassociation, denial or resignation, all of which suggest a negative response to illness and therefore treatment regimes. In addition, the family risks becoming totally immersed in the illness. The professional, therefore, is in a prime position to help families adapt to illness, giving accurate information about the illness, practical advice on management and equipment, and as necessary informing others.

Training of professionals

The giving of practical, accurate advice assumes that the professional is knowledgeable about the child's condition and, if not, is prepared to be honest about this and obtain the information needed. In addition, knowledge of the

Activity 25.3

Victoria is 7 years old. She lives with her mother, brother James aged 4 years, and sister Anne aged 9 years. Her father does not live with the family but visits most weekends. Both maternal and paternal grandparents live a long distance away. Victoria and her sister attend school, which is within 10 minutes' walking distance of home; James attends a nursery school three mornings each week.

Victoria was diagnosed as having cystic fibrosis soon after birth. Her nursing needs require her mother to perform physiotherapy twice daily (more often if she has a chest infection), administer medication at meal times, attend out-patient clinics every 3 months and take sputum specimens as necessary. In addition, Victoria's failure to thrive has necessitated the need for nasogastric overnight feeding.

1. List all of the aspects of daily life which will be affected by the care Victoria requires.
2. List all of the people who may be involved in Victoria's care and daily life.
3. Think of yourself in the role of Victoria's mother:
   a. What will you do if you are offered a full-time job in a career you have always wished to pursue?
   b. You are invited out for the evening; your estranged husband is unable to baby-sit; who will you get to care for the children?
4. Think of yourself in the role of Victoria. In particular, think of the things you liked to do when you were 7 years old:
   a. What things would you be prevented from doing?
   b. How would you manage with the apparent lack of choices you have?

Keep your ideas in mind as you read on.

community in which the family lives is paramount in order to give holistic care. The debate about appropriate training of nurses in this role continues (Whiting 1994). The appropriateness of a district nurse or health visitor who has not had paediatric training is questionable. Although general practitioners offer medical support, much of the support needed requires nursing skills and the education of carers to undertake them. In the recent past, sick children were either not discharged from hospital or returned to hospital frequently for what was perceived by paediatric staff as appropriate support and advice. More recently, paediatric community services have increased in number making 'appropriate support' available at home for the families of sick children (While 1991).

Provision of equipment

Carers have identified the provision of equipment as the worst practical problem which they face (Jennings 1989). Where an authority decides that a piece of equipment should be provided as part of NHS treatment, it should be provided free of charge, under Section 1 of the NHS Act 1977. However, which authority (e.g. community trust or acute unit) should decide, and therefore whose responsibility it is, is not made clear. For example, is the provision of a nebuliser for a child with asthma to prevent admission to hospital, the responsibility of the community health team, family health services authority, or the hospital? A lack of understanding by professionals not familiar with specific care has led to misunderstandings of what equipment is required. For example, a primary health care professional, who had been allocated the care of a child with a tracheostomy, budgeted for the use of one suction catheter per week, clearly appreciating neither the frequency of need for suction nor up-to-date suction procedures (anecdotal from a patient). It is therefore imperative that, prior to discharge, the responsibility for equipment and on-going supplies is clarified. It is important to remember that equipment in the community is not as readily available as it is in hospitals. It may take 10 working days to acquire appropriate items. Phoning a community nurse or GP on a Friday afternoon and expecting him or her to take responsibility for provision of equipment the next day causes frustration for all.

Educational facilities

School and nursery placements can cause considerable anxiety for a parent of an ill child. Some children with a physical and/or mental handicap will need 'statementing'. This is a process whereby an educational psychologist assesses the child's needs, drawing on as much information as possible from the professionals and carers involved (see Ch. 21). The local education authority is obliged to provide an appropriate school placement, according to the results of the assessment. Those children who do not require 'special schooling' but need extra support in a mainstream school will also be assisted by statementing. Those who have a medical condition, such as diabetes, do not normally need extra help in school. However, for the safety of the child, the school staff need to be informed of specific care which the child may require in school, e.g. snack times and the treatment of hypoglycaemia. The responsibility for informing the school staff lies with the parents. However, if the child is newly diagnosed and the parents therefore lack knowledge, the information that is passed on may not be correct. Consequently, it is most appropriate for a paediatric community nurse to act as educator in these situations, and it may be appropriate even when parents are very knowledgeable.

Relieving the parents

Parents of sick children, like all parents, need to get out from time to time, but who can be trusted to care for a sick child? This is an increasing concern now that more sick children are being cared for at home. The NHS and Community Care Act 1990 identifies the needs of carers as a vital part of care, stating that provision must be made for their support. The sitting services provided are individual to each area and would require investigating locally with social services departments. These parents may not be able to ask a neighbour to help, because of their child's special needs. Respite care is also of concern; admission to hospital care is inappropriate. Most areas should have appropriate respite facilities, which will require investigating locally.

Coordination of services

Many professionals are involved in the care of a child with a chronic illness. These include GP, practice nurse, health visitor or school nurse,

nurse specialist, consultant (of which there may be more than one), physiotherapist, occupational therapist, speech therapist, clinical psychologist, paediatric community nurse, educational psychologist, teachers, social workers, volunteers — the list may be longer or shorter. With so many professionals involved, and with lots of appointments to keep and opinions to take in, the family is in danger of becoming confused. In these circumstances it is vital that someone takes a lead role in coordinating the various services. In order to minimise family confusion, it is helpful for the professionals to identify each other's roles and be aware of what information has been given; thus vigilance in communication is vital.

TRANSFER FROM PAEDIATRIC TO ADULT CARE

The transition from paediatric to adult care is a difficult time for the family as well as the young person. Adult care traditionally is geared toward the individual ill person taking responsibility for his or her own care. In paediatric care the emphasis is more often on the main carer undertaking the role of responsibility.

All adolescents and young adults go through psychological crises, which were identified by Erikson in 1959 as:

- identity versus confusion
- intimacy versus isolation (Revell & Liptak 1991).

Young people with a chronic illness not only have these crises to contend with but also the psychosocial aspects of their illness.

When does paediatric care end?

Where paediatric care ends and adult care begins seems to be arbitrary and dependent on the beliefs of the individual professionals involved. The change over usually occurs between the ages of 16 and 20 years. Perhaps the best indication that a chronically ill child should move into adult care is his or her wish to do so. The transition can be made easier if all parties clearly identify the differences it will make to the care received, and the effects of loss of contact with those perceived to have known the child all his or her life. These effects can be alleviated by the paediatric and adult consultants and nurses holding combined clinics, so that the adult team can develop relationships with the adolescent/young adult in the paediatric setting. Alternatively the paediatric team members can attend the adult clinic with the young person. It is worth noting that some young people do not attend any facility for regular management after leaving paediatric care. Dunning (1993) suggested that this may be due to the inappropriateness of services.

Parental reactions

The effects on the family may be profound; the main carer will need increasingly to 'let go' and give the responsibility of care to the young person. Many parents find this difficult with a well child and, in these circumstances, the illness will become an extra obstacle.

Talking through the feelings of guilt, resentment, frustration and sometimes anger with the parent and young adult separately may allow the individuals to come to terms with their feelings. This can lead to reconciliation if the professional is able to assist in a dialogue that facilitates understanding of each other's point of view.

Peer group pressure

Many young adults are exposed to, and take part in, the cultural behaviours of their peer group. This may include experimental behaviours such as smoking, drinking, sexual activity and drug taking. Whilst schools and parents undertake (in most cases) to inform children from an early age about the dangers of these activities, the particular effects on the ill child may not have been discussed. Such effects will include reactions with prescribed medications. In addition, whilst it may be difficult to get information regarding particular illnesses and these activities, consideration should be given to the consequences of such behaviours. Suggested sources of information include drug dependency units, who publish information on the specific effects of different 'street drugs' and alcohol, health education departments and specific illness support groups.

It may be necessary to encourage the carers and young adult to discuss these issues together, or individually. Without this information, the young adult cannot make an informed choice.

For example, a diabetic who, unaware of the likely consequences, drinks alcohol at a party, dances vigorously and then has sex may become hypoglycaemic. The danger then lies in the reactions of friends, who may not give life-saving glucose because they believe that the symptoms of slurred speech, dizziness, erratic behaviour, collapse, and so on, are due to the alcohol consumed.

Genetic counselling

Many chronic illnesses are the consequence of abnormal genes, and the affected individual will need genetic counselling in order to make informed choices with regard to family planning. This subject should be broached before the development of a sexual relationship, and may then need to be raised with the individual's partner.

If you now look back to Activity 25.5, you may find that some of the questions it raises have been left unanswered. This is because each individual situation must be assessed within its own context, and answers may lie within the morals and ethics of society, the family and professional thinking.

CONCLUSION

Child care and the development from dependent baby to independent adult encompasses many complex issues. The influences of culture, society, economy and environment affect both the lay and professional views. Where a child has a chronic illness, these issues are highlighted and the influences on the child and family are extended due to professional interventions. It is therefore the role of the professional to be knowledgeable, non-judgemental, practically supportive, and holistic in order to give appropriate support. In this way, children with chronic illness will be assisted in adapting to the illness, enabling them to develop within their peer group into independent well-adjusted adults.

REFERENCES

Bibace R, Walsh M E 1980 Development of children's concepts of illness. Pediatrics 66(6): 912–917

Bradford R 1991 Staff accuracy in predicting the concerns of parents of chronically ill children. Child: Care, Health and Development 17: 39–47

Bury M 1991 The sociology of chronic illness: a review of research and prospects. Sociology of Health and Illness 13(4): 0141–0158

Canam C 1993 Common adaptive tasks facing parents of children with chronic conditions. Journal of Advanced Nursing 18: 46–53

Dunning T 1993 Moving to adult care. Practical Diabetes 10(6): 226–229

Eiser C 1985 Changes in understanding of illness as the child grows. Archives of Disease in Childhood 60: 489–492

Helman C 1990 Culture, health and illness. Butterworth-Heinemann, Oxford

Holden C 1990 Home enteral feeding. Paediatric Nursing 2(July): 18–21

Holden C 1991 Home parenteral nutrition. Paediatric Nursing 3(3): 13–18

Jennings P 1989 Tracheostomy care—learning to cope at home. Paediatric Nursing 1(October): 13–15

Kendrick R 1993 Giving intravenous therapy at home. Paediatric Nursing 5(1): 22–24

Knafl K A, Deatrick J A 1986 How families manage chronic conditions: an analysis of the concept of normalisation. Research in Nursing and Health 9: 215–222

McEvilly A 1991 Diabetic home care. Nursing Standard 6: 20–21

Mishel M 1991 Uncertainty in illness theory: a replication of the mediating effects of mastery and coping. Nursing Research 40(4): 236–240

Nevin M, Nevin M 1992 Help the parent and you help the child. Paediatric Nursing 4(1): 25–27

NHS Act 1977 HMSO, London

NHS and Community Care Act 1990 HMSO, London

Revell G M, Liptak G S 1991 Understanding the child with special health care needs: a developmental perspective. Journal of Pediatric Nursing 6(4): 258–267

Rundahl Hauck M 1991 Cognitive abilities of preschool children: implications for nurses working with young children. Journal of Pediatric Nursing 6(4): 230–235

Stein R, Jones Jessop D 1984 Does pediatric home care make a difference for children with chronic illness? Pediatrics 73(6): 845–853

Swanwick M 1990 Knowledge and control. Paediatric Nursing 2 (June): 18–20

Swanwick M 1993 Bringing up baby. Paediatric Nursing 5(4): 20–23

Vehvilainen-Julknen K 1992 Client–public health nursing relationships in child health care: a grounded theory. Journal of Advanced Nursing 17: 896–904

While A 1991 An evaluation of a paediatric home care scheme. Journal of Advanced Nursing 16: 1413–1421.2

Whiting M 1994 Meeting needs: RSCNs in the community. Paediatric Nursing 6(1): 9–11

FURTHER READING

Barriball K L 1993 Measuring the impact of nursing interventions in the community: a selective review of the literature. Journal of Advanced Nursing 18: 401–407

Gallo A M et al 1992 Description of the illness experience by adolescents with chronic renal disease. ANNA Journal 19(2): 190–193

Haste F H, Macdonald L D 1992 The role of the specialist in community nursing: perceptions of specialist and district nurses. International Journal of Nursing Studies 29(1): 37–47

Meeropol E 1991 One of the gang: sexual development of adolescents with physical disabilities. Journal of Pediatric Nursing 6(4): 243–250

Patterson J M et al 1990 The impact of family functioning on health changes in children with cystic fibrosis. Science Medicine 31(2): 159–164

Powell C, Grantham-McGregor S 1989 Home visiting of varying frequency and child development. Pediatrics 84(1): 157–164

CHAPTER CONTENTS

In working through the contents of this chapter the student is introduced to the care of the critically ill child and his or her family, and the role of the paediatric intensive care nurse.

The chapter aims to:
- identify the needs and care required by the critically ill child in the paediatric intensive care unit, including the standards necessary to allow for optimum care and recovery
- outline the methods the nurse will use, in partnership with the family, to give the individual child the intensive care specific to his or her needs
- describe the role of the nurse during transport of the critically ill child
- review the need for organ donation and the effects of brain stem death on the family, and discuss the role of the nurse in helping the parents and family throughout the process of organ donation
- summarise the change from the normal parent–child relationship to the unfamiliar role of the parent of the critically ill child and identify family responses and coping strategies and implications for the nurse
- list stressful situations in the critical care setting and outline the nurse's responses and coping strategies.

THE PAEDIATRIC INTENSIVE CARE UNIT

The critically ill child has special medical and emotional needs, and therefore requires care from medical and nursing staff who have been specially trained in paediatric intensive care. This care is best provided in a paediatric intensive care unit (PICU), which offers a facility especially designed, staffed and equipped for the treatment and management of critically ill children from 4 weeks of age to adolescence, who are referred regardless of speciality category.

Types of intensive care

Level 1: High-dependency care

The child needs close monitoring and observation but does not require assistance from life-support machines; for example the recently extubated child, the child undergoing close postoperative observation with ECG, oxygen saturation or respiratory monitoring and who may be receiving supplementary oxygen and intravenous fluids or parenteral nutrition. This level of care requires a nurse-to-patient ratio of at least 0.5 : 1 (PICS 1992).

Level 2: Intensive care

The child requiring continuous nursing supervision who is intubated and is ventilated. Some unintubated children may also fall into this category, such as those with acute upper airway obstruction, whose condition is unstable and who may be receiving nebulised adrenaline. This level of care requires a nurse-to-patient ratio of at least 1 : 1 (PICS 1992).

Level 3: Intensive care

The child needs intensive supervision at all times, requiring additional complex and regular nursing and therapeutic procedures (Fig. 26.1). This category would include ventilated patients who are undergoing peritoneal dialysis or receiving intravenous infusions of vasoactive drugs or inotropes and patients with multiple organ failure. Level 3 intensive care requires a nurse-to-patient ratio of at least 1.5 : 1 (PICS 1992).

Provision of paediatric intensive care

Bed requirements and admissions

Because intensive care is expensive in terms of manpower and resources, it is essential to centralise paediatric intensive care facilities so that they may be used in the most efficient and cost-effective way. The facilities will only be employed effectively if all staff can retain their skills and are exposed continuously to the clinical and technical problems which may arise. The Paediatric Intensive Care Society standards (1992) recommend that a PICU should have at least four beds and admit a minimum of 150 patients a year. All PICUs should be based at a children's hospital or major paediatric centre. Those children requiring intensive care who present at other hospitals should undergo initial assessment and stabilisation and then be transferred to a designated PICU.

Facilities required

A PICU must be able to provide facilities for artificial ventilation, invasive cardiovascular monitoring, renal support, intracranial pressure monitoring, and complex intravenous nutrition and drug scheduling. There should be a comprehensive selection of monitoring and other equipment suitable for use over the entire paediatric age range, including a blood gas machine within or adjacent to the unit. Facilities must be available within the hospital to perform all routine haematological and biochemical tests on very small samples of blood, and there should be ready access to expert microbiological, biochemical and haematological advice together with an availability of all necessary blood products. There should be immediate access within the hospital to all routine radiological and imaging facilities, including ultrasound and CT scanning, and an emergency out-of-hours service.

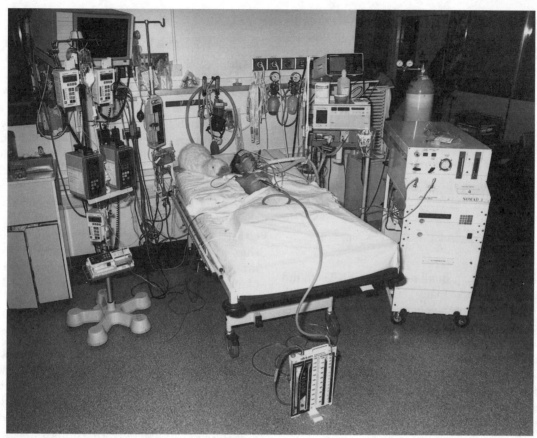

Figure 26.1 Child receiving level 3 intensive care.

Multidisciplinary team

The special needs of the critically ill child demand a high level of medical and surgical expertise from a multidisciplinary team; the unit should be staffed by paediatric intensivists and PICU-trained nurses, with input from other relevant specialities including paediatric medicine and surgery, microbiology, radiology and subspecialities such as urology, cardiology, neurology, orthopaedics, and haematology. In addition, there should be close involvement of appropriate non-medical and support staff, such as physiotherapists, radiographers, pharmacists, dietitians, transplant coordinator, parenteral nutrition team, ECG and EEG technicians, medical physics officer, and ventilator/general equipment technician.

Particular attention must also be given to the psychological and emotional needs of the child and the family, and there will need to be a support team which should include social workers, health visitors, parent support teams and clergy.

Transfer services

Each PICU should provide a fully equipped transport team, including a doctor and senior nurse from the PICU, which is available 24 hours a day for the safe retrieval and transfer of critically ill children from other units and hospitals.

Standards

Advances in practice and provision of paediatric intensive care have led to significant improvements in the prognosis of critically ill children.

Conditions which were once fatal can now be treated. Many children who would previously have sustained permanent disability may now make a complete recovery. To maintain and improve the outcome for critically ill children the Paediatric Intensive Care Society has established specific standards and guidelines for paediatric intensive care, detailing staffing (medical, nursing and other), equipment required, structure and design of units, services such as engineering, management policies, parental visiting, and data collection and audit (PICS 1992).

Limitations of present provision of paediatric intensive care

As there are only a small number of PICUs in the United Kingdom, many critically ill children undergo treatment in general intensive care units which cater predominantly for adults; in these units, children may be nursed in an open-plan area alongside adults undergoing intensive care. Some hospitals also manage critically ill children in part of a general paediatric ward (Intensive Care Society 1984, 1990). Both of these arrangements have serious disadvantages, such as:

* Lack of registered sick children's nurses with experience and training in intensive care.
* Medical staff involved in the care of these children may not have experience or training in paediatric intensive care.
* The equipment for monitoring and treating critically ill children may be inadequate.
* Children's wards may be located at some distance from other departments in the hospital and, in the event of an acute emergency, immediate availability of anaesthetic and other appropriate help cannot always be guaranteed.
* The needs of the critically ill child cannot be met in adult-centred units. Children need unrestricted access and visiting by parents and family members and require physical, emotional and psychological understanding by the multidisciplinary team involved in giving care, e.g. physiotherapists, dietitians, pharmacists.

Priorities of care

Each child receiving intensive care is an individual requiring care that is specific to his or her needs. Care is organised and prioritised according to physical illness, emotional, psychological, social and cultural circumstances and age.

The Activities of Living model of Roper et al (1983) is a useful way of looking at the care required by the critically ill child (Punton 1983). (Although they do not allow for cardiac function and output, this will be included.) Each child, depending on the severity and type of acute/chronic illness, requires variable degrees of specialised care by the nurse and family in partnership, in each of the activities of living. The main priority is to restore the child to his or her own level of independence in as short a time as possible.

Maintaining a safe environment

All staff in the PICU should be registered children's nurses who have experience in paediatric intensive care or have obtained relevant training. Every shift should have enough trained nurses to enable one-to-one nursing, with the appropriate numbers of extra nurses to comply with the PICS standards. Drug administration must be carried out according to UKCC and local policy, including appropriate training for competency and accountability in i.v. administration to ensure safe administration and elimination of mistakes. All staff should have an up-to-date working knowledge of all emergency procedures. Measures to ensure the safety of patients include:

* the provision of cot sides to prevent the child falling out of bed
* ensuring that endotracheal tubes, intravenous and intra-arterial lines and all drainage systems are secure and well fixed.

Adequate and appropriate sedation and pain relief should be given. The work area should be kept clean and tidy, with well-positioned and properly used equipment, and particular attention should be paid to preventing infection

Box 26.1 **Methods of communicating**

- Verbal—even though children may not be able to respond, they may still hear what is being said and what is going on around them; therefore it is important that the nurse explains all procedures and care, and encourages the parents to talk to their child
- Nonverbal—using sign language and mime
- Visual—using pictures and keywords
- Audible—story tapes, message tapes and favourite music
- Tactile—touching, cuddling, stroking as appropriate

and maintaining isolation from potential or actual infection.

Communicating

Communication between the child, the family and the staff of the unit is important. Children, according to their age, can communicate their needs through verbal and nonverbal cues. Depending on the severity of their illness and the need for airway management, sedation and/or paralysis, children may be unable to communicate in these ways. The parents and nurses can use the methods listed in Box 26.1 to help children to feel comfortable in their new environment and understand what is happening to them.

Families can react to the intensive situation by withdrawing, becoming angry or aggressive or seeming to act in inappropriate ways. The nurse needs to give support and encouragement to the families to enable them to feel comfortable in communicating with their child and feel involved in the caring.

Communication is just as important between the staff in the unit, including the multidisciplinary team, during ward rounds and in nursing handovers. Details of each child's history, medical condition, social circumstances and nursing care are discussed.

Breathing

The normal respiratory rate and pattern for the child's age should be well known to the nurse, who is able to observe for any deviation or change. Continual observation, assessment and monitoring of respiratory function will include:

- respiratory rate, pattern and sounds
- air entries and respiratory effort
- depth and symmetry of respiration
- colour of skin
- continuous oxygen saturation
- arterial blood gases
- type and amount of secretions.

When the child is mechanically ventilated, there should be frequent observation and recordings of:

- oxygen concentration
- mode and rate of ventilation
- peak airway pressure
- mean, positive end expiratory pressure (PEEP)
- minute volume.

When mechanical assistance is not necessary, oxygen may be given by face mask or nasal cannulae. To assist breathing and gas exchange with a secure airway, continuous positive airways pressure (CPAP) can be given via a nasopharyngeal airway (neonates and small babies) or endotracheal tube. Mechanical ventilation is delivered via an oral/nasal endotracheal or tracheostomy tube.

Fixation of airway is by taping or the use of metal frames and headbands, using specialised systems (e.g. minilink) to prevent tube movement. Patency is ensured by regular suction and clearing of secretions, physiotherapy to help clear secretions and prevent chest infection, and frequent repositioning of the child to enable the best lung function and assistance with sputum removal.

Cardiac output and function

Frequent assessment, monitoring and recording is important to detect changes and enable a quick response to maintain the optimum cardiac function and output. Routine observations will include:

- heart rate and rhythm
- blood pressure—systolic, diastolic and mean
- central venous pressure

- atrial and pulmonary artery pressures
- colour of skin, lips, and nail beds
- core and peripheral temperature difference
- renal function—including a check for the presence of oedema, particularly the eyes, face and dependent parts of the body.

To ensure adequate cardiac function and output, there must be continual maintenance of normal circulating blood volume, and prevention of electrolyte disturbances whilst replacing volume loss. Medications and drug infusions are given as prescribed, observing for and acting on any adverse effects.

Eating and drinking

Adequate hydration is maintained with the prescribed amount of fluids via the oral, nasogastric, nasojejunal, gastrostomy or intravenous route. Most children will have a nasogastric tube passed to allow feeding to be delivered safely. Milk feeds can be prescribed and prepared by the dietitian, who can add extra calories, electrolyte and other supplements to help in absorption. If there is a problem with enteral feeding, for example due to intolerance or surgery, parenteral nutrition will be required. This type of feeding creates problems as it requires a dedicated central venous line or lumen of a multi-lumen catheter, with no interruption by other drug infusions. Particular care is required to prevent the introduction of organisms, as the high level of dextrose provides a good culture medium for bacteria, increasing the risk of sepsis. The pharmacist, as with the dietitian, should review the feeding regime daily and adjust the calorie, electrolyte and other supplements according to the patient's needs and the doctor's prescriptions.

Eliminating

Maintaining the balance of input and output is an essential component of intensive care. Correct hourly charting and calculation of fluid balance is important, and consideration must be given to all types of fluid loss from the patient. These include:

- Urine—collected via nappies, urine bags, catheter and bedpan/urinal. Measure output hourly and take daily sample for urinalysis. Take samples twice weekly for culture and sensitivity if the child is catheterised or infection is indicated. Diuretics and restricted fluids can influence the amounts of urine passed.
- Bowels—note frequency and type of stool passed. Send sample for culture if there is any diarrhoea or other indication of infection.
- Nasogastric drainage—note type and amount of drainage, give prepared feed as soon as possible if not contraindicated, and use prophylactic anti-ulcerative medication if prescribed.
- Wound drainage—may require replacement with blood, plasma or plasma substitutes.
- Insensible losses—occur with pyrexia, when the amount of insensible loss requires approximation, and particularly with air-flow beds, when the amount of insensible loss may increase by at least 50% of the expected loss.
- Secretions from oropharynx/nasopharynx—may be profuse and contribute to overall fluid balance.
- Blood loss from arterial line sampling for blood tests—can add up to a substantial amount particularly in babies and may require regular top-up blood transfusions.
- Peritoneal dialysis/haemofiltration are methods to increase the amount of fluid elimination from the patient who has inadequate urine output.

Personal cleansing and dressing

In intensive care it is important to keep the children clean and fresh in order to reduce contamination of lines and wounds from body fluids and secretions, maintain personal hygiene and make the child look as normal as possible, although it can be difficult with invasive monitoring and intravenous lines. Parents can be encouraged to help with bed bathing, nappy changing, and the care of mouth, eyes, nose, hair and nails; they often enjoy supplying their own child's clothing. Linen is changed regularly and checks made on the skin of pressure areas. The dressings of wounds and intravenous sites are changed as required, and swabs should be taken for culture and sensitivity testing if there is any indication of infection.

Controlling body temperature

The critically ill child often has difficulty in maintaining core and peripheral body temperatures within the normal range. It is usual to nurse the child naked to allow for monitoring, fluid input, drainage systems and wound care. To increase and maintain core and/or peripheral temperature use cotton wadding, extra blankets, bootees, socks, cotton mittens and hats, overhead heaters and space blankets. To cool the child, nurse exposed, sponge with tepid water and use a fan to cool the surrounding air, and give antipyretic medicine. Ice packs or a cooling blankets must be used with extreme care to avoid the danger of peripheral shut-down occurring with peripheral cooling. Consideration must be made of the relatively large size of the child's head, which leads to greater temperature loss. Keep the environment at a stable temperature, if possible using air conditioning.

Mobilising

All children require regular turning, positioning and support of their limbs and body and require passive limb exercises if iatrogenically or pathologically paralysed; this should be coordinated with other nursing care.

When children are awake and their condition permits, the use of baby seats, reclining chairs, and floor mats can provide a change from the bed and encourage more movement. Allow the child to adopt a preferred position if permissible. The physiotherapist and occupational therapist can be involved in encouraging the child's interest in toys and games which can help to improve muscle tone, strengthening muscles and reducing lung problems.

Working and playing

The main 'work' of the critically ill child is to get better. Depending on the age of the child, the type and severity of the illness and the need for medical intervention to maintain and support body systems, the length of time and amount of effort spent 'working' will vary, and not every child will improve. The child who is not heavily sedated needs stimulation, and the nurse and family can provide this by spending time talking, reading books and encouraging the child to play with mobiles and toys. Television and video tapes and games can pass the time for older children.

Expressing sexuality

All children and their parents must be treated sensitively and respectfully in regards to their privacy. Older children who are nursed in an open unit may be embarrassed by their lack of clothing and their need for help with cleansing and bodily functions. Cultural beliefs and customs should be respected. If any clothing is able to be worn, it is important that it should be sex-appropriate.

Sleeping

Children in intensive care require as much rest as possible. Nursing care should be coordinated, with minimal handling of the child. A defined night and day routine should be followed, dimming ward lights at night and giving adequate and appropriate sedation. The child should be free of pain, positioned and supported comfortably, and provided with any special comforters such as a dummy or special toys, blanket, etc. Soft music may help to reduce the irritating noise of the unit, and control of the individual and environmental temperature can improve resting opportunities. For older children, a working clock helps to give their day more meaning.

Dying

The dying child must have adequate pain relief and measures should be taken to ensure that there is no suffering. Privacy must be ensured for the parents and family to say goodbye to their child and to mourn in the manner they wish. All families require support from either professional support services or from family members. The nurse should be aware of the unique and individual needs of families at this time and make every effort to meet these needs compassionately.

Activity 26.1

A 9-month-old baby is admitted to the PICU for ventilation. Plan the care of this baby, clearly indicating how the parents can be involved in the care.

If the parents appear reluctant to be involved, describe ways in which you can encourage their participation.

Managing and organising care in the PICU

There are many ways of organising care in a PICU and the method chosen can depend on factors such as the number of beds available, nursing staff numbers and skill levels, geographic location of beds and local policies. Many units are moving away from task- and patient-allocation methods of dividing work to allowing nurses to be accountable for their practice, with the use of primary/team nursing and models of nursing. Two documented methods of using primary nursing in a PICU are the Co-primary Nursing method (Kaplow et al 1989) and the Family Nurse Team (Dutko & Malan 1987). It is very important that paediatric nurses strive to help all children to achieve their full potential. To realise this aim, a useful model of nursing should be one that facilitates holistic care within the context of the family. Purcell (1993) described both the Biomedical model and the Partnership model, and concluded that a combination of both could provide a useful framework, which would provide a standard of care acceptable to the child and family, and one that is both realistic and holistic. The Activities of Living model (Roper et al 1983) can be useful when adapted to individual intensive care situations.

THE ROLE OF THE TRANSFER NURSE

The principles of safe transport

The guiding principles of safe transport of critically ill children are:

• thorough assessment, resuscitation and stabilisation before transfer
• appropriate monitoring during transfer by suitably trained accompanying staff using appropriate equipment (Doyle et al 1992).

These principles of safe transport between hospitals apply equally to transfers between theatres, recovery rooms, resuscitation areas, general paediatric wards and diagnostic areas.

The transfer nurse

The transfer nurse should be an experienced senior member of the paediatric intensive care team, who has undergone further specific training in inter-/intrahospital transport of the critically ill child. This training may be formal, or by in-service experience with the support of a trained transfer nurse.

The composition of the transfer team may vary from situation to situation and should match the nature and severity of the child's illness. The team should always include experienced and trained senior medical staff from a pool of paediatric intensivists.

The PICU should aim to have all senior nurses trained in the transport of the critically ill child so that continuity can occur as the transfer nurse becomes the child's nurse in the receiving unit.

Referral

There should be a clear line of communication between the referring hospital and the receiving hospital. Referrals should be consultant to consultant and clearly documented (Box 26.2).

When the PICU is alerted with this information, the transfer nurse is able to collect and check the equipment for the transfer and arrange the receiving bed-space.

Box 26.2 **Information required at time of referral (Dorman 1994)**

- Date and time of referral
- Name of doctor taking the call
- Referring hospital, ward and doctor
- Demographic data: name, age, date of birth, address
- Clinical history
- Clinical status on admission
- Treatment
- Current clinical status
- Reason for referral
- Accepted or refused (with reasons)
- Treatment advice given
- Further telephone calls

Equipment

Admissions to the PICU range in age from premature babies to teenagers. Thus a wide range of equipment is needed (see Box 26.3), although with planning it can be made portable enough for two people to carry. It is important that the nurse becomes familiar with the equipment, the layout of the kits and the additional equipment needed for each transfer. Units differ as to which member of the team is responsible for the daily and post-transfer checking of the equipment. The check includes making sure that all equipment is present and working, all battery-powered equipment is fully charged, and drugs have not reached their expiry dates. Drugs that are normally refrigerated are added at the last minute and discarded at the end of the journey if not used.

Patient and family care

On arrival, the nurse introduces herself to the patient and to the nurse who is caring for the child before transfer. An initial handover should be undertaken, in which the transfer nurse receives information about the child's condition and particular medical and nursing needs, special equipment and details of the family. Once the medical staff have been assisted in the initial examination, resuscitation and stabilisation as necessary, the nurse's priority is to meet and support the family and allow them time to visit their child before transportation.

Box 26.3 **Suggested equipment for transport of the critically ill child**

Airway
Facemasks
Oropharyngeal airways (sizes 000–3)
Endotracheal tubes (sizes 2.5–6.5 mm uncuffed, 6.0–8.5 mm cuffed)
Minitracheostomy kit
Nasogastric tubes
Laryngoscopes with a range of curved and straight blades
Magill forceps
Suction catheters

Breathing
Ayre's T piece
Self-inflating bag
Portable ventilator
Oxygen masks
Nasal cannulae
Chest drains
Heimlich valves

Cannulation
Venous cannulae (18–24 G)
Central venous cannulae
Arterial cannulae (22 G)
Intraosseous needles

Drugs
Sedatives
Analgesics
Muscle relaxants
Anticonvulsants
Inotropes
Diuretics
Antibiotics
Resuscitation drugs

Electrical equipment
To measure:
- ECG
- invasive blood pressure
- CVP
- pulse (oximeter)
- temperature
- non-invasive blood pressure
Defibrillator

Fluids
20% dextrose
10% dextrose
5% dextrose/0.18% saline
5% dextrose/0.225% saline
5% dextrose/0.45% saline
Colloid solution
Syringe drivers

The family are introduced to the transfer team, and the reasons for the need for specialised care are explained. Any problems and worries that the family may have are discussed, particularly if there is already a relationship with the referring hospital due to the child having spent time there as an inpatient. If so, the move can be stressful and the parents anxious about leaving a trusted and secure environment for one that is unknown to them. If the child has been recently admitted, the family will also be anxious and may not have had much time with their child since admission.

The procedure for the transfer of their child is explained, and the family are given appropriate information and the chance to have their questions answered. Arrangements are made for the parents to make their own way to the receiving hospital; it is impossible for them to travel in the ambulance because all available space is taken up by equipment, the transfer team and the paramedics. A study by MacNab (1992) found that most parents would prefer to travel with their sick or injured child, but even when there is space available, the transport team tend to discourage parents from accompanying the child because of their concern that the parents will make care more difficult to perform or will be distressed if an emergency procedure becomes necessary.

As the parents make their way to the receiving hospital, it is essential that they travel safely, driving if able, or with the help of family and friends. A map is helpful, and they should be given instructions not to follow the ambulance and a contact telephone number for the PICU. The family are reassured that they will be met and looked after in the PICU until the ambulance arrives and, once their child has been admitted to the unit, stabilised and made comfortable, they will then have immediate priority to visit.

Communication

Prior to leaving the referring hospital, ensure that a copy of the medical and nursing notes, referral letter and X-rays are available to accompany the child.

Arrangements are made with the ambulance control centre for return, with a police escort if necessary, giving details of equipment, accompanying personnel, and stability of the child.

The PICU is alerted regarding the estimated time of arrival, condition of the child, medical and nursing requirements, and family arrangements and needs.

Safety and comfort for transport

Prior to departure, a final assessment should be made of the patient and a check made that all battery-operated equipment is charged and working. Table 26.1 gives guidelines for the many aspects of transport that must be considered when planning the move.

Transportation

The most efficient means of getting to and from the referring hospital should be used. Road, sea and air transfers are all possible but each has problems; the distance, weather, accessibility and potential instability of the patient will all dictate the mode of transport.

The transfer nurse must consider all the known potential difficulties associated with the move, the pretransport severity of the illness and the current condition of the patient and be prepared to deal with the unknown problems that may occur and those which could be avoided (Tompkins 1990).

Admission to the PICU

On arrival at the receiving hospital, the patient is transferred to the waiting bed-space. The appropriate mode of ventilation is continued, and monitoring, and particular procedures are initiated as necessary. To maintain continuity, the transfer nurse remains as the patient's bedside and primary nurse.

Once the child has been stabilised, the transfer nurse updates the nurse in charge of the unit. It is then her priority, whilst continuing to monitor and record observations, to allow the family to visit and explain to them, in conjunction with the medical staff, the procedures, progress of treatment and nursing care required.

Completing the transfer

All nursing documentation should be finalised and placed in the notes. The transfer equipment is checked, restocked, and recharged as necessary.

The family are shown the waiting rooms and telephones, the visiting policy is explained and accommodation arranged. An information booklet for the hospital and the PICU is given to the parents.

The referring hospital should be informed of the safe arrival of the child and family.

ORGAN DONATION

Transplantation has developed rapidly with multi-organ donation now commonplace and widely accepted by professionals and the public alike. Though much has been achieved, the biggest challenge that remains is how to increase the numbers of transplants taking place (Gore et al 1989). Surveys and audit have revealed that 94% of families of potential donors are being asked about organ donation and therefore there is limited room for expansion (Gore et al 1991, Gore et al 1992). Why do we need to approach relatives for donation? For two reasons, firstly to give bereaved parents and family choice, meaning and comfort, and secondly to prevent avoidable deaths of potential recipients. Asking the parents to consider organ donation after they have been told that their child is dead does not make it worse, but it may make it better. The distressed family may find meaning in donation and should be given the choice and opportunity to decide; it is not always possible to tell how someone feels inside from what they show outside. Giving the parents choice prevents the detrimental consequences of not asking, and it may be that they are able to fulfil the child's wishes. The nurse may get satisfaction from helping the family to have a good death and helping someone else to live.

Who should be asked?   All parents or legal guardians of suitable donors.

By whom?   Medical and nursing staff who have been trained in how to do it well and are prepared to cope with reactions.

When?   After the first set of brain stem death tests, when the initial intensity of grief has abated, in time to obtain the decision before the second set of tests.

Where?   In a separate, private room where the family can be alone to grieve and consider donation without interruption.

Brain stem death

Brain stem death is defined as 'the irreversible loss of the capacity for consciousness, combined with irreversible loss of the capacity to breathe' (Pallis 1984). These functions depend on the integrity of the brain stem. There is evidence to show that for a patient with severe structural brain damage, if all the brain stem death criteria are satisfied, asystole will inevitably follow within a few days despite continued ventilation (Jennett et al 1981).

Testing for brain stem death

Brain stem death is confirmed when it is impossible to elicit any brain stem reflexes (see Box 26.4). Tests for brain stem death are done when:

- the child is comatose and mechanically ventilated for apnoea
- the diagnosis of structural brain damage has been established or the immediate cause of the coma is known
- drugs have been excluded as a cause of coma, neuromuscular blockade has been demonstrably reversed
- hypothermia does not exist
- there is no endocrine or metabolic disturbance (BPA 1989).

Table 26.1 Guidelines for transport (adapted from Tompkins 1990)

Principle	Questions	Actions
Know the estimated time of journey and mode of transport	How long?	Estimate oxygen usage during transport and allow for delays
	Are portable monitors charged?	Continual check of battery-operated equipment to ensure charged and working Determine connections in the transport suitable for the use of oxygen, suction, and monitoring
Evaluate patient stability	Is the patient stable enough for the transfer? Does the risk of transfer outweigh the benefits?	Anticipate potential emergencies and associated equipment needs
Maintain airway	Is the airway secure?	Secure endotracheal tube with tape well-anchored around tube and face Manually hold the endotracheal tube when moving patient
	Is the airway patent?	Instil saline and suction endotracheal tube prior to transfer Ensure adequate suction catheters, saline, and functioning suction unit
	Are alternative airways available?	Equipment bag should include a self-inflating bag with valve, correct size of mask, extra endotracheal tubes, nasal cannulae and oxygen masks for delivery of supplemental oxygen
Monitor continuously	What should be monitored?	Monitor ECG and respiration and oxygen saturation for all patients Monitor arterial pressure, central venous pressure, and ICP, pulmonary artery catheters if applicable Monitor airway pressure if ventilated Take vital signs every 15 minutes Include a check of neurological function
	What other monitoring is necessary?	Use non-invasive blood pressure monitoring, temperature
Maintain i.v. access	Is the i.v. line operating?	Check catheter site and blood return If any i.v. line is in question, insert a new line before leaving
	Is the i.v. line secure?	Ensure i.v. line is anchored to the skin and protected from dislodgement
	What about fluid regulation?	Have plasma or plasma substitutes available for boluses as necessary Use syringe drivers to deliver fluids
Consider immobilisation	How, what and when to immobilise?	Consider drug therapy to immobilise child if there is any doubt about maintaining airway Immobilise combative or active patients to protect them from injury Use of restraints when necessary
	Does the patient have a neck or back injury?	Maintain C-spine precautions for all children with suspected head or neck injury Use of neck collar or sandbags

Table 26.1 Continued

Principle	Questions	Actions
	Are there any other items that need to be secured?	Secure drainage systems to the bed or stretcher
Consider temperature regulation	How should body temperature be maintained?	Use of portable incubator Cover with sufficient cotton wadding blankets Use of silver swaddlers, and head coverings
Consider medications	What medications should be available?	Emergency drugs: adrenaline, atropine, sodium bicarbonate, 50% dextrose, ready to use Narcotics, sedatives, anticonvulsants, relaxants. Particular drugs required for patient's illness
Transfer team nutrition	How hungry and thirsty will the team get?	Cans of drink, Mars bars and sandwiches can make the transfer more comfortable for the team

Preparing the family for brain stem death

Whilst the medical and nursing staff are involved in struggling to save the child's life, the family are balancing hope for cure with preparation for the possibility of death. When death is probable or certain, the aim of intervention needs to shift from saving life to that of a good death and promoting good grief for the family (Le Poidevin 1987). The nurse needs to establish a rapport with parents, keeping them informed of what is being done. Wherever possible, the parents should not be alone; efforts should be made by the nurse to contact other family members and friends so that they can comfort each other at this time. Communication is very important. Always look the parents in the eye, speaking slowly, softly and gently, using plain words and always telling the truth. Try not to overprotect the parents from unpleasant reality; do not give false hope or mixed messages; the better prepared they are, the easier the adjustment at death. Keep them informed step by step of what is happening: 'He has a severe head injury, the brain damage is serious'; 'We will do all we can, but his life is in danger'.

Encourage the parents to express their thoughts and feelings: invite and answer questions; volunteer information; do not always wait to be asked; find out what they understand; clarify and repeat again what they find difficult to understand.

The nurse should always be present when the doctor is informing the family about brain stem death and the probability of death, in case the parents do not fully understand what they are being told and need further explanations. Always explain brain death in plain language. For example: 'Pressure in the upper brain is squeezing down and squashing the brain stem; it is permanently damaged beyond repair. That means that he will never again be conscious, be able to breathe or have a heartbeat of his own and he will never recover.' The extent of technology makes the concept of brain stem death difficult

Box 26.4 Reflexes involving brain stem function (BPA 1989)

1. No pupillary response to light
2. No corneal reflex
3. No vestibulo-ocular reflex (caloric test)
4. No doll's eye reflex
5. No motor response to pain—in the Vth nerve distribution
6. No gag reflex in response to suction through endotracheal tube or tracheostomy
7. Apnoea persists despite a rise in $PaCO_2$ to greater than 50 mmHg (6.6 kPa) against a background of a normal PaO_2

for the family to understand and come to terms with, because, though the spirit has gone, the body lives on, maintained by machinery. Box 26.5 lists questions that are often asked by parents of children with irreversible brain stem damage, and provides suggestions for answers.

Once the parents understand brain stem death, then is the time to give them the option of organ donation.

Approaching the parents about possible organ donation

The parents will need time to adjust to the pronouncement of brain death and to think about the option of organ donation. Exactly how and when this delicate subject is broached is a matter of fine judgement requiring experience and tact. The nurse who has developed a trusting and solid relationship with the family is often the most appropriate person to make the approach for donation. The nurse requires certain qualities and skills which include:

- a thorough knowledge of organ donation and transplantation including the legal implications

- the ability to communicate clearly, in a kind, sensitive, sincere and professional manner
- the ability to tolerate distress without becoming too attached or overwhelmed
- the ability to acknowledge her own emotional response to distress and deal with it.

The nurse's own feelings of comfort in approaching the parents must be considered before entering into highly sensitive discussions with grieving families, and those nurses who feel unable to be involved in these situations must not be made to feel that they have failed.

The nurse should take the family away from the intensive care unit to a quiet and secluded sitting room for any discussion. Time should be given for the family to discuss the matter amongst themselves privately without interruptions. Some families will be able to give an answer immediately; if they are undecided, it is best to give a further hour for reflection and then ask for a decision. (Parents who behave aggressively when first asked, quite often change their minds given time; thus the importance of broaching the subject of organ donation early.) If they agree, thank them; if they give a firm refusal, apologise for causing distress, but give the reason why the question had to be asked. Some families may have firm religious or personal opposition to the concept of organ donation and this should be respected.

The parents will have specific concerns regarding the donation procedure such as the length of time it will take (this depends on what organs are to be donated). They may only agree to donate particular organs and may worry about disfigurement (they can be assured that all wounds are closed as for any surgical incision, and that there are no visible signs of disfigurement).

Caring for the family throughout the process of organ donation

It is important for the nurse at this time of intense grief to allow the family to experience their feelings fully. All parents will react in different ways and must be treated appropriately. The common stages of grief that will be seen include denial, anger, bargaining, depression and acceptance, which the nurse should see as being normal and expected. Despite the atmosphere of the intensive care unit the nurse should do all she can to promote a warm and caring environment where the parents and family can be encouraged to spend time with their child and participate in his or her care. It can be very helpful if the child is given to the parents to hold. A lock of hair, hand and footprints, and photographs can be taken by the nurse and given to the parents at an appropriate time. The nurse should be as sensitive as possible to the family's needs and do as much as can be done to ease their distress. Encouraging them to talk about their child can help the nurse to view her patient more comprehensively and will enable the family to deal with the dying process in a personal and humane way. Parents and family members are encouraged to say good-bye to their child after the second set of tests for brain death, which is the legal time of death (Pallis 1983). Some parents will never comprehend the concept of brain death and, especially in cases of organ donation (following theatre), they need to see their child without the ventilator and with no heartbeat. If they do not have this opportunity, they may always feel that they 'left' their child in the ICU and, despite the funeral, the child is not dead, because they last saw the child 'alive'. The family should be offered the opportunity to visit their child in the chapel of rest after donation. The child can be dressed in clothes brought by the parents and viewed or held for as long as is needed. Time spent in this way can help the parents begin to take in the reality of their loss.

Family support following organ donation

Bereavement support after donation is an essential part of assisting the donor family in working through the grieving process. The intensity and duration of this period is affected by factors which include the circumstances surrounding the death (whether sudden or anticipated), the particular religious faith and beliefs of the family, and their previous exposure to death. Many go through the phases of grief at different speeds with very different time-tables; special events and memories, such as birthdays, may stimulate a return to the grieving process for many years after the death. Grief is specific and unique to each individual and situation, although different people in grief frequently share common feelings and concerns. Donor families deal not only with death but with the different emotions that donation brings.

Without adequate support, many survivors will never recover. Therefore it is important for nurses to realise that the way in which they behave around the time of death does influence the family, and recognise their responsibility to offer caring, compassionate and knowledgeable support which will contribute towards healthy long-term adjustment in bereavement (Johnson 1992). The nurse works closely with the local professional support team of the clergy, health visitor, general practitioner and social worker. One of the family's main supports following organ donation is the transplant coordinator, employed by the health authority. The role of the transplant coordinator includes education, organisation of the donor referral system, and informing and supporting the families and staff involved in donation. Prior to transplant, their experience is invaluable, as they are more able to answer parents' questions and give help to inexperienced nurses. Once donation has occurred, the transplant coordinator makes contact with the family and visits them as often as is wished. The parents of the donor are able to receive general information on any of the transplant operations that subsequently take place. A letter of appreciation from the local transplant unit not only allows the unit to thank the family for their generosity at a time of great personal sadness, but also allows the recipients and their own families to express their gratitude to the donor family.

Families can be guided toward established organisations such as CRUSE (the National Organization for the Bereaved and Their Children) and Compassionate Friends.

Activity 26.2

As a nurse dealing with organ donation, what support do you feel you could offer the grieving family? Who would be your local professional support team? What established organisation could be of help in this situation?

The nurse's role

Many nurses find themselves unprepared to assume the management of the patient's family so that they can more easily and effectively come to terms with their child's death and consider the possibility of organ donation. It is important that the nurse be provided with more detailed advice, training and guidance on managing the family in the many aspects of such a situation.

Training for nurses can include learning to manage the emotions of families. With sensitivity, self-awareness and planning, the nurse can help them to express and contain feelings safely, and encourage discussion of painful reality honestly and openly. Some nurses may find themselves afraid and unsure of the emotions displayed and are worried that they will be overwhelmed. It may be that their worries are about particular emotions, such as being attacked by angry relatives, or breaking down in tears when the family are sobbing. Nurses can learn to manage emotions, both in themselves and the families, so that they are able to have greater control over emotional reactions and can prevent them from getting out of hand. Inadequacy, guilt at failure to save life and fear of emotional release are all often felt by nurses dealing with death.

Learning to deal with emotions is as important a clinical skill in terminal care as in active treatment and may be more appropriate; aiming to help the child and family to have a good death is as valid as striving for a cure.

Learn to:

- be aware of, recognise and accept you own feelings; use role play, analysis, discussion or write them down

- develop confidence in your own ability to release emotional tension without being irreparably damaged or destroyed; if you know the depths of your own feelings you are less likely to be afraid of the feelings of others
- develop the ability to release/contain your own feelings in a controlled, direct and open way
- accept support from others who will listen, accept and comfort you without being critical or inhibiting
- give support and share your knowledge with colleagues once you have gained confidence and experience.

FAMILY SUPPORT
Family life changes

Children are very special people in the lives of their parents, whose main concern is to meet their needs, give them understanding, love, support and protection, and provide a stable environment in which their children can develop and mature. Whilst any admission to hospital is a distressing experience, admission to the PICU causes a radical change from the normal parent–child relationship to the unfamiliar role of the parent of the critically ill child. This new role has emotional and psychological implications and demands on the parents and the family.

Admission to the PICU may:

- precipitate a crisis within even the most organised family unit
- disrupt the family's ability to provide support and stability for their child and other family members
- change the caring role that is familiar to parents, removing certain duties and responsibilities, creating uncertainty and causing anxiety and stress
- prevent the parents from being able to demonstrate their love and care at a time that it is needed most
- cause conflicting demands among the parents, the sick child, siblings, and the work role
- create feelings of inadequacy, and helplessness in the parents because of the highly specialised care by skilled care givers

- affect the way siblings and friends react to the parents, their new role and the situation they are now in (Daley 1984, Rennick 1986, Farrell 1989, Carnevale 1990).

Family responses and coping strategies

Identifying family needs

To care for the family within the intensive care setting, we need to identify and understand their needs. This includes appreciating those needs which differ according to the social, educational, ethnic, cultural and religious backgrounds of the families. Identifying sources of stress and stressors that cause the most distress, gives some insight into the needs of the parents and the measures which would best meet these needs. This enables the parents to become more involved in the care and support of their child and gives value and importance to their role as parents of the critically ill child.

Studies by Miles & Carter 1982, Daley 1984, McIvor & Thompson 1988, Kirschbaum 1990, and Farrell & Frost 1992 have identified many categories of parental needs. The five most common needs described include:

1. To receive as much accurate and honest information about their child's condition as is possible. (The need to know what is happening, why it is happening and what the likely course of events is to be during the time of the child's admission.)
2. To be with their sick child. (To spend as much or as little time as they feel is right for them.)
3. To participate in their child's physical, emotional and psychological care. (Parents who are accustomed to providing total care wish to continue to participate, despite the PICU environment and the gravity of the child's illness.)
4. To feel assured that their child is receiving the most appropriate and highest level of care possible. (Included in this is the parents' need to feel that there is hope; the assurance that their child is receiving the best care may reinforce this feeling and also develop parental trust.)

5. The parents' own personal and support needs. (Included in these is a place to sleep and rest, refreshments and to have family members nearby.)

Identifying stress

Carnevale 1990 identified 17 different themes relating to sources of stress or stressors.
Grouped into five categories they are:

1. *Parental role conflict*—refers to thoughts and feelings pertaining to an inability to parent
2. *Concern for child*—refers to concern for the child's well-being, including the physical condition as well as the feelings of the child
3. *Environment*—involves the level of activity, noise, lights, and people in the environment, including significant changes in the environment such as transfer to a ward
4. *Friends*—refers to the particular behaviours of friends that cause distress
5. *Siblings*—includes the feelings and perceptions of other children in relation to the situation.

Miles & Carter 1982 examined some of the other aspects of the PICU which caused stress to parents. These include:

- Their child's appearance, i.e. the presence of restraints, intravenous infusions, drainage tubes, bruises, oedema and the child's nakedness.
- Their child's behaviour, i.e. confusion, agitation, unresponsiveness, pain and loss of body control.
- Nursing procedures. Much of the nurse's contact with the child involved procedures such as commencing intravenous infusions, nasopharyngeal/tracheal suction, nursing observations, etc.
- Staff communications. Parental anxiety is increased by the medical/nursing team communication styles. For example, the nurse spoke too quickly, used technical jargon, failed to inform the parents adequately of any changes that may have occurred in their child's condition, or sent parents out of the unit without any explanation.

• Staff behaviours. The parents were concerned regarding the medical/nursing team constantly rushing round, inappropriate joking, lack of gentleness in the giving of care to the sick child and acting in a remote way or appearing apprehensive.

Identifying coping strategies

Coping mechanisms are necessary to enable the parents to deal with their critically ill child and the PICU. A study by Carnevale (1990) found no consistent relationship between types of stressors and the strategies used to cope with each stressor.

The coping strategies most commonly seen are:

• Thoughts and feelings. (Anger, resentment and bitterness over losing control of their child, and inability to assume responsibility. Scary thoughts and difficulty in concentrating on the child and not the machines, denial and eventual resignation to 'waiting it out'.)
• Actions to staff, family and friends. (Trying to be in on decisions and learning medical terms quickly to sound sensible. Making the staff their community in whom they soon develop personal interests. Family relationships and friendships may become strained and individuals withdrawn as the family react to the crisis.)
• Social support. (Drawing on family members, friends and parent support groups for encouragement, support and contact. Such people provide someone to listen, to take a break from the unit with, and to spend time with the child to allow the parents time together.)
• Direct actions. (Particular behaviour that alters the environment favourably, such as reading the charts.)
• Environmental. (Having a place to stay close by, a telephone and refreshments.) (Broome 1985, Carnevale 1990.)

Involving the parents

The nurse can help the parents to feel involved with the care of their child and maintain close contact by asking them to help with basic

Case study 26.1 Ryan's parents' story

The day of Ryan's operation was, to say the least, nerve-racking. The waiting was the worst part. When we went to the PICU we were asked to wait as they were not ready for us; it seemed like forever. No matter how well prepared you are, or how many times your child has been in hospital, the initial shock of seeing him just lying there with drips and lines all over the place is just too much; all I could do was cry. Having a child in intensive care is like being on a roller-coaster, with its highs and lows. You could have a good day, then a bad day, but the good ones made up for the bad. It was very difficult to be strong when he was not responding, but if we do not have faith, what hope does he have? I thank the staff for their persistence in trying everything possible to keep Ryan alive. We try to take part as much as possible in his care and feeding as we feel it helps in understanding what is involved in caring for a critically ill child, and it also helps bonding with Ryan.

nursing tasks such as eye and mouth care, daily bed bathing, cleaning the napkin area, keeping the hair brushed and tidy, and massaging the skin with moisturising cream when dry.

Passive exercises can be taught to the parents by the physiotherapist, and stroking and caressing can be beneficial to both parent and child. The parents can be encouraged to bring in the child's own toiletries, suitable clothes that the child may be able to wear and special, familiar blankets, sheets and toys that can make the environment seem a little more friendly.

Reading and telling stories, listening to tapes made by friends and family and familiar music can all help the parents to feel that they are able to make a worthwhile contribution to the care of their critically ill child.

Displaying a photograph of their child and/or family may give parents the subconscious feeling that they are showing staff that this child belongs to them, not to the PICU, and allow them to share control over the present alien situation and the very different way in which the child appears at present.

Parents of newly born babies have a special need to get to know their child. The nurse needs to be supportive of the family who have not anticipated such a joyous event ending in this way.

Implications for nurses

The PICU nurse has a major caring responsibility to assist the parents of the critically ill child to adapt and respond to the changes in the parental role that their child's admission to a PICU will demand. To be effective, the nurse must have some understanding of the effects that a PICU can have upon the parents and implement those measures and strategies that meet the parents' needs. If these needs can be met, then the parents will be able to adapt to their new role, become involved in the continuing care of their child and, with encouragement, gain the knowledge and confidence to be more supportive and help promote recovery.

It is important that the nurse is able to encourage an environment in which the participation of the parents in the care of their child is seen as an essential component of care. Parental conflict with professional staff is documented as a major source of stress (Carnevale 1990), so the nurse must be prepared to consider the following strategies to help resolve conflicts between nurses and parents and to achieve the best possible outcome for sick children and their families:

- Constant review of the nurse's existing practice and behaviour toward families (discussion about the individual parent's role, feelings and specific needs, and implementing appropriate outcomes).
- Enhancement of the nurse–parent relationship. (Understanding the parents' need for the reciprocation of the trust they place in the nurse to be demonstrated by words and actions that show sensitivity to their need for full participation in the care of their child. The use of suggestion, where the nurse may anticipate areas of possible concern and enable parents to talk by prompting. For example: 'I know that a lot of parents in your situation worry about…')
- Identifying those policies that may prevent parental participation (visiting hours, inappropriate parent–child separation).
- Introducing the parents to other health professionals who may facilitate particular coping strategies (social worker, chaplain, family information and support coordinator, and health visitor).
- Implementation of educational programmes to help all nurses to develop their knowledge and skills in working with parents.

The effectiveness of the nursing interventions can be evaluated by documenting changes in the parental role performance and the level of anxiety shown. When parental needs are met, the critically ill child, family and the nursing staff benefit from an improved parental role performance, reduced parental stress and enhanced parent–staff relationships.

NURSES' RESPONSES AND COPING STRATEGIES

When children are cared for in as near ideal conditions as possible, it can bring great satisfaction for the nurse, compensating for the emotional stress and frustration felt with many of the difficult situations and experiences of intensive care. In response to the many critical situations (see Box 26.6) and the lack of control felt over them, professional attitudes and behaviour can change in negative ways. Some of these characteristics are:

- labelling patients
- feeling unappreciated and guilty
- a sense of failure
- intolerance of colleagues and patients
- hating going to work
- cynicism and dislike of patients
- frequent minor illnesses and a high level of absenteeism
- exhaustion and sleep disturbances

Activity 26.3

What could you do to lessen the distress felt by parents on the admission of their child to your PICU? Identify specific family needs and ways in which you could best meet these needs in your own situation.

- withdrawal and isolation
- lack of concentration
- weight loss or gain and eating disorders
- overdependence on stimulants like cigarettes and alcohol (adapted from Swaffield 1988).

This is the danger for all who are in the caring professions, and one to which those who are in authority give the least amount of attention. They do not realise that nurses, the care givers, can lose hold of their ideals and faith (Iveson-Iveson 1983).

Coping strategies

Burning-out starts when nurses (or their superiors) take no action to deal with the early signs of stress. A vicious circle starts, with more and more work being done and less and less being achieved. Depression about feeling depressed, and the buildup of symptoms of over-stress, make it harder and harder to summon the energy to do something about them (Swaffield 1988).

Some existing coping strategies that are common to most nurses and frequently seen in the ICU are:

- complaining
- talking about others
- smoking
- showing emotions
- callous or off-hand behaviour
- hysterical inappropriate laughter (tension relief).

Nurses are protecting themselves with these 'coping strategies', which mask the real problems. Even when the person using them knows that they are unhealthy and counterproductive, they are hard to part with.

Stress is an individual thing whether it occurs in one person or the whole unit, so solutions must be suitable and will require hard work to maintain. There is major benefit in using both group and personal remedies to stress, and they can only improve the work environment and the individual nurse's job satisfaction.

> **Box 26.6   Stressful situations in intensive care**
>
> **Death and dying**
> - Providing for the needs of the dying child and family
> - Prolonged illness of the child requiring intensive family support
> - The nurse's own feelings and the expression of them to the family
> - The family's reaction and ability to deal with death
> - The religious, ethnic and cultural aspects of dying and death
> - The nurse who frequently looks after the dying patient
> - New staff and students who have no experience in nursing a dying patient
>
> **Crisis situations**
> - The suddenness of emergencies
> - More than one crisis at the same time
> - The variety of different emergency situations such as trauma, cardiac arrest, SIDS
> - The frequent requirement to make rapid and independent decisions
> - Rapid increase in admissions and discharges
>
> **Relationships with family**
> - Dealing with individual family situations (single, separated, unsupported, extended families)
> - Families with difficult financial circumstances
> - Unfamiliar religious, ethnic and cultural differences
> - The demanding and intense family
>
> **The long-term patient**
> - Little or no progress
> - Poor prognosis
> - Irritable, unsettled and demanding patients
>
> **Communication and decision-making**
> - The medical staff may tend to deal only with the technical details of medical management and put less emphasis on the nurse's more direct involvement with the patient and the family
> - Decisions about major factors, for example resuscitation, have not been reached when needed and cause anguish in crisis situations
> - Nurses tend to be more sensitive to emotional issues than medical staff
>
> **Seasonal illness trends**
> - High levels of bed occupancy during the winter influx of respiratory illness
> - Rapid turnover of patients
> - With high levels of bed occupancy there is the need for the nurses working on the unit to do overtime

Group remedies

- Counselling—which must be 100% confidential, and separate from nursing management or personnel department.

Activity 26.4

Look at your own life experiences. In what ways have you personally responded to difficult and stressful situations? What strategies did you use to cope with these situations? In what ways does your own experience help you in caring for children and their families in the PICU?

• Informal group support—an atmosphere in which individuals can joke, chat, offer sympathy, admit to feeling stressed without losing face, and share feelings with others in the same position.
• Formal group support—regular meetings to discuss individual cases or client groups, individual nurse's problems and difficult issues. These should be focused round work problems—not amateurish group therapy.
• Feedback from patients/relatives—a big satisfaction to nurses which should be encouraged. Where appropriate, it may be helpful to seek news of patients who have been discharged or referred on.
• Feedback from management on what is expected, and praise when it is achieved.
• Support from managers—regular contact, and an 'open door' for staff with problems or suggestions, either individually or collectively.
• Somewhere to unwind during working hours.
• Training, basic and post-basic, in understanding stressful areas of care (e.g. death and dying), in stress management, and in interpersonal skills.
• Overload avoidance—rotating stressful jobs, making sure all breaks are taken, encouraging time out of the unit where possible, and watching for staff who are overworking.
• Flexible organisation—hours and shift patterns which suit staff, and a chance to take short breaks at minimum notice and plan holidays.
• Management of change—lots of (genuine!) consultation, listening to people's worries, and full preparation before change is made.
• Action on poor standards—quality assurance methods, with coherent action on problems that are identified.

• Guidelines (local or national) on disputed procedures and roles (adapted from Swaffield 1988).

Personal remedies

Learn to be realistic and accept your limitations and emotions; everybody has them. Accept that feeling stressed is natural; learn about your individual stress symptoms and when you get them; seek the cause and try to take action.

Have realistic goals; change the things that you can change and accept those that you cannot. Do not try to sort out problems which belong to someone else; deal with your own priorities and ask for help when you need it. Make use of others with skills that can help you with patient problems (social worker, health visitor, occupational therapist, etc.).

Look at further training—short courses and study days—in areas you find difficult to deal with. Seek out someone with expertise and ask for their help.

Look after yourself. Eat well, and exercise regularly. Cultivate interests and friends outside of nursing.

REFERENCES

British Paediatric Association (BPA) 1989 Working party report on the diagnosis of brain stem death in children. BPA, London
British Paediatric Association (BPA) 1993 The care of the critically ill child. Report of a multidisciplinary working party on intensive care. BPA, London
Broome M 1985 Working with the family of a critically ill child. Heart and Lung 14(4): 368–372
Carnevale F A 1990 A description of stressors and coping strategies among parents of critically ill children—a preliminary study. Intensive Care Nursing 6: 4–11
Daley L 1984 The perceived immediate needs of families with relatives in the intensive care setting. Heart and Lung 13(3): 231–237
Dorman T 1994 Transport of the critically ill child. Care of the Critically Ill 10(2): 80–83
Doyle E, Freeman J, Hallworth D, Morton N S 1992 Transport of the critically ill child. British Journal of Hospital Medicine 48(6): 314–319
Dutko I, Malan M 1987 The family nurse system: a variation in primary nursing. Dimensions in Critical Care Nursing 6(5): 293–302
Farrell M 1989 Parents of critically ill children have their needs too! A literature review. Intensive Care Nursing 5: 123–128

Farrell M, Frost C 1992 The most important needs of parents of critically ill children: parents' perceptions. Intensive and Critical Care Nursing 8: 130–139

Gardner D, Stewart N 1978 Staff involvement with families of patients in critical care units. Heart and Lung 7: 105

Gore S M, Hinds C J, Rutherford A J 1989 Organ donation from intensive care units in England. British Medical Journal 299: 1193–1197

Gore S M, Taylor R M R, Wallwork J 1991 Availability of transplantable organs from brain stem dead donors in intensive care units. British Medical Journal 302: 149–153

Gore S M, Cable D J, Holland A J 1992 Organ donation from intensive care units in England and Wales: 2 year confidential audit of death in intensive care. British Medical Journal 304: 349–355

Guidelines Committee of the American College of Critical Care Medicine, Society of Critical Care Medicine and American Association of Critical Care Nurses Transfer Guidelines Task Force 1993 Guidelines for the transfer of critically ill patients. Critical Care Medicine 21: 931–937

Intensive Care Society (ICS) 1984 Standards for intensive care units. ICS, London

Intensive Care Society (ICS) 1990 Standards for intensive care units. ICS, London

Iveson–Iveson J 1983 Banishing the burnout syndrome. Nursing Mirror 156(18): 43

Jennett B, Gleave J, Wilson P 1981 Brain death in three neurosurgical units. British Medical Journal 282: 533–539

Johnson C 1992 The nurse's role in organ donation from a brainstem dead patient: management of the family. Intensive and Critical Care Nursing 8: 140–148

Kaplow R, Ackerman N, Outlaw E 1989 Co-primary nursing in the intensive care unit. Nurse Manager 20(12): 41–42, 46

Kasper J, Nyamathi A 1988 Parents of children in the paediatric intensive care unit: what are their needs? Heart and Lung 17(5): 574–581

Kirschbaum M 1990 Needs of parents of critically ill children. Dimensions of Critical Care Nursing 9(6): 344–352

Le Poidevin S 1987 The management of bereaved relatives and approaching the next of kin about organ donation. Unpublished handout from the Psychiatry Department, London Hospital Medical College, London

MacNab A 1992 Paediatric inter-facility transport. The parents' perspective. Social Work in Health Care 17(3): 21–29

McIvor D, Thompson F J 1988 The self perceived needs of family members with a relative in the intensive care unit. Intensive Care Nursing Journal 4: 139–145

Miles M S, Carter M C 1982 Sources of parental stress in the ITU. Journal of the Association for the Care of Children's Health 11(2): 65–69

Paediatric Intensive Care Society (PICS) 1992 Standards for paediatric intensive care. Available from: Stonehart Subscription, c/o Care of the Critically Ill, Hainault Road, Little Heath, Romford, Essex, RM6 5NT, Tel: 0181 597 7335

Pallis C 1983 The ABC of brain stem death. British Medical Association, London

Pallis C 1984 Brain stem death: the evolution of a concept. In: Morris P J (ed) Kidney transplantation, 2nd edn. Grune & Stratton, London, pp 101–127

Philichi L 1989 Family adaption during a pediatric intensive care hospitalization. Journal of Pediatric Nursing 4(4): 268–276

Punton S 1983 A model for nursing. Nursing Times 79(9): 24–27

Purcell C 1993 Holistic care of a critically ill child. Intensive and Critical Care Nursing 9(2): 108–115

Rennick J 1986 Re-establishing the parental role in a pediatric ICU. Journal of Pediatric Nursing 2: 40–44

Roper N, Logan W, Tierney A J (eds) 1983 Using a model for nursing. Churchill Livingstone, Edinburgh

Swaffield L 1988 Burnout. Wallchart. Nursing Standard 2(14): 24–25

Tompkins J 1990 Intrahospital transport of seriously ill or injured children. Pediatric Nursing 16(1): 51–53

FURTHER READING

Bailey R 1985 Coping with stress in caring. Blackwell Scientific Publications, Oxford

Bond M 1993 Stress and self-awareness: a guide for nurses. Heinemann Nursing, Oxford

Carter B (ed) 1993 Manual of paediatric intensive care nursing. Chapman & Hall, London

Chalmers H 1988 Using models series: choosing a model. Edward Arnold, London

Goldman A 1994 Care of the dying child. Oxford Medical Publications, Oxford

Hazinski M F 1992 Nursing care of the critically ill child, 2nd edn. C V Mosby, St Louis

McCann Flynn J, Pardue-Bruce N 1993 Introduction to critical care skills. Mosby Year Book, St Louis

Smith J B 1983 Pediatric critical care. Delmar Publishers, Albany NY

USEFUL ADDRESSES

Compassionate Friends
53 North Street
Bristol BS3 1EN
Tel: 0117 966 5202
Helpline: 0117 953 9639

CRUSE
126 Sheen Road
Richmond
Surrey TW9 1UR
Tel: 0181 940 4818
Helpline: 0181 332 7227

27

Terminally ill children

Jayne Taylor   Karen Skilbeck   Sally Huband

One of the most frequent fears expressed by children's nurses is the fear of caring for a terminally ill child. Nowadays childhood death in the United Kingdom is relatively rare and in some ways this makes it harder (see Ch. 3). The expectation is that children will survive and parents expect to die before their children. The death of a child affects us all, whether we have direct dealings with the family or whether we hear of the death through the media.

In working through the contents of this chapter the student is introduced to the needs of dying children and their families. Concepts of death are explored and the effects of a terminal illness on family functioning are discussed. Principles of palliative care are outlined.

The chapter aims to:
- discuss the emergence of death as a concept during childhood
- explore the effects of terminal illness on the child and the family
- discuss the needs of dying children and their families
- discuss the principles of palliative care.

CHILDREN'S CONCEPTS OF DEATH

All children, whether well or sick, will at some time during their childhood years experience death. It may be the death of a pet, an elderly

461

relative or a family friend, or it may be a television character or a fictional person or animal in a book.

Children will often have the ability to talk in quite sophisticated language about death. They will discuss funerals, cremations and burials and may use terms such as 'passed on', 'passed away', 'gone to sleep' or 'gone to heaven'. It is important that we look beyond these outward signs of knowledge and understanding, which can be deceptive, and try to appreciate what children really understand by death.

Exploring children's concepts of death is not a simple task. It is a sensitive area and one with which many adults have difficulty. Exploring death with children means facing up to our own mortality and being faced with questions to which we do not have answers. Children's concepts of death will also be influenced by their previous experiences, which may have been painful. They may have lost a relative, friend or pet who they were close to and the way in which significant adults have handled the situation will affect their response.

The age at which a child develops a concept of death will vary from child to child. Some attempts have been made to correlate the developing concept with chronological age (Table 27.1) and this can be useful even if there are likely to be individual variations. Lansdowne & Benjamin (1985) in their study of children aged from 5–9 years old, found that 60% of the children studied had a complete or almost complete concept of death. By the age of 8 or 9 years almost all of the children had a complete concept. Up to the age of 5, it is difficult to assess children's understanding, partly due to their restricted use of language. Gonda & Ruark (1984) suggest that children between the ages of 2 and 5 years find it difficult to accept the finality of death and see it as a reversible process.

Nurses who are caring for children with terminal illness need to have some insight into the child's concept of death in order to respond to them appropriately. Young children are direct in their approach and it can be an area of concern to the nurse that she may be questioned by them

Table 27.1 Development of the concept of death and dying

Age	Stage
Under 2 years	The stage of animism. If everything is alive, there is little concept of death. The child is more frightened of separation. Adults can reassure children by maintaining their security and ensuring that they are not left alone
2–5 years	Children may have had their first experience of death, seeing a dead bird or losing a pet. They see death as reversible and have little insight into its finality
6–9 years	First understanding that death is irreversible. It tends to be seen as violent. Children may be frightened of changes to their body
10 years and over	Children are capable of abstract thought and are aware of the possible consequences of death for those left behind
Adolescence	An adult's concept of death is developed

about their impending death. It is almost instinctive that we wish to protect children from anything which may frighten them and there can be few more frightening concepts than that of death and dying. In the past, adults were often not told the truth about their terminal illness. Nowadays professionals are aware that people have the right to be told the truth about their own illnesses and that most of them will appreciate honesty. Children also have a right to the truth

Activity 27.1

Think of young children you have known who have experienced death, either of a person or a pet. How did they respond and how were they helped to come to terms with their loss?
  Discuss with a friend how you would respond to:

1. a child of 3 who is terminally ill and says her teddy has died
2. a child of 6 who asks you whether he is dying.

and parents can be helped to answer their children's questions honestly and appropriately.

 For further reading, see Stickney (1982), Varley (1984), Wilhelm (1985), Wells (1988) and Lindsay (1994/5).

The concept of death in terminally ill children

The extent to which dying children develop an understanding of their own mortality is clearly even more complex and sensitive than the general understanding which develops in well children. Ross-Alaolmolki (1985) suggests that dying children develop a more complete concept of death earlier than well children, particularly in relation to the finality of death. Bluebond-Langner (1989) also suggests that dying children view death differently. She writes: 'When a child is dying, his or her experiences are very different from other children of the same age, and hence the accepted developmental model of children's view of death is not as applicable for the dying child as it would be for healthy children'.

The awareness of impending death in dying children is a peculiar phenomenon in that these children have often not been formally told that they are dying. The awareness that they are dying appears to develop instinctively (Bluebond-Langner 1989). Nurses need to be aware that because dying children may not discuss impending death, this does not mean that they are unaware of the terminal nature of their illness. This awareness may be demonstrated through their play or in their drawings.

Bluebond-Langner describes the process of becoming aware of impending death in children who have not formally been told that they are dying, as one of discovery. She describes five stages of developing awareness in children:

1. knowing that they have a serious illness
2. learning the names of their medication and side effects
3. learning the purposes of various treatments
4. putting together several sources of information to come up with the whole picture of relapses and remissions
5. developing an understanding of the terminal prognosis of the illness.

When children reach this stage, Bluebond-Langner suggests that a change in behaviour can be observed. The children may get frustrated with adults who continue to pretend and who try to give them false hopes. They also demonstrate an urgency in their behaviour and do not like to waste time. Bluebond-Langner writes: 'these children were having their time cut short and they knew it'.

THE EFFECTS OF TERMINAL ILLNESS ON THE CHILD AND FAMILY

The child

Psychological dysfunctioning is not an uncommon finding in children who have a terminal illness. Stein et al (1989) found that 40% of their sample of children with life-threatening illness had psychological difficulties. They were anxious and unhappy and had emotional or behavioural problems. Bluebond-Langner (1989) found that terminally ill children in her study frequently displayed anger and would withdraw at times. She described this type of behaviour as disengagement and suggested it to be a way of rehearsing for the final separation which comes with death. The children also displayed a reluctance to talk about other children who had died and became angry when long-term plans were discussed. Papadatou (1989) found similar problems in relation to dying adolescents and long-term plans. These young people need help to 'discard their unfulfilled dreams, expectations and goals' which involves open and honest discourse. Letting go of long-term aspirations is a difficult but necessary part of the grieving process. These adolescents need to focus on shorter-term goals, which, whilst they are not the same, can bring some hope and optimism to their lives.

Terminal illness does not only have potentially negative psychological effects on children; it also

Case study 27.1 Andrew

Andrew, aged 14 years, has had leukaemia for the last 2 years and is now in the terminal stages of the disease. He has been admitted to the ward as his pain is not controlled. Andrew has also lost his hair as a result of chemotherapy.

On admission, Andrew presents as a very angry young man. His relationship with his parents and his 11-year-old sister is strained and his parents are finding it difficult to cope with his moodiness and anger.

During the next few days, his nurse develops a rapport with him and at a ward meeting where his case is being discussed, gives the following information concerning Andrew.

- He is angry with his parents because he feels that they have not been honest with him. His father is always talking of his plans for Andrew's future, when Andrew knows that he is dying.
- He is angry with his sister, but does not really understand why. He feels it is so unfair that he is ill and she is healthy.
- He wants to know what will happen to his belongings when he dies. He has a computer that he is particularly attached to and would like it to go to one of his close friends but is frightened that his parents will give it to his sister who will not appreciate it.
- He wants to go home and does not see why he should stay in hospital when he is not able to be cured. As both of his parents are working, he wonders if one of the reasons they do not take him home is because they would have to take time off work.
- He wants to see some of his close friends but does not like the cap his parents have bought him to cover his head and he feels that his friends will laugh at him as the cap is not 'cool'.

Activity 27.2

With a group of friends, discuss how the information given by the nurse in Case History 27.1 might be used in order for Andrew's care to be adjusted to meet his needs.

Might it be appropriate for some children and adolescents to have a say in what happens to their possessions after their death?

months and years with periods of remission followed by relapses. The families may have had to be involved in decisions to stop curative therapy in favour of palliative care.

The parents

Stein et al (1989) in their study of children with life-threatening illness found that 45% of the mothers and 27% of the fathers in their sample had psychological difficulties as measured by the General Health Questionnaire. All of the mothers identified by Stein et al had been prescribed tranquillisers within the 12-month period preceding the study. Lawler et al (1966) found that many mothers were clinically depressed and experienced constant thoughts about death. A proportion of the mothers had frequent fantasies about funerals and cemeteries. Marital relationships also appeared to be adversely affected by the presence of a dying child. The parents may have problems in spending time alone together as there can be difficulties in arranging for someone else to care for the child. There may also be financial problems, with parents having to take time off work and find money for fares to visit the child in hospital. Friends may find it difficult to be supportive as they may be frightened, not knowing how to respond or what to say.

Siblings

There is also the potential for the presence of a terminally ill child to adversely affect healthy siblings, who according to Bluebond-Langner (1989) live in 'houses of chronic sorrow'. They

has physical effects as a result of the disease process and/or therapeutic interventions. Children may need to be hospitalised at regular intervals and this can be seen as curtailing valuable 'living time'. They may have to cope with pain, with hair loss or with other distressing symptoms.

The family

The families of children with terminal illness are subjected to enormous stress. Often they face the uncertainty of whether the child will live or die, and if death is inevitable, they do not know when it will happen. Children may live several

Case study 27.2 Susan

Susan is 5 years old and is terminally ill with a brain tumour. She was discharged from hospital 1 week ago and the paediatric community nurses have been asked to visit and assess the family's needs. Susan's mother, a part-time primary school teacher, has taken time off work to look after her and her father is also very involved with Susan's care. The family is experiencing some financial problems as a result of Susan's illness and have had to cancel their usual summer holiday; Susan is not well enough to go away and also they feel that this year they do not have any money for holidays.

Susan's mother has been getting increasingly tired and anxious, and when the community nurse visits, she breaks down and says that she is not sure whether she will be able to care for Susan at home, although she would like to and feels that Susan will be happier.

The following problems have occurred:

- Susan wakes frequently at night so the parents have had little sleep. They have decided to take it in turns to sleep in the same room as Susan.
- Susan's pain does not seem to be well controlled and her mother says she cannot bear to see her in pain.
- Simon, Susan's 7-year-old brother, is being very difficult. He is very close to Susan and they have always been good friends. However, recently he has become very jealous and says that it is not fair, Susan gets all the attention and all the presents. He does not understand why they cannot go to Wales for their usual summer holiday. He has taken to waking at night and will go into Susan's room and wake whichever parent is sleeping there. He has also started to wet his bed again, something he has not done for over 3 years.

may find that their parents have little time to spend with them and are preoccupied with the ill child and their own anxieties. Healthy siblings may be denied information as parents either try to protect them from bad news or are unable to put their own emotions into words. Older siblings are more prone to adverse effects than younger siblings. They worry about the possibility of family breakdown and feel particularly isolated from the family (Stewart et al 1992). Younger children in the egocentric stage of development may feel that they are the cause of the illness. 'I hate you and wish you would die,' is not an unusual comment from children in the middle of an argument or struggle for supremacy. The child who has thus expressed

Activity 27.3

With a group of friends, discuss ways in which the needs of the family described in Case History 27.2 might be met.

himself, may then feel that he has caused his sibling's illness. Bluebond-Langner (1989) describes how children may feel jealous of their dying sibling and angry that their 'playmate' is going to desert them. They may seem insensitive on hearing of the actual death of a sibling: 'Good, now I can have all his toys'. This must not be taken at face value; they are likely to be feeling the pain and loss acutely and are looking for a tangible way of coping.

Significant others

It is also important to remember the other significant people who are likely to be affected by the impending death of a child. The child's friends, grandparents and other close relatives, step-parents and teachers can all experience the extreme stress and uncertainty associated with dying children and may need support and help to come to accept a poor prognosis.

THE NEEDS OF DYING CHILDREN AND THEIR FAMILIES

In the previous section of this chapter we have explored the possible effects of terminal illness on the child and the family. These effects result in the development of specific needs in these children and their families which can be defined as physical, psychological and social. Nursing activity should focus on meeting such needs and enabling dying children and their families to develop adaptive ways of coping.

This is a complex task because the lives of these children and their families are inextricably interwoven. The coping behaviour of each individual family member will affect other members of the family unit.

The child

There is very little literature which looks specifically at the psychological needs of dying children and their ways of coping. Graham (1985) suggests that needs will vary according to:

- the type of the disorder
- the age of onset
- the nature of medical treatment
- the presence or absence of stigma associated with the disorder.

Whilst this is useful it does not provide any great insight into the needs of these children or their ways of coping.

Rossman (1992) undertook a study on healthy school-aged children and their perceptions of stress and their strategies of coping. In the absence of any studies on ill children, this study is worth considering. Rossman classified coping strategies into categories which include:

- distress
- distraction/avoidance
- use of peers
- self-calming
- anger.

These five categories of coping strategy are considered below; Box 27.1 gives a brief scenario to illustrate each strategy.

Distress

This first category described by Rossman is identified as a cathartic behaviour which can elicit aid from others. Mattsson (1972) suggests that, in relation to sick children, distress provides an outlet for feelings such as sadness, anxiety and impatience. Bluebond-Langner (1989), who observed signs of distress in dying children's drawings and conversations, also noted that such behaviour would elicit care from adults. The distress of dying children clearly needs an outlet, and nurses along with play therapists, psychologists and parents can enable children to find a medium through which to displace their frustrations.

Box 27.1   Scenarios that illustrate Rossman's five categories of coping strategy

Distress
Amy is terminally ill and is known to be very distressed. She is anxious and tearful. The play therapist is working with Amy and enables her to express her feeling in drawing and painting. She is also enabled to express some of her anxieties by using dolls as an intermediary.

Distraction/avoidance
Mark is 10 years old and is aware that he is very ill and likely to die. He can no longer play football which was his passion. He has, however, become absorbed in playing games on the family computer. When his friends visit, he no longer talks to them about football but tries to get them interested in his computer.

Peers
Alison, aged 14 years, is terminally ill with cystic fibrosis and is being cared for in hospital, as her mother is on her own and is unable to care for her at home. The hospital have made her cubicle as homely as possible and her friends have been encouraged to visit. They have been able to give her a considerable amount of support. However, 3 days before her death, Alison states that she does not wish her friends to visit any more.

Self-calming
Martin is being taught relaxation exercises to help him cope with his pain. Since he has started using this technique he has required less analgesia and appears less stressed.

Anger
Patricia is being cared for at home. She has a very close relationship with her mother, but suddenly has an angry outburst against her. Her mother is very distressed but is helped to understand Patricia's feelings and arranges for a friend to stay with Patricia whilst she goes out for a while. When she gets home again, Patricia apologises for her outburst and is her usual loving self.

Distraction/avoidance

The second category of coping strategy usually involves the child in avoiding stressful thoughts, often by denial, and in the avoidance of stressful actions by a variety of means including self-distraction. Avoidance by denial can be used by ill children in both adaptive and maladaptive ways (Bruce 1986). The adaptive use of denial can help children who face an uncertain future to maintain a degree of hope and still strive for potentially unobtainable goals (Mattsson 1972). Whilst it is important that children are not given false hope, it is also important that they are given some aspirations for the future, even though this may be extremely limited. The maladaptive use of denial may involve the child in denying realistic dangers and in non-compliance with treatments.

Distraction can also help children cope with the stress of impending death. Mattsson (1972) suggests that ill children will compensate for specific limitations by pursuing activities which are still within their capability.

Use of peers

Rossman's third category relates to the use of peers for emotional assistance, help with problems and support through activities. There is little evidence that dying children will use peers in coping, possibly because contact with peers may become less frequent as they approach death. It is important, however, to recognise that peers fill a place in the lives of children that neither parents, nurses nor siblings can fill, and if the dying child wishes to spend time with peers it is right that this wish is fulfilled. Hospital departments should, if the child wishes, encourage peer visits and allow the dying child and his peers the privacy to talk and if necessary to say goodbye. If the child is being cared for at home, the child's friends can be encouraged to continue to visit and may be able to lighten the atmosphere.

Self-calming

Rossman's fourth category of self-calming is rarely referred to in relation to dying children. However, McGuire & Dizard (1982) advocate the use of relaxation techniques with children in pain, and Garmezy & Rutter (1985) discuss teaching children relaxation techniques as a way of preventing stress. As alternative therapies such as relaxation and guided imagery and meditation become more socially and medically acceptable, more work in this field is likely to be undertaken with dying children.

Anger

The fifth category described by Rossman is anger, which like distress may be used to elicit aid from others. Angry behaviour is identified in several studies relating specifically to ill and dying children. Bluebond-Langner (1989) found that dying children used anger to disengage other people and create distance. When situations became unbearable, angry outbursts from the dying children provided parents with an excuse to leave followed by a reunion. It is interesting to speculate that perhaps these children feel a need to rehearse their deaths and allow their parents to start to separate from them. Older children may also need space and privacy at times, although the child must be the one who sets the agenda for time alone as some children may perceive parental absence as rejection.

The family

Much more is known about the needs of the families of dying children and their ways of coping than is known about the needs of the children themselves. The stages can be discussed under the headings identified by Kubler-Ross (1969) in her work with dying adults:

- denial
- anger
- bargaining
- depression
- acceptance.

These different stages of parental reaction are considered below with those that precede acceptance being illustrated by the scenarios in Box 27.2.

Denial

The use of denial by adults with terminal illness is well documented by Kubler-Ross. Mattsson (1972) found that parents often displayed denial and disbelief, particularly around the time of diagnosis. This denial led parents to 'shop around' other medical and non-medical sources in the hope that someone might dispute the original diagnosis and prognosis. Denial in the parents of ill children can be seen as a response to the fear and uncertainty that they face around the time of diagnosis. It can give them valuable space, and the shopping around provides

---

Box 27.2   Examples of possible parental responses to terminal illness in a child

Denial

Mary has been told that her son James has a brain tumour and is unlikely to survive. When she returns home she tells her husband that the hospital must have got James' results muddled with another child's. She insists on a second opinion which is arranged and confirms the original diagnosis. Mary is still unable to accept the diagnosis. The staff realise she is still in the stage of denial and take time to repeat the information until she is able to acknowledge the diagnosis.

Anger

John has been diagnosed as having a terminal illness. The parents were asked to come and see the consultant by one of the staff nurses on the ward and are given the news. Following this, they express extreme anger towards the nurse and say that she is not fit to be looking after John. They also say that the consultant should have diagnosed John's condition sooner and that they are thinking of taking legal advice. The sister on the ward reassures the staff nurse that the parents are angry at the diagnosis and need to express it in some way. After a few days they are calmer and apologise for the way in which they have reacted.

Bargaining

Amy's parents are told that she is terminally ill. They plead with the doctor that she should survive until after Christmas. They go to church for the first time for years and ask the priest to pray for them. They promise that they will come to church regularly, if only Amy gets better.

Depression

Martin's mother visits her GP and tells him that she cannot cope with his illness any more. She cannot stop crying, her house is in a mess and the other children distraught. Her GP arranges for her to have practical support in the house and visits her on a regular basis to see how she is coping.

---

distraction. Kubler-Ross suggests that denial is only a temporary response which should lead at least to partial acceptance ultimately. Parents cannot be hurried through this stage. It is difficult for professionals to offer support for families who are in the denial stage but, eventually, denial will no longer be a realistic strategy for parents.

Anger

Kubler-Ross sees anger as a stage through which adults pass when they can no longer deny

illness. Anger is often projected towards doctors and nurses, perhaps because it is less emotionally traumatic to be angry towards someone who is detached. Kubler-Ross warns health care professionals that they should try to understand the reasons for such anger and not take it personally.

Bargaining

Kubler-Ross describes this as the attempt to postpone; it has to include a prize for good behaviour and usually has self-imposed deadlines. The parent may promise to be a better person, to say regular prayers, or may ask that the child should survive until a particular birthday or Christmas.

Depression

This stage comes when the illness and prognosis can be denied no longer. Parents will describe feelings of extreme exhaustion, they may have periods of uncontrollable weeping. They are unable to function in their normal way. For siblings, this can be a traumatic period. In the words of one young child: 'When my Mummy is sad, she can't be a proper Mummy any more.' The parent is unable to respond to the needs of others. Some parents will become depressed enough to require medical intervention.

Acceptance

At this stage the prognosis is accepted and parents can be helped to move forward.

Not all parents will go through all of these stages; they may go through them in a different order and there can be no time limit. Some parents may have reached the period of acceptance before the child dies, some may still be in denial. The length of the illness can be a factor in determining this. Nor is the list exhaustive. Parents may express feelings of *failure*. They may say that the first duty of parents is that their child should survive, so that if the child is terminally ill, they have failed. Others may express feelings of *guilt*. They may remember that they did not always follow the advice of health professionals in the past and feel that they are now being punished and the illness is the result. These parents need to be reassured that they did not cause their child's illness.

Parents need to be kept fully informed of their child's condition. Many will express feelings of *loss of control* and can be helped by being given back some control. For some parents, being actively involved in the treatment and care of their child can be therapeutic. More terminally ill children are now cared for at home and, with support from paediatric community nurses, the parents can be helped to care for their child until the child's death. This can also be helpful to the siblings, who can also be involved in the caring. They can help by playing with the sick child, or by fetching things or by providing company.

Nurses need to be aware of the wide range of emotions and reactions that can be encountered when working with families of terminally ill children. They are often worried about what they should say. There are no magic words to comfort parents at a time like this. Professionals can help by listening and supporting, by involving parents and by empathising with them. The Child Bereavement Trust is a newly formed organisation which provides training for nurses and other health professionals working with bereaved parents.

PRINCIPLES OF PALLIATIVE CARE

This chapter has so far focused on the psychological effects of terminal illness and the coping strategies of children and their families. Some of the physical implications also need to be addressed, as psychological support will be ineffective if the child is in pain and the parents anxious about physical symptoms.

Sutherland et al (1993) define palliative care as: 'Care which is provided when curative treatment is not possible or appropriate, and which personalises the care of the whole child and family, focusing on the relief of physical, emotional, social and spiritual distress and aiming for the best possible quality of life'.

Pain control

The aim of pain control should be that the child should be pain free and comfortable at all times. Most children have a real fear of injections so these should be avoided if at all possible.

Oral analgesia. This is usually effective in the early stages and should be given regularly to prevent pain. Morphine syrup given 4-hourly can be effective and the dose adjusted as necessary.

Patient-controlled analgesia (PCA). Analgesia can also be given either intravenously or subcutaneously via a pump. This prevents the child being given frequent injections and is usually well tolerated (see Ch. 9).

Radiotherapy. In some instances palliative radiotherapy can help to control pain; however, it is important that both the child and the parents understand that the aim of the treatment is to control the pain and not to cure the disease.

Steroids. Children with brain tumours may benefit from being given dexamethazone to reduce the intracranial pressure and so relieve some of the symptoms.

Massage, aromatherapy and hypnotherapy. Some children may benefit from a combination of traditional analgesia and alternative therapy. The use of the latter is still in its infancy but is worth considering.

Factors that may exacerbate pain

There are many other factors which can contribute to the amount of pain felt by the child and so should be minimised or prevented.

Nausea and vomiting. The use of opiates can cause nausea and vomiting. Anti-emetics should be given prior to meals and the effects monitored. A vomit bowl and tissues should be kept near the child, who should be given the opportunity to rinse the mouth after any vomiting.

Constipation. Terminally ill children will often become constipated due to a combination of factors. Many analgesic drugs cause constipation as a side effect. The child is likely to be less mobile than usual, and may be eating and drinking less. The first approach should be to try to increase the amount of roughage in the diet but this may well be impossible if the child's appetite is poor. The fluid intake should be encouraged and the child kept as mobile as possible. Children may also prefer to be carried to the toilet, rather than use a bedpan or commode. If these measures fail, aperients or suppositories can be used.

Sore or infected mouths.   Children who have had chemotherapy may also have mouth ulcers or oral thrush (see Ch. 24). It is important to treat the child's mouth effectively as this will encourage him to eat and drink, which in turn enhances his feeling of well-being.

Positioning.   Children who are less mobile than usual will need to be well supported and to have their position altered so that they do not become stiff or develop pressure sores.

Fatigue.   The child may not be sleeping well at night and may need periods of rest during the day. Small children will often fall asleep even if there are people making a noise in the surrounding area but older children need to be given quiet periods.

Other considerations

Palliative or curative.   Sometimes it is right that treatment is given to the dying child which may at first consideration seem inappropriate. The child who has developed a urinary tract infection will be more comfortable if the urinary infection is treated with antibiotics. The child dying from cystic fibrosis may need oxygen and physiotherapy. To deny him physiotherapy when to him it is part of his normal routine may well cause distress. Sometimes it is difficult to separate the curative from the palliative; in the case of the dying child, the first principle should be the relief of distressing symptoms, and if the treatment provides relief, there should be no conflict of views.

HOME OR HOSPITAL?

In the past, most terminally ill children would have been cared for in hospital, mainly because there was little support for them in the community. With the increase in paediatric community nursing teams and the advent of paediatric Macmillan nurses in some parts of the country, more children are being cared for at home. Most children feel more secure in their home, surrounded by their families, their friends and familiar toys. The child can remain at the centre of family life, provided that the family is well supported. Families must know where they can turn to for help and must be reassured that admission to hospital can always be arranged if they find that they cannot manage. It is important, however, that the parents are not made to feel that they have failed.

If the child does have to be cared for in hospital, the family will need to feel welcomed at all times of day and night. Facilities need to be provided for them to stay and areas need to be as homely as possible. Over the last few years, some children's hospices have been opened, the first being Helen House in Oxford. There are few of these, however, and they are only likely to cater for the needs of those families who live near at hand. They aim to provide respite care as well as caring for children and families in the terminal stages, if this is what the families wish.

AFTER THE DEATH OF THE CHILD

Support for the family should not cease at the time of death. Many parents are young and have not had to deal with a death before. They may need to be helped to register the death and gently steered towards funeral directors who will be able to give them all the information they require. Parents often appreciate staff who have cared for their child attending the funeral or sending flowers. In some areas, cards are sent on the anniversary of the death. There are support groups who can provide much needed help. These are usually made up of other parents who have lost children and can appreciate the feelings in a way that others cannot. Parents will often comment that they need to talk about the child who has died, but friends and relatives may shy away from this, finding it too difficult and worried that they may upset the parents. Support groups can give parents the opportunity to talk.

Nurses who have cared for terminally ill children can also feel bereaved after the death and many units will provide support groups for the staff so that these feelings can be explored and support offered.

I think it is helpful to warn parents or other newly bereaved people that other people's pious platitudes can be insensitive and hurtful; however close the relationship between two people may be, they may grieve differently; and that the healing of grief is a very long, slow process. It is never complete; parents will never 'get over' the death of their child.

Mother Frances Dominica 1987

REFERENCES

Bluebond-Langner M 1989 Worlds of dying children and their well siblings. Death Studies 13: 1–16
Bruce T 1986 Emotional sequelae of chronic inflammatory bowel disease in children and adolescents. Clinics in Gastroenterology 15: 89–104
Dominica Mother F 1987 Reflections on death in childhood. British Medical Journal 294
Garmezy N, Rutter M 1985 Acute reactions to stress. In: Rutter M, Hersov L (eds) Child and adolescent psychiatry, 2nd edn. Blackwell Scientific Publications, Oxford
Gonda T A, Ruark J E 1984 Dying dignified. The health professional's guide to care. Addison-Wesley, Menlo Park CA
Graham P J 1985 Psychosomatic relationships. In: Rutter M, Hersov L (eds) Child and adolescent psychiatry, 2nd edn. Blackwell Scientific Publications, Oxford
Kubler-Ross E 1969 On death and dying. Macmillan, New York
Lansdowne R, Benjamin G 1985 The development of the concept of death in children aged 5–9 years. Childcare and Development 11: 13–20
Lawler R, Nakielny W, Wright N 1966 Psychological implications of cystic fibrosis. Canadian Medical Association Journal 94: 1043–1052
McGuire L, Dizard S 1982 Managing pain in the young patient. Nursing 12(8): 52, 54–55
Mattsson A 1972 Long term physical illness in children: a challenge to psychosocial adaptations. Journal of Pediatrics 77: 571–578
Papadatou D 1989 Caring for dying adolescents. Nursing Times 85(18): 28–31
Ross-Alaolmolki K 1985 Supportive care for families of dying children. Nursing Clinics of North America 20(2): 457–467
Rossman B B R 1992 School-age children's perceptions of coping with distress: emotion regulation and the moderation of adjustment. Journal of Child Psychology and Psychiatry 33: 1373–1397
Stein A, Forrest G C, Woolley H, Baum J D 1989 Life threatening illness and hospice care. Archives of Disease in Childhood 64: 697–702
Stewart D A, Stein A, Forrest G C, Clark D M 1992 Psychosocial adjustment in siblings of children with chronic life-threatening illness. Journal of Child Psychology and Psychiatry 33: 779–784
Sutherland R, Hearn J, Baum D, Elston S 1993 Definitions in paediatric care. Health Trends 25(4): 148–150

FURTHER READING

Baum J D, Woodward R N 1990 Listen my child has a lot of living to do. Oxford University Press, Oxford
Bluebond-Langner B 1978 The private worlds of dying children. Princeton
Foster S, Smith P 1987 Brief lives. Arlington Books, London
Kubler-Ross 1983 On children and death. Macmillan, New York
Lindsay B 1994/5 Like skeletons or ghosts. Developing a concept of death and dying. Child Health 2(4): 142–146
Pincus L 1981 Death and the family. Faber & Faber, London
Stickney D 1982 Water bugs and dragonflies. Explaining death to children. The Pilgrim Press, Berwick on Tweed
Varley S 1984 Badger's parting gifts. Picture Lions, London
Wells R 1988 Helping children cope with grief. Facing a death in the family. Sheldon Press, London
Wilhelm H 1985 I'll always love you. Hodder & Stoughton, London

USEFUL ADDRESSES

Support groups
Bereaved Parents Helpline
16 Canons Gate
Harlow
Essex

The Child Bereavement Trust
1 Millside
Riversdale
Bourne End SL8 5ED

The Compassionate Friends
53 North Street
Bristol BS3 1EN
Tel: 01179 539 639

CRUSE
Cruse House
126 Sheen Rd
Richmond
Surrey TW9 1UR

SANDS
Argyle House
29–31 Euston Rd
London NW1 2SD

Children at risk

Nicola M. Eaton

This chapter introduces students to the identification and care of children who are at risk of abuse or neglect.

The chapter aims to:
- describe the use of child protection registers to identify children at risk
- distinguish between different forms of child abuse, i.e. physical, sexual or psychological, and passive or active
- discuss Munchausen syndrome by proxy—a very subtle form of child abuse
- consider the care of children who attend accident and emergency departments
- provide examples of cultural and religious practices that may place children at risk
- describe the particular health needs of travelling families
- discuss the role of other health professionals in the care of these children
- emphasise the need for communication and cooperation between all the health professionals involved to ensure that the most effective strategies are implemented.

INTRODUCTION

Children may be at risk for many reasons such as the environment in which they live, war, pollution, or from the adults who care for them, as in cases of child abuse and neglect. This chapter aims to introduce some of these topics, review some of the literature and provide points for discussion. The children's nurse must be aware of social, legal, religious and cultural issues involved in identifying and caring for children who are at risk. The nurse must also understand the role of other health professionals in this caring process and, in the light of this, the concept of a case conference relating to the child at risk is discussed.

IDENTIFYING THE CHILD AT RISK

It is the responsibility of all members of a society to protect children, as they are the future of that society and are vulnerable. All health, social and educational professionals have a particular responsibility to be vigilant where those weaker members of society are liable to exploitation. In the United Kingdom, health visitors and social workers are particularly involved in the surveillance of normal and disadvantaged children. Other health professionals become involved when the child is ill or handicapped in any way.

All health authorities are obliged to keep child protection registers which identify children in need of extra professional attention. In April 1991, 45 200 children were on child protection registers in England—a rate of 4.2 per 1000 population below the age of 18 years. The main reasons for being on the register were:

- Grave concern—47%
- Physical abuse—20%
- Sexual abuse—12%
- Neglect—12%
- Emotional abuse—6% (Meadow 1993).

A child is placed on the register after a case conference when the child is deemed to have been abused or to be at risk of future abuse. The categories now used are:

1. Neglect, physical abuse and sexual abuse
2. Neglect and physical abuse
3. Neglect and sexual abuse
4. Physical abuse and sexual abuse
5. Neglect (only)
6. Physical abuse (only)

7. Sexual abuse (only)
8. Emotional abuse (only).

(This revised list takes into account the requirements of the Children Act 1989.) 'Grave concern' as a category was withdrawn, except in cases where there has been no recent review or re-categorisation (Welsh Office 1993).

The identification of this 'at-risk' population results in many professionals providing much-needed surveillance and probably averts many problems.

THE ABUSED CHILD

Meadow (1993) defines the abused child as one who is 'treated in a way that is unacceptable in a given culture at a given time' (p. 1). What constitutes child abuse may vary between generations, between cultures and even between subcultures. The first legislation to protect children in the United Kingdom appeared in 1889, 67 years after the introduction of legislation to protect animals (Meadow 1993).

Professional agencies such as social services departments or the National Society for the Protection of Children (NSPCC) are notified of suspected cases of abuse in as many as 4% of children under 12 years old. In 1986, the NSPCC reported a yearly incidence of 0.57 cases of child abuse per 1000 children (Meadow 1993).

It has been noted (Kelly 1988) that children with (among other things) physical handicaps and developmental delays seem to be at increased risk of abuse. The child may be at risk of abuse for many reasons, some of which occur when normal parenting patterns break down. Both boys and girls are abused, with the younger ones being more at risk, partly because they are most vulnerable and partly because they cannot

Activity 28.1

Find out about local agencies involved in child protection and how to access them.

Table 28.1   A classification of abuse with examples of major forms (Stratton 1988)

	Physical abuse	Psychological abuse	Sexual abuse
Active	Non-accidental injury Poisoning	Emotional abuse	Incest Rape
Passive	Failure to thrive Poor health care	Neglect Lack of affection	Failure to protect

seek help anywhere. Children under 2 years old are more at risk of physical abuse. Death from this is rare after the age of 1 year (Meadow 1993). Abuse may be physical, psychological or sexual, and either active or passive. Parents who abuse their children do not fall into any specific category. They may be any social class, ethnic group or age. As few causal factors have been identified, there are no ways to predict accurately which adults will abuse their children (Roberts 1988). However, they may be people who are impulsive, aggressive and violent and have often themselves been the victims of abuse (Kaufman & Zigler 1987). Stratton (1988) classifies child abuse as in Table 28.1.

Physical abuse (non-accidental injury)

Child abuse is what is said to have occurred when the parent has intentionally injured the child. So when does slapping and hitting as punishment become abuse? It is necessary to be careful to distinguish between true abuse and non-abuse injuries such as bruising and other skin discoloration, and bleeding or bone disorders, especially in young babies and children. Although the number of reported cases of abuse appears to be on the increase, it may be that health professionals are more alert to this

Activity 28.2

Discuss with colleagues your attitudes to parents who abuse children and how the issue might be dealt with sympathetically.

diagnosis (Creighton 1988). The child who repeatedly appears at the GP's surgery or the casualty department with different injuries may be an abused child. Fractured skull or limbs are other signs of physical abuse, especially when the history of the injury is vague or inconsistent.

The term 'battered baby' was coined by Henry Kempe in 1962 and has been well publicised since. It can include burns and scalds, but most of the abuse is violent and short term, although it may be repetitive (Meadow 1993). The term more commonly used now is non-accidental injury (NAI).

Speight (1993) suggests that NAI is not a diagnosis but a symptom of disordered parenting. The aim of treatment is to identify or diagnose and cure (if possible) the disordered parenting. Meadow (1993) lists seven pointers to diagnosing NAI. They are:

1. There is a delay in seeking medical advice.
2. The story of the accident may be vague or change at each telling or from person to person.
3. The account of the injury is not compatible with the injuries observed.
4. The emotional response of the parents is abnormal—abusing parents tend to be more preoccupied with their own problems.
5. The behaviour of the parents is abnormal; they may, for example, become abusive and refute accusations that have not been made.
6. The child's interaction with the parents may be abnormal and the child's appearance may be sad, withdrawn or frightened.
7. The child may say something which is indicative of abuse, such as, 'Daddy said he wouldn't do it again'.

Classic non-accidental injuries include finger-tip bruising (fingertip-shaped and -spaced bruises on the body), cigarette burns, adult bite marks, lash marks and a torn frenulum. Other indicators may be subdural haemorrhage and retinal haemorrhages.

Emotional and psychological abuse

This type of abuse may be very difficult to detect and prove. Indeed, Azar et al (1988) suggest that it is more serious than physical abuse. Adults who emotionally abuse their children may reject, isolate, terrorise, ignore or corrupt the child. There is an idea that emotional abuse may lead on to mental health problems in later life.

Sexual abuse

Sexual abuse of children is defined as:

the involvement of dependent, developmentally immature children and adolescents in sexual activities they do not truly comprehend, to which they are unable to give informed consent and that violate the social taboos of family roles.

(Beezley-Mrazek & Kempe 1981)

It occurs in children of all ages and may be suspected when the child's behaviour is odd; for example, girls who are precocious or 'act up' to adult males. The adult involved in sexual abuse initiates sexual activity for his or her own satisfaction. In about 85% of cases the children are abused by someone they know, often a member of the family. The child becomes confused, may feel guilt, shame and fear and believe that they are responsible in some way. The adults may have threatened them that if they tell they will be taken away. Mothers sometimes collude in sexual abuse, although some may genuinely not know of its occurrence.

Other indicators of child sexual abuse can be seen in the behaviour of the children. Some become withdrawn, have disturbed sleep, become aggressive, or undergo behavioural changes that lead to the formation of inappropriate relationships. Loss of self-esteem appears to be the most pervasive consequence of sexual abuse and adolescents may become anorexic, self-mutilating, suicidal or aggressive, or turn to prostitution (Bentovim et al 1988). It has also been noted that some children display inappropriate sexual knowledge through play or pictures.

Munchausen syndrome by proxy

This is a very subtle type of child abuse which may be difficult to diagnose. The parent (and very occasionally other adults, as possibly in the case of Beverley Allitt, a nurse caring on a children's ward, who was convicted of murder and attempted murder in 1993) victimises the child by presenting him or her with a history of a fictitious illness. The medical profession then, based on this information, subject the child to a series of diagnostic procedures and therapeutic interventions. The child is usually normal and healthy although Gale & Horner (1992) document a case involving a handicapped adopted child.

Since 1977 when the first case of this syndrome was identified and reported (Meadow 1977), there have been other reports in the literature. According to Gale & Horner (1992), in all the reported cases the perpetrator has been the mother rather than the father; however, as shown by the Allitt case, the person responsible may be unrelated to the child. There are two issues here: the welfare of the child and the mental problem of the mother. The mother has often had training in a health-related field, often nursing or paramedical and often involving children, and is therefore able to give quite detailed but false histories which can be impressive. She appears to be very loving and concerned about the child and stays with him or her during all procedures and all the time spent in hospital. The mother forms strong relationships with other parents on the ward and also with members of the hospital staff who may have sympathy for her; she manipulates them, often very successfully to the extent that they find it very hard to believe that the mother is harming her own child. Although the mother appears to be loving and concerned, she has her own problems. She often has a high level of insecurity, uncertainty, loneliness and depression and may have a low self-esteem. She appears to thrive in a medical setting and on the attention she and the child receive. This mother may herself have been emotionally deprived or abused in childhood (Sigal et al 1989).

Incidents such as producing specimens contaminated with blood (often the mother's own or from a wound elsewhere on the child) or causing the child to suffer brief periods of asphyxiation and reporting it as apnoea, fiddling with equipment such as drips, and administering drugs including laxatives and diuretics to produce symptoms are just some of the reported actions of the mother in these cases.

The child is usually young (rarely over 6 years

Activity 28.3

Find out your ward or department's policy in a suspected case of child abuse.

---

according to Senner & Ott 1989) and unable to tell other adults what is happening. He may display behaviour inappropriate to his age, become hyperactive or display fear and negativism. The child may see the mother's love as dependent upon the illness (Crouse 1992). It is only after long and close observation that the true picture can be revealed.

How may this syndrome be recognised?

Gale & Horner (1992) give a list of warning signs (see Box 28.1) and suggest that the greater the number of these which appear over a prolonged timespan the more likely it is that this syndrome is occurring.

Every ward which admits children should have procedures in place for dealing with suspected child abuse. Interactions between the parents and child should be observed and the child not left alone with them. Record keeping needs to be particularly good as the nurse might be later required to give evidence in a court.

THE CHILD IN ACCIDENT AND EMERGENCY DEPARTMENTS

Accidents account for the highest number of deaths in children aged 1 to 14 in the United Kingdom. At least 3 million children are treated in accident and emergency (A&E) departments each year (Lancaster 1993). Boys are more likely to be injured than girls (except in passive accidents such as car accidents) and those children who are in economically deprived families are more likely to have accidents. The age of the child is relevant to the injury; for example, babies and small children fall and injure themselves in the home, while older children are more likely to be injured climbing trees or falling or being

---

> **Box 28.1   Warning signs of Munchausen syndrome by proxy (Gale & Horner 1992, p. 28)**
>
> 1. Common fabrications: bleeding, neurologic, fevers, biochemical chaos, feculent vomiting, rashes, glycosuria.
> 2. Unexpected persistent or recurrent illness.
> 3. Discrepancies between clinical findings and history.
> 4. The working diagnosis of 'a rare disorder'.
> 5. An experienced physician states: 'I've never seen a case like this before'.
> 6. Signs and symptoms do not occur in mother's absence.
> 7. A very attentive mother who refuses to leave child alone.
> 8. The child has frequent intolerance to all forms of treatment.
> 9. Mother is less concerned about her child's illness than are the medical professionals.
> 10. Seizures do not respond to appropriate treatment.
> 11. Mother has previous medical or nursing experience.
> 12. Mother has a history of illnesses similar to that of the child.
> 13. The child experiences multiple hospitalisations.
> 14. The mother perpetrates the fraud.
> 15. The mother is willing to have her child undergo diagnostic procedures and medical treatments, often invasive in nature.
> 16. There is multiple physician involvement.
> 17. Father is typically uninvolved in the care of the child.
> 18. There is usually a poor marital relationship between parents.

knocked from bicycles. Children aged between 1 and 14 are more likely to be injured as pedestrians (Levene 1992). 95% of children under 10 years old who attend A&E departments do so between 9 a.m. and 9 p.m. (Lancaster 1993), and the guidelines issued by the DoH (1991a) recommend that there is a qualified paediatric nurse available 24 hours a day in all accident and emergency departments. This is important if children are to get optimum care. Researchers have suggested that non-children's nurses underestimate the amount of distress children experience in this situation (Powell 1991, Gay 1991) and Burton (1993, p. 107) describes how the A&E department can be 'a deeply frightening and traumatic experience' for a child. There are strange noises, odd smells and atmosphere, and people in uniforms, along with the trauma of seeing other patients in distress. This, in addition to the trauma of an injury or illness, contributes to making it an extremely stressful situation. Burton describes a philosophy of care which involves communicating with and gaining the trust of the child and family; this might involve time-consuming procedures such as play with toys and equipment to gain trust and information. Specific issues such as undressing can become traumatic—children may see their clothes as a link with home and will be reluctant to part with them. Honesty is all important—if it will hurt then the child should be warned. Children also enjoy achieving badges for bravery. The parents should be allowed to stay with their child at all times and should be

Activity 28.4

What special provision is made for children in your local A&E department, if any? Consider how this may be improved.

Imagine that you have been asked to provide a plan for a new paediatric A&E department. List, in priority order, what facilities are necessary.

given written instructions about the specific care of their child after discharge (e.g. advice on head injury, care of plaster of Paris, etc.).

Lancaster (1993) presents a case for a specific child A&E department staffed by children's nurses. She cites the particular skills of the children's nurse that help to identify non-accidental injuries, due to their knowledge of the many factors involved (see Box 28.1).

A small research study was performed by Gay (1992) which looked at pain and anxiety in children attending A&E departments, as perceived by them, their parents and the nurses looking after them. The study suggested that nurses tend to underestimate the amount of pain experienced by young children and so do not instigate pain relief or coping mechanisms. Anxiety was acknowledged by most nurses to be present but not many implemented strategies, some as simple as telling children what was to happen and allowing them to see the instruments to be used, to reduce anxiety.

The statistics on numbers of children attending A&E departments and the reasons for those

Table 28.2 Reasons for visits to accident and emergency departments according to age group in the study performed by Gay (1992)

Reason for admission	Number of children admitted for each reason Age in years				
	2–4	4–7	7–12	12–16	Total
Lacerations	4	6	2	2	14
Sprains and fractures	1	2	7	5	15
Dog bites	0	0	2	1	3
Burns	1	0	1	0	2
Total	6	8	12	8	34

Activity 28.5

Find out the most popular days and times for child attenders at your local A&E department.

visits are not well detailed in the United Kingdom. However, based on the small numbers in Gay's study it is possible to get an idea of the types of injuries and ages of children to whom they occur (Table 28.2).

A study performed by Bolton & Storrie (1991) looked at inappropriate attendance of children in A&E departments and suggested educational methods of reducing these. They found that the most commonly presenting diagnoses were problems related to the digestive tract (34.5%; diarrhoea and vomiting the main one) and the respiratory tract (26.8%; viral illness and upper respiratory tract infection being the most common here). Various suggestions were made in relation to educating parents about using the A&E department more sensibly.

Dove & Kobryn (1991) describe the use of a computer system which enables staff to record attendances at the A&E Department at the University Hospital in Nottingham. The intention is to enable early detection of frequent attenders in the casualty department who may have been victims of abuse. The computer is also linked to the Nottinghamshire 'Children at Risk' register and gives an audible and visual warning when details are entered which indicate that a child has attended three or more times during the last 12 months. Confidentiality is maintained through the use of passwords and different levels of access.

Paediatric nurse practitioners

Some enlightened hospitals have introduced paediatric nurse practitioners into A&E departments. This can help in situations where the children (with their parents) attend the department without first consulting a GP. Kobryn &

Pearce (1991) describe the introduction of a nurse practitioner into an A&E department. They define the nurse practitioner (who has had specific training to extend the nurse's role) as one who is:

a nurse specialist who has a sound nursing practice base in all aspects of accident and emergency nursing with additional preparation and skills in physical diagnosis, psychosocial assessment, the prescribing of care and preventative treatment.

(Kobryn & Pearce 1991, p. 11)

The qualifications for this role also require that the nurse is a Registered Sick Children's Nurse, has worked in A&E for 3 years and is at 'F' grade or above.

Some of the conditions that are dealt with by nurse practitioners in children over the age of 1 year include plaster of Paris checks, removal of sutures, minor abrasions, superficial animal bites, removal of splinters, and wasp and bee stings. The parents are given the choice about their child seeing a nurse practitioner, and referrals are made to the doctor as necessary. The role also includes administering analgesia, such as paracetamol, prior to the doctor seeing the child who has sustained minor burns and scalds and abrasions, and has a pyrexia. This reduces distress if there is waiting time.

Some of the benefits reported by Kobryn & Pearce (1991) in their study included:

- greater satisfaction of patients due to reduced waiting times
- parents' reports of finding it easier to talk to a nurse
- slightly reduced workloads for medical staff
- greater job satisfaction for the nurse practitioner.

Activity 28.6

Describe how the role of paediatric nurse practitioner might be implemented in your local A&E department.

When a child dies

One of the most distressing events in an accident and emergency department is the child who is brought in dead or who dies while in the department. This calls for particularly sensitive care and actions on the part of the nurses involved. Burton (1993) provides some guidelines for use in the case of parents whose child has suffered a cot death (also called sudden infant death syndrome or SIDS). Burton suggests that one nurse should be assigned to stay with the parents at all times. This nurse should keep the parents informed and help them to contact family and friends and make other arrangements such as care of siblings. A private room should be made available and the parents should be able and encouraged to see and hold the baby/child and be alone if they wish. Listening is important —parents may repeat over and over the events leading up to the accident or death and may say it is their fault. Parents should be encouraged to come back and talk to staff as often as they want. They also need to be given written instructions about the necessary legal procedures, such as registering the death and removal of the body.

Nurses involved, especially students, may need support too, and after any situation of such distress it is necessary to have a 'debriefing' session where all concerned can discuss their feelings and receive support, and review strategies of care with a view to improving care. These sessions can be formal or informal and a counsellor may be involved if necessary.

CULTURAL ISSUES

Female circumcision or female genital mutilation (FGM) is thought to affect up to 75 million women and children world-wide according to the United Nations Organization (1981). It is common in countries such as Indonesia, Malaysia, Yemen and also in immigrant communities in Europe. FGM may be performed when the baby is a few days old (as in Ethiopia) or at any age up to 7 years old (in Egypt) to adolescence in West Africa. It may involve excising the clitoris completely, cutting the hood of the clitoris, or more radically, removing the clitoris, labia majora and minora and sewing up the sides of the vulva leaving only a small hole. Anaesthetics, cleansing agents and sterile instruments are seldom used. Some immediate complications of this surgery include the usual postoperative complications of shock and haemorrhage, but also injuries to adjacent organs, urine retention and death. Long-term complications may involve chronic pelvic inflammation, renal problems, chronic and extended periods, endometriosis, and painful intercourse. Problems also occur during pregnancy and delivery, including recurrent urinary tract infections, difficulty in performing vaginal examinations, bad tears and problems with episiotomies, and vaginal delivery may be impossible (Trevelyan 1994).

In the United Kingdom, up to 10 000 girls are thought to be at risk of FGM, which presents a problem to health professionals. They may know that the ritual is being carried out, but may be afraid of accusations of racism if they attempt to prevent it. It is thought to be a cultural/religious practice which is 'traditional' and difficult to alter. There are no health benefits from FGM and it is not a legal practice in the United Kingdom.

Female genital mutilation is just one, rather extreme, example of conflict between and within cultures. Other examples of this are female children who may be at risk of malnutrition and other forms of neglect in cultures in which boys are highly valued. There is evidence that in these cultures boy babies are breast-fed for longer and more often taken for medical care than girls (Trevelyan 1994).

Activity 28.7

Discuss with colleagues your views on female circumcision, examine your attitudes and describe how you might deal with a Somali family with daughters.

TRAVELLING FAMILIES

Children living in nonconventional families or in nonconventional situations are potentially at risk if their health is neglected. Examples of this are health problems encountered by gypsies and other travelling families. These are a large population who are 'disadvantaged in health and health care' (Save the Children 1983). Education authorities have a long history of concern for the special needs of traveller children and innovative programmes to solve some of these problems have been devised. Health authorities do not seem to have addressed their responsibilities in the same way. Issues of site safety, cleanliness, use of GP services and dental care are of concern. Statistics show that gypsy and traveller families have more children than the national average, perinatal mortality is above average and there are more low birth weight babies born. These families make greater use of A&E departments for accidents.

Pahl & Vaile (1986) carried out a study, by questionnaire, in Kent of traveller and gypsy families. They checked on child development monitoring and found that most children (80%) had had the appropriate examinations by the age of 1 year. However, this high rate fell off dramatically for subsequent examinations. Immunisation uptake was generally poor. This study was carried out by health visitors who were working with the families and there may have been some bias in the reporting and accuracy of this information. To reduce some of the problems of health care, travellers should carry their own medical records. Some health authorities have appointed special health visitors for travelling families and these appear to increase the uptake of immunisations.

Activity 28.8

What problems might the children of traveller families have with attending hospital as either inpatients or outpatients?

RELIGIOUS ISSUES

Children may be at risk due to religious beliefs. Jehovah's Witnesses, for example, do not allow blood transfusions for themselves or for their children and Christian Scientists do not approve of any traditional medical care. Medical practitioners are legally obliged to gain consent from parents of children under the age of 18 years before any medical intervention (except in an emergency situation). However, when children are 16 or older they can give their own consent in line with the Family Law Reform Act of 1969 (Dimond 1990). Conflict may arise when children of 16 or 17 wish either to give or withhold consent in opposition to their parents' wishes. Dimond (1990) gives examples of this situation and suggests that the medical practitioner is in a difficult situation.

WORKING WITH OTHER PROFESSIONALS

Nurses involved in the care of sick children will come into contact with other professionals who are also involved in the children's welfare. These other professionals include school teachers, health visitors, social workers and general practitioners. As nurses and other professionals work more closely together in protecting children at risk of injury, for example in child abuse, there must be greater cooperation and understanding of each other's roles. Both the Department of Health's document *Working Together* (DoH 1991b) and the Cleveland report (Butler-Sloss 1988) emphasised the collaboration which needs to exist particularly between nurses and social workers. One mechanism whereby this cooperation might occur is through the medium of the case conference.

Case conferences

An important role for all professionals involved in case conferences is that of making decisions based on shared information. Decision making is an important skill in the repertoire of the children's nurse and has been studied in many ways. The central issue in the process is how to acquire, process and use information. Many decision-making theories are explained in the literature and a specific example of one used in relation to child health nursing is described by Lauri (1992). Nurses are familiar with problem solving: the nursing process is a form of problem solving and involves decision making. Most models contain steps such as:

1. define the problem
2. assess needs
3. prioritise these needs
4. plan alternative interventions
5. implement the interventions
6. evaluate.

Nurses working with children and their families interact quite closely and all members are involved in decision making. Collaborative decision making will promote the child's and family's health and well-being. The nurse needs to be able to understand the family and see them and their problems in the context of their total situation.

Lauri (1992) suggests that the decision-making process should include the six phases above in three main modules:

• assessment
• prioritising needs
• implementing interventions.

The first module, assessment, involves collecting information about the family and child's health status, past and present, and the developmental stage of the child. This leads to the generation of possible predictions regarding needs. The second stage, prioritising needs, takes place in the presence of the family and involves reassessing the family's current situation as well as their health behaviour. This then leads to a collaborative planning of the appropriate interventions. The third stage, implementing interventions, allows for continued evaluation of the nursing interventions selected.

Lauri (1992) describes the development of a computer simulation program which follows this model. She found that computer simulations are useful teaching tools and reveal interesting factors in the decision-making processes which nurses use. The nurses studied appeared to be influenced in their decision making by the developmental stage of the child rather than the family situation they observed at the time of a visit.

Case conferences are an important forum for all health professionals involved in the decision making in a particular case. Each professional is expected to keep records and report findings to the conference. The child involved may be on a child protection register which all health authorities are obliged to keep. Periodic reviews of these children and families take place. It is important that nurses keep accurate and timely reports on all their visits to these families.

Warner (1993) discusses the development of a pack designed to help nurses to record information in a format which makes case information presented at case conferences understandable by all professionals involved. There are five forms which prompt the nurse to record details such as the family details, a report on the nurse's contact with the family and child and their cooperation and environment, a list of critical incidents which may highlight non-accidental injury and other risks to the child. The other forms record a map of the skin and a case conference summary. The purpose of this last document is for each participant to record the decisions made at the case conference. This enables decisions to be implemented as soon as possible. Warner reports that the nurses who use this pack have gained in confidence in all aspects of report writing and case presentation.

Activity 28.9

Ask to attend the case conference of a child and his family with whom you have been involved. Devise a set of questions and write a report following the case conference.

CONCLUSION

The information presented above is a relatively small cross-section of the issues involved when considering the child at risk. Nurses working with well and sick children need to be vigilant and work to protect children. The legal issues have only been mentioned in passing here but the nurse should act as the advocate of the child in collaboration with the parents. The nurse must also remember and abide by the professional code of conduct which involves being accountable and responsible for his or her own actions. Children should at all times be protected from risks and their health and well-being safeguarded.

REFERENCES

Azar S T, Barnes K T, Twentyman C T 1988 Development outcomes in abused children; consequences of parental abuse or a more general breakdown in caregiver behaviour? Behaviour Therapist 11: 27–32

Beezley-Mrazek P, Kempe C H 1981 Sexually abused children and their families. Pergamon Press, Oxford

Bentovim A, Elton A, Hildebrand J, Tranter M, Vizard E 1988 Child abuse within the family: assessment and treatment. Wright, London

Bolton K, Storrie C 1991 Inappropriate attendances to A&E. Paediatric Nursing 3(2): 22–24

Burton R 1993 The child in accident and emergency: a philosophy of care. In: Glasper E A, Tucker A 1993 Advances in child health nursing. Scutari Press, London

Butler-Sloss 1988 The report of the enquiry into child abuse in Cleveland 1987. HMSO, London

Children Act 1989 HMSO, London

Creighton S J 1988 The incidence of child abuse and neglect. In: Browne K, Davies C, Stratton P (eds) Early prediction and prevention of child abuse. Wiley, Chichester

Crouse K 1992 Munchausen syndrome by proxy: recognizing the victim. Pediatric Nursing 18(3): 249–252

Department of Health (DoH) 1991a Guidelines on the welfare of children and young people in hospital. HMSO, London

Department of Health (DoH) 1991b Working together under the Children Act 1989. HMSO, London

Dimond B 1990 Legal aspects of nursing. Prentice Hall, London

Dove A, Kobryn M 1991 Computer detection of child abuse. Nursing Standard 6(10): 38–39

Gale C A, Horner M M 1992 Another case of Munchausen by proxy? Journal of Clinical Nursing 1: 27–32

Gay J 1991 Caring for children in A&E. Paediatric Nursing 3(7): 21–23

Gay J 1992 A painful experience. Nursing Times 88(25): 32–35

Kaufman J, Zigler E 1987 Do abused children become abusive parents? American Journal of Orthopsychiatry 57: 186–192

Kelly S J 1988 Physical abuse of children: recognition and reporting. Journal of Emergency Nursing 14: 82–90

Kobryn M, Pearce S 1991 The paediatric nurse practitioner. Paediatric Nursing 3(5): 11–14

Lancaster N 1993 The right staff. Paediatric Nursing 5(2): 22–24

Lauri S 1992 Using a computer simulation program to assess the decision making process in child health care. Computers in Nursing 10(4): 171–177

Levene S 1992 Preventing accidental injuries to children. Paediatric Nursing 4(9): 12–14

Meadow R 1977 Munchausen syndrome by proxy: the hinterland of child abuse. Lancet ii: 343–345

Meadow R (ed) 1993 ABC of child abuse, 2nd edn. BMJ, London

Pahl J, Vaile M 1986 Health and health care among travellers. Report published by University of Kent, Canterbury

Powell C 1991 A better service. Paediatric Nursing 3(7): 18–20

Roberts J 1988 Why are some families more vulnerable to child abuse? In: Browne K, Davies C, Stratton P (eds) Early prediction and prevention of child abuse. Wiley, Chichester

Save the Children 1983 The health of traveller mothers and children in East Anglia. Save the Children Fund, London

Senner A, Ott M 1989 Munchausen syndrome by proxy. Issues in Comprehensive Pediatric Nursing 12: 345–357

Sigal M, Gelkopf M, Meadow R 1989 Munchausen by proxy syndrome: the triad of abuse, self-abuse, and deception. Comprehensive Psychiatry 30(6): 527–532

Speight N 1993 Non-accidental injury. In: Meadow R (ed) 1993 ABC of child abuse, 2nd edn. BMJ, London

Stratton P 1988 Understanding and treating child abuse in the family context: an overview. In: Browne K, Davies C, Stratton P (eds) Early prediction and prevention of child abuse. Wiley, Chichester

Trevelyan J 1994 A woman's lot. Nursing Times 90(15): 49–50

United Nations Organization 1981 Women: challenges to the year 2000. United Nations, New York

Warner U 1993 Improving input in case conferences. Nursing Standard 7(22): 33–34

Welsh Office 1993 Child protection register. HMSO, London

FURTHER READING

Blumenthal I 1994 Child abuse: a handbook for health care practitioners. Edward Arnold, London

Peder P, Duncan S, Gray M 1993 Beyond blame: child abuse tragedies revisited. Routledge, London

Journals
Child Abuse and Neglect: The International Journal
Child Abuse Review

USEFUL ADDRESSES

Child Accident Prevention Trust
4th Floor
Clerk's Court
18–20 Farringdon Lane
London EC1R 3AU

End Physical Punishment of Children Campaign
(EPOCH)
77 Holloway Road
London N7 8JZ

National Society for the Prevention of Cruelty to
Children (NSPCC)
42 Curtain Road
London EC2A 3NH

Royal College of Nursing (RCN) Child Protection Special
Interest Group
20 Cavendish Square
London W1M 0AB

Royal Society for the Prevention of Accidents
Cannon House
The Priory
Queensway
Birmingham B4 6BS

Appendices

Girls: preterm–2 years

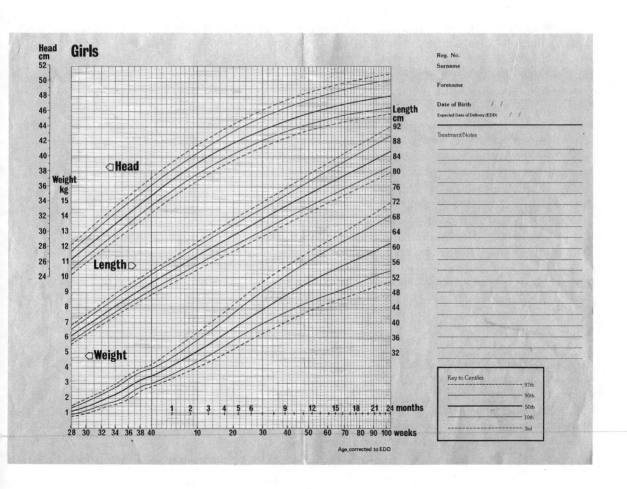

Girls: birth–20 years

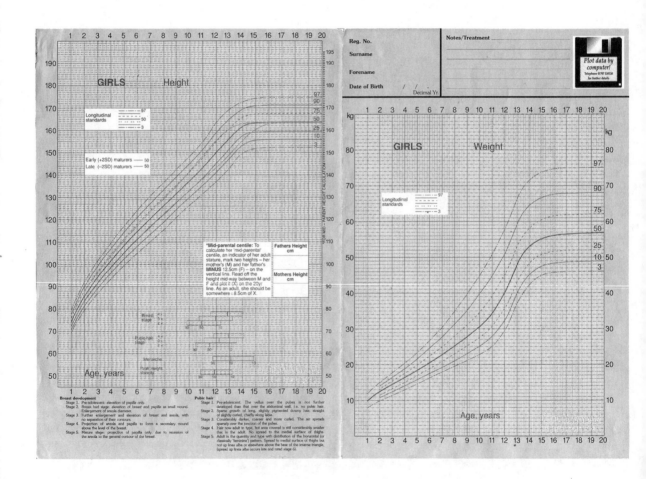

Boys: preterm–2 years

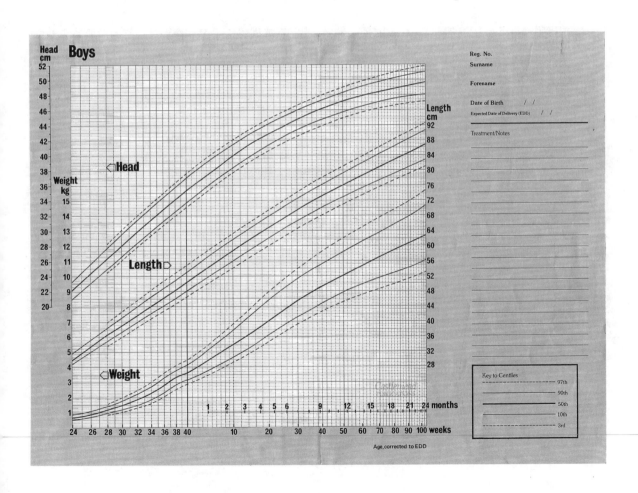

Boys: birth–20 years

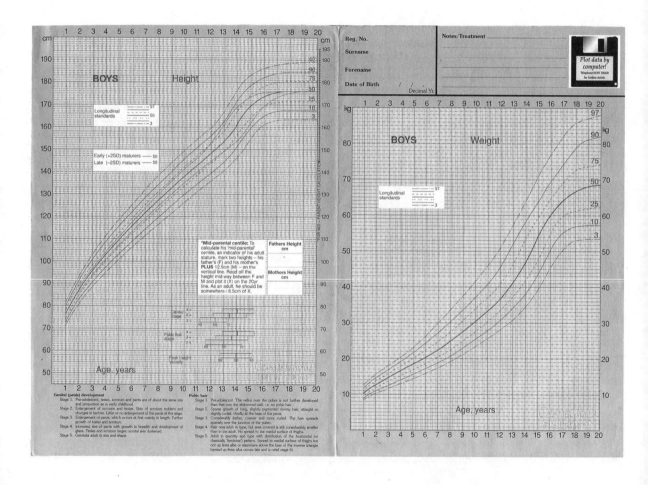

Index

Page numbers in bold type indicate main discussions of a topic. Page numbers in italics refer to information in Boxes, Figures and tables.

Index